The Medicinal Uses of Cannabis and Cannabinoids

The Medicinal Uses of Cannabis and Cannabinoids

Edited by

Geoffrey W Guy

BSc, MB BS, DipPharmMed, MRCS Eng, LRCP, LMSSA

Executive Chairman, GW Pharmaceuticals, Salisbury, Wiltshire, UK

Brian A Whittle

BPharm, MSc, PhD, FRPhS

Scientific Director, GW Pharmaceuticals, Salisbury, Wiltshire, UK

Philip J Robson

MB, MRCP, FRCPsych
Senior Research Fellow, Department of Psychiatry, Oxford University
and Medical Director, GW Pharmaceuticals, Salisbury, Wiltshire, UK

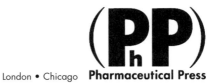

London • Chicago **Pharmaceutical Press**

Published by the Pharmaceutical Press
Publications division of the Royal Pharmaceutical Society of Great Britain

1 Lambeth High Street, London SE1 7JN, UK
100 South Atkinson Road, Suite 206, Grayslake, IL 60030-7820, USA

© Pharmaceutical Press 2004

Text design by Barker/Hilsdon
Typeset by Gray Publishing, Tunbridge Wells, Kent, UK
Printed in Great Britain by TJ International, Padstow, Cornwall

ISBN 0 85369 517 2

A catalogue record for this book is available from the British Library

Contents

Foreword xi
Preface xiii
Acknowledgements xvi
About the editors xvii
Contributors xix
Introduction xxi

1   **History of cannabis as a medicine**   1
     Cannabis, the plant 9
     Effects of legislation on research 11
     References 13

2   **Growth and morphology of medicinal cannabis**   17
     Cannabinoids and cannabis anatomy 20
     Cannabis life cycle 22
     Optimisation of cannabinoid production 23
     Why does the plant produce cannabinoids
           and terpenes? 27
     The value of sinsemilla 28
     Propagating medicinal cannabis 29
     The growing environment 42
     Phototropy and photonasty 45
     Quality, safety and efficacy: meeting EU Good Agricultural
           Practice guidelines 48
     The way forward – the great outdoors? 50
     References 54

3   **The breeding of *Cannabis* cultivars for pharmaceutical
     end uses**   55
     The position of medicinal *Cannabis* breeding 55
     Goals and strategies of the pharmaceutical
           breeding programme 56
     Germ plasm resources 60

Current breeding achievements   63
Future developments   67
References   68

**4   The evolution of *Cannabis* and coevolution with the
      cannabinoid receptor – a hypothesis   71**
Origin of the association   72
Cannabis taxonomy and evolution   73
The species debate   74
Biotypes and cannabinoid profiles   78
Cannabis and cannabinoid receptors   80
The evolutionary arabesque   82
The enigma of animal receptors and plant ligands   84
Deconstructing 'exogenous ligands'   86
Plant ligands and 'the great leap forward'   87
Evidence for coevolutionary adaptations in
      CB receptors   88
Evidence for coevolutionary adaptations in
      plant ligands   89
Coevolution makes good medicine   91
Conclusions and future directions   93
References   94

**5   Receptors and pharmacodynamics: natural and synthetic
      cannabinoids and endocannabinoids   103**
Cannabinoid CB_1 and CB_2 receptors   104
Endogenous ligands for CB_1 and CB_2 receptors   107
Other agonists for CB_1 and CB_2 receptors   114
Chirality of cannabinoids   117
CB_1 and CB_2 receptors antagonists   120
Other cannabinoid receptor ligands   124
Other cannabinoid receptors?   125
Conclusions   128
References   129

**6   Therapeutic potential of cannabis and cannabinoids in
      experimental models of multiple sclerosis   141**
Cannabis as a therapeutic in MS   142
Symptom control   143
Immunomodulation   150
Neuroprotection   152
References   155

7   **Natural cannabinoids: interactions and effects**   165
           Background references   167
           Pain   169
           Anxiety   172
           Depression   177
           Alcohol dependence   178
           Spasticity   179
           Schizophrenia   182
           Epilepsy   185
           Antioxidant effects   187
           Anti-inflammatory effects   191
           Conclusions   195
           References   197

8   **Metabolism and pharmacokinetics of**
           cannabinoids   205
           Metabolism of Δ^9-THC, cannabidiol, cannabinol and
               Δ^9-tetrahydrocannabivarin in humans   208
           Metabolism *in vitro* in humans   209
           Hepatic cytochrome P450s (CYPs) responsible for
               phase 1 metabolism of cannabinoids   211
           Inhibition and induction of oxidative metabolism in the liver
               by cannabinoids   212
           Pharmacokinetics by different routes of
               administration   216
           Routes of administration for CBD and CBN   220
           Conclusion   220
           References   221

9   **Clinical studies of cannabis-based medicines**   229
           Review of existing clinical evidence for therapeutic
               potential   230
           GW Pharmaceuticals patient database   241
           Delivery systems for cannabis medicinal extracts   242
           Practical issues in initiating a clinical research
               programme   245
           Recently completed human research   254
           Future directions for clinical research   260
           References   262

10   Cannabis in the treatment of chronic pain   271
History   272
Understanding pain   274
Pain assessment and management   280
Starting to study cannabis medicines for pain   282
Influence of cannabis on driving   296
Final comments   296
References   297

11   The forensic control of cannabis   301
Analytical aspects of cannabis control   303
Trends in potency of cannabis   304
Analytical techniques   306
Determination of cannabinoids in body fluids
      for forensic purposes   312
Interpretation of cannabis use in a forensic
      context   316
Cannabis and driving   324
Quality control of analytical procedures   324
Conclusions   325
References   325

12   A review of cannabis and driving skills   329
Forensic control of cannabis and driving   329
Laboratory studies of cognition and motor
      performance   330
Retrospective analyses of traffic collisions   336
Prospective driving studies   344
Medicinal cannabis and driving   363
References   366

**13   International control of cannabis: changing
attitudes**   369
A case study: the United States   370
Social turmoil of the 1960s and a new
      symbolism   378
International legislation   385
The Conventions and cannabis use   393
What types of cannabis reform are possible?   395
Do international treaties allow cannabis-based
      medicines to be legally available?   398

What evidence must a country have to make
        cannabis available as a medicine?   398
What legal changes are necessary to permit
        the use of medicinal cannabis?   400
Separating the issues of cannabis use   403
Separating medicinal and recreational cannabis
        use   405
What may drive a change in a nation's attitudes
        towards cannabis?   406
Relative influence of factors   416
Where are we now?   417
Ending thoughts   424
References   424

14   **Development of cannabis-based
        medicines: risk, benefit and serendipity**   **427**
Cannabis as a medicine   428
The historical legacy   431
Regulatory route   438
Quality   442
The dosage form   446
Safety   450
Efficacy   453
Risks, benefits and serendipity   460
References   463

Glossary   467

Index   473

The colour plate section is between pages 232 and 233.

Foreword

The history of human beings' use of cannabis is long and turbulent. In antiquity, cannabis was used to treat a wide variety of diseases, but because it affects cognition, it has been used as a mood-altering drug. Its potential for other than purely therapeutic purposes led to restriction of its use during the twentieth century and its withdrawal as a medicine under the 1961 and 1971 Narcotic Conventions. Despite proscription, unauthorised use for medical purposes continued. Bona fide claims by patients such as those suffering from multiple sclerosis and pain unresponsive to morphine and other analgesics were increasingly given as mitigating circumstances in cases of possession of cannabis. This presented a problem to the judiciary in sentencing, and threatened to bring the law into disrepute.

In 1997, Her Majesty's Government set up a House of Lords Committee to report on the scientific evidence for the medicinal use of cannabis. The conclusions of the Select Committee on Science and Technology were that clinical trials of cannabis for the treatment of multiple sclerosis and chronic pain should be mounted as a matter of urgency and it is gratifying to see that this has been done in a timely manner. The committee also recommended research into alternative modes of administration and it is interesting to see that progress has been made on this front.

Rehabilitation of cannabis as a prescription medicine is a multifaceted problem. Like any new medicine, the case must be made for approval on grounds of quality, safety, efficacy and need. However, in addition to the description of the development of a prescription medicine from a botanical drug, the authors have taken account of the regulatory, international legislative, social and ethical problems attending the use of material which was formerly regarded as a drug of abuse. A start has been made on the tortuous path of disentangling the essentials from anecdotal reports on the use of cannabis, and applying rigorous scientific method to clinical trials demonstrating safety and efficacy.

All this would be of academic interest but little practical value if the prescription medicine could not be used by the patient groups most in need. A review of the legislative control of cannabis through the years indicates the way in which a prescription medicine based on cannabis can be re-introduced into the canon of acceptable therapeutic treatments.

The original prohibition of cannabis arose from social pressure as much as safety concerns. It is heartening that the scientific evidence on which a rational reappraisal of cannabis as a prescription medicine can be made has been forthcoming. Patients with intractable disease will welcome this. They are often afflicted in their prime, and availability of an effective and safe prescription medicine will, in turn, lead to an improved quality of life. It is also refreshing to see that the derivation of the first prescription medicine based on whole cannabis represents a return to the roots of science – medicinal plants.

Mr Alan MacFarlane
March 2004

Preface

Cannabis has a long history of use both as a medicine and as a recreational drug. The written records of its use span more than five millennia and it has frequently been the focus of interest by regulatory authorities of one kind or another who have sought to control its use. During the last century cannabis moved from being a frequently prescribed item for a variety of therapeutic conditions, through a period of increasing opposition to its use because of its potential for abuse, to the point where its use was completely withdrawn in the mid-twentieth century. The reasons for this demotion of cannabis as a prescription medicine to its present position as a proscribed drug of abuse are legion. They include scientific, clinical, sociological and forensic concerns. Until recently, lack of understanding of the mechanism of action, abuse potential and apprehension about its use as a gateway drug have conspired to bring it into disrepute.

In the last 10 years, the realisation that cannabis alleviates modalities of pain untouched by morphine-like analgesics and that it is one of the few agents that can prevent or reverse the wasting in patients with AIDS and cancer has rekindled interest in cannabis as a medicine. In parallel, the discovery of cannabinoid receptors and endocannabinoids as intercellular signalling agents has re-established the basis for restoration of cannabis as a medicine.

Another strand in the research on cannabis is the programme supported by the National Institute for Drug Abuse (NIDA). NIDA has funded research into cannabinoids, synthetic analogues, antagonists and their mode of action. Although the primary purpose of this research was to discourage the use (both recreational and clinical) of cannabis, it has nevertheless laid the foundation for a better understanding of phytocannabinoids and endocannabinoids in terms of their structure and function. The range of pharmacological effects displayed by cannabinoids is remarkable and helps to explain its use in many human disorders.

Recently, there has been a resurgence of interest in cannabis as a medicine for the treatment of conditions unresponsive to other types of therapy. In the last 20 years an increasing number of patients with severely debilitating diseases such as multiple sclerosis have used street material to obtain symptom relief. As a Class C substance (Schedule I in the USA) its medical use is still illegal in most states, but in the UK the judiciary have increasingly taken a lenient attitude towards people who were using marijuana for the treatment of disease. This threatened to bring the law into disrepute and in 1997 the UK Government asked the House of Lords Select Committee on Science and Technology to advise on its future course of action with regard to cannabis. One of their key recommendations was that the UK Government should encourage research that, when evaluated by the regulatory authority, could lead to a prescription medicine. The way would then be open for re-scheduling medicinal cannabis. In parallel, there has been a growing campaign to legalise cannabis both for medicinal and recreational use.

This book documents the research leading to the registration of a cannabis-based medicine and also describes the blossoming research into the basic science behind cannabis and cannabinoids. In addition to a time perspective on the use of cannabis, there are also chapters on the genetic pedigree of cannabis and the breeding of specific chemovars. The system of plant husbandry used to produce pharmaceutical-grade cannabis herb is described.

A striking new development in cannabinoid research is the recognition that within the body there is an endocannabinoid system that interacts with the same receptors as the plant cannabinoids and produces related effects. Endocannabinoid receptors can be detected in the tissues of most phyla from Hydra onwards, and they appear to constitute an additional intracellular messenger system. The phylogenetic history of cannabis in relation to pest competitors and human consumption is also described, touching on the complex social, legislative and therapeutic interactions between humans and the use of the plant as medicine.

Research in this field is moving rapidly and the current state of research on cannabis extracts used as medicines is outlined. The constituents of cannabis and the endocannabinoids, together with the compounds derived from them, continue to be of interest both to academic workers and the pharmaceutical industry, and have opened up a new area of research. From a practical and strategic perspective chapters address the development work required to produce medicines from cannabis and the risks that are inherent in this exercise. There is growing evidence that the clinical benefits of cannabis are more than just the sum of the pharmacological effects of the individual constituents, and an account is given of the clinical work that complements the pharmacological studies.

Development of safe and effective medicines also requires consideration of other issues, including health regulation, forensic science and international initiatives required to change legislation. There is also a need to change the attitude of health professionals to cannabis and cannabinoids as medicines. The first step in this process involves demonstrating the scientific credentials of cannabis and cannabinoids. Data are brought together from recent clinical and preclinical work and related to the attitudinal, political and legislative changes that are long overdue. The regulatory history is dealt with *in extenso* because it provides the background to the current situation. The discussion of the risks and benefits flowing from reinstatement of a cannabis-based prescription product looks forward to evidence-based changes in regulatory approval and legislative re-scheduling.

Dr Brian Whittle
March 2004

Acknowledgements

We are grateful to the Pharmaceutical Press for their invitation to write the book, and to Paul Weller, Lorraine Parry and Louise McIndoe for their help and encouragement.

Grateful acknowledgment is given to Jan Harris, Steph Harris, Emma Brierley and Julia Sampson for their editorial help in preparing the manuscript.

Peter Smith and David Potter produced the excellent photographs and we acknowledge the care and precision of the accurate botanical illustrations of plant materials produced by Valerie Bolas.

The support of the Home Office has been of singular and critical importance, without which GW Pharmaceuticals would not have been able to expedite progress in the project in such a timely manner. We are grateful to the Medicines and Healthcare products Regulatory Agency for helpful discussions.

About the editors

Dr Geoffrey W Guy, BSc, MB BS, DipPharmMed, MRCS Eng, LRCP, LMSSA, Executive Chairman of GW Pharmaceuticals plc.

Dr Guy founded GW Pharmaceuticals in 1998. He is a physician with over 20 years' experience in pharmaceutical development covering new chemical entities, biotechnology products, plant-based medicines and drug delivery systems. Dr Guy has been the physician in charge of over 350 clinical studies including first dose in humans, pharmacokinetics, pharmacodynamics, dose ranging, controlled clinical trials and large-scale multicentred studies and clinical surveys.

Dr Guy gained a BSc in pharmacology from the University of London in 1976, an MB BS at St Bartholomew's Hospital in 1979, an MRCS Eng and LRCP London in 1979, an LMSSA Society of Apothecaries in 1979 and a Diploma of Pharmaceutical Medicine from the Royal Colleges of Physicians in 1984. Dr Guy is a member of the editorial board of the *Journal of Cannabis Therapeutics*.

Dr Brian A Whittle, BPharm, MSc, PhD, FRPhS, Scientific Director of GW Pharmaceuticals plc.

Dr Whittle is a co-founder of GW Pharmaceuticals. He is a fellow of the Royal Pharmaceutical Society, the Linnean Society and the British Institute of Regulatory Affairs. He is a Qualified Person under the provisions of Directive 73/319/EEC and Directive 81/85/EEC and oversees the scientific development of the Research and Development programme at GW Pharmaceuticals.

He was awarded a BPharm degree from the University of Nottingham in 1954, a PhC Diploma by the Pharmaceutical Society in 1954, and an MSc by the University of London in 1963.

Dr Philip J Robson, MB, MRCP, FRCPsych, Medical Director of
GW Pharmaceuticals plc.

Dr Robson joined GW Pharmaceuticals as Medical Director in January
2000, having for the previous ten years been a Consultant Psychiatrist
in Oxford and Senior Clinical Lecturer in the Oxford University
Department of Psychiatry.

Dr Robson has been interested for many years in the therapeutic
potential of cannabis and cannabinoids. In 1996 he was commissioned
by the Department of Health to carry out a critical review of the relevant scientific literature, and in 1998 was called on to submit both
written and verbal evidence to the House of Lords Science and
Technology Committee investigation into cannabis.

In addition to his duties as Medical Director of the company,
Dr Robson is also a Senior Research Fellow in the Department of
Psychiatry at the University of Oxford.

Contributors

Alex Allan PhD
Merit Scientist Drugs and Toxicology, Forensic Alliance Limited, F5
Culham Science Centre, Abingdon, Oxfordshire, UK

David Baker PhD
Department of Neuroinflammation, Institute of Neurology, University
College, London, UK

Etienne de Meijer PhD
Head of Plant Breeding, GW Pharmaceuticals, Porton Down
Science Park, Salisbury, Wiltshire, UK

Geoffrey W Guy BSc, MB BS, DipPharmMed, MRCS Eng, LRCP, LMSSA
Executive Chairman, GW Pharmaceuticals, Porton Down Science
Park, Salisbury, Wiltshire, UK

David Hadorn MD
Former health policy adviser to the New Zealand Ministry of
Health and the British Columbia Ministry of Health. Former
adviser to the California Attorney General's Task Force on Medical
Marijuana

Gabrielle Hawksworth PhD
Professor of Molecular Toxicology, Department of Medicine and
Therapeutics, University of Aberdeen, Foresterhill, Aberdeen, UK

Karen McArdle BSc (Hons)
Department of Medicine and Therapeutics, University of Aberdeen,
Foresterhill, Aberdeen, UK

John M McPartland DO, MSc, ABFP
Head of Graduate Programme, Faculty of Health and
Environmental Science, UNITEC, New Zealand. Clinical Assistant

Professor of Family Medicine, University of Vermont. Adjunct Assistant Professor of Biomechanics, Michigan State University, USA

Alice Mead JD, LLM
Special Counsel, Medical Affairs (North America), GW Pharmaceuticals, Porton Down Science Park, Salisbury, Wiltshire, UK

Richard E Musty PhD
Department of Psychology, University of Vermont, Burlington, Vermont, USA

William Notcutt MB, ChB, FRCA
Consultant in Anaesthesia and Pain Management, James Paget Hospital, Great Yarmouth, and Honorary Senior Lecturer, School of Health Policy and Practice, University of East Anglia, UK

Roger Pertwee PhD
Professor of Neuropharmacology, Department of Biomedical Sciences, Institute of Medical Sciences, University of Aberdeen, Foresterhill, and Director of Pharmacology, GW Pharmaceuticals, Porton Down Science Park, Salisbury, Wiltshire, UK

David Potter
Director of Botanical Research and Cultivation, GW Pharmaceuticals, Porton Down Science Park, Salisbury, Wiltshire, UK

Philip J Robson MB, MRCP, FRCPsych
Senior Research Fellow, Department of Psychiatry, Oxford University and Medical Director, GW Pharmaceuticals, Porton Down Science Park, Salisbury, Wiltshire, UK

Ethan Russo MD
Clinical Assistant Professor, Department of Internal Medicine, University of Washington; and Adjunct Associate Professor, Department of Pharmaceutical Sciences, University of Montana, USA

Brian A Whittle BPharm, MSc, PhD, FRPhS
Scientific Director, GW Pharmaceuticals, Porton Down Science Park, Salisbury, Wiltshire, UK

Introduction

This is a book about the development of plant-based prescription medicines. It is not an apology for unauthorised use of cannabis herb for treatment of clinical conditions, nor does it enter the debate on decriminalisation. The authors, each a worker in at least one aspect of cannabis research, have sought to capture current developments in the field and put them into perspective. The chapters are designed to be complete in themselves to enable readers from different backgrounds to dip into the text as their particular interest dictates. They are intended as a reference source on horticultural and technological, clinical, regulatory, sociological, legal, political and ethical issues. There is, of necessity, overlap in the content of some of the chapters, which reflects the complexity of cannabis therapeutics. This is kept to a minimum, consistent with providing context.

The style of the authors is as varied as the content of their chapters and the editors have not sought to impose a rigid stylistic framework on the contributors. Each author brings a special expertise to their individual accounts, and in the process a number of self-perpetuating myths have been shaken, if not rocked to their foundations. No apology is made for this approach. When commissioning this book, the Royal Pharmaceutical Society asked for a wide-ranging volume addressed to a broad constituency of healthcare professionals. The perceived need was for a balanced account of the scientific case for cannabis and the way that this informs decisions on regulatory control and professional advice to patients.

Much has been written on the chemistry and basic pharmacology of cannabis. The prime focus of this book is the therapeutic evaluation of cannabis as a medicine. This is appropriate because of the neglect of clinical research in favour of preclinical studies over the last few decades. Emphasis on the negative aspects of cannabis as a recreational drug and medicine, mainly based on unauthorised use of smoked herb of indifferent quality, has made it difficult to achieve an objective risk benefit analysis. An attempt has been made in this book to redress this imbalance by providing data both on the therapeutic use of cannabis and the adverse events that may attend its use. Intoxication with cannabis is a function of dose and a major breakthrough in safe usage of cannabis-based medicines is the ability to titrate dosage to obtain symptom relief within the bounds of an acceptable degree of change in cognitive function. The therapeutic utility of non-psychoactive plant components has become an exciting possibility.

Although the selection of areas for study has been dictated to some extent by history, recent political pressures have forced a re-evaluation of the issues of increasing or decreasing control of cannabis in the face of increasing (claimed) use as a medicine. This is the background to the setting up of the House of Lords Select Committee on Science and Technology in 1997. It was anticipated that one of the larger pharmaceutical companies would pick up the baton and use its vast drug development machinery to bring the project to fruition. Two major problems emerged. First, established 'Big Pharma' is not comfortable generally with development of phytomedicines from starting materials that have a history of abuse. It prefers established drug development paradigms in which research is carried out to define the 'active constituent'. This can then be treated as a new chemical entity (NCE). This approach is also thought to maximise Intellectual Property Rights (IPR). In practice, the advantages of new chemical or new therapeutic use patents may not afford more protection than patents on methods of preparation of plant medicines. There is a trade-off between IPR gain and the longer development time required for NCE-based products. The time taken to develop a prescription medicine from an NCE is approximately twice that required for development of a botanical drug.

Second, in an environment where opinion is divided on the ethics of developing a cannabis-based product, the boards of major companies probably reflect this dichotomy. In a situation where there are arguments for and against developing a prescription product from a drug with a history of misuse, caution usually prevails. The response of shareholders is assumed to be conservative and this tends to inhibit innovation. These strictures do not apply in a company set up specifically to carry out this development. This is further strengthened by a determination to develop the medicine using a plant extract rather than an NCE. It therefore fell to GW Pharmaceuticals to shoulder the task of developing the first true cannabis-based medicine. This book records the technological and clinical problems that have been encountered in this development.

The exercise has also had spin-off in a number of other ways. Devices which afford a high degree of security in dispensing drugs with abuse potential have been developed, and they appear to have application outside the immediate fields of cannabis therapeutics. The opportunity has been taken to define, in a rigorous manner, the genetic make-up of the plants, using conventional plant breeding practices. Advanced growing techniques have been introduced to maximise yield and ensure consistency of the biomass. This has added a new dimension to quality control of botanical drugs. New methods of extraction and administration have followed and these technological developments are the subject of individual chapters.

An attempt has been made to represent the breadth of the contributions made by the various scientific disciplines that have coalesced to produce a convincing argument to support a therapeutic role for cannabis-based medicines.

The interdisciplinary nature of the research and development programme for any new prescription medicine requires examination of scientific and other issues in appropriate detail. At scientific conferences on cannabis, the emphasis is on preclinical work. Very few papers to date have been presented on clinical work and this book seeks to correct this imbalance. Each chapter is intended to provide a reference source for the various types of professional whose work is impacted by cannabis.

Cannabis has a history of use extending back to antiquity, but this aspect of cannabis has received extensive coverage elsewhere. Chapter 1 provides a short summary of its history and gives a time-line of major events in its long history. For much of the twentieth century cannabis was banned as a medicine, and clinical research was not carried out. This type of research is a necessary preliminary to reinstatement of cannabis as a prescription medicine.

Paradoxically, the prohibition of the therapeutic use of cannabis and the associated lack of clinical research deflected government-funded research towards the search for novel compounds. It was reasoned that synthetic compounds which had some of the useful pharmacological actions of cannabinoids, but not the euphoric actions of tetrahydrocannabinol, would not be subjected to the restrictions imposed under the Narcotics Conventions. Success in this quest would render cannabis unnecessary and further justify its proscription. The investigation of the mode of action and structure of compounds with cannabis-like activity has opened up a whole new chapter in physiology and pharmacology.

After several millennia of use, we are only now beginning to understand the pharmacology and pharmacodynamics of phyto-cannabinoids and the endocannabinoid systems. Cannabis is emerging from half a century when its clinical use has been prohibited and may once again come to occupy a central role in the therapeutic armamentarium. It is particularly exciting that many of its potential applications focus on intractable diseases for which available treatments are only partially effective or dangerously toxic. This book brings together the strands which make up this complex and fascinating story.

1

History of cannabis as a medicine

Ethan Russo

Thousands of years ago in Central or North-East Asia, someone stumbled upon the knowledge of cannabis as medicine. Perhaps it was first ingested because of its sweetly intoxicating aroma or perhaps because an unusual mental change was perceived when hemp was burned. We cannot say with authority, but today cannabis is one of the most versatile medicines available, although only potentially so, due to its prohibited legal status. Here we will review the recorded history of cannabis use as a therapeutic agent. Further details can be found in the historical reviews by Merlin (1972), Abel (1980), Mechoulam (1986), Aldrich (1997) and Russo (2001b, 2002).

It has been claimed that cannabis was used by the Bylony Culture in Central Europe 7000 years ago (Kabelík *et al.*, 1960), but the earliest well-documented evidence of cannabis use is from China, where carbon-14 dating has confirmed it from 4000 BCE (Li, 1974). The first record of therapeutic use is in the *Shen Nong Ben Cao Jing* or *Pên-tsao Ching*, a traditional herbal written in the first or second century, but which was based on the oral traditions passed down from the Emperor Shên-nung in the third millennium BCE. Hemp seed was a common Chinese foodstuff at this time, but its psychoactive effects and hallucinatory potential were also noted, along with an ability to allay senility (Shou-zhong, 1997). Julien documented the legend of Hua-Tho, a second-century emperor who was given a hemp-based anaesthetic during surgery (Julien, 1849). Folk art depicts him as playing chequers during the operation!

In Ancient Egypt, hieroglyphic data, fabric and pollen remains provide evidence of cannabis use as a fumigant, as a salve to treat ophthalmologic conditions and as a suppository to increase vaginal contractions (Mannische, 1989). Similar uses from 29 medical citations and a few obscure ones ('hand of a ghost') attributed to superstitious afflictions were recorded in the Sumerian and Akkadian medical literature of 2000 BCE, which was later collected in the Assyrian Library of the Assyrian king Ashurbanipal (Thompson, 1924, 1949; Russo, manuscript in preparation). Clear written documentation of *bhang* as one of five sacred herbs to allay anxiety is noted in the *Atharva Veda* (11.6.15) in India in the second millennium BCE. The Ayurvedic tradition of using cannabis extends to at least the early pre-Christian centuries (Chopra and Chopra, 1957; Dwarakanath, 1965), with a strong case for smoked medicine being made by certain authors (Walker, 1968; Oman, 1984), supported by documentation of the Ayurvedic 'smoke-roll' and even modern techniques of rolling a hashish cigarette with no pipe or paper (Clarke, 1998). Archaeological smoking paraphernalia with cannabinoid residues has also been found in remains from fourteenth-century Ethiopia, pre-dating the Columbian conquest (van der Merwe, 1975). However, some early cannabis clinical claims remain controversial, as is the reported finding of carbonised cannabis metabolites in a fourth-century tomb in Ancient Judea, said to be from inhaled material used as an aid to childbirth (Zias *et al.*, 1993).

Less debate surrounds the Ancient Greek and Roman sources, where the term 'cannabis' was employed explicitly. Herodotus reported that the ritual use of burned cannabis as part of the funeral rites of the Scythian nomads of the Asian plains in the fifth century BCE caused them to dance and sing (Herodotus, 1998, Book 1, Verse 202). Physical proof of this Scythian rite has been unearthed more recently (see Artamonov, 1965; Rudenko, 1970).

Subsequent classical authors also noted the medicinal effects of cannabis. In the first century CE, Dioscorides published his *Materia Medica*, in which cannabis seed was recommended for the treatment of otalgia (Dioscorides, 1968). Pliny (1951) also noted the use of cannabis root to treat cramped joints, gout and burns around the same time. Galen, in the second century CE noted the gastrointestinal effects of cannabis, and that it could be psychoactive when taken in excess (Brunner, 1973). As evidenced in the above citations, cannabis and its various parts were employed orally, topically, via inhalation, by vaginal suppository and by clyster. Certainly, the evidence supports an early empirical knowledge of the versatility and pharmacokinetics of this phytomedicinal.

For the next thousand years Europe was largely silent about cannabis, with rare exceptions – a recurrent theme in cannabis therapeutics this author has dubbed *cannabis interruptus* (Russo, 2001b). According to archaeological and pollen records, cannabis came to the British Isles during the Roman era (Dark, 2000), becoming an important grain, fibre source and medicinal. Two early herbal citations are noteworthy: the first is from the ninth century in the *Old English*

Herbarium Manuscript V, translated from Anglo-Saxon (Pollington, 2000, p. 301):

> (1) For wounds take this plant which one calls 'chamepithys' and another name 'hemp', pound it and lay it onto the wound; if the wound be very deep then take the sap and wring it into the wound. (2) For pain of the innards take the same plant, give it to drink, it takes away the pain.

Subsequently, although hemp was one of many ingredients in a 'holy salve' described as 'partly Irish' in the tenth-century medico-religious text the *Lacnunga* (Grattan and Singer, 1952, p. 123), it remained for the dominant Arabic culture of the era to advance cannabis therapeutics (Lozano, 2001). Sabur ibn Sahl in ninth-century Persia described the use of a multi-herbal preparation containing the juice of cannabis tops, which was instilled into the nostrils to treat a variety of pains, including migraine, and to preserve pregnancy (Kahl, 1994; Russo, 2001b, 2002). Many Arabic writers preserved the Greek knowledge but a few, including Avicenna, Al-Biruni and Maimonides, extended the list of indications to include digestive ills, treatment of parasites, dandruff, and obstetrical and gynaecological ailments (Russo, 2002). Little notice was paid to these developments in the West, aside from the attribution of homicidal urges to hashish-crazed assassins by Marco Polo and others, which modern study later proved to be apocryphal (Aldrich, 1970). The first known government sanction on the herb occurred at the behest of King al-Zahir Baybars at the close of the thirteen century (Hamarneh, 1957), but it was singularly ineffective.

A famous treatise on agriculture penned by Abu al-Fadl Radi ad-Din al-Ghazzi al-'Amiri, who lived in Damascus between 1457 and 1529 (Hamarneh, 1957), described cannabis with considerable vitriol yet acknowledged a medical role:

> It causes sudden death or madness, hectic fever, consumption, dropsy, dyspnea, trembling, fatigue, pallidity, cirrhosis of the liver and darkens the vision. It depraves the body and defiles religion. Most physicians agree that it is intoxicating, as quoted from Ibn al-Baitar's Jami' and this was confirmed by ash-Shailh Abu Ishaq in his at-Tadhkira fil-Khilaf, and an-Nawari in Sharh al-Muhadhdhab. They approved small doses for medical treatment.

Meanwhile, in Europe, cannabis therapeutics began to emerge once more, but faced challenges. Hildegard von Bingen, a twelfth-century abbess, musician, visionary and herbalist, described cannabis in her *Physica* (Fankhauser, 2002). But after the Papal Bull of Innocent VIII in 1484, cannabis became associated with witchcraft and its use went underground (de Pasquale and Costa, 1967). Rabelais resurrected it under a pseudonym in his *Gargantua et Pantagruelion* in the mid-sixteenth century (Rabelais, 1990).

Most European herbalists echoed the Classics when citing the indications for cannabis, but a few English authorities extended them (see review by Crawford, 2002): Gerard in 1597 recommended cannabis for jaundice and colic (Gerard and Johnson, 1975); Langham and Harper (1633, p. 306) observed that when properly prepared as a drink the seed was effective 'to make thee merry, fierce, hardy to fight, and comely to see'; Culpeper noted the benefits of cannabis for inflammation of the head in 1649 (Culpeper, 1994); Salmon (1710) cited benefits for cramps and contractures; and Short (1751, p. 138) claimed benefit for enuresis or, more prosaically, 'pissing the bed'. Even Linnaeus acknowledged an analgesic effect in his *Materia Medica* (Linné, 1772).

Garcia da Orta was perhaps the first European to explicitly describe the psychoactivity of Indian hemp in 1563 (da Orta, 1913), and eventually this knowledge spread to cognoscenti such as Robert Burton, who in 1621 acknowledged *bange* as an ecstatic agent benefiting depression (Burton, 1907). British explorers soon recognised the plant taxonomically as cannabis, but noted the distinctiveness of Indian hemp and the variability of its effects upon its users. Thomas Bowery and his sailing companions noted its ingestion and smoking in India in the late seventeenth century (Bowrey and Temple, 1905, p. 79):

> And it Operates according to the thoughts of fancy of the Partie that drinketh thereof, in Such manner that if he be merry at that instant, he Shall Contine Soe with Exceedinge great laughter for the before mentioned Space of time, rather overmerry then Otherways, laughinge heartilie at Every thinge they discerne; and, on the Contrary, if it is taken in a fearfull or Melancholy posture, he Shall keep great lamentation and Seem to be in great anguish of Spirit, takeinge away all manly gestures or thought from him.

After the Napoleonic invasion of Egypt, another round of prohibition was attempted, and was again unsuccessful. French scientists took notice, but it was not until O'Shaughnessy, a physician in India who carried out work between 1838 and 1840, that Indian hemp truly came into its own in Western medicine (O'Shaughnessy, 1838–1840). O'Shaughnessy used an ethanolic extract of cannabis as the active pharmaceutical ingredient (API) and clinical trials carried out recently have reverted to the use of extracts, albeit prepared with different solvents. O'Shaughnessy listened to local lore, then effected animal studies and human trials to demonstrate the efficacy of cannabis extracts in the frequently fatal diseases of tetanus and cholera, and in providing a more peaceful passage to inevitable demise in rabies. Soon *Cannabis indica* and extracts were exported to Great Britain and an enthusiastic bout of experimentation extended to Europe and America. This led to a rediscovery of cannabis indications, such as for migraine in England (Clendinning, 1843), neuropathic and musculoskeletal pain in Ireland (Donovan, 1845), mental illness in France (Moreau, 1845), and as an aid to parturition (Churchill, 1849), as first noted in the Ancient Middle East. This model of pragmatic research with plant medicines fell out of favour during the pharmaceutical revolution of the twentieth century, but has been revisited recently.

The existence of the historic use of a botanical in medicine provides a presumption of sufficient safety and efficacy to justify the investigation of the botanical drug. A safe and effective dose can be determined using the appropriate research methodology of the day. Investigation of active principles, a research model that fits in with modern pharmacological research and development practice, can then follow after confirmation of activity in clinical studies. This is not an absolute requirement before clinical investigation.

In nineteenth-century Europe, the *literati* seized upon the 'new' substance, and it is known that it contributed to the writings of Gautier, Baudelaire and Dumas, of Le Club des Hachichins in Paris. In America, Fitz Hugh Ludlow (*The Hasheesh Eater*, 1857) and Louisa May Alcott (*Passionate Play*, 1869) also exercised their literary imaginations with cannabis.

At the same time, cannabis became more firmly established in American medicine for a large variety of indications after an extensive report in Ohio (McMeens, 1860). Subsequently, the great physicians of the age supported its medicinal use. Sir John Russell Reynolds described the use of cannabis extract for more than a generation (Reynolds, 1868) for treating medical conditions ranging from insomnia to the dysmenorrhoea that affected his most famous patient, Queen Victoria. Other celebrities employing cannabis therapeutically included Silas Weir Mitchell (1874), Sydney Ringer (1886) and Sir William Gowers (1888). Many useful lessons emerged, among them the unique ability of cannabis to treat neuropathic pain, its anti-anorectic benefits, the requirement for individual dose titration, a rather disturbing difficulty with quality control and an 'opiate-sparing' effect.

By the end of the century, cannabis was in widespread use as a prescription medicine, and appeared in the form of solid extracts, tinctures, cigarettes for asthma, corn plasters and as an ingredient in a large array of patent medicines (Fankhauser, 2002). It is fascinating to consider that cannabis was often combined with opium and capsicum extracts; it has been argued that this empirical experimentation and manipulation of the endogenous cannabinoid, opioid (endorphin) and vanilloid (capsaicin) systems in the nineteenth century provided better outpatient analgesia than we have at our disposal today. In each instance, these plants (*Cannabis sativa, Papaver somniferum, Capsicum annuum*) were required to elucidate the nature of analgesia and our endogenous neurotransmitter functions. Thus cannabis informed our discovery of endocannabinoids, the poppy our knowledge of endorphins and enkephalins, and the chile pepper our awareness of the endovanilloid system.

Despite its continued recommendation by physicians (Osler and McCrae, 1915; Fishbein, 1942) and scientists (Dixon, 1923), cannabis faced an onslaught of prohibitive legislation in the early twentieth century, leading to its elimination from pharmacies across the globe despite the endorsement of various commissions (see Figure 1.1). In the UK, cannabis continued to be available clinically until 1971 when it was reclassified as a Class B drug and banned under the Misuse of Drugs Act. Cannabis use became a social issue, whose 800-year-old controversy dogged it everywhere, leading to increasingly stringent international controls. Medical utility and research endeavours unfortunately thus fell by the wayside, while the focus remained solely on its abuse potential, which had rarely been a serious issue over the previous century of therapeutic application.

In 1964, tetrahydrocannabinol, or THC, the main psychoactive component of cannabis, was isolated and synthesised in Israel by Raphael Mechoulam's team (Gaoni and Mechoulam, 1964). In 1972, the National Institute on Drug Abuse (NIDA, USA) began funding studies on cannabis with the intent of demonstrating its deleterious effects. Due to this, however, many adverse event allegations were advanced, including its effects on gynaecomastia, chromosome damage, addiction and cognitive deterioration (Zimmer and Morgan, 1997; Russo *et al.*, 2002). Chronic use studies in Costa Rica, Jamaica and Greece, which were funded by the NIDA, refuted the claims, and were largely ignored (Rubin and Comitas, 1975; Stefanis *et al.*, 1977; Carter, 1980). This crisis led to opportunity, however, as important pathophysiological benefits were soon noted for cannabis as a musculoskeletal and neuropathic analgesic, as an anti-inflammatory, an immunomodulatory, an antiemetic and as an appetite stimulant for patients with AIDS (British Medical Association, 1997). Cannabis was vigorously touted for use by patients with a diverse list of intractable clinical conditions

Cannabis use, Bylony culture, Central Europe
    Chinese hemp by ^{14}C dating
        Chinese Emperor Shên-Nung prescribes cannabis
        Cannabis pollen, Egypt
        Sumerian/Akkadian cannabis use
ANCIENT CULTURES   *Atharva Veda, bhang* for grief
        Ebers Papyrus, Egypt,
        obstetrical use

5000	4000	3000	2000	1000	BCE

Hemp textiles, Gordion, Turkey
  Bhang described in *Avesta* of Zoroaster, Persia
  Hemp seeds as food of Buddha
    Qunnapu, Babylonian incense
      Herodotus, cannabis as Scythian funerary
      Preserved cannabis fruits, Wilmersdorff, Germany
      Ayurvedic medical use of cannabis
ANCIENT CULTURES II   Tombs of Pazyryk, Scythian hemp/burned cannabis
        Diodorus Siculus, use in Egypt

700	600	500	400	300	200	100	0	BCE

Pliny, *Natural History,* fibre/food/medicine
  Dioscorides' *Herbal*, cannabis for otalgia
    Cannabis anaesthesia in China
      Galen, cannabis for GI complaints, inebriant
        Burnt cannabis in cave, Judea, obstetrical aid
          Tantric use of cannabis in India
            Sabur ibn Sahl, parenteral analgesic, Persia
            Old English Herbarium, arthritis/burns
CLASSICAL/MEDIEVAL   Hildegard von Bingen,
         Physica
         King Baibars,
         prohibition

0	100	200	300	400	500	600	700	800	900	1000	1100	1200	1300	CE

Cannabis metabolites in pipes, Ethiopia
  Garcia da Orta, India, psychoactive/anti-anorectic
    Rabelais, *Gargantua et Pantagruel*
      Li Shih-Chen, *Mu Bencao Gang*, China
      Gerard, *The Herball,* jaundice/fluxes
        Robert Burton, *Anatomy of Melancholy*, ecstatic
        Parkinson, *Theatrum Botanicum*, England
        Culpeper, *Complete Herbal*
        Persian *Makhzan Al-Adwiya*
RENAISSANCE   Salmon, *Botanologia*, gout/colic
        Short, *Medicina Britannica*
        Linnaeus, *Materia Medica*

1300	1400	1500	1600	1700	1800 CE

Figure 1.1 Cannabis time line by Ethan Russo, MD. *Continued over page.*

Napoleon in Egypt, prohibition
O'Shaughnessy in India, rabies/tetanus
Moreau, *Du Haschich et de l'Alientation Mentale*
Christison, Scotland, arthritis/labor
Reynolds, Queen Victoria's physician
Ringer, book chapter on
cannabis
19th CENTURY   India Hemp Drugs
Commission
Dixon, smoked for
pain/work/appetite

1800 1810 1820 1830 1840 1850 1860 1870 1880 1890 1900 CE

Harrison Act
Osler, cannabis best for migraine
Fishbein, cannabis in labor
Panama Canal Zone Commissions
Marihuana Tax Act (USA)
LaGuardia Commission (USA)
Single Convention Treaty, UN
Mechoulam, isolation and synthesis of THC
Wooton Report (UK) recommends medical
availability
Controlled Substances Act (USA)
LeDain Commission (Canada) for
decriminalisation
Misuse of Drugs Act (UK)
Shafer Commission (USA) for
decriminalization/research
Noyes, cannabis analgesia
20th CENTURY   Chronic use studies, Costa Rica, Jamaica
Marijuana and Health (USA)

1910 1920 1930 1940 1950 1960 1970 1980 CE

Judge Young (FDA) recommends Schedule II status
Central cannabinoid receptor (CB_1) discovered
Endogenous cannabinoid, anandamide isolated
Grinspoon, *Marihuana, the Forbidden Medicine*
Peripheral cannabinoid receptor (CB_2) discovered
2-arachidonylglycerol (2-AG) discovered
Prop. 215 in California legalizes medical use
BMA Report, rescheduling/research
House of Lords Report
'Entourage effect' described
Institute of Medicine (USA)
Jamaica for
decriminalisation
RECENT EVENTS

Medical use/
Canada

1988 1989 1990 1991 1992 1993 1994 1995 1996 1997 1998 1999 2000 2001 CE

Figure 1.1 *Continued.* Cannabis time line by Ethan Russo, MD.

that were unresponsive to conventional pharmacotherapy (Grinspoon and Bakalar, 1997). At this point, however, even medical users remained subject to arrest in most societies.

In 1988, a cannabinoid receptor (CB_1) was found in the brain (Howlett *et al.*, 1988), and in 1992, anandamide (from *ananda*, Sanskrit for 'bliss'), the first central endogenous cannabinoid, was characterised (Devane *et al.*, 1992). Subsequently, a peripheral receptor (CB_2) was discovered on immune cells (Munro *et al.*, 1993), and, after 5000 years of medical usage, the biochemical basis of cannabis therapeutics became understandable at last.

Cannabis, the plant

Debate continues as to the number of cannabis species in existence. Some authorities identify three: *Cannabis sativa*, *C. indica and C. ruderalis* (Schultes *et al.*, 1974), while others recognise only *sativa* (Small and Cronquist, 1976) (Plate 1). The issue has recently been exhaustively revisited with support for a single heterogeneous species based on taxonomic, morphological and genetic parameters (Merzouki, 2001). For further information, see Chapter 4, where an account of the taxonomy and history of cannabis from an evolutionary perspective is given.

To date there are several facts regarding cannabis use that are clear. Cannabis originated in Central to Eastern Asia and with hops (*Humulus lupulus*) and it is a member of the Cannabaceae (or Cannabidaceae, in older taxonomic classifications) family. All strains (or 'species') crossbreed indiscriminately, which is of critical import in its husbandry, as windborne pollination from hemp strains will render a medicinal crop all but useless. Maximal potency in cannabinoid production results only when the female flowering tops remain unfertilised. This cultivation technique has been known in India for more than 2000 years, and is used to produce the product *ganja*, known in North America as *sinsemilla*, which is Spanish for 'without seed'.

Cannabis vegetative growth is optimised in bright light and long day-length, while flowering and fruiting requires a cycle of 12 hours or less exposure (Clarke, 1981) (see Chapter 2 for discussion of cannabis propagation). Medical chemovars (varieties distinguished by content of useful metabolites, rather than morphological characteristics) are produced from genetically select seeds, or preferably by clonal propagation with adequate legroom. Ultraviolet exposure and perhaps altitude favour THC production (Pate, 1994). Selective breeding provides the capability to cultivate clones favouring production of single specific cannabinoids, whether they are THC, cannabidiol (CBD) or tetrahydrocannabivarin (THCV) (Whittle *et al.*, 2001). These C21 or C22 compounds, including carboxylic acid precursors, are unique to the species and bind to endocannabinoid receptors much as the endogenous compound anandamide (Pertwee and Ross, 2002).

Cannabinoid concentration is not uniform throughout the plant biomass; cannabinoids are present in the leaves but are most abundant in the unfertilised flower head, the bracts and, to a lesser extent, in glandular trichomes on the leaves that store resin. The head of the glandular trichome is a cellulose envelope containing resin; when harvested and compacted this constitutes 'hash'. Fibre strains of hemp are best cultivated in dense stands, favouring them over weeds, and allowing development of long strands of cellulose. In both cannabis fibre and seed strains, THC production is low to negligible, while CBD production is maximised. Hemp as a textile was extremely popular in previous ages until the era of synthetics and is currently staging a comeback. So, too, is the hemp seed industry, on account of its product's yield of high protein and essential fatty acids (EFAs), linoleic (LA), linolenic (LNA) and the pharmaceutically important gamma-linolenic acid (GLA) (Wirtshafter, 1997; Pate, 1999).

The terpenophenolic cannabinoids have been assigned a variety of numbering systems, thus THC may appear in the literature as Δ^1-THC (the monoterpenoid system, favoured in Europe), or Δ^9-THC (the dibenzopyran system, preferred in North America). These systems have arisen due to the fact that the open ring in the cannabinol series gives rise to different numbers for substituents than the dibenzopyran system (see Chapter 8, Figure 8.1). Medically important effects of cannabis are also attributable to its terpenoid essential oil content with possible contributions from its flavonoid and phytosterol components (McPartland and Russo, 2001). This raises a critical issue: there is increasing evidence that the biological effects of cannabis are not produced by THC alone, but rather, that the herbal synergy of the whole cannabis extract yields pharmacological results greater than the sum of its parts. This barrage of phytocannabinoids is directly analogous to the orchestrated effects of the various endocannabinoids and their 'inactive' precursors in endogenous systems, dubbed the 'entourage effect' (Mechoulam and Ben-Shabat, 1999). Seemingly, humans and cannabis have coevolved for thousands of years and the neurochemical and psychopharmacological interactions that have developed provide fascinating possibilities for further investigation.

Cannabis research has been confounded by various scientific and political challenges. Vernacular cannabis in the USA is THC rich, but virtually lacking in CBD (Gieringer, 1999). The cannabis produced by the NIDA, the sole legal research supplier in the USA, is not assayed for CBD (Russo *et al.*, 2002), and this low potency product does not represent the pinnacle of therapeutic possibilities for phytotherapy. In Europe, in contrast, a reliance on North African and Middle Eastern strains (referred to collectively as 'Moroccan' cannabis) provides chemovars that are richer in CBD, yielding heterogeneous medicinal effects. CBD modulates the 'high' of THC, inhibits its hepatic metabolism to the more psychoactive 11-OH-THC, and provides its own anti-inflammatory, antianxiety, antipsychotic and anticonvulsant benefits (McPartland and Russo, 2001). New possibilities attend investigation of South African and South-East Asian cannabis strains with their rich endowment in THCV. These strains are purported to produce analgesic effects with a shorter half-life and have less hangover effects than THC. The weight of the current evidence supports the concept that cannabis will meet its full therapeutic potential as a botanical product rather than as a single new chemical entity (NCE).

Effects of legislation on research

Cannabis has been regulated by a variety of national and international treaties and laws including the Marihuana Tax Act (USA, 1937), the Single Convention Treaty (United Nations, 1961), the Misuse of Drugs Act (UK, 1971) and the Controlled Substances Act (USA, 1970). These have inhibited cannabis research and therapeutics (Abrams, 1998; Russo *et al.*, 2002), and are in striking contradistinction to the recommendations of various commissions studying the issue (see Figure 1.1). In essence, cannabis is identified internationally as an addictive and dangerous drug with no therapeutic utility. The way that legislation has extensively shaped attitudes to the use of cannabis in modern medicine, and the generation of evidence that would allow a reappraisal of utility, are dealt with in Chapter 13. Legislation trumps science, *pro tem*, but research that scientifically supports the use of therapeutic cannabis-derived medicines may change the law eventually.

In the USA in particular, the NIDA has conducted research solely designed to demonstrate the deleterious effects of cannabis, while barely allowing the study of potential benefits. Thus, natural THC in cannabis is a Schedule I substance provoking incarceration, while the identical compound, synthetically manufactured and placed in a sesame oil capsule licensed as Marinol ('dronabinol'), can be prescribed legally and was downgraded to Schedule III in 1999.

Fortunately for the therapeutic potential of medicines derived from cannabis, both for treating diseases where current treatments are not satisfactory and for diseases with unmet clinical needs, challenges are being raised to these concepts and are beginning to appear in Europe. Encouraged by progress by the British Medical Association (1997) and the House of Lords Select Committee on Science and Technology (2001) and with support from Home Office licensing and the Medical Control Agency, clinical studies of cannabis by the Royal Pharmaceutical Society and GW Pharmaceuticals have been initiated (Whittle *et al.*, 2001). These studies will investigate with modern methods the considerable anecdotal evidence supporting the popular usage of clinical cannabis (Grinspoon and Bakalar, 1997; Gieringer, 2001).

Once more, contrasts are evident. In the UK, thanks largely to the indefatigable Clare Hodges, who has campaigned for and highlighted the need for cannabis to be medically available for patients with multiple sclerosis, the treatment of pain and spasm in multiple sclerosis is the lead indication for clinical cannabis investigation. In the USA, in contrast, interest in AIDS (Russo, 2001a) and cancer chemotherapy (Musty and Rossi, 2001) are paramount.

What seems evident is that cannabis is addressing the unmet clinical aims for many patients with intractable clinical problems, whether neuropathic, musculoskeletal and cancer-associated pain, arthritis, head injury, stroke, migraine, asthma, nausea, epilepsy, glaucoma or long-neglected areas of obstetrics and gynaecology (Russo, 2002). The knowledge that cannabinoid effects are integral to our human physiology and are tonically active in the nervous system makes further clinical research essential, and it would be short-sighted to ignore the essence of our own being. The disadvantages must coexist with the advantages. Acute THC intoxication may impair short-term memory, but forgetting is as essential to mental function as remembering (Hampson and Deadwyler, 2000) in order to avoid the chaos of a mind lost in tumultuous disorder. This medical research is not the attack of 'legalisers' or 'cannabis carpetbaggers', but is motivated by the highest ideals of medicine: those of providing relief and longer life to those in pain and suffering. This becomes increasingly possible with cannabis, which is a source of food, fibre, fuel and pharmaceuticals, and could be said to be Nature's most versatile botanical treasure.

References

Abel E L (1980). *Marihuana, the First Twelve Thousand Years*. New York: Plenum Press.

Abrams D I (1998). Medical marijuana: tribulations and trials. *J Psychoactive Drugs* 30(2): 163–169.

Alcott L M (1869). *Perilous Play*. Frank Leslie's Chimney Corner, February 3.

Aldrich M R (1970). Cannabis myths and folklore. Doctoral dissertation, State University of New York at Buffalo, Buffalo.

Aldrich M R (1997). History of therapeutic cannabis. In: Mathre M L, ed. *Cannabis in Medical Practice: A Legal, Historical and Pharmacological Overview of the Therapeutic Use of Marijuana*. Jefferson, NC: McFarland.

Artamonov M I (1965). Frozen tombs of the Scythians. *Sci Am* 212(5): 101–109.

Bowrey T, Temple R C (1905). *A Geographical Account of Countries round the Bay of Bengal, 1669–1679*, 2nd series, no. 12. Cambridge: Hakluyt Society.

British Medical Association (1997). *Therapeutic Uses of Cannabis*. Amsterdam: Harwood Academic Publishers.

Brunner T F (1973). Marijuana in ancient Greece and Rome? The literary evidence. *Bull Hist Med* 47(4): 344–355.

Burton R (1907). *The Anatomy of Melancholy*. London: Chatto and Windus.

Carter W E (1980). *Cannabis in Costa Rica: A Study of Chronic Marihuana Use*. Philadelphia: Institute for the Study of Human Issues.

Chopra I C, Chopra R W (1957). The use of cannabis drugs in India. *Bull Narc* 9: 4–29.

Churchill F (1849). *Essays on the Puerperal Fever and Other Diseases Peculiar to Women*. London: Sydenham Society.

Clarke R C (1981). *Marijuana Botany: An Advanced Study*. Berkeley, CA: And/Or Press.

Clarke R C (1998). *Hashish!* Los Angeles, CA: Red Eye Press.

Clendinning J (1843). Observation on the medicinal properties of *Cannabis sativa* of India. *Medico-Chirurgical Trans* 26: 188–210.

Crawford V (2002). A homelie herbe: Medicinal cannabis in early England. *J Cannabis Ther* 2(2): 71–79.

Culpeper N (1994). *Culpeper's Complete Herbal*. London: W Foulsham.

da Orta G (1913). *Colloquies on the Simples and Drugs of India*. London: Henry Sotheran.

Dark P (2000). *The Environment of Britain in the First Millennium AD*. London: Duckworth.

de Pasquale A, Costa G (1967). Sull'attivita' farmacologica della canape indiana. Istituti di Farmacologia e di Farmacognosia dell'universita' di Messina 5: 173–184.

Devane W A, Hanus L, Breuer A *et al.* (1992). Isolation and structure of a brain constituent that binds to the cannabinoid receptor. *Science* 258(5090): 1946–1949

Dioscorides P (1968). *The Greek Herbal of Dioscorides*. Translated by J Goodyer and R W T Gunther. London, New York: Hafner Publishing.

Dixon W E (1923). Smoking of Indian hemp and opium. *BMJ* 2(1179–1180).

Donovan M (1845). On the physical and medicinal qualities of Indian hemp (*Cannabis indica*). *Dublin J Med Sci* 26: 368–402, 459–461.

Dwarakanath C (1965). Use of opium and cannabis in the traditional systems of medicine in India. *Bull Narc* 17: 15–19.

Fankhauser M (2002). History of cannabis in Western medicine. In: Grotenhermen F, Russo EB, eds. *Cannabis and Cannabinoids: Pharmacology, Toxicology and Therapeutic Potential.* Binghamton, NY: Haworth Press: 37–51.

Fishbein M (1942). Migraine associated with menstruation. *JAMA* 237: 326.

Gaoni Y, Mechoulam R (1964). Isolation, structure and partial synthesis of an active constituent of hashish. *J Am Chem Soc* 86: 1646–1647.

Gerard J, Johnson T (1975). *The Herbal: or, General History of Plants,* the complete 1633 edition. NY: Dover Publications.

Gieringer D (1999). Medical cannabis potency testing project. *Bull Multidisciplinary Assoc Psychedelic Studies* 9(3): 20–22.

Gieringer D (2001). Medical use of cannabis: Experience in California. In: Grotenhermen F, Russo E, eds. *Cannabis and Cannabinoids: Pharmacology, Toxicology, and Therapeutic Potential.* Binghamton, NY: Haworth Press: 153–170.

Gowers W R (1888). *A Manual of Diseases of the Nervous System.* Philadelphia: P Blakiston Son & Co.

Grattan J H G, Singer C J (1952). *Anglo-Saxon Magic and Medicine. Illustrated Specially from the Semi-pagan text 'Lacnunga'.* London, New York: Oxford University Press.

Grinspoon L, Bakalar J B (1997). *Marihuana, the Forbidden Medicine,* revised and expanded edition. New Haven: Yale University Press.

Hamarneh S (1957). Pharmacy in medieval Islam and the history of drug addiction. *Med Hist* 16: 226–237.

Hampson R E, Deadwyler S A (2000). Cannabinoids reveal the necessity of hippocampal neural encoding for short-term memory in rats. *J Neurosci* 20(23): 8932–8942.

Herodotus (1998). *The Histories.* Translated by R Waterfield and C Dewald. Oxford: Oxford University Press.

House of Lords Select Committee on Science and Technology (1998). *Cannabis: The Scientific and Medical Evidence.* The House of Lords Session 1997–8, 9th report. London: Stationery Office.

House of Lords Select Committee on Science and Technology (2001). *Therapeutic Uses of Cannabis, with Evidence.* London: Stationery Office.

Howlett A C, Johnson M R, Melvin L S, Milne G M (1988). Nonclassical cannabinoid analgetics inhibit adenylate cyclase: development of a cannabinoid receptor model. *Mol Pharmacol* 33(3): 297–302.

Julien M S (1849). Chirugie chinoise. Substance anesthétique employée en Chine, dans le commencement du III-ième siecle de notre ère, pour paralyser momentanement la sensibilité. *C R Hebd Acad Sci* 28: 223–229.

Kabelík J, Krejeí Z, Santavy F (1960). Cannabis as a medicament. *Bull Narc* 12: 5–23.

Kahl O (1994). *Sabur ibn Sahl: Dispensatorium parvum (al-Azrabadhin al-Saghir).* Leiden: E J Brill.

Langham W, Harper T (1633). *The Garden of Health,* 2nd edn. London: Thomas Harper.

Li H-L (1974). An archaeological and historical account of cannabis in China. *Econ Bot* 28: 437–448.

Linné C A (1772). *Materia Medica per Regna Tria Naturae*. Lipsiae et Erlangae: Wolfgang Waltherum.

Lozano I (2001). The therapeutic use of *Cannabis sativa* L. in Arabic medicine. *J Cannabis Ther* 1(1): 63–70.

Ludlow F H (1857). *The Hasheesh Eater: Being Passages from the Life of a Pythagorean*. New York: Harper.

McMeens R R (1860). *Report of the Ohio State Medical Committee on* Cannabis indica. White Sulphur Springs: Ohio State Medical Society.

McPartland J M, Russo E B (2001). Cannabis and cannabis extracts: Greater than the sum of their parts? *J Cannabis Ther* 1: 103–132.

Mannische L (1989). *An Ancient Egyptian Herbal*. Austin: University of Texas.

Mechoulam R (1986). *Cannabinoids as Therapeutic Agents*. Boca Raton, FL: CRC Press.

Mechoulam R, Ben-Shabat S (1999). From gan-zi-gun-nu to anandamide and 2-arachidonoylglycerol: the ongoing story of cannabis. *Nat Prod Rep* 16(2): 131–143.

Merlin M D (1972). *Man and Marijuana; Some Aspects of their Ancient Relationship*. Rutherford, NJ: Fairleigh Dickinson University Press.

Merzouki A (2001). El cultivo del cáñamo (*Cannabis sativa* L.) en el Rif, Norte de Marruecos, taxonomía, biología y etnobotánica. Doctoral dissertation, Departamento de biología vegetal, Universidad de Granada, Granada, Spain.

Mitchell S W (1874). Headaches, from heat-stroke, from fevers, after meningitis, from over use of brain, from eye strain. *Med Surg Reporter* 31 (July 25, August 1): 67–70, 81–84.

Moreau J J (1845). *Du Hachisch et de L'aliénation Mentale: Études Psychologiques*. Paris: Fortin Masson.

Munro S K, Thomas K L, Abu-Shaar M (1993). Molecular characterization of a peripheral receptor for cannabinoids. *Nature* 365(6441): 61–65.

Musty R E, Rossi R (2001). Effects of smoked cannabis and oral delta-9-tetrahydrocannabinol on nausea and emesis after cancer chemotherapy: A review of state clinical trials. *J Cannabis Ther* 1(1): 29–42.

Oman J C (1984). *The Mystics, Ascetics, and Saints of India*. New Delhi: Cosmo Publications.

O'Shaughnessy W B (1838–1840). On the preparations of the Indian hemp, or gunjah (*Cannabis indica*); their effects on the animal system in health, and their utility in the treatment of tetanus and other convulsive diseases. *Trans Med Phys Soc Bengal* 71–102: 421–461.

Osler W, McCrae T (1915). *The Principles and Practice of Medicine*. New York, London: Appleton and Company.

Pate D (1994). Chemical ecology of cannabis. *J Int Hemp Assoc* 2: 32–37.

Pate D W (1999). Anandamide structure–activity relationships and mechanisms of action on intraocular pressure in the normotensive rabbit model. Doctoral thesis. University of Kuopio, Kuopio, Finland.

Pertwee R G, Ross R A (2002). Cannabinoid receptors and their ligands. *Prostaglandins Leukot Essent Fatty Acids* 66: 101–121.

Pliny (1951). *Pliny: Natural History*, Vol. 6. Translated by W H S Jones. Cambridge, MA: Harvard University.

Pollington S (2000). *Leechcraft: Early English Charms, Plant Lore, and Healing*. Hockwold-cum-Wilton, Norfolk, UK: Anglo-Saxon Books.

Rabelais F (1990). *Gargantua and Pantagruel*. Translated by B Raffel. New York: Norton.

Reynolds J R (1868). On some of the therapeutical uses of Indian hemp. *Arch Medic* 2: 154–160.

Ringer S (1886). *A Handbook of Therapeutics*, 11th edn. New York: W Wood.

Rubin V D, Comitas L (1975). *Ganja in Jamaica: A Medical Anthropological Study of Chronic Marihuana Use*. The Hague: Mouton.

Rudenko S I (1970). *Frozen Tombs of Siberia; the Pazyryk Burials of Iron Age Horsemen*. Berkeley: University of California Press.

Russo E B (2001a). *Cannabis Therapeutics in HIV/AIDS*. Binghamton, NY: Haworth Press.

Russo E B (2001b). Hemp for headache: An in-depth historical and scientific review of cannabis in migraine treatment. *J Cannabis Ther* 1(2): 21–92.

Russo E B (2002). Cannabis treatments in obstetrics and gynaecology: A historical review. *J Cannabis Ther* 2(3–4): 5–35.

Russo E B, Mathre M L, Byrne A *et al.* (2002). Chronic cannabis use in the Compassionate Investigational New Drug Program: An examination of benefits and adverse effects of legal clinical cannabis. *J Cannabis Ther* 2(1): 3–57.

Salmon W (1710). *Botanologia. The English herbal: or, History of Plants*. London: I Dawkes.

Schultes R E, Klein W M, Plowman T, Lockwood T E (1974). Cannabis: An example of taxonomic neglect. *Botanical Museum Leaflets of Harvard University* 23: 337–367.

Short T (1751). *Medicina Britannica*, 3rd edn (reprinted). Philadelphia: B Franklin and D Hall.

Shou-zhong Y (1997). *The Divine Farmer's Materia Medica: A translation of the Shen Nong Ben Cao Jing*. Translated by Y Shou-zhong. Boulder, CO: Blue Poppy Press.

Small E, Cronquist A (1976). A practical and natural taxonomy for cannabis. *Taxon* 25: 405–435.

Stefanis C N, Dornbush R L, Fink M (1977). *Hashish: Studies of Long-term Use*. New York: Raven Press.

Thompson R C (1924). *The Assyrian Herbal*. London: Luzac and Co.

Thompson R C (1949). *A Dictionary of Assyrian Botany*. London: British Academy.

van der Merwe N K (1975). Cannabis smoking in 13th–14th century Ethiopia. In: Rubin V, ed. *Cannabis and Culture*. The Hague: Mouton Publishers.

Walker B (1968). *The Hindu World; An Encyclopedic Survey of Hinduism*. New York: Praeger.

Whittle B A, Guy G W, Robson P (2001). Prospects for new cannabis-based prescription medicines. *J Cannabis Ther* 1(3–4): 183–205.

Wirtshafter D (1997). Nutritional value of hemp seed and hemp seed oil. In: Mathre M L, eds. *Cannabis in Medical Practice*. Jefferson, NC: McFarland and Company.

Zias J, Stark H, Sellgman J *et al.* (1993). Early medical use of cannabis. *Nature* 363(6426): 215.

Zimmer L E, Morgan J P (1997). *Marijuana Myths, Marijuana Facts: A Review of the Scientific Evidence*. New York: Lindesmith Center.

2

Growth and morphology of medicinal cannabis

David Potter

Hemp (*Cannabis sativa* L.) is an extraordinarily versatile plant that has been highly valued since Neolithic times or even earlier. When ancient civilisations exchanged the hunter-gatherer lifestyle for that of the mixed farmer, cropping became dominated by wheat, maize and rice, but many other seed crops were also grown for food, and hemp was one of them. Archaeological remains of the Lianghzu culture in China indicate that hemp seed was being consumed between 3300 and 2300 BCE (Nelson, 1996).

Hemp is unique amongst cultivated crops for its versatility, providing a source of food, medicines, fuel, oil, paper, building materials and textiles. In recent times, the additional use of cannabis as a recreational drug has led the Establishment to regard it as harmful in many ways to the fabric of society. Sadly, this fibrous plant's non-recreational uses have often been forgotten as a consquence. How humans discovered the narcotic effects of cannabis is a matter of conjecture (see Chapter 1). It has been suggested that when early farmers separated hemp seeds from the resinous inflorescences their fingers became covered in sticky resin – the plant's richest source of cannabinoids. Chewing the sticky resin off the fingers, or flicking the resin onto a smoky fire, could have resulted in sufficient cannabinoids being ingested or inhaled to cause mind-altering results (Clarke, 1998).

Although still popular in China, hemp seed for human consumption is currently an undervalued minor crop in the Western world, but enthusiasm is developing (Calloway, 2002). The seeds produce a highly valuable oil in abundance, which is rich in healthy polyunsaturates and has a range of pharmaceutical, industrial and nutritional uses. Hemp seed frequently finds its way into commercial bird food and many cannabis plants found in British gardens allegedly arrived there from discarded birdcage sweepings. The seed is also widely bought by freshwater fisherman for use as bait; it is said that roach are especially attracted to it (Wheildon, 2000). Contrary to some suggestions, the seed does not drug the fish into a submissive state as the seeds do not contain the drug. Indeed, if it did, homing pigeons would not be able to consume large quantities before accurately finding their way many miles home over open seas.

The stems of hemp provide some of the strongest natural fibres known. Archaeological remains from China show these fibres were spun to make textiles to produce a strong rope as long ago as 2800 BCE (Bosca and Karus, 1998). This use spread to other continents, with European naval history and hemp production being firmly intertwined. Indeed, the word canvas is derived from cannabis. The Vikings used hemp for rope and sail cloth manufacture, and if their boats were not the first to introduce the material to the east coast of America, then Columbus's were when he sailed there in 1492. In addition to the sail cloth and rope, Columbus's charts, maps, logs and bibles would also have been made of hemp (Herer, 1994). Britannia could not have ruled the waves without hemp materials. So important was this crop to Henry VIII that he introduced a fine of five gold sovereigns for farms not growing hemp. Queen Elizabeth I in 1563 decreed that every farm of 60 acres or more had to have at least one acre devoted to the growing of hemp (Drugs of Dependence, 1996). To meet the rope and canvas demands of its defensive and mercantile fleets, the seventeenth-century Dutch built windmills to crush hemp stalks and speed hemp production.

Paper from hemp fibres was possibly first produced in China in about 100 BCE. Today, hemp is still made into speciality papers, including those used to produce banknotes and tobacco rolling papers. Euro banknotes are printed on paper with a high hemp fibre content.

The Ancient Greeks and Romans knew of the great value of hemp. Pausanius (second century BCE) was apparently the first Roman to write of hemp, and when the Greek physician Pedacius Dioscorides wrote of it in *De Materia Medica* (3: 165) in the first century CE he was the earliest to record its medicinal value using the name *Kannabis* (Nelson, 1996).

Today, the binomial *Cannabis sativa* L. bears the suffix L. in acknowledgement of the taxonomist Carolus Linnaeus, who defined the genus *Cannabis* in his *Species Plantorum* of 1753. Linnaeus studied the plant's flowering behaviour by growing it on his windowsill and wrote of the narcotic effects of the resin. Although Linnaeus is frequently credited as the first user of the name *Cannabis sativa*, the name had been used much earlier by Leonhardt Fuchs in his herbal *Kreuterbuch* of 1543 (Figure 2.1) (Fuchs, 2002).

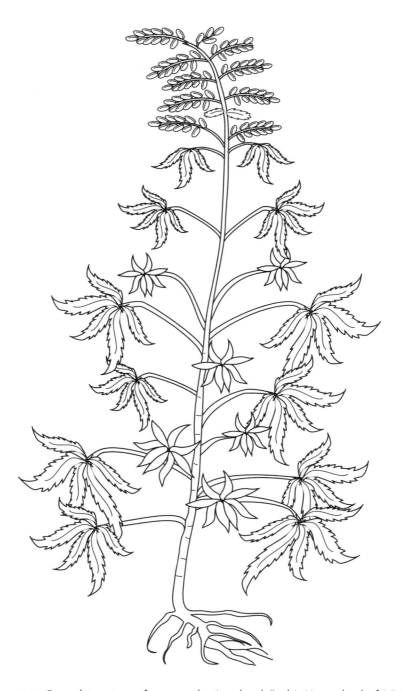

Figure 2.1 *Cannabis sativa* as first named in Leonhardt Fuch's *Kreuterbuch* of 1543.

Cannabinoids and cannabis anatomy

This book focuses on the cannabinoids – a range of well over 60 terpenoid compounds found exclusively in cannabis. Cannabis also contains other groups of metabolites that are potentially of biological interest, including terpenes, flavonoids and carotenoids. In his herbal of 1653 Nicholas Culpeper recommended a decoction of cannabis roots as an anti-inflammatory and a relief against pains in the joints caused by gout. If there was any genuine efficacy in this treatment we can now say that this could not have been attributable to cannabinoids. Analysis of the various parts of the plant confirms that the major source of cannabinoids is the female flower. Cannabinoids are not detected in the roots. The concentration of the cannabinoids tetrahydrocannabinol (THC) and cannabidiol (CBD) in various parts of the plant are shown in Table 2.1. The varieties referred to in this table are given the code designations of G1 and G5. These chemovars (varieties distinguished by content of useful metabolites) are GW Pharmaceuticals plc's primary sources of THC and CBD.

Male flowers were not analysed in this study. In a separate study these have been found to contain minimal amounts of cannabinoids. The untrimmed and manicured female flower samples used in this analysis are shown in Figure 2.2a and b. While the appearance of cannabis is cosmetically important for recreational cannabis, the whole of the aerial parts (less stem) are used for the preparation of extracts for medicinal products.

Table 2.1 Comparison of the cannabinoid content of a range of cannabis plant tissues

Plant tissue	Cannabinoid content (% of dry weight)	
	Variety G1 THC[a]	Variety G5 CBD[b]
Seeds	0.0	0.0
Roots	0.0	0.0
Stems	0.3	0.5
Leaves	0.8	1.0
Mature unseeded female flowers	15.2	7.7

[a]THC + THCA.
[b]CBD + CBDA.
'Manicuring' the mature G1 female flower to remove the less THC-rich bracts and stalks increased the THC content of the remaining material by 3.0%. Figure 2.2 shows this sample before and after the manicuring process.

(a)

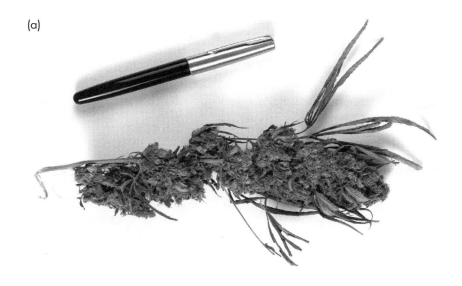

(b)

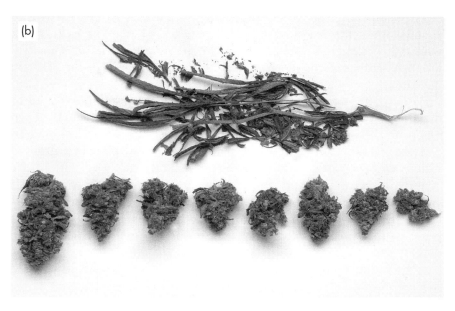

Figure 2.2 (a) Dried mature cannabis inflorescence. The material has not been 'manicured' and the less potent small leaves remain attached. (b) The same inflorescence after manicuring, as if for recreational use. The leaves and central stalk have been removed and the less potent tips to the bracts have been trimmed. The trimmings or 'trash' (above) here lies separated from the most potent material – the 'stash'. A range of alternative street names is used to describe this process. (Photos courtesy of Peter Smith.)

The objectives of the recreational drug grower and the medical grower are different. As this table shows, the richest sources of cannabinoids are the leaves and flowers. These are the only plant tissues worth harvesting for the production of THC and CBD-based medicines. Before discussing the method of producing cannabis material of suitable quality for medicinal use, we need to understand a little of the botany of cannabis.

Cannabis life cycle

Cannabis originates from Central Asia, but now the species is almost as widespread as the human race itself. Plants can be found growing outdoors from the Equator to the edges of the Polar Regions.

Cannabis is an annual herb. As with the hop, *Humulus* sp., the only other member of the family Cannabaceae, cannabis is a 'short day plant'. This means that the plant grows vegetatively through the long days of summer. Only when the day length falls, signalling the end of summer, does the plant start to flower. The point in the calendar at which flowering is induced marks the critical day length. This will differ according to the geographical and genetic origin of the plant in question.

There are exceptions to the above rule. Plants established close to the Equator experience minimal natural changes in day length. Such plants are slow to flower, commencement of flowering being more directly related to the age of the plant. Conversely, plants naturalised well away from the Equator, like the Finnish oilseed variety Finola, are adapted to grow in a very short growing season. The genetics of this variety have strongly programmed the plant to flower at the first opportunity. Even in a warm glasshouse, with lamps burning 24 hours per day, this variety will flower as soon as the first few leaves have developed.

Cannabis is, in most cases, a dioecious plant. That is to say, the species produces separate male (staminate) and female (pistillate) plants (Plate 2) with females tending to slightly outnumber the males. The sole function of the male plant is to pollinate the females. The male plants generally commence flowering slightly before the females. Over the next few weeks the males produce abundant anthers that split open, enabling passing air currents to transfer the released pollen to the receptive females. Varieties of cannabis grown for fibre would normally be harvested soon after pollination. At this stage the fibres still consist of cellulose primarily and are soft and pliable. Hemp intended for textile purposes is harvested at this stage. Later the stems become progressively lignified. Large, lignified hemp stems have been used as reinforcement for plastic composites in car manufacture, and even as reinforcement for concrete. For medicinal and drug type cannabis the final weeks of the growth cycle are the most important.

Soon after pollination, the male plants wither and die, leaving the females maximum space, nutrients and water to produce a healthy crop of viable seeds. Depending upon growing conditions and the level of pollination the female plant may take weeks or months to complete its life cycle.

Optimisation of cannabinoid production

It is during the last few weeks of life that the female plant is most active in the production of cannabinoids and terpenes. The plant will produce variable inflorescences, these being complex clusters of flowers and bracts. Close examination of these inflorescences reveals the individual flowers, which are fairly insignificant to the naked eye. Each flower consists of a furled specialised single leaf – the calyx – within which is housed the ovary (Figure 2.3).

Protruding from each calyx are two pistils (each comprising a fused style and stigma). These are white, pink or yellowy green in colour and up to 20 mm long. The pistil's function is to trap passing pollen. Within minutes of landing on the pistil the pollen can germinate, its pollen tube then migrating to the ovule where fertilisation is completed.

Each calyx is covered in minute sticky organelles – the stalked glandular trichomes (Plates 3–6). Although the individual trichomes are only just visible to the naked eye, in vast numbers they make a striking presence, covering the flowers in a layer of white 'frosting'. Viewed in strong daylight, these trichomes sparkle like drops of dew, giving the cannabis plant a unique beauty. By reflecting the light so spectacularly, the trichome-surrounded flowers must clearly derive some protection from the scorching sun.

When viewed through a hand lens, each trichome resembles a golf-ball (the resin head, also known as the glandular head) sitting on a tee (the trichome's stalk) (Figures 2.4–2.6). Brushing the plant will rupture some of these resin heads, immediately releasing the distinctive heavy, aromatic smell of the essential oils containing terpenes such as limonene and myrcene. Traces of many other terpenes and terpenoids contribute

Stem section

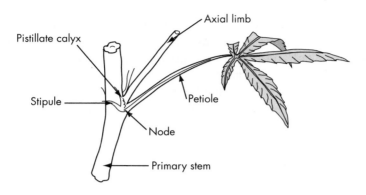

Pistillate calyx

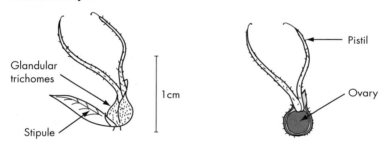

Figure 2.3 Cannabis pistillate calyx structure and location during early stages of plant development.

to the characteristic aroma of cannabis. Up to 70 compounds of this type are present, albeit many of them in very small quantities. In addition to these volatile compounds, the trichomes are extremely rich in cannabinoids, which are themselves odourless. Separated from the dried plant by shaking and sieving, or similar methods, these trichomes constitute the prime ingredients of hashish.

Resinous stalked glandular trichomes are most abundant in the flowers, but significant numbers are sometimes also found on the uppermost leaves. Trichome production reaches its peak in the late flowering stage, and this gives an indication of the optimum time to harvest the plant. Elsewhere on the foliage and stems the plant also develops smaller sessile (unstalked) glandular trichomes, also known as peltate trichomes. These also release essential oils when touched, but as the

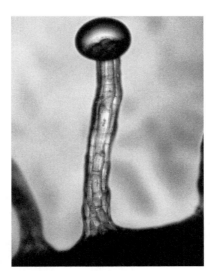

Figure 2.4 A capitate stalked glandular trichome. In this photomicrograph the trichome was dry mounted. The secretory cells appear as dark organelles at the base of the trichome glandular head. (Photomicrograph courtesy of David Potter.)

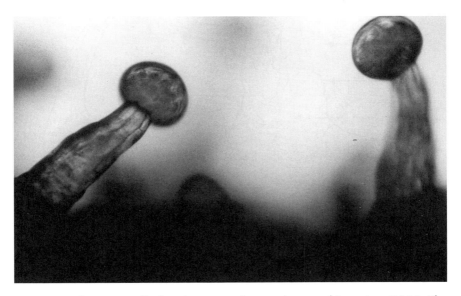

Figure 2.5 Capitate stalked trichomes on the purple cannabis variety G116. The naturally pigmented secretory cells are clearly visible within the glandular head. See also Plate 7. (Photo courtesy of David Potter.)

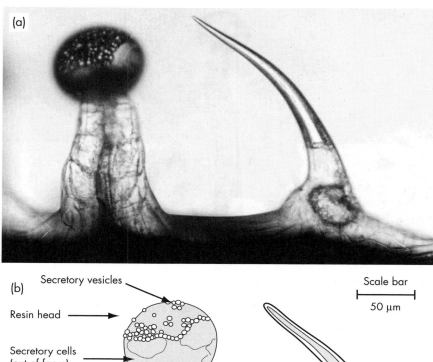

Figure 2.6 Photograph and diagram of a glandular stalked trichome (left) and cystolithic non-glandular trichome (right). (Photo courtesy of David Potter; illustration by Valerie Bolas.)

fragrance generally differs from that of the oils in the stalked glandular heads near the flowers, the exact function of these organs is perhaps different.

Why does the plant produce cannabinoids and terpenes?

The biological function of cannabinoids remains a great mystery. Most if not all the cannabinoid production and storage appears to occur within the glandular trichomes, with the secretory cells within the trichome's glandular head being the exact site of production. These glandular trichomes are found in the greatest quantity in the flowers – the part of the plant most important to ensuring the survival and spread of the species. The compounds appear to afford the plant some protection against bacteria and fungi (McPartland *et al.*, 2000). Some cannabinoids are antioxidants and free radical scavengers. They have been credited with protecting the flowers against damage caused by ultraviolet light (Pate, 1999). It has also been suggested that a predator would become intoxicated before eating too much of the cannabis plant. This role as a deterrent contradicts the observation that, at least in humans, cannabis is an appetite stimulant.

Cannabinoid content varies in different landraces but the high cannabinoid content of modern varieties is purely due to plant breeding. The most potent of modern varieties can contain more than 10 times the cannabinoid content of wild varieties. Indeed, many of the increases in cannabinoid yield have been achieved within the last 25 years (Clarke, 1998). The House of Lords Select Committee on Science and Technology 1997–98 Ninth Report stated that a 'joint' smoked today may contain more than six times the THC of a 1970s reefer (House of Lords Select Committee on Science and Technology, 1998).

The true cannabinoid content of ancient hemp can only be guessed. Comparison of THC and CBD contents of modern material and wild or cultivated crop forms gives an indication of the possible difference. However, modern day 'wild' populations of cannabis have become affected by stray seed and pollen from cultivated forms (Table 2.2).

Unlike the cannabinoids, which are unique to cannabis, volatile terpenes are found in a wide range of species including pine and cedar, where they are known to deter insect attack. Indeed, plant resins containing terpenes have been used to good effect in mummification, preserving corpses against insect attack for centuries. The unsavoury smelling terpenes in cannabis would render the plant unpalatable to all but the most determined feeder (Sumner, 2000). Terpene-rich glandular trichomes, similar to those found in cannabis, are extremely common throughout the flowering plant kingdom – perhaps most notably in the Labiatae (= Lamiaceae – the mint family). In addition to limited studies showing that the terpenes in the Labiatae species repel mammalian

Table 2.2 Comparison of the THC and CBD content of some recreational/medicinal, fibre and wild *Cannabis* varieties. (% w/w in dry seedless female flower material)

Variety[a]	Use	THC (% w/w)	CBD (% w/w)
GW Pharmaceuticals G1	Medicinal	16.2	0.7
GW Pharmaceuticals G5	Medicinal	0.2	7.4
White Widow	Recreational	17.6	0.8
Hindu Kush	Recreational	17.6	0.7
Northern Lights	Recreational	16.4	1.0
Chinese hemp	Fibre	2.6	0.1
Imported hemp	Fish bait	1.7	1.2
Cannabis sativa ssp. *ruderalis*	Roadside weed	0.3	3.0

[a]In all cases, when grown from seed, great variation was found in the cannabinoid content and profile of plants of the same variety. The results shown here are for one typical plant of each variety.

predators, there are many more reporting that these compounds are generally repellent to insect pests (Hallahan, 2000).

The value of sinsemilla

Growers of the most potent cannabis have long known the value of growing the females in a totally pollen-free environment – the so-called sinsemilla technique. This is a Spanish-derived term meaning 'without seeds'. Once pollinated, the plant's energy is diverted from flower and trichome production to seed development. Being an annual, once the plant is in seed-setting mode final senescence follows. In the absence of pollen, the female plant will continue to produce new flowers for a finite time but each pistil can only remain viable for a few days or weeks.

Recognising the 'sinsemilla effect', knowledgeable users of herbal cannabis will generally frown at material containing seeds. As well as spoiling the taste and texture of the cannabis, seeds denote a less than perfect growing technique and probably only a modest THC content.

Life finds a way

Ethan Russo (2002) has described cannabis as the most useful plant on earth, and 'nature's highest expression of unrequited female botanical passion'. Occasionally, these 'passionate' female plants react strongly to being reared in the total absence of males. After weeks of no success with the opposite sex, and apparently faced with the prospect of not being able to produce seed, cannabis females sometimes take matters into their own hands. Starved of males for too long, some female cannabis flowers will develop hermaphrodite tendencies and suddenly produce male florets that release pollen to make self-fertilisation possible. Growers of all-female crops may thus find unexpected seeds setting in their crops. Such growers disposing of their used compost in grandmother's garden should be aware that unexpected seeds might be included (Plate 8).

Pollen produced from normal male plants, which carry both X (female) and Y (male) chromosomes, will produce approximately equal proportions of pollen carrying each type of chromosome. Fertilising females (which naturally carry only X chromosomes) with pollen from males will allow seed to set, which when germinated will give rise to approximately 50/50 male and female plants. Pollen produced from females will only carry the female X chromosome. All progeny from the cross made with this pollen will be female. Masculinisation can be induced by chemical means. This feat can be used to good effect by the plant breeder (Raman, 1998).

Propagating medicinal cannabis

Medicinal cannabis must be of consistent quality. In striving to produce cannabis of uniform high quality commercially, the pharmaceutical company needs to ensure that the correct plant material is selected for the propagation process. At the same time, the correct environment has to be found in which this material can be propagated, carefully harvested and stabilised by prompt drying. These processes are examined in turn.

Selecting plant varieties for cannabinoid production

The history and the essential processes involved in the selection and propagation of quality cloned materials are outlined in Tables 2.3 and 2.4.

Selecting and cloning seedlings

The production of uniform high-quality material is dependent upon the bulk production of 'cloned' plants; that is to say, all plants are derived from cuttings taken from a few select 'mother plants'. Being genetically

Table 2.3 Procedure used by GW Pharmaceuticals to identify and produce THC and CBD clone lines of high purity, yield and quality, commencing with seed samples imported from HortaPharm BV

Date	Activity
1993–1998	High-THC and high-CBD varieties produced at HortaPharm BV, Holland
19 August 1998	Seeds of high-THC and high-CBD HortaPharm varieties arrive in GW glasshouse
24 August 1998	All varieties sown in seed trays
3–8 September 1998	1600 seedlings potted up into individual labelled pots
25 September 1998	All obviously weak plants destroyed. All healthy plants sampled. Analysis of each plant's cannabinoid profile commences
22 October to 16 November 1998	Cuttings taken from all plants and retained in 24-h day-length area to keep vegetative
16 November 1998	All seed-derived plants switched from a 24-h to a 12-h day-length regime to induce flowering, thus enabling male and female plants to be identified
23–30 November 1998	All male seed-derived plants identified and destroyed. All cuttings produced from plants now known to be male are also destroyed
26 November 1998	Planting of rooted female cuttings (clones) commences
30 December 1998	Harvesting of seed-derived plants commences. Agronomic qualities of the plants at harvest is recorded
11 March 1999	Harvesting of clone-derived plants commences
March 1999	Cannabinoid profile data and agronomic data are compared. Having started with 1600, plants derived from the best 32 clone lines are selected for detailed glasshouse trials. All remaining plant material is destroyed
August 1999	Following detailed glasshouse trials the 32 clone lines are reduced to 10. (All botanical raw material used in the clinical trials is derived from these 10 lines)
September 1999 to date	Continuous waves of mother plants raised for the procurement of cuttings for medicinal cannabis production

Table 2.4 Propagation and botanical raw material production

Propagation/production stage	Day-length (h)	Light intensity	Humidity[a] Temp (°C)	Duration (weeks)
Mother plants grown sufficiently to produce >30 cuttings per plant	24	High	Moderate 25	6–8
Cuttings taken, rooting powder applied and placed in peat plugs	24	Low	High 25	2
Rooted cuttings potted-up in proprietary compost and vegetative growth nurtured	24	High	Moderate 25	3
Flowering induced and plant grown to maturity	12	High	Moderate 25	8
Crop harvested and dried before flowers and leaves stripped from stems	n/a	Minimal	Low 20	1

[a]High humidity = >85%; moderate humidity = 60–85%; low humidity = <60%.

identical, all the cloned plants have the potential to exactly replicate the characteristics of the mother plant. The qualities the grower would look for to ensure regulatory acceptability and commercial viability include:

- High rate of cannabinoid production
- High yield of cannabinoid per unit area
- High level of purity of the desired cannabinoid (purity as used here defines the consistency of cannabinoid content as a ratio)
- High inflorescence to leaf ratio (the 'harvest index')
- Natural resistance to pests and diseases
- Sturdy growth capable of bulk plant handling
- Ease of harvesting
- Minimal production of anthers on female plants.

Ongoing research into cannabis breeding indicates that batches of seed may eventually be produced that reach levels of uniformity only achieved at present using cloned material. However, cloned material has other advantages over plants grown from seed. In the first weeks of growth, plants grown from seed develop in a vegetative form, with decussate phylotaxy (Figure 2.7a). Leaves and axial limbs form in symmetrical pairs on the stem, the internodes between these limbs being relatively long. The plant's development stage reaches the 'GV point' at which growth switches from the vegetative form to the generative form (Figure 2.8). Branches now appear on alternate sides of the stem rather

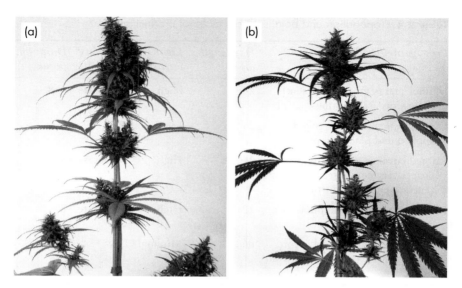

Figure 2.7 (a) A female cannabis plant grown from seed. The plant has maintained a vegetative or decussate phylotaxy (leaf arrangement) right through to the flowering stage. Notice that the side branches appear as symmetrical pairs on either side of the main stem. (b) A female cannabis plant grown from a cutting. The phylotaxy is generative. Notice that the side branches are no longer symmetrical, but appear on alternating sides of the stem. (Photos courtesy of Peter Smith.)

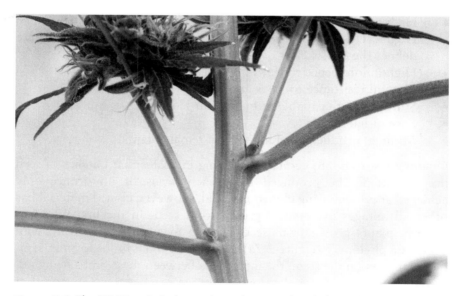

Figure 2.8 The 'GV Point'. At this point on the stem, the phylotaxy has just switched from vegetative to generative.

than in pairs (Figure 2.7b). The internodes between these branches are much shorter than during the vegetative phase. Whether cuttings are taken from cloned or seedling material, the phylotaxy of cloned material will always be the alternate type with shorter internodes.

Whether grown from seed or cuttings, cannabis plants will generally produce the same quantity of cannabinoid per unit area. However the plants grown from cuttings will be shorter, easier to handle and will produce less waste stem material (de Meijer, personal communication).

The improvement in uniformity of cannabinoid content that GW Pharmaceuticals achieved by growing plants from cuttings can be seen

Table 2.5 Comparison of uniformity of cannabinoid profile in 24 cloned and seed-sown plants of varieties G1 and G5

	Cannabinoid[a] (%)			
	THC	CBD	CBG	THCV
CBD variety G5				
Cloned	3.5	90.4	6.0	
	3.7	90.9	5.4	
	3.7	92.7	3.7	
	3.7	92.4	3.8	
	3.6	91.4	4.9	
	3.6	91.4	4.9	
Seeded	4.2	91.4	4.4	
	4.3	91.7	3.9	
	4.0	92.6	3.5	
	4.1	89.1	6.8	
	4.2	90.3	5.5	
	4.1	92.1	3.9	
Variety G1				
Cloned	94.5	3.6	1.5	0.5
	94.6	3.3	1.8	0.4
	94.5	3.0	2.1	0.4
	93.9	3.6	2.0	0.4
	93.9	3.8	1.8	0.4
	94.5	3.4	1.7	0.4
Seeded	82.8	13.1	3.7	0.4
	91.5	4.5	4.0	0
	90.8	5.0	4.2	0
	90.1	5.3	4.3	0.3
	94.8	1.4	3.8	0
	94.8	0.8	4.4	0

[a]For each cannabinoid, data for carboxylated and decarboxylated were combined.

in Table 2.5 and Figure 2.9. These data show that the THC content was much more variable than the CBD. This reflects the fact that the high-THC (for brevity referred to as THC cannabis) variety G1 was produced by crossing varieties from very different habitats, each producing plants with strongly contrasting characteristics. The high-CBD (for brevity referred to as CBD cannabis) variety, however, was crossed from two European parents with similar growth forms.

This variability is a great problem for the illegal grower who relies upon cannabis grown from seeds bought commercially. Despite the fact that such seeds can trade for more than £5 each (US$8 or 8 euros), yields and cannabinoid profiles of plants grown from seeds within the

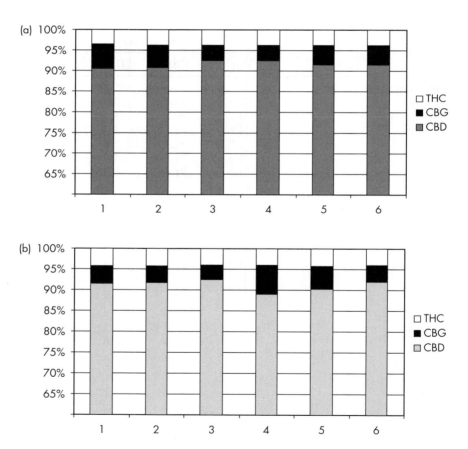

Figure 2.9 Comparison of cannabinoid profiles in cloned and seed-sown plants. (a) Six cloned plants, variety G5. (b) Six plants grown from seed, variety G5. (c) and (d) *continued opposite.*

same packet can vary greatly. If used for medicinal purposes, the pharmacokinetics of these plants could similarly vary.

For the production of the THC material, GW Pharmaceuticals started with seeds of improved strains of cannabis closely related to the variety Skunk no. 1. This was bred by HortaPharm BV in Amsterdam from the same parentage of (Afghani × Mexican) × Colombian genetics. The first crop of Skunk no. 1 was grown in Holland in 1984.

Skunk no. 1 was the first true stable hybrid in Holland's marijuana world, changing the course of cannabis development in the Netherlands (Rosenthal, 2001). Skunk no. 1 was the first of many similar hybrids

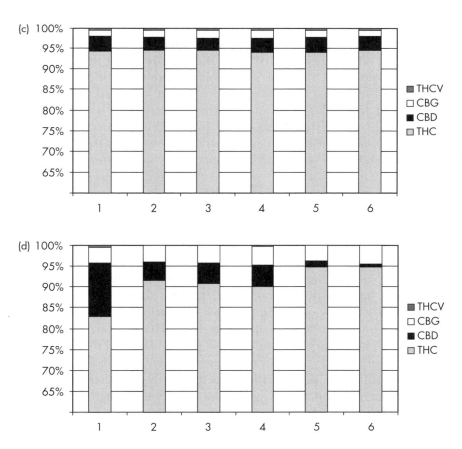

Figure 2.9 *Continued.* Comparison of cannabinoid profiles in cloned and seed-sown plants. (c) Six cloned plants, variety G1. (d) Six plants grown from seed, variety G1.

that subsequently raised the THC levels of commercially available Dutch herbal cannabis to unprecedented levels.

In addition to a high THC content. Skunk no. 1 had many other qualities that made it important in the history of cannabis breeding. In the 1970s the most potent and sought-after recreational cannabis plants in the United States were of the type we regard as *Cannabis sativa* L. subsp. *sativa*. To produce the favourite varieties of that era, such as Original Haze and Purple Haze, the most potent but late-flowering plants from Colombia, Panama or Thailand were crossed with earlier maturing plants from Mexico. Unlike its Colombian relative, when grown outdoors in central California, Purple Haze grew and matured quickly enough for it to be harvested at peak perfection in October, before the weather deteriorated. These '*sativa*' varieties commonly grew to over 2 m, making these illegal plants rather conspicuous when grown outdoors and difficult to handle in a glasshouse.

Skunk no. 1 was produced as a result of a breeding programme to cross these outdoor California '*sativa*' plants with those of the *Cannabis sativa* L. subsp. *indica* type. Seeds of the '*indica*' type had arrived from Afghanistan and included various genetic landraces that were grown to produce cannabis resin. Although of lower THC content than their Californian '*sativa*' relatives, these plants had some highly desirable qualities – a much shorter stature and a much quicker maturation rate. Skunk no. 1 was a highly successful result of this breeding programme. This totally new variety retained the high THC content of its '*sativa*' parents but also inherited the '*indica*-derived' short growth habit and early maturation rate. Not only that, but the variety 'bred true', meaning that when self-pollinated the plant set seed that retained the desirable qualities of the parent. As a result, Skunk seeds could be swiftly produced and passed on to new growers. Being of such short stature, these Skunk plants were easily handled in the glasshouse; and for the cannabis producer, with this variety, new opportunities grew (Connell Clarke, 2001).

GW Pharmaceuticals propagated 400 THC plants from its first seed batch. Laboratory analysis of these plants identified those with the highest cannabinoid concentration and purity. Detailed agronomic studies identified the plants with the best growth characteristics. These combined studies led to 10 individual genotypes being selected for repeat glasshouse trials. From these 10, five were finally recommended for the bulk production of quality medicinal cannabis for clinical trials. Mirroring this process for the selection of CBD material, 1200 plants derived from a selection of European landraces were grown, of which the best four were finally selected.

Maintenance of mother plants

Once potted up and grown in continuous bright light (75 W/m^2 PAR (photosynthetically active radiation)) at 25°C in optimised compost, a rooted cutting will reach a height of 2 m in 12 weeks (Figure 2.10). This plant is then capable of being heavily pruned; the removed branches being cut up to produce up to 80 cuttings per mother plant. If well kept, over the next 10–15 weeks the trimmed mother plant will regrow to produce at least two more flushes of cuttings. The vigour of the mother plant then wanes, and the plant is destroyed to make way for younger mothers.

Taking cuttings

With the right combination of vigorous plant material, favourable glasshouse conditions and horticultural skills, greater than 95% success

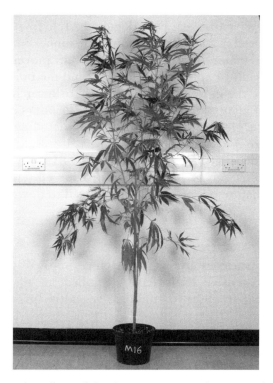

Figure 2.10 A 'mother plant' of the CBD variety G5. This 12-week-old plant is 2 m tall and will produce enough vegetative material for an initial wave of at least 50 cuttings. (Photo courtesy of Peter Smith.)

is regularly achieved when rooting cuttings. Best results are achieved when cuttings are taken from a rapidly growing mother plant.

As fresh material wilts within minutes of being removed from the plant, it is best to work quickly. Branches of the mother plant are removed where there are sufficient numbers of axial buds developing, these being the new growths that develop just above the nodes where the petioles are attached to the stem (Figure 2.11a). The largest leaves are removed or partly trimmed, as these will cause the cutting to lose too much water through transpiration. The branch is then cut into sections, each supporting only one axial bud (Figure 2.11b). Larger cuttings incorporating more than one bud are a waste of valuable mother plant material. These larger cuttings have been found to produce plants with the same yield at harvest (Wilkinson, personal communication). To encourage good root growth, at least 5 cm of stem is left attached below each bud. Normally the stem will be 5–8 mm in diameter and only slightly pliable.

The cutting is then placed in rooting powder and immediately plunged into a very moist peat plug (Figure 2.11c). To minimise wilting, the cutting is placed in a small clear-polythene tunnel on wet fine gravel. High humidity is maintained by restricting the air movement within the tunnel. Roots begin to appear after 7 days, and the polythene is raised slightly to allow the cuttings to acclimatise to lower humidity before potting up. The plants are exposed to light 24 hours/day throughout this period. After 14 days, the cuttings are rooted sufficiently to be potted up (Figure 2.11d).

To reduce dependency upon mother plants, the lower side branches of young plants can be removed to provide cuttings. This is best performed just before plants have been induced to flower.

Potting up

Some cannabis varieties are very exacting in their growing media requirements. Extensive trials have identified an ideal mix, which contains sufficient fertiliser to stimulate vegetative growth and flower production.

Rooted cuttings are plunged into the compost to a depth where the lowest leaf sits just above the surface. If two or more buds have developed, the weaker buds are removed, leaving the strongest bud intact, thereby preventing the plant from developing a forked shape. In the drive to produce uniform plants, all the specimens are encouraged to grow with just one main stem.

Vegetative growth period

For the first three weeks after potting, plants are grown in continuous bright light. With no night time breaks during this period the plant grows to around 50 cm and establishes a healthy root system. Increasing the vegetative growth period beyond three weeks produces taller plants but these do not flower on the lower branches due to the inability of light to penetrate the increased foliar canopy above. The slight increase in final yield of cannabinoid does not justify an extra week's delay in the vegetative phase.

Flowering period

After three weeks the lighting is switched to a 12-hour light and 12-hour dark regime. Having established themselves in an unreal 'land-of-the-midnight-sun' with subtropical temperatures, the plants experience the immediate arrival of the autumn equinox. For a short-day plant (i.e. late summer/autumn flowering) like cannabis, the response is dramatic. As mentioned earlier, such plants have an in-built inductive photoperiod, this being the critical daylength at which flowering will commence. This critical daylength varies according to the latitude from which the variety was derived. The varieties used by GW Pharmaceuticals flower within 5 days of the daylength switch.

The inflorescences increase in size over the next six weeks, becoming white with myriad receptive stigmas. The unfertilised stigmas then start to senesce to an orange/brown colour. After eight weeks in flower, the bulk of stigmas have senesced and the rate of cannabinoid biosynthesis in the selected varieties slows rapidly. Increasing the length of the flowering period by 10% would only increase yield by around 3%. Economics dictates that harvest has arrived (Figure 2.11e).

In both the THC and CBD-rich varieties the other cannabinoid found in appreciable quantities was cannabigerol (CBG). Whereas the ratio of THC to CBD was remarkably uniform in each variety, the CBG levels showed rather more variation. This is because THC and CBD are both relatively stable final products of separate branches of the cannabinoid biosynthetic pathways. CBG however is an intermediate in these pathways and is convertible to THC, CBD or CBC according to the enzyme make-up of the plant in which it is found. The proportion of CBG is slightly higher in immature flowers. This suggests that all plants should be harvested at around the same growth state if the concentration of CBG in successive batches of botanical raw material is to be kept constant.

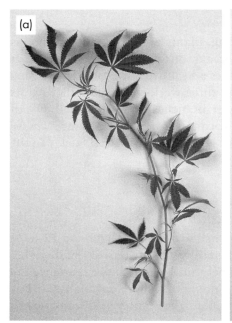

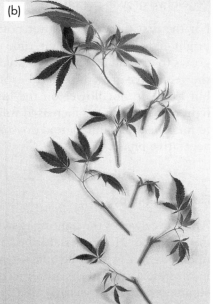

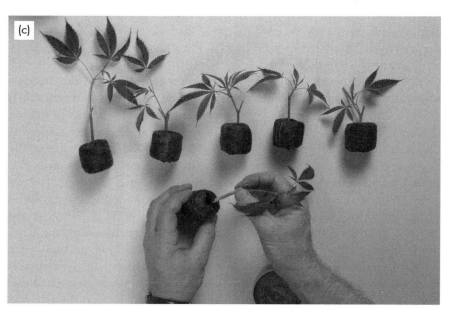

Figure 2.11 (a) A side branch removed from the mother plant for the production of cuttings. (b) The same branch, cut into small pieces each with one axil bud. (c) The branch produces six viable cuttings. Each is dipped in rooting powder before being placed in a moist peat plug. (d) and (e) *continued opposite.*

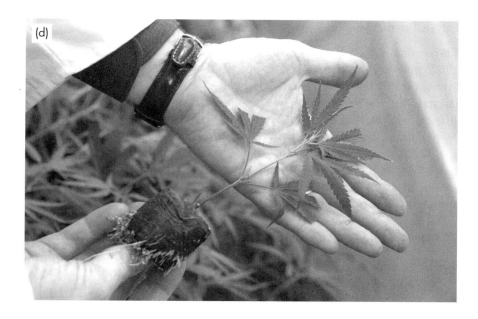

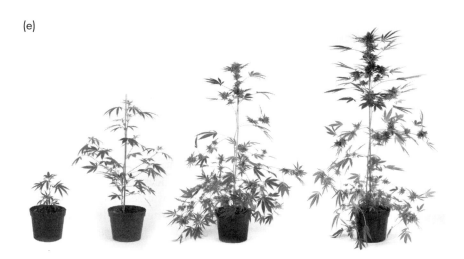

Figure 2.11 *Continued.* (d) After 14 days in a high humidity propagation zone over 95% of cuttings have produced healthy roots and are ready for potting. (e) THC medicinal cannabis variety G1, 1, 4, 7 and 10 weeks after cuttings are potted. Plants are harvested after 11 weeks. (Photos courtesy of Peter Smith.)

Harvest and drying

Harvesting is a simple, but aromatic, operation. Plants are cut just below the lowest branch and moved as quickly as possible to a dark dry room. Almost immediately after harvest, a slow but steady deterioration in the cannabinoid content commences. This deterioration is accelerated in the presence of light. Drying therefore takes place in the dark, but when some light is necessary for inspection of the crop yellow light is used as this has been found least damaging to the cannabinoids (Plate 9).

Drying the crop as quickly as possible reduces the cannabinoid losses, and this is achieved by keeping the plants in a stream of dehumidified air. Plants are crisp to the touch in less than 7 days.

Processing

Despite the low cannabinoid content of the leaves, all aerial parts of the plant apart from the main stem are retained for cannabinoid extraction. This botanical raw material can be seen in Plates 10a and 10b. The THC and CBD content of these materials is approximately 15% and 8% respectively. Although this level of THC potency greatly exceeds the typical content of illegally produced samples seized by the US police, it perhaps sounds modest compared to the values often quoted by suppliers of cannabis to the Dutch Coffee Shops. However, it should be realised that this material is a mixture of potent dry flowers and less cannabinoid-rich leaves and flower-stalks. In the hands of an experienced marijuana supplier, this botanical raw material would be carefully processed, the leaves and stalks being put aside and the bracts removed from the inflorescences to leave the highly prized dried flowers. This final process is called 'manicuring'. Figure 2.2 shows an 11 g inflorescence before and after manicuring. Manicuring produced 3 g of trimmings, leaving 8 g of top grade material with a greatly increased THC concentration.

This highly labour-intensive grading and manicuring process is not cost effective to the bulk producer of medicinal cannabis. Although processing the flowers and leaves *en masse* reduces the cannabinoid concentration of the harvested material, it does not affect the quality of the extracted material which is later purified to bring cannabinoid contents above 90% purity.

The growing environment

To maintain the quality of plant material through the year, the growing environment has to be kept as uniform as possible. With sufficient investment, temperature can be reliably controlled by heat energy being pumped into the growing environment in winter and chilled air on the hotter summer days. A greater challenge is the provision of suitable and sufficient light intensity, especially if attempting the task in northern Europe, 50–55 degrees north.

Let there be light

The most potent outdoor drug varieties of cannabis are adapted to grow at latitudes of 40 degrees or less, where light intensity levels are much higher than in northern Europe. When propagated outdoors cannabis is an annual plant, growing through the brightest months of the year. If aiming to propagate quality cannabis all year round, the European grower needs therefore to recreate very high light levels, week in – week out.

In the UK glasshouse trials GW Pharmaceuticals plc found that cannabis yields are strongly correlated to light intensity. Indeed yields were seen to increase linearly as light levels were steadily raised to a level above which horticultural staff welfare would be compromised. Following these trials, the production glasshouse was fitted with sufficient supplementary light fittings to maintain average daily irradiance levels at 75 W/m^2 PAR throughout the year. This is equivalent to a natural sunlight intensity of 31 000 lux, which exists naturally around midday inside the glasshouse in a UK summer. (*Note:* Intensity of solar radiation is commonly measured in lux and includes the spectrum of wavelengths between 300 and 3000 nm. The horticulturalist is wise to concentrate on photosynthetically active wavelengths only. These have a spectrum of wavelengths between 400 and 700 nm only and account for approximately 45% of the total light energy.)

During the early stages of this research, the first trial crops of medicinal cannabis were grown in a glasshouse with relatively inefficient high-pressure mercury vapour lamps (see Figure 2.12). High pressure sodium (HPS) and metal halide lamps were found to be more efficient (see Figure 2.13).

Light emitted from metal halide lamps is a very pure white, whereas that from HPS lamps is the familiar orange colour of street lighting. GW Pharmaceuticals compared metal halide and high-pressure sodium lamps in growth-room trials. Cannabis plant quality and yield proved to be equal when grown under either type of light. Newly purchased metal halide lamps are slightly more efficient than high-pressure sodium fittings in converting electrical energy into photosynthetically usable light energy. However, metal halide lamps rapidly fade while

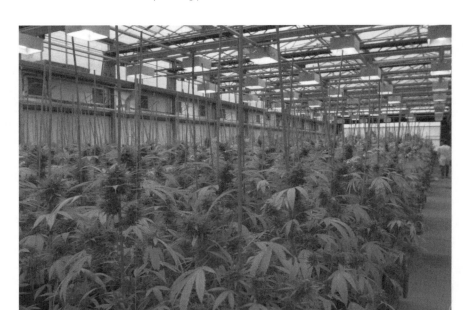

Figure 2.12 First experimental crops of medicinal cannabis were grown under inefficient mercury vapour lamps. (Photo courtesy of Peter Smith.)

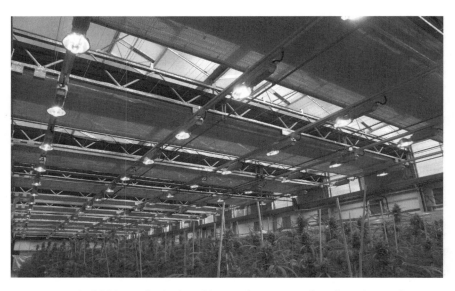

Figure 2.13 In 2001 regular high yielding uniform crops of medicinal cannabis were grown under a complex array of high-pressure sodium lamps, shades and blinds which enable uniform light intensity to be delivered all 12 months of the year. (Photo courtesy of Peter Smith.)

sodium lamps continue to perform well for long periods. In a medicinal cannabis production facility, where uniformity of product is important, the ability of the HPS lamp to deliver uniform light intensity made this lighting system the preferred option.

There was a dramatic improvement in the quantity and uniformity of cannabis yields following the substantial investment in high-energy supplementary lighting (Figure 2.14). This shows the mean average yields of crops of dry herbal cannabis (flowers + leaves) in the glasshouse before and after the HPS lighting installation. The average natural light levels falling on the glasshouse roof are also shown for comparison.

The benefits of high light levels on early plant growth are shown in Figure 2.15. The three high-THC plants on the left were grown under continuous light for three weeks in a growth room. Metal halide lamps produced a uniform round-the-clock irradiance of 75 W/m^2 PAR. The three plants on the right were grown in the glasshouse when mid-day irradiance levels peaked at 75 W/m^2 PAR but then fell to a minimum of 15 W/m^2 PAR through the night time under mercury vapour lamps. Temperature was 25°C in both environments.

The plants in the bright light produced a far greater number of side branches. These would later develop a significant number of THC-rich flowers. Plants that flowered in poor light only produced substantial flowers at the top of the plant, and these were much smaller than those in bright light.

For maximum yields, high light levels are also essential during the flowering stage. Plants grown in high light levels produce much larger flowers containing a higher concentration of cannabinoids. In high light levels, substantially more light energy penetrates the plant canopy to reach the lower branches. The flowers on the lower branches produce worthwhile flowers only if there is sufficient light penetration.

Phototropy and photonasty

These two Greek-derived terms relate to the direction of plant growth in response to light. Although a full understanding of these responses is not essential to the grower of medicinal cannabis, the curious behaviour of cannabis does deserve a brief description.

Phototropism or phototropy can be defined as a directional plant growth response to a light stimulus. Most of us will have germinated garden plants on the windowsill before planting them outside. Just as

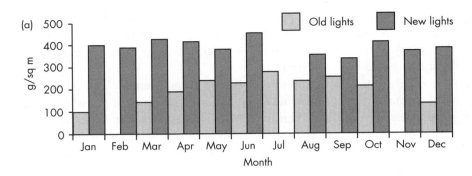

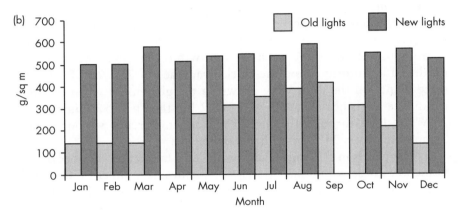

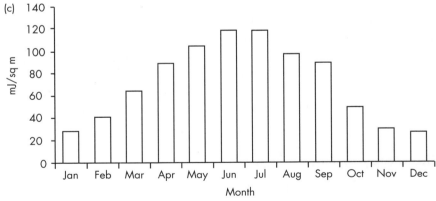

Figure 2.14 Effect of light installation on yield. (a) CBD botanical raw material (BRM). (b) THC BRM. In 2000 the poor-quality light from the mercury vapour lamps resulted in a large seasonal variation in yield (Old lights). In 2001 the new high-pressure sodium lamps provided uniform year-round high-light conditions (New lights). As a result, uniform high yields were achieved throughout the year. (c) Daily glasshouse light levels 2000, 7 a.m to 7 p.m.

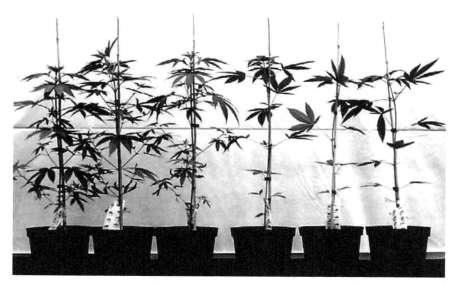

Figure 2.15 Effects of light on leaf development. The plants on the left received high light; those on the right received low light.

Linnaeus would have observed when he grew cannabis this way, such plants stray from the vertical and grow towards the light. In addition to this type of phototropic response, some plants grown in the GW Pharmaceuticals glasshouse under a mixture of mercury vapour and HPS ancillary lamps responded by remaining upright but orienting their younger, fully expanded leaves to face the sodium light fittings.

Photonastism or photonasty is a growth response to light that is not directly correlated to the direction of that light. Well-known examples of this are the closing of daisy flowers and clover leaves as evening approaches. During the earlier growth stages, come sunset or 'lights-out' the upper leaves of the young cannabis plant will drop from a near-horizontal aspect to a more vertical angle. This is illustrated in Figure 2.16 which shows a plant 5 minutes before being plunged into darkness and again 45 minutes later. The temperature was kept constant during this period.

To intercept maximum light energy during the day the plant needs to orientate the bulk of its leaves in the horizontal position. With no significant light available at night time, the cannabis plant droops its upper leaves. A clear benefit of this is that any light showers of rain will then fall unheeded to the soil to be taken up by the roots. Had this rain remained on the upper foliage, much of it would have evaporated and been lost by the plant.

(a)

(b)

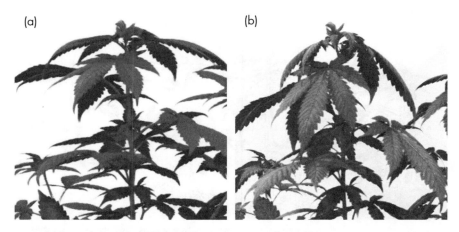

Figure 2.16 Photonasty effects. (Photo courtesy of David Potter.)

Quality, safety and efficacy: meeting EU Good Agricultural Practice guidelines

When producing the medicinal cannabis crop, regard must be paid to regulatory requirements. Growers need to be mindful of such documents as: *Good Agricultural Practice of the Working Group on Herbal Medicinal Products* of the European Medicines Evaluation Agency (Europam, 2003). These have to be read in conjunction with the Medicines Control Agency *Rules and Guidance for Pharmaceutical Manufacturers 1997* (Medicines Control Agency, 1997).

Essentially, the growers have to ensure that the bacterial and fungal contents of their crops do not exceed specified limits. Crops have to be grown and stored in such a way as to minimise any damage to the medicinal ingredients, and in a suitably controlled manner such that similar batches could be reproduced. The facilities used for the propagation and storage have to be kept as clean as is practicable. The growing environment and irrigation systems need to be kept free of pesticides wherever possible. If pesticides are used, the crop has to undergo rigorous testing to prove the absence of unacceptable chemical residues. Harvest conditions should be such that the crop is at the correct stage of development, and any contamination with dirt, moisture or incorrect plant species is avoided.

Growing the crop in a tightly controlled glasshouse environment makes it easier to meet these exacting standards, but specific precautions still have to be put in place.

Microbiological safety

While the crop is grown as 'organically' as possible, nutrition is supplied in the form of mineral additives. Although the risk is low, poultry manure and fish-blood-and-bone are avoided as unacceptable sources of potentially pathogenic bacteria. The growing environment is kept free of birds and vermin. The plants are irrigated with water of drinking quality. Contamination of plant material at harvest is minimised by prompt transfer to the drying room. Bacterial and fungal bioburden is reduced during decarboxylation and cannabinoid extraction processes, but their earlier presence in high numbers would be unacceptable. Similarly, the presence of unacceptable toxins such as aflatoxin is prevented by prompt drying.

Pesticide residues

All botanical material at GW Pharmaceuticals has been produced without the use of pesticides. The growth medium is derived from a pesticide-free environment and the use of these chemicals is not permitted in the immediate vicinity of the glasshouse.

Pest and disease control

Grown outdoors for fibre, the hemp crop has seen a resurgence in recent years. The organic lobby understandably advocates field hemp, as the crop has few natural predators or disease problems and therefore needs little intervention with pesticides. Grown in the balmy conditions of the glasshouse however, conditions swing in favour of certain insect pests and fungi (McPartland *et al.*, 2000). Overcoming the pressures of pests and diseases necessitates the two-pronged attack of prevention and cure.

Prevention of pest attack

Glasshouse pests and diseases of cannabis arrive in a number of ways. Many are windborne and their entry is limited by placing filters within the air inlet channels. Roof vents need shielding with very fine netting. Ideally the glasshouse should be kept at positive pressure; airborne intruders will thereby meet a head wind if attempting to fly into the glasshouse. Insects can hitch a ride on clothing as individuals enter the glasshouse. Staff are therefore issued with separate work attire, and visitors given protective clothing.

The main diseases of glasshouse cannabis experienced to date are grey mould (*Botrytis cinerea*) and powdery mildew (*Sphaerotheca macularis*). The former strikes in the last two weeks of growth, causing great damage to the inflorescences. The disease proliferates in conditions of high humidity. Many cannabis varieties with Afghan genetics are especially susceptible to the disease, no natural resistance having developed in their arid home environment. *Botrytis* infestations are prevented by lowering the glasshouse humidity, and keeping air moving in the crop canopy, or by avoiding susceptible cannabis varieties.

Powdery mildew is less prevalent when growing the plants in high light conditions. Avoiding moisture stress and excess nitrogen fertiliser is recommended to reduce the chance of attack.

Whenever diseases do strike, the affected material has to be removed and destroyed. The infected plants do not meet the required quality standards, and the disease may have altered the chemical profile of the plant material. The infected material can also act as a source of infection for the rest of the crop.

Once diseased or infested plants are identified, routines need to be established whereby personnel do not handle healthy plants having just worked on the affected material.

Cure

Although limited use of pesticides is permitted in the *Good Agricultural Practice Guidelines*, GW Pharmaceuticals has totally avoided their use so far. Mostafa and Messenger (1972) listed 272 insect and arachnid pests of cannabis. McPartland *et al.* (2000) describe about 150 of these in *Hemp Diseases and Pests* and reported spider mites to be the most damaging. Two pest species have proved a substantial problem in the GW crop: spider mite (*Tetranychus* spp.) and onion (tobacco) thrip (*Thrips tabaci*). Small populations of these pest species are permanently present in the glasshouse. The infestations are kept in check with the help of biological control methods, appropriate species of predatory mite being regularly introduced into the crop. Routine close monitoring of the crop is essential to identify and eradicate plant material infested with spider mites before damage spreads.

The way forward – the great outdoors?

This chapter has often emphasised the requirement for uniform growing conditions in the production of a high-quality cannabis-based medicine.

In contrast, many medicines are produced from plants grown in much more variable outdoor situations. Examples are:

- Morphine from opium poppy (*Papaver somniferum*)
- Taxol from Pacific yew (*Taxus brevifolia*)
- Vinblastine and vincristine from Madagascar periwinkle (*Catharanthus roseus*).

However, these plants are all grown to enable single ingredients to be extracted and purified. Cannabis-based medicines are more complex, containing a mixture of cannabinoids, terpenes and flavonoids. These interact together synergistically in a way that is not fully understood (McPartland *et al.*, 2000). Current research will determine just how variations in the growing conditions affect the ratios of these active ingredients.

In addition to variabilities in growing conditions, the outdoor environment presents other problems:

- Just one crop is produced each year
- Harvest date and conditions are unpredictable
- There are large seasonal variations in yield
- Drying a single large crop presents logistical difficulties
- The crop is more likely to be exposed to chemical spray drift and pollution
- It is difficult to ensure the security of the crop
- Some diseases and pests are more likely to occur
- Biological control systems are less easy to use
- The crop is vulnerable to storm damage
- There is increased likelihood of bacterial and fungal contamination from soil, birds and delays in drying, etc.

To test the feasibility of growing such crops, the first experimental outdoor crops of all-female high-CBD medicinal cannabis were grown in southern England in 2000 and 2001. In 2000 the single crop was harvested in excellent conditions in late September. Crops were grown on two farms in 2001 and poor light levels in September delayed the maturation of the crop until the middle of October. Rain and long dew periods approaching the harvest date encouraged high levels of *Botrytis* fungus. Despite the plants looking of good quality when visibly inspected, in both seasons, the level of fungi approached or exceeded the permitted level for a pharmaceutical crop (Figure 2.17).

To reduce some of the above difficulties associated with growing an outdoor crop, in 2001 a batch of 800 plants was grown in polythene

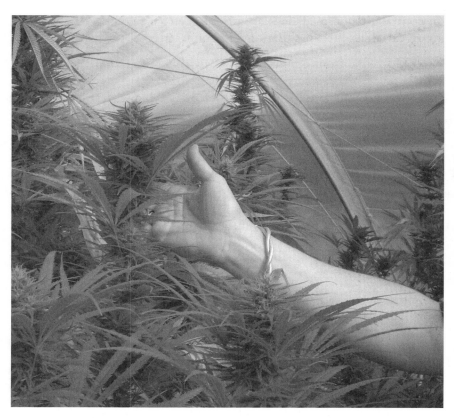

Figure 2.17 A first experimental crop of medicinal CBD variety G5 grown outdoors under polyethylene in 2001. Despite its good appearance, levels of fungal contamination approached unacceptable levels. (Photo courtesy of David Potter.)

tunnels designed for propagating strawberries. The variety used was the same as that regularly grown in the glasshouse. The crop was harvested in early October, and CBD concentrations in the herb were found to be approximately equal to that in the glasshouse crop. The purity of CBD compared with other cannabinoids was the same as the glasshouse crop. This again demonstrates that cannabinoid profile is genetically fixed and not affected by growing conditions. However, limited analyses suggest that the terpene profile and content of the crop was different to that of the same chemovar grown in the glasshouse. The material could not, therefore, be regarded as being of the same quality. More research is required to fully understand how, or indeed if, this change of terpene profile affects the efficacy, safety and quality of the drug substances derived from it.

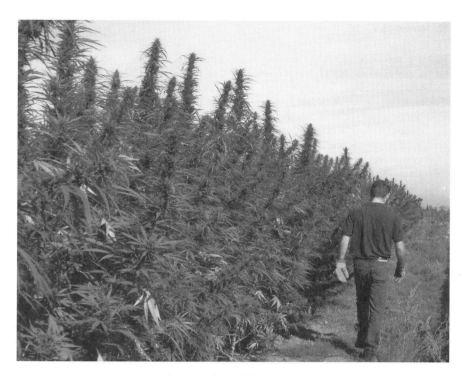

Figure 2.18 An experimental UK outdoor all-female medicinal CBD cannabis crop. *Botrytis* fungus caused major spoilage of the crop in the last days before harvest. (Photo courtesy of David Potter.)

Although this 2001 crop achieved the microbiological safety level for a pharmaceutical crop, a similar crop produced in 2002 was almost decimated by *Botrytis* fungus (Figure 2.18). The problems of growing the cannabis outdoors in northern Europe are made worse when using all-female material. Grown in the absence of males, female crops flower for longer, thus extending their season further into the wet autumn months when fungi are more likely to attack. Perhaps the plant breeder can resolve this problem by producing earlier flowering varieties that yield equally well.

Having invested in highly sophisticated and well-controlled growing conditions, and using these facilities to grow carefully developed and selected plant varieties, it has proved possible to produce a botanical drug substance (BDS) with provenance and a pedigree. This has allowed the generation of a specification for the regulatory dossier. Many exciting cannabis-based medicines will follow and a key player in this advance will be the cannabis plant breeder.

References

Bosca I, Karus M (1998). *The Cultivation of Hemp: Botany, Varieties, Cultivation and Harvesting*. London: Chelsea Green Publishers.

Calloway J C (2002). Hemp as food at high altitudes. *J Indust Hemp* 7(1): 105.

Clarke R C (1998). *Hashish!* California, USA: Red Eye Press.

Connell Clarke R (2001). Sensemilla heritage – what's in a name? In: King J, ed. *The Cannabible*. Berkeley, California: Ten Speed Press: 1–24.

Drugs of Dependence (1996). Drugs of Dependence 9 (Amendment) Bill 1996. *Hansard* (Australia) 15 May, p. 1238.

Europam (2003). Guidelines for Good Agricultural Practice (GAP) of medicinal and aromatic plants. http://www.europam.net/GAP.htm (accessed January 2004).

Fuchs L (2002). http://info.med.yale.edu/library/historical/fuchs/222–3.gif (accessed 28 November 2002).

Hallahan D L (2000) Monoterpenoid biosynthesis in glandular trichomes of labiate plants. In: Callow J A, ed. *Advances in Botanical Research incorporating Advances in Plant Pathology*, Vol 31: *Plant Trichomes*. London: Academic Press: 77–111.

Herer J (1994). *The Emperor Wears No Clothes: The Authoritative Historical Record of the Cannabis Plant, Marijuana Prohibition & How Hemp can still Save the World*. London: Knockabout Comics.

House of Lords Select Committee on Science and Technology (1998) *Cannabis: The Scientific and Medical Evidence*. The House of Lords Session 1997–8, 9th report. London: Stationery Office: chapter 6, para 6.1.

McPartland J M, Clarke R C, Watson D P (2000). *Hemp Diseases and Pests: Management and Biological Control*. Oxford: CABI Publishing.

Medicines Control Agency (1997). *Rules and Guidance for Pharmaceutical Manufacturers 1997: Orange Guide*. London: The Stationery Office.

Mostafa A R, Messenger P S (1972). Insects and mites associated with plants of the genera *Argemone, Cannabis, Glaucium, Erythroxylum, Eschscholtzia, Humulus*, and *Papaver*. Unpublished manuscript, University of California, Berkeley.

Nelson R A (1996). Hemp and history – history of cannabis: the original unabridged text of *The Great Book of Hemp*. http://www.rexresearch.com/hhist/hhicon%7E1.htm (accessed January 2004).

Pate D (1999). Food products. In: Ranalli P, ed. *Advances in Hemp Research*. Binghamton, NY: Haworth Press: 21–42.

Raman A (1998). *Cannabis. The Genus Cannabis*. London: Harwood Academic: 33.

Rosenthal E (2001). *The Big Book of Buds*. Hardknocks Factory.

Russo E (2002). Pot pioneer. *Cannabis Culture* 36. http://www.cannabisculture.com/articles/2302.html (accessed December 2003).

Sumner J (2000). *The Natural History of Medicinal Plants*. Portland, Oregon: Timber Press.

Wheildon T (2000). *Complete Guide to Fishing Skills*. London: Caxton Editions.

3

The breeding of *Cannabis* cultivars for pharmaceutical end uses

Etienne de Meijer

This chapter gives an overview of GW Pharmaceuticals' plant breeding programme. It focuses on those aspects of *Cannabis* breeding that are specific to the development of optimised cultivars for pharmaceutical raw material production. The following subjects will be discussed: the position of this work in the wider spectrum of *Cannabis* breeding, goals and strategies, relevant germ plasm resources, present achievements and expected future developments.

The position of medicinal *Cannabis* breeding

The domestication of *Cannabis* has been directed at the optimised production of distinct plant components such as bark fibre, seed, the psychoactive, dried floral tissue (marijuana) and the extracted psychoactive resin (hashish) (Zohary and Hopf, 1994). Today there are two main 'schools' of *Cannabis* breeding: fibre hemp breeding and the breeding of recreational drug strains. Fibre hemp breeding used to be targeted primarily at yield and quality of bark fibre. Straw yields and bark fibre contents were increased, and the associated fibre quality parameters were monitored and kept within limits. Secondary concerns in the recent past were the development of monoecious cultivars with better uniformity, and the breeding of cultivars resistant to hemp broomrape, various insect pests and nematodes (Becu *et al.*, 1998; Bócsa, 1998). Nowadays, most of the fibre hemp breeders seem to be involved in projects aimed at reducing the psychoactive potency of fibre cultivars from negligible to zero (e.g. Anonymous, 1996; Virovets, 1996).

Breeders of *Cannabis* for the production of recreational drugs ignore the fibre characteristics and select varieties that are rich in THC. Earliness, taste, fragrance and 'the type of high' also appear to be primary points of concern (Rosenthal, 2001). Drug strains were traditionally grown in the (sub)tropics, but nowadays a range of cultivars has been developed for the popular indoor cultivation market (Frank and Rosenthal, 1978; Clarke, 1993; Rosenthal, 2001). A large number of clonal cultivars, as well as their pure or cross-bred seed offspring, are available. Due to legislation, most breeders of recreational drug *Cannabis* are forced to operate in obscurity. Their numerous cultivars are published in counter-culture journals and seed catalogues, but they are generally not named and registered in accordance with official guidelines (Snoeijer, 2002).

Although high fibre content and significant psychoactive potency are not necessarily mutually exclusive (de Meijer *et al.*, 1992), there is no evidence of serious breeding for multipurpose strains. Neither has a conscious exchange of *Cannabis* germ plasm between fibre and drug breeding programmes been reported.

The genetic optimisation of *Cannabis* for the strict medicinal utilisation of its constituent cannabinoids is an unprecedented branch of breeding. This type of activity was initiated at HortaPharm B.V., in the Netherlands in the early 1990s. Since 2001, the HortaPharm programme has continued at GW Pharmaceuticals in the UK. Pharmaceutical *Cannabis* breeding, being aimed at efficient cannabinoid production, is inherently more closely related to the breeding for recreational drugs than to fibre hemp breeding. However, it differs from the breeding for recreational drugs in being focused on a wider range of cannabinoids than just THC, and in being fairly indifferent to traits such as taste and smell. It is also much more eclectic in its choice of breeding sources, as many individual genotypes, selected from non-drug strains, have shown to be of potential interest due to their unusual cannabinoid composition.

Goals and strategies of the pharmaceutical breeding programme

The primary and long-term goal of GW Pharmaceuticals' breeding programme is to enable the constitution of any desired, single or multicomponent cannabinoid profile in an efficient, well-performing cultivar. As far as cultivars with multicomponent profiles are concerned, it has been concluded that for regulatory reasons it is more attractive to establish a certain ratio of active compounds already in a single raw material source, than to blend raw materials from different sources. The term 'desired cannabinoid profile' can relate to various compositions of the pentyl cannabinoids tetrahydrocannabinol (THC), cannabidiol (CBD), cannabichromene (CBC) and cannabigerol (CBG) as well as their respective homologues with a propyl side chain (THCV, CBDV, CBCV and CBGV), and perhaps even of some of their degradation products (cannabinol (CBN), cannabielsoin (CBS) and cannabicyclol (CBL)).

Of course, it is not the role of plant breeding to decide which compositions will eventually be of pharmaceutical interest. 'Well-performing' refers to features such as: high yielding, convenient to grow, reproducible, uniform and stable. 'Convenient to grow' can be specified as being endowed with a good vigour, a fairly short and determined generative cycle, a compact habit, and a reasonable resistance to pests. Also, built-in means of intellectual property protection, such as triploid sterility, a high level of heterozygosity and the presence of conspicuous morphological markers, are appreciated traits. Some of these characteristics are easier to realise and maintain in a clonal cultivar; others in cultivars grown from seed. It is more a logistic and agronomic than a plant breeding issue to decide which cropping system is preferable for a certain application.

For a systematic approach to the programme's primary target (i.e. the development of cultivars that efficiently produce cannabinoids in well-defined compositions), it is necessary to consider the yield of a certain cannabinoid per crop area unit as a complex trait comprising the following independent components:

1. The total amount of above ground, dry biomass (at maturity).
2. The weight proportion of inflorescence leaves and bracts (the 'harvest index').
3. The total cannabinoid content in the floral fraction.
4. The proportion of the particular cannabinoid, in the total cannabinoid fraction (the 'purity').

Vigour and photosynthetic efficiency, plant architecture and the density and metabolic efficiency of the resin glands determine components 1, 2 and 3, respectively. These are evidently polygenic traits unrelated to specific metabolic pathways, and are heavily affected by environment. Together they determine the 'cannabinoid quantity'. Heterosis breeding, in particular, can greatly affect the contribution of these three components, but they are also an agronomic concern. One single genotype shows enormous phenotypical plasticity for components 1, 2 and 3 under the influence of environmental factors such as photoperiod regime, light spectrum, light intensity, nutrient levels and cultivation system (cuttings or seedlings). Component no. 4 is the chemotype (chemical phenotype) in the narrow sense of cannabinoid ratio and reflects the 'cannabinoid quality'. It depends solely on the metabolic pathways followed by a certain genotype to convert common precursors into specific end-products; it behaves as a qualitative trait, and is hardly affected by environment (de Meijer *et al.*, 2003).

Therefore, the manipulation of chemotype is the exclusive territory of plant breeding. At the beginning of the breeding programme it was postulated that line selection (repeated, selective self-fertilisation) would be an effective technique to create uniform, homozygous lines that accumulate only one predominant cannabinoid in high proportions. This has since been confirmed. The given goal and the described concept of cannabinoid accumulation has led to a general breeding procedure of first one facultative, then two fixed, and then again one facultative step. The first facultative step is a basic cross. Often, the germ plasm sources for cannabinoids other than THC are non-drug *Cannabis* types with a less favourable phenotype for drug production (mainly low values for the yield components 2 and 3). As a consequence, when employing such materials, it is standard to perform a basic cross of the selected non-drug plant with a high yielding THC individual. A basic cross may also be required to introgress additional traits such as improved fertility, the ability to artificially revert sex or a morphological marker gene. Then, with the resulting cross progeny, up to five cycles of line selection should be performed to produce homozygous, single cannabinoid breeding parents. Subsequently, the resulting inbred parental lines are mutually crossed, and the performance of the several hybrids is evaluated in a combining ability trial.

On the basis of such an evaluation, those parental combinations that give the most desired progenies according to quantitative yield (components 1, 2 and 3) and quality criteria (component 4) can be identified. A final and facultative step in the breeding process is the production of triploid homologues of the best hybrids. This is achieved by making tetraploid clonal versions from parental inbred lines, and then using these to repeat the most profitable crosses in a $4n \times 2n$ form.

Line selection (i.e. repeated self-fertilisation) in a dioecious species requires the possibility of artificially induced sex reversion. The same applies to the initial basic crosses and final heterotic crosses, where only female genotypes are crossed to produce unisexual (100% female) offspring. Such a technique is available and has been optimised for mass-scale application in the breeding programme (Figure 3.1). Apart from the avoidance of sexual dimorphism in progenies, the exclusive use of female genotypes has an additional benefit. It enables efficient selection

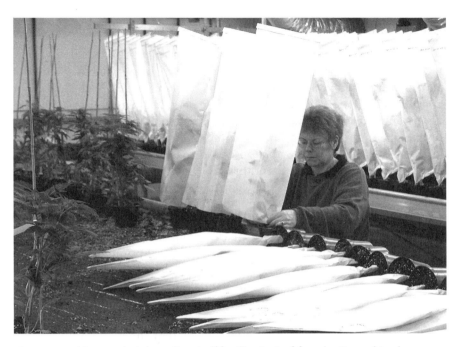

Figure 3.1 Mass-scale inbreeding (self-fertilisation) of female *Cannabis* plants.

of both parents of a hybrid. Since the quantitative yield components 2 and 3 are only fully expressed in female individuals, the selection of dioecious, male cross parents remains a matter of intuition rather than objective measuring.

An adequate metaphor for the described breeding strategy is provided by the common daily procedure in a paint shop. The line selection work will eventually result in a fairly limited number of homozygous parental lines, genetically fixed to produce just one of the cannabinoids in the highest possible purity (comparable to basic colour pigments). On request, these lines can be crossed (which is, due to co-dominant inheritance, comparable to blending) in order to produce a range of hybrid progenies with distinct, predictable cannabinoid compositions (comparable to the infinite variation in custom-made paints). Like paint, the hybrids, with their specific chemical profiles, can at any time be reproduced in any quantity by simply maintaining the parental lines, together with the chemotypical combining ability data (the computerised blending formulas).

Germ plasm resources

All *Cannabis* populations can cross readily and produce fertile hybrids, whereas they are reproductively isolated from other genera. *Cannabis* can, therefore, in terms introduced by Harlan and de Wet (1971), be considered as one isolated primary gene pool, albeit a very heterogeneous one, due to its dioecious, cross-breeding nature, its cosmopolitan distribution, and its long history of adaptation to distinct human utilisations. De Meijer (1998) proposed a further subdivision of this gene pool on the basis of natural and practical criteria, which is useful for an adequate specification of the many different *Cannabis* subgroups. Group indications derived from this classification will be used here to specify the various sources relevant to the GW breeding programme.

Because of a long history of divergent selection, *Cannabis* drug strains differ from fibre, seed and wild or ruderal populations in having a somewhat higher floral fraction with dramatically higher total cannabinoid content (the polygenic yield components 2 and 3). The proportion of a certain dominant cannabinoid in the total cannabinoid fraction (the monogenic component 4) is not necessarily different for drug or other strains. The only difference is that the dominant cannabinoid in drug strains is usually THC and in most of the others it is CBD. Exceptions occur: hashish landraces usually comprise individuals with high CBD levels and Far Eastern fibre and seed hemp plants may have very substantial THC proportions.

The other, so-called minor cannabinoids can frequently be found at low purity (up to 10% of the total cannabinoid fraction) and, rarely, in higher proportions, in all kinds of populations. The low frequency of naturally occurring individuals with substantial purity levels for the minor cannabinoids may be due to reduced fitness associated with such chemotypes. Prior to the stage of active breeding, HortaPharms'/GW Pharmaceuticals' programme was aimed at the selection and maintenance in a clone library of a range of individual plants with relatively high purity values for just one single cannabinoid, irrespective of its identity. Regardless of taxon, geographical provenance, crop-use type or domestication status, many source populations were screened for this purpose.

Per cannabinoid, the most relevant germ plasm sources are discussed below.

Δ^9-THC

Numerous potent, pure THC marijuana cultivars are commercially available on the recreational seed market in the Netherlands, and latterly, also in Canada and Switzerland (e.g. Rosenthal, 2001). Mostly, these are full-sib cross combinations of a fairly limited number of parental materials that were developed from the 1970s onward (de Meijer, 1998). The majority of these basic strains were selected in the US, either from single landrace sources or from multihybrid progenies made with different landraces. Important and currently used parents from single landrace origin are: Afghani and Hindu Kush (*indica*, hashish types) and the *sativa*, marijuana types: Durban, Thai, Hawaiian, South African, Mexican and Colombian. Important hybrids are Skunk, Haze, Northern Lights and more recently developed strains like Blueberry and White Widow. Ancestries of these are described by de Meijer (1998) and Rosenthal (2001).

Under optimal indoor conditions, the current best THC strains are claimed to produce up to 500 g/m^2 of dry marijuana with THC contents up to 20% (Rosenthal, 2001). This implies that THC yields of nearly 100 g/m^2 have been achieved, which, if it is true, is impressive for a secondary metabolite, the function of which for the plant itself is still a mystery. Nevertheless, since, next to THC content, additional traits like smell, taste and colour play a role in the appreciation of materials, breeding for the recreational market is still a very dynamic business. Cultivars are continually released and replaced probably just for the sake of commerce itself. For the pharmaceutical breeding programme, the modern THC cultivars can be used to contribute good productivity traits in basic crosses with plants having fairly pure minor cannabinoid profiles, but poor yield characteristics.

CBD

A rich source for pure CBD individuals is some fairly resinous fibre hemp landraces from Turkey. Population average cannabinoid contents can be up to 4.5% (de Meijer, 1994), and individuals with contents up to 7% and CBD proportions of 95% can be selected. Hashish landraces from Afghanistan and Pakistan also form a self-evident source. Unlike marijuana strains, hashish landraces usually show segregation for chemotype and comprise individuals with pure THC, pure CBD and mixed THC/CBD profiles.

CBC

The purest CBC lines in the programme are derived from different sources such as an Afghani hashish landrace, a Korean fibre landrace and a Chinese seed landrace. The productivity traits in these source populations are generally poor and total cannabinoid contents do not exceed 2% in the best individuals. Also, in plants naturally occurring in these source populations, the CBC purity is fairly low, with 57% as the highest value so far found.

CBG

CBG is the common precursor for THC, CBD and CBC. Significant accumulation of CBG therefore requires the presence of a non-functional allele in the homozygous state at the locus that controls the CBG conversion (de Meijer *et al.*, 2003). Fournier *et al.* (1987) reported on a single individual, with a CBG purity of 97%, which was detected during the multiplication of monoecious fibre hemp. The French fibre cultivar 'Santhica', which is claimed to be absolutely devoid of THC (Anonymous, 1996), is probably derived from this individual. Although registered for breeders' rights, 'Santhica' has never been released on the market, nor have its pedigree or cannabinoid composition been revealed. Fortunately, at least one other source for CBG mutants is now identified, this time an Italian fibre strain. The latter materials have been introduced into GW Pharmaceuticals' breeding programme in 2002.

Tetrahydrocannabivarin (THCV)

Tetrahydrocannabivarin (THCV) can be found in substantial proportions in a wide range of materials. In the GW programme, inbred lines have been derived from South African marijuana landraces, Chinese seed hemp and THC drug strains. Plants from the latter group are convenient to work with as they already have reasonable production characteristics. In the course of the line selection programme for THC homozygotes occasionally certain individuals suddenly showed a significant proportion of THCV. The most plausible explanation for this is an apparently easily occurring mutation at the locus that controls the first specific step in the cannabinoid biosynthesis, the addition of geranylpyrophosphate with olivetolic acid or divarinolic acid. When divarinolic acid is added instead of the more common olivetolic acid, CBGV is formed instead of CBG, which consequently converts into THCV, instead of THC.

CBDV, CBCV and CBGV

No natural sources with substantial proportions over 10% purity have yet been traced. However, it seems feasible to derive CBDV, CBCV and CBGV lines through the inbreeding of THCV × CBD hybrids, THCV × CBC hybrids, and THCV × CBG hybrids, respectively.

Current breeding achievements

The applied procedure of selective inbreeding is effective in increasing the chemotypical purity of the different breeding lines. Parental plants containing two cannabinoids in substantial proportions yield inbred generations (S_1s), showing a fairly clear-cut segregation for cannabinoid composition (Figure 3.2). As Table 3.1 shows, already in the S_1 generation, cannabinoid purity arrives at a fixed level, reflecting the simple Mendelian mechanism of chemotype inheritance. However, inbreeding is continued at least until the S_4 or S_5 generation in order to obtain homozygosity for the polygenic yield-related traits.

For each target cannabinoid, the maximal achievable proportion (purity) in the total cannabinoid fraction appears to be specific. For

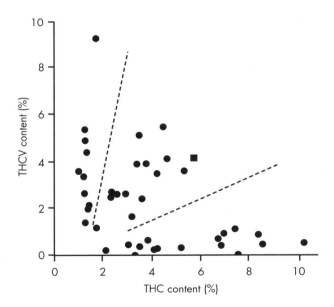

Figure 3.2 THCV versus THC content of a single plant with a mixed THCV-THC chemotype (square symbol) and its segregating, inbred S_1 progeny (circle symbols). The dashed lines separate the three chemotypical segregant groups. All the plants considered had a (THCV + THC) proportion over 94% of the total cannabinoid fraction.

Table 3.1 The development of THCV purity in a progeny derived from a basic cross, subjected to four cycles of line selection. The bold ciphers denote the specific individuals that have been crossed (parents) or self-fertilised (F_1 and $S_1–S_4$) to obtain the subsequent generation

Generation	Code of selected individual	THCV proportion in the total cannabinoid fraction (%)
1st Parental clone, selected from 'California orange'	55.7.1	39.9
2nd Parental clone, selected from 'Thai'	55.22.7	0.5
$F_1 (S_0)$	97.2.71	41.5
S_1	97.2.71.16	79.5
S_2	97.2.71.16.5	83.5
S_3	97.2.71.16.5.14	83.1
S_4	97.2.71.16.5.14.6	82.2

THCV it is circa 83% (Table 3.1), for CBC it is found to be 76%. Both THC and CBD can reach proportions up to 98%. However, it is remarkable that even after five cycles of inbreeding, purity never arrives at a perfect 100%.

Several conspicuous, discrete morphological markers have been found in the many different S_1 generations that were evaluated. Examples so far observed are the so-called Duckfoot leaves (joined leaflets, previously indicated as 'Pinnatifidofillia' by Crescini (1956), a mild form of chlorophyll deficiency in stems and leaves, triple instead of pairwise leaf arrangement and dwarfism. On the basis of segregation ratios, these markers appear to be monogenic, recessive traits. Markers with a neutral or minor effect on productivity and quality could play a role in technical, intellectual property protection.

An expected problem, appearing in some lines during line selection, is a strong decrease in fertility. Normally, there are alternative sufficiently fertile sister plants to get around this obstacle. However, specifically in CBD inbred materials, a strong drop in fertility was found to be almost general. A solution to this problem is to perform, prior to line selection, a basic cross of the CBD starting materials with a highly fertile and vigorous THC individual.

The breeding process is currently most advanced for the pure THC materials. Several S_4 inbred lines have been obtained and were mutually crossed. The hybrid seedling progenies, the parental lines (seedlings) and the current best THC reference clones have been evaluated for the relevant yield and quality characteristics. As an example, Table 3.2 shows the performance of just two parental lines, their hybrid F_1 and, as a reference, GW Pharmaceuticals' THC production clone G1, M1.

The hybrids' THC yield by far exceeds that of its parents. A large heterosis effect is found for each of the quantitative yield components: above ground dry matter, floral proportion and total cannabinoid content. Being the cross-combination of two pure THC parents, the F_1s' THC proportion can, of course, hardly deviate from the mid-parent value. For crosses between chemically contrasting lines, this qualitative component is a much more exciting trait (de Meijer *et al.*, 2003).

The production clone G1, M1 is also outyielded by the hybrid. For a more adequate comparison of clonal standards and an elite subset of newly made hybrids, a trial is now being prepared with the object of comparing new hybrids grown as seedlings with new hybrids grown as clones and references grown as clones. This test will elucidate the effect of the mode of cultivation on the performance of a fixed genotype and the effect of genotype on the performance of clones.

An unexpected finding in the trial evaluating the several new THC seedling hybrids and the reference clones was that the variability (calculated as coefficient of variation) for the yield components was often similar and in some cases even lower within hybrid seedling progenies

Table 3.2 Yield components and the resulting THC yield for two parental inbred lines and their cross progeny

	Above ground dry matter (g/m²)	*Floral proportion (g/g)*	*Total cannabinoid content (g/g)*	*Δ^9-THC proportion (g/g)*	*Δ^9-THC yield (g/m²)*
1st parental inbred line (S₄, 100% ♀), selected from 'Haze'	609	0.34	0.1233	0.93	23.9
2nd parental inbred line (S₄, 100% ♀), selected from 'Thai'	167	0.34	0.1684	0.92	8.8
F_1	708	0.51	0.2915	0.95	99.6
G1, M1	650	0.75	0.1500	0.98	71.7

The F_1 values are calculated as averages for two reciprocal F_1s. Both parents and the F_1 were grown as seedlings. For comparison, the bottom line gives the performance of the reference clone G1, M1.

than within clones. The variation within a clone can only be attributed to environmental variation, whereas the variation in a seedling progeny is a consequence of both environmental and genetic variation. Clearly, the genetic variation in seedling progenies from S_4 parents is very small. It is very likely that cuttings originating from different parts of a mother plant have such differences in potential from the outset that in a competitive crop situation the variability in performance eventually exceeds that of hybrid seedlings. Their high level of uniformity, their high productivity and the less laborious crop establishment make certain hybrid seedling progenies a serious alternative to clonal cultivars.

Ten different series of triploid hybrid progenies were grown together with their diploid homologues in a pollen-saturated environment. Seed set per plant and subsequently seed viability in germination tests were evaluated as parameters for fertility (Table 3.3). The resulting fertility was calculated as the product of these two parameters. The fertility values for the diploids were set at 1 and those of the corresponding triploids were expressed as relative to these diploid values. As expected, the triploid plants showed a reduced seed set, reduced seed viability and therefore a lower calculated fertility.

However, none of the triploid progenies was perfectly sterile, and within a progeny there was considerable variation for the level of fertil-

Table 3.3 Fertility parameters of triploid progenies

Diploid, parental S_4 line	Tetraploid clonal parent	No. of triploid F_1 plants tested	Relative no. of seeds	Relative seed viability	Relative fertility[a] (min)-avg-(max)
94.5.2.30.1.2	55.46.1 (4n)	1	0.15	0.58	0.09
55.18.2.44.5.1	55.46.1 (4n)	12	0.25	0.60	(0.02)–0.15–(0.26)
55.22.7.2.2.31	55.46.1 (4n)	12	0.54	0.93	(0.08)–0.50–(0.75)
55.24.4.34.7.24	55.46.1 (4n)	3	0.29	0.74	(0.15)–0.21–(0.25)
55.27.1.11.24.2	55.46.1 (4n)	4	0.20	0.74	(0.04)–0.15–(0.22)
55.28.1.4.12.2	55.46.1 (4n)	11	0.29	0.77	(0.05)–0.24–(0.65)
55.28.1.82.4.20	55.46.1 (4n)	4	0.31	0.84	(0.17)–0.26–(0.32)
92.73.2.13.11.1	55.46.1 (4n)	12	0.21	0.78	(0.03)–0.16–(0.28)
92.76.5.6.3.16	55.46.1 (4n)	6	0.41	0.67	(0.07)–0.29–(0.83)
92.76.9.23.27.1	55.46.1 (4n)	1	0.30	0.76	0.22

The values are relative to those of diploid homologues with identical genetic background, i.e. progenies from the same parental S_4 lines, but now crossed with the diploid clone 55.46.1. The corresponding relative values for diploid homologues are set at 1.
[a]The relative fertility is calculated as the product of the relative number of seeds × the relative seed viability.

ity. The lowest relative fertility values of single individuals (0.02 and 0.03) still correspond to about 40–60 fertile seeds per plant. However, it must be emphasised that these figures relate to an absolutely worst-case scenario. The test plants were fairly tall, placed in low density and subjected to turbulent pollen-saturated air throughout the flowering period. The observed variation in fertility within triploid progenies could partly be due to the fact that the used tetraploid parent was a non-inbred clone. The tentative conclusion of this first trial is that it is at least feasible to select triploid production clones with strongly reduced fertility that will be hard to employ for illegal further breeding.

Future developments

On the basis of results achieved so far it appears feasible and therefore only a matter of time to largely realise the general goal of the pharmaceutical breeding programme by classical methods. However, it would not be wise to ignore the possibilities offered by 'molecular breeding', especially where these could offer solutions that are really beyond the classical approach.

A self-evident and the least radical application of molecular techniques would be marker-assisted breeding. By now, a number of sex-linked DNA markers are available for *Cannabis*, and markers closely linked to alleles controlling the synthesis of certain cannabinoids will probably follow soon (de Meijer *et al.*, 2003). This last group of markers could play a role in the breeding programme, although the current gas chromatographic determination of chemotype is quite competitive for the screening of massive numbers of plants. Quantitative trait loci (QTL) markers closely associated with the polygenic yield-related traits, in particular, the total cannabinoid content, would be of much more additional value. Of similar neutral emotional impact to the use of markers is the application of DNA fingerprinting as a tool in the protection of intellectual property.

As far as genetic modification is concerned, the first step is the identification of truly desirable genetic improvements that remain un-realised after the possibilities of classical breeding have been spent. The following topics seem to be eligible: better, if not perfect, purity of the target cannabinoids, synthesis of cannabinoids novel to the existing natural ones, plants with an obstructed cannabinoid synthesis ('knock-outs') to serve as the perfect placebo in clinical trials and the insertion of resistance genes against insect pests, especially spider mites.

The strategic question of whether or not it is a wise decision to implement genetically modified *Cannabis* as a pharmaceutical raw material is beyond the scope of this chapter. Genetic modification for pharmaceutical application might be less emotionally charged than it is for food and fodder crops. In the author's personal opinion, the improvement of purity for those target cannabinoids whose proportions do not reach the arbitrary threshold of 95% in the total cannabinoid fraction is the only problem in pharmaceutical *Cannabis* breeding important enough to consider addressing by genetic modification. However, for the compounds concerned (mainly CBC and the propyl cannabinoids) it should first be decided if there is sufficient pharmaceutical interest to make such an investment worth the effort.

References

Anonymous (1996). Nouvelles variétés de lins et chanvre. *Semences et Progrès* 96: 110–111.

Becu D M S, Mastebroek H D, Marvin H J P (1998). Breeding for root knot nematode resistance in hemp. *Proceedings of Bast Fibrous Plants Today and Tomorrow*. St. Petersburg: 149.

Bócsa I (1998). Genetic improvement: conventional approaches. In: Ranalli P, ed. *Advances in Hemp Research*. New York, London: The Haworth Press: 153–179.

Clarke R C (1993). Indoor *Cannabis* breeding. In: Cervantes J, ed. *Indoor Marijuana Horticulture*. Portland, OR: Van Patten: 250–274.

Crescini F (1956). La fecondazione incestuosa processo mutageno in *Cannabis sativa* L. *Caryologia* 9: 82–92.

de Meijer E P M (1994). Diversity in cannabis. PhD thesis, Wageningen University.

de Meijer E P M (1998). *Cannabis* germplasm resources. In: Ranalli P, ed. *Advances in Hemp Research*. New York, London: The Haworth Press: 133–151.

de Meijer E P M, van der Kamp H J, van Eeuwijk F A (1992). Characterisation of *Cannabis* accessions with regard to cannabinoid content in relation to other plant characters. *Euphytica* 62: 187–200.

de Meijer E P M, Bagatta M, Carboni A *et al.* (2003). The inheritance of chemical phenotype in *Cannabis sativa* L. *Genetics* 163: 335–346.

Fournier G, Richez-Dumanois C, Duvezin J, Mathieu JP, Paris M (1987). Identification of a new chemotype in *Cannabis sativa*: cannabigerol-dominant plants, biogenetic and agronomic prospects. *Planta Med* 53: 277–280.

Frank M, Rosenthal E (1978). *Marihuana Groeiboek*. Drachten: Woord Noord/Educare B.V.

Harlan J R, de Wet J M J (1971). Towards a rational classification of cultivated plants. *Taxon* 20: 509–517.

Rosenthal E (2001). *The Big Book of Buds*. Oakland, CA: Quick American Archives.

Snoeijer W (2002). *A Checklist of Some Cannabaceae Cultivars, Part A: Cannabis*. Division of Pharmacognosy, Leiden/Amsterdam Center for Drug Research.

Virovets V G (1996). Selection for non-psychoactive hemp varieties (*Cannabis sativa* L.) in the CIS (former USSR). *J Int Hemp Assoc* 3: 13–15.

Zohary D, Hopf M (1994). *Domestication of Plants in the Old World*, 2nd edn. Oxford: Clarendon Press: 126–127.

4

The evolution of *Cannabis* and coevolution with the cannabinoid receptor – a hypothesis

John M McPartland and Geoffrey W Guy

The title and topics in this chapter reiterate themes expressed by our mentors Richard Schultes and Raphael Mechoulam (Schultes, 1970; Mechoulam *et al.*, 1991). Herein we review the natural history of *Cannabis*, especially the accelerated changes it has undergone since its association with humans. Next we examine the phylogenetic history of the cannabinoid receptor, including the pivotal influence of exogenous ligands. This pair of natural histories will be interpreted through the lens of evolutionary theory, particularly in terms of coevolution.

Ehrlich and Raven (1964) coined the term coevolution to describe reciprocal adaptations between plants and animals leading to their interdependence. The concept of coevolution has itself evolved. It is now interpreted broadly, from cases of casual cohabitation to those of absolute interdependence. The term encompasses interactions ranging from seasonal associations (such as in pollination and seed dispersal) to life-long obligate parasitism. Coevolution arises along the continuum of 'life' – between nucleotide sequences within a genome, between cells of a multicellular organism, between individual plants and animals, or between populations of organisms on a global 'Gaia' scale (McEno, 1991).

Coevolution often begins with mutualism (Pirozynski and Hawksworth, 1988). Mutualism occurs when two species benefit from their interactions. For example, we nurture a plant's growth (cultivation) and disperse seeds (zoochory); the plant provides us with fibre, oil and medicaments. Once a pair of species improves each others' evolutionary fitness, then traits that favour their association become sustained, genes become selected, and coevolution arises. The time scale involves millennia. Coevolution can engage taxa of different rank with asymmetric evolution rates, such as *Cannabis* and *Homo sapiens,* in which 'arrays of populations reciprocally affect each others' evolution' (Pirozynski and Hawksworth, 1988).

Origin of the association

No one knows exactly where *Cannabis* originated. DeCandolle (1884), a past master of ethnobotany, reported 'the species has been found wild, beyond a doubt, to the south of the Caspian Sea, near the Irtysch, in the desert of Kirghiz, beyond Lake Baikal.' Vavilov (1926), perhaps our best expert on *Cannabis* origins, described plants 'of a primeval character' growing in the Altai mountains and western Siberia. McPartland *et al.* (2000a) proposed a *Cannabis* origin in the rich alluvial soil surrounding the southern Altai or Tien Shan mountains (Figure 4.1). Hence it was somewhere in Central Asia that *Homo sapiens* first encountered *Cannabis.* Humans migrated from Africa into Central Asia at least 1.75 million years ago (Vekua *et al.,* 2002). Given this time frame, it seems conservative to estimate that humans first used *Cannabis* 12 000 years ago (Abel, 1980).

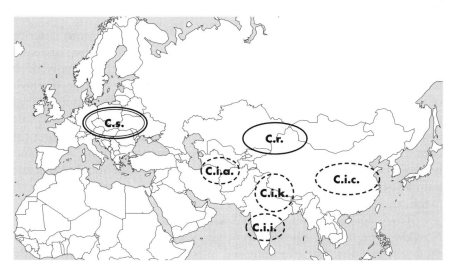

Figure 4.1 Distribution of *Cannabis* biotypes prior to the age of Herodotus. C.r. = *Cannabis ruderalis*; C.s. = *Cannabis sativa* ssp. *sativa* and *Cannabis sativa* ssp. *spontanea*; C.i.k. = *Cannabis indica* ssp. *kafiristanica*; C.i.i. = *Cannabis indica* ssp. *indica*; C.i.a. = *Cannabis indica* ssp. *afghanica*; C.i.c. = *Cannabis indica* ssp. *chinensis*.

Who first cultivated cannabis? Most of our crops are associated with classic civilisations: the Incas and Aztecs with potatoes and maize, Egyptians with wheat, and the Chinese with rice. It has been proposed that cannabis was associated with a lost civilisation, a Shangri La or Shambala of Central Asia (McEno, 1991). Alternatively, cannabis may have been domesticated by nomads, independent of erstwhile civilisations. Nomadic cultivation is supported by the simultaneous historical appearance of cannabis in several locations (China, India, Persia, Europe). The Altai and Tien Shen mountains flank the Central Asian steppes, a Neolithic 'nomad belt' stretching from the Black Sea to Mongolia. The Scythians, a Neolithic tribe of migrants, emerged from this territory at the dawn of history. '*Cannabis ruderalis*' seeds have been unearthed from Scythian tombs in the Altai mountains (Rudenko, 1970). Herodotus (1906 reprint, written ca. 450 BCE) documented the Scythians carrying hemp seed to Europe; the Scythians also migrated to India and China, where they may have transported cannabis germ plasm. After cannabis was carried across Eurasia, geographically isolated human communities began selecting plants for diverse purposes – for food (seed and seed oil), fibre and medicaments. These isolated areas of cannabis cultivation gave rise to the fantastic variety of plants we see today.

Cannabis taxonomy and evolution

Within the plant order Urticales, Endlicher (1837) created a separate family, the Cannabaceae, for *Cannabis* and her sister genus, *Humulus* (hops). Subsequently, Bentham and Hooker (1880) moved *Cannabis* to the Urticaceae (the nettle family), and Engler and Prantl (1889) transferred it to the Moraceae (the fig family). Most contemporary taxonomists assign *Cannabis* to the Cannabaceae (e.g. Thorne, 1992) or the Moraceae (e.g. Greuter *et al.*, 1993). The Urticaceae designation has fallen out of common use, although Schultes (1970) considered *Cannabis* more closely allied to the Urticaceae than to the Moraceae.

Fossil records of *Cannabis* are lacking, so the epoch when it evolved must be inferred from fossils of related plants. Whether *Cannabis* is more closely allied with the Moraceae or the Urticaceae bears directly upon this question – fossils suggest that the Moraceae is a much older family than the Urticaceae (Collinson, 1989). Unfortunately, this 'family feud' has not been answered satisfactorily with morphological and phytochemical analyses (Schultes, 1970). Another set of data, host plant–parasite relationships, may offer clues. Many obligate parasites coevolve with their host plants, eventually becoming dependent on single species or single families. Parasite phylogeny accordingly mirrors host phylogeny and this has become known as 'Fahrenholtz's Rule'. McPartland and Nicholson (2003) compared a monograph of *Cannabis* parasites (fungi, nematodes and insects) with lists of parasites that attack other plants. Seven obligate parasites of *Cannabis* were shared by hosts in the Urticaceae, whereas no obligate parasites of *Cannabis* were shared by hosts in the Moraceae. These results suggest that *Cannabis* shares a sister group relationship with the Urticaceae (whose convincing fossil record begins in the Oligocene epoch, 34 million years ago), instead of the Moraceae (with a fossil record dating to the early Eocene, 56 million years ago). Thus the Cannabaceae lineage evolved no earlier than 34 million years ago.

The species debate

Most taxonomists consider *Cannabis* a one-species genus, *C. sativa* L. 1753. The polyspecies concept began when Lamarck described *Cannabis indica* in 1785. Lamarck described plants collected in southern India as 'very distinct' from *C. sativa*, morphologically and phytochemically. The polyspecies debate began 20 years later, when Persoon rejected Lamarck's species and reduced it to a synonym of *C. sativa* (McPartland, 1992). Schultes *et al.* (1974) recognised three species: *C. sativa*, *C. indica* and *Cannabis ruderalis* Janischevsky 1924. McPartland *et al.* (2000a) described four biotypes: *C. sativa*, *C. indica*, *C. ruderalis* and *Cannabis afghanica* Vavilov 1926. Hillig (2004a) recognised two major gene pools, which corresponded to a revised circumscription of *C. sativa* and *C. indica*, based on a genetic analysis of 157 *Cannabis* accessions collected from around the world. A third putative gene pool that corresponded to *C. ruderalis* was given tentative recognition, although it was based on an analysis of only five germ plasm accessions. Hillig's working hypothesis offers some surprises, such as the presence of 'cryptic' biotypes within the concept of 'hemp' (a term applied to *Cannabis* cultivated for its fibre). The next seven subsections of this chapter examine the putative *Cannabis* biotypes described by Hillig (2004a).

Cannabis ruderalis

C. ruderalis, often called 'wild hemp', is considered a primeval biotype, unmodified by domestication. This biotype is not cultivated, although feral populations have been harvested for fibre (Vavilov, 1957) and drugs (Clarke, 1998). *C. ruderalis* plants grow in the proposed ancestral home of *Cannabis*, covering approximately 140 000 hectares in Kazakhstan, and 6000 hectares in Kyrgyzstan (International Narcotics Control Board, 1996). *C. ruderalis* also ranges north into western Siberia (Schultes *et al.*, 1974).

Cannabis sativa ssp. sativa

This taxon represents classic European hemp. Although *Cannabis* probably originated in Central Asia, *C. sativa* has existed in Europe for a long time; central European archaeologists have unearthed hemp seeds dating to 5500 BCE (Renfrew, 1973). Over millennia, humans have maximised European hemp fibre for its quality, length and ease of harvest by selecting plants for height, lax branching, hollowness of stalk and rettability. This selection evolved from an unconscious to a conscious process (Small and Cronquist, 1976). *C. sativa* has also been selected for seed production (Wirtshafter, 1997; Pate, 1999a). The *C. sativa* gene pool exhibits greater genetic diversity than the *C. indica* gene pool (Hillig, 2004a). Cultivation of European *C. sativa* spread to the New World (Chile) by 1545, and North America (Nova Scotia, Canada) by 1606 (Dewey, 1914). It became naturalised in North America by 1852, colonising large areas of alluvia in eastern Canada and the USA (McPartland, 1992).

Cannabis sativa ssp. spontanea

This biotype includes ruderal plants from eastern Europe and western Asia. Its genetic characteristics interdigitate somewhat with *C. sativa* ssp. *sativa* and *C. ruderalis*; the biotype requires further sampling and analysis (Hillig, 2004a). It may represent the primeval biotype into which genetic traits from cultivated *C. sativa* ssp. *sativa* have introgressed and merged. The resultant hybrids express a range of morphological variation.

Cannabis indica ssp. kafiristanica

Several investigators believe that humans were originally attracted to cannabis for its unique psychoactive qualities, not for its fibre or seed. Reininger (1946) even argued that 'Use of *Cannabis* for fiber occurred rather late'. The Scythians, the first people known to utilise cannabis, were aware of its psychoactive properties. Herodotus (1906 reprint) recorded the Scythians crowding into small tents to burn cannabis: 'They enjoy it so much they howl with pleasure'. Hillig (2004a) assigned this putative taxon to ruderal drug plants from Nepal and northern India. *C. indica* ssp. *kafiristanica* may represent the ancestral source of cultivated *C. indica* ssp. *indica*, based on genetic evidence (Hillig, 2004a) and a shared cannabinoid profile (Hillig and Mahlberg, 2004).

Cannabis indica ssp. indica

C. indica ssp. *indica* has been cultivated for millennia as a drug plant in India. This biotype, like *C. indica* ssp. *kafiristanica*, is relatively tall (not as tall as *C. sativa* biotypes), with narrow leaflets. *C. indica* ssp. *indica* is subtropical, with a long growing season and a tolerance for rainfall and dampness. *Ganja* (a Sanskrit term for cannabis) spread from India to South-East Asia, especially Burma and Thailand. *Ganja* may have been carried to Africa via Zanzibar by 200 CE (DuToit, 1980). Bantu tribes near Zanzibar (in Tanzania and Mozambique) spread *riamba* (a linguistic variant of *ganja*) to Angola, Zambia and Zaire, and eventually all the way south to the Cape, long before the arrival of Europeans (Schleiffer, 1979). *C. indica* ssp. *indica* was introduced into the New World when the Portuguese shipped East African slaves to Brazil in 1549. According to Rubin (1975), the *civilizados* and their seed-smuggling slaves introduced the Maué and other Amazonian tribes to *diamba* (a variant of African *riamba*). The abolition of slavery in Jamaica in 1834 led to the introduction of *ganja* on that island, when English landowners imported servants from India, who brought seeds (Clarke, 1998). Mexican 'marihuana' was first described in 1886, and moved to the Gulf region of the United States (Texas, Louisiana) by 1910 (Walton, 1938). Old police photographs of cannabis confiscated in Louisiana show plants with *indica* morphology (Walton, 1938). Increased border interdiction during the late 1960s became a catalyst for increased US domestic cultivation. Breeders in California developed several hybrid cultivars of *C. indica* ssp. *indica*, exampled by 'Haze', a multihybrid with parentage from Colombia, Mexico, Thailand and southern India (de Meijer, 1999). 'Durban' from South Africa is another well-known *C. indica* ssp. *indica* landrace.

Cannabis indica ssp. afghanica

McPartland *et al.* (2000a) assigned this putative taxon to broad-leafleted *Cannabis* plants cultivated for drug production. Hillig (2004a) called these plants 'C. *indica* sensu Schultes *et al.* (1974) and Anderson (1980)', pending further taxonomic characterisation. This biotype evolved in Afghanistan and western Turkmenistan (Clarke, 1998), a cold and arid region that favoured plants with short height and a short growing season. Unlike C. *indica* ssp. *indica*, the dense flowering tops of C. *indica* ssp. *afghanica* do poorly in high humidity – they retain moisture and easily succumb to 'bud mould' caused by *Botrytis cinerea* and *Trichothecium roseum* (McPartland *et al.*, 2000a). The cannabinoid-rich gland heads of *afghanica* trichomes readily detach from their stalk cells. This trait enabled the development of a unique procedure for manufacturing hashish – separating gland heads from the rest of the plant by passing dried flowers over a screen or sieve. Hashish manufactured by this method could only have evolved in a cool, arid climate (Clarke, 1998). In warm or damp environments, the screen becomes gummed with cannabinoid resins from ruptured gland heads (hashish made in India from C. *indica* ssp. *indica* is gathered by hand-rubbing of plants). Thus, the cold, arid environment favoured unique plants as well as a unique harvesting technique, resulting in the evolution of sieved hashish. C. *indica* ssp. *afghanica* germ plasm was smuggled into the US in the early 1970s (S. Selgnij, personal communication, 1984), leading to the development of several inbred cultivars. Examples include 'Afghani No. 1' and 'Hindu Kush', both incestuously bred in California (de Meijer, 1999). 'Skunk No. 1' is a cross of C. *indica* ssp. *afghanica* and C. *indica* ssp. *indica* (from Mexico and Colombia). 'Northern Lights No. 1' is one-quarter C. *indica* ssp. *indica* (from Thailand) and three-quarters C. *indica* ssp. *afghanica* (de Meijer, 1999).

Cannabis indica ssp. chinensis

This taxon represents classic Chinese hemp, cultivated primarily for fibre and seed. Specimens of Chinese hemp fibre are 5200–6200 years old (Li, 1974), approximately the same age as European archaeological specimens. Chinese hemp is often lumped with European hemp and labelled C. *sativa*. This is erroneous – the two biotypes differ by morphology (Dewey, 1914) and by cannabinoid profile (Small and Beckstead, 1973; de Meijer *et al.*, 1992; Hillig and Mahlberg, 2004). New research demonstrates that C. *indica* ssp. *chinensis* shares more genetic similarities with drug plants (C. *indica* ssp. *indica*, C. *indica* ssp. *afghanica*, C. *indica* ssp. *kafiristanica*) than with European hemp (C. *sativa* ssp. *sativa*) (Hillig, 2004a). C. *indica* ssp. *chinensis* germ plasm spread to the New World (Kentucky, USA) by the late 1800s (Dewey,

1914). The two hemp gene pools (*C. sativa* ssp. *sativa* and *C. indica* ssp. *chinensis*) were hybridised by Lyster Dewey at the US Department of Agriculture (Dewey, 1914), and more recently by Ivan Bócsa in Hungary (de Meijer, 1999).

Whether or not the seven putative taxa are species, subspecies or varieties remains to be determined. Whatever their taxonomic rank, they are frequently confused and misnamed in the literature. The narrow-leafleted drug biotype is misnamed *C. sativa* and the broad-leafleted drug biotype is misnamed *C. indica* ssp. *indica* or *C. ruderalis* (e.g. Schoenmakers, 1986). Taxonomists lump the narrow-leafleted drug biotype with the broad-leafleted drug biotype (e.g. Small and Cronquist, 1976; de Meijer, 1999). Even Schultes *et al.* (1974) lumped these biotypes together, judging from an inspection of his herbarium specimens at Harvard (McPartland, 1997; McPartland and Nicholson, 2003). Unfortunately, broad-leafleted cannabis from Afghanistan has come to typify *C. indica*, especially in the eyes of marijuana breeders. This is inaccurate. Lamarck (who named *C. indica*) was entirely unfamiliar with Afghan cannabis. His taxon refers to the biotype from India (*indica*). Photographs of Lamarck's original specimens – with narrow lanceolate leaves, not broadly oblanceolate leaves – are illustrated by Schultes *et al.* (1974) and Small and Cronquist (1976).

Despite a wide diversity of forms within *C. indica* (including ssp. *kafiristanica*, *indica*, *afghanica* and *chinensis*), the *C. indica* gene pool is narrower than that of *C. sativa*, suggesting that a founder effect may have bottlenecked the genetic base of *C. indica* (Hillig, 2004a). It remains to be determined whether *C. indica* and *C. sativa* segregated before or after the advent of human selection pressure. Their geographical ranges may have been contiguous and then separated by an ice-age glaciation event. The genus *Humulus* (hops) exhibits similar geographic discontinuities between different species in North America, Europe and Japan.

Biotypes and cannabinoid profiles

Mechoulam and Gaoni (1967) defined 'cannabinoids' as a group of C_{21} terpenophenolic compounds uniquely produced by cannabis. Subsequent development of synthetic cannabinoids (e.g. CP55,940) has blurred this definition, as has the discovery of endogenous cannabinoids (e.g. anandamide, a derivative of arachidonic acid), defined as 'endocannabinoids' by DiMarzo and Fontana (1995). To clarify the terminology, Pate (1999b) proposed the term 'phytocannabinoids' to designate the C_{21} compounds produced by cannabis.

Phytocannabinoids are formed in epidermal glandular trichomes by the condensation of a terpenoid (e.g. geraniol) with a phenol (e.g. olivetolic acid or phloroglucinol), yielding cannabigerol (CBG) (Taura *et al.*, 1995; Fellermeier and Zenk, 1998). CBG is subsequently transformed by a variety of enzymes and degradations into over 60 different phytocannabinoids, primarily tetrahydrocannabinol (Δ^9-THC and Δ^8-THC), cannabidiol (CBD), cannabichromene (CBC), CBG-monomethyl ether (CBGM), and several propyl analogues such as cannabidivarin (CBDV) and tetrahydrocannabivarin (THCV). In living plants these compounds exist predominately as their carboxylic acid derivatives. The primary psychoactive ingredient is Δ^9-THC (Gaoni and Mechoulam, 1964), whereas CBD may prove to be the primary medicinal agent for treating many human conditions (Mechoulam *et al.*, 2002). THC degrades to cannabinol (CBN) after prolonged storage or exposure to light and heat. CBN arises in old hashish, and it was the first cannabinoid successfully isolated by nineteenth-century chemists (Wood *et al.*, 1899).

Research by de Meijer *et al.* (2003) suggested that CBG is converted to THC or CBD by different isoforms of the same synthase enzyme, corresponding to two alleles B_T and B_D, respectively. The gene sequence for the synthase enzyme is available (see www.ncbi.nlm.nih.gov/entrez/query.fcgi GenBank accession number E33090), and has been genetically engineered into tobacco plants (Shoyama *et al.*, 2001). THC concentration and the frequency of the B_T allele are significantly higher in *C. indica* biotypes than in *C. sativa* and *C. ruderalis* (Hillig and Mahlberg, 2004). Chinese hemp (*C. indica* ssp. *chinensis*) expresses a cannabinoid profile similar to drug plants (*C. indica* ssp. *indica*, *afghanica* and *kafiristanica*) and dissimilar to European hemp (*C. sativa* ssp. *sativa*). Chinese hemp produces more THC than European hemp (Chapter 3); the THC:CBD ratio in Chinese hemp averages 2.5:1, whereas European hemp expresses a 1:3 ratio (Hillig and Mahlberg, 2004). Levels of CBG, THCV and CBDV are also higher in *C. indica* biotypes than *C. sativa* biotypes; CBGM is particularly unique to *C. indica* ssp. *chinensis* (Hillig and Mahlberg, 2004).

Quantitative differences and THC:CBD ratios provide useful chemotaxonomic markers for distinguishing between the *C. indica* biotypes – in *C. indica* ssp. *indica* the total phytocannabinoid content can reach 14% in manicured seedless flowering tops (K Hillig, personal communication, 2002), and a THC:CBD ratio of 100:1 is not unusual.

In *C. indica* ssp. *afghanica* the total phytocannabinoid content can reach 25% (McPartland and Russo, 2001), with a THC:CBD ratio ranging from 2:1 to 1:2 in *afghanica* hashish (Clarke, 1998). In *C. ruderalis*, the total phytocannabinoid content is usually less than 1%, and the primary phytocannabinoid is CBD (Beutler and Der Marderosian, 1978). If *C. ruderalis* is the primeval *Cannabis* biotype, then the preponderance of CBD may be an ancestral or 'palaeontological' trait.

Different *Cannabis* biotypes produce different responses in humans. The psychoactivity of *C. indica* ssp. *indica* has been described as 'energetic, light, clear, and high', whereas *C. indica* ssp. *afghanica* is described as 'soporific, dull, stupefying, narcotic, with a delayed onset' (Clarke, 1998). These distinctive effects may be due to different CBD:THC ratios, or due to other unique phytocannabinoids (e.g. THCV, cannabidivarin), or due to terpenoid variation (McPartland and Mediavilla, 2001), segregating by biotypes identified by genetic studies (Hillig, 2004a) and cannabinoid variation (Hillig and Mahlberg, 2004). Terpenoids are polymers composed of repeating units of isoprene (C_5H_8). Cannabis produces over 100 terpenoids, primarily monoterpenoids (with C_{10} templates) and sesquiterpenoids (C_{15} templates) (Ross and ElSohly, 1996). Collectively, terpenoids are called the essential oil or volatile oil of the plant. The unique smell of cannabis comes from its volatile terpenoids, not its phytocannabinoids. Field-cultivated cannabis yields about 1.3 L of essential oil per ton of fresh weight plants, or up to 18 L/ha in sinsemilla crops (Mediavilla and Steinemann, 1997). In general, *C. indica* biotypes expressed a more uniform terpenoid profile than *C. sativa* biotypes, reiterating the founder effect that may have narrowed the genetic base of *C. indica* (Hillig, 2004b). *C. indica* ssp. *indica* produced relatively high levels of *trans*-β-farnesene, and *C. indica* ssp. *afghanica* could be discriminated by high levels of guaiol, eudesmol and bulnesol (Hillig, 2004b).

Cannabis and cannabinoid receptors

Many botanists speculate that the phytocannabinoids initially evolved as toxins to deter herbivores and pathogens. Phytocannabinoids do indeed have pesticidal capabilities; they can kill fungi and stunt the growth of some animals (McPartland, 1984, 1997). But some time during the existence of cannabis, this evolutionary strategy was diverted – the phytocannabinoids became *attractive* to some animals; the 'botany of desire' elucidated by Pollan (2001).

Phytocannabinoids primarily affect animals by activating specific G protein-coupled receptors (GPCRs) called cannabinoid (CB) receptors. Two CB receptors have been identified. CB_1 receptors predominate in the central nervous system (they may be the most common neuroreceptors in the brain), whereas CB_2 receptors prevail in immune cells (B cells, monocytes, T cells, etc.) and immune tissues (tonsils, spleen, etc.). Recent studies indicate the presence of a third CB receptor (Breivogel *et al.*, 2002) and perhaps a 'CBD-like' receptor (Jarai *et al.*, 1999; Pertwee *et al.*, 2002). Taken together, CB receptors are nearly ubiquitous and arise in all organs and body tissues.

Signals from CB receptors are transduced by G proteins. G proteins are intracellular 'mobile units'; they amplify signals from the receptor and activate a variety of ion channels and enzymes. At least three families of G proteins are associated with CB receptors: Gi, Go and Gs (Glass and Felder, 1997). All GPCRs use common pools of G proteins, so when many CB receptors are activated, they sequester the pool of available G proteins (Vasquez and Lewis, 1999). CB receptors thus have the potential to 'bully' other GPCR neuroreceptors, by stealing their signalling mechanisms, preventing the other neuroreceptors from transmitting their messages.

Evidence suggests that CB receptors are phylogenetically ancient, because CB receptor homlogues are found in many animal species, including (in descending phylogenetic order) other mammals, birds, amphibians, fish, sea urchins, molluscs, leeches and even primitive *Hydra vulgaris* (reviewed by McPartland and Pruitt, 2002). The nucleotide sequences of genes encoding these CB receptors vary from species to species, due to accumulated mutations. Their percentage identity with the human CB sequence is proportional to the evolutionary distances between the organisms. For example, the CB_1 gene from the rhesus monkey (*Macaca mulatta*) is 100% identical to the human CB_1 sequence, whereas the CB_1 gene from the leech (*Hirudo medicinalis*) shares only 58% identity with human CB_1. McPartland and Pruitt (2002) used these divergences to construct a CB receptor gene tree (Figure 4.2). The CB gene tree provides a 'molecular clock' for the timing of evolutionary events. The tree is rooted by an ancient CB gene, which underwent a duplication event that gave rise to present-day CB_1 and CB_2. Calibrating the CB gene tree with palaeontological evidence indicates that the duplication event that gave rise to CB_1 and CB_2 occurred at a date over 600 million years ago. By this analysis, CB receptors evolved well before *Cannabis*, which is certainly not more than 34 million years old. It is intriguing to consider that dinosaurs probably expressed CB receptors, but they became extinct before *Cannabis* evolved.

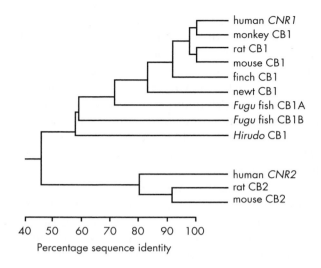

Figure 4.2 The cannabinoid receptor gene tree, based on similarities between 12 cloned gene sequences.

The evolutionary arabesque

As with all chicken-and-egg questions, the story of CB receptors and cannabis began long before the current pair of protagonists appeared in evolutionary time. It is probable that both CB receptors and cannabis had evolutionary predecessors. CB receptors evolved from an older, primordial 'proto-CB' receptor. The proto-CB receptor was probably a membrane protein, with an ancient lineage that includes GPCRs and ligand-gated ion channels (LGICs). LGICs are older than GPCRs; they appeared about 1.2 billion years ago, with the rise of multicellularity (Chiu *et al.*, 1999). Present-day LGICs include NMDA, AMPA and iGluR glutamate receptors, vanilloid receptors (VR1 or TRPV1), glycine receptors, nicotinic acetylcholine receptors, one of the serotonin receptors (5-HT$_3$), and one of the γ-aminobutyric acid receptors (GABA$_A$). The first GCPRs evolved 1.0 billion years ago (Peroutka and Howell, 1994). Present-day GCPRs include CB$_1$ and CB$_2$, and receptors for adenosine, dopamine, adrenaline (epinephrine) (alpha- and beta-adrenergic receptors), acetylcholine (muscarinic but not nicotinic receptors), serotonin (all 5-HT classes except 5-HT$_3$), glutamate (metabotropic glu receptors), GABA$_B$, ACTH, CCK, VIP, FSH, LH, TSH, opioids, substance P, parathyroid hormone, calcitonin, glucagon, oxytocin, lysophosphatidic acid and melanocortin. The leech CB receptor gene – which is the oldest CB gene (in evolutionary terms) to be sequenced to date – contains a stretch of sequence that resembles a gene for melanocortin receptors (Elphick, 1998). However, the *overall* sequences of CB_1 and CB_2 are most closely related to lysophosphatidic acid receptors, such as EDG-1 (Fredriksson *et al.*, 2003).

The evolution of receptor genes is driven by gene duplication events. Most duplicated genes experience a brief period of relaxed selection early in their history, undergoing mutational changes within a few million years (Lynch and Conery, 2000). If the mutated gene codes for a new receptor that improves an organism's survival, the mutation (*and* the new receptor *and* the organism) persists and reproduces. In other words, receptor genes survive if they improved their host organism's evolutionary fitness. Nonetheless, over the past billion years, some receptors may have served a biological need that does not currently exist. If such a need was *episodic* (such as improved survival in episodic epidemics or other environmental challenges), the receptor could persist as a 'vestigial receptor', analogous to an appendix. CB receptors may be vestigial; we do not know their exact physiological function. Transgenic 'knockout mice' that lack CB_1 receptors have been generated, and they survive and reproduce, but they suffer increased morbidity and premature mortality (Zimmer *et al.*, 1999). CB_1 knockout mice show greater aggression, anxiogenic-like behaviour, depressive-like behaviour, anhedonia, and they develop fear of newness (Martin *et al.*, 2002). Their very survival probably depends on the recruitment of other vestigial or 'redundant' receptor systems.

If the need for a receptor is no longer episodic but completely absent, then the receptor's gene would eventually degenerate, or the gene could mutate to express a new receptor with a new function. A mutated receptor often develops an affinity for a new ligand, because it is not under evolutionary constraints to maintain coupling with the original ligand (Baker, 1997). The original ligand, 'orphaned' by the mutated receptor, may then face degeneration, unless it links with another receptor and/or another function. Evidence suggests that this scenario transpired with CB receptors and their ligands, to be discussed shortly. Over evolutionary time we see a waxing and waning of receptors, driven by duplications and mutations, resulting in sorting events (extinctions) or new structures and new functions (Maddison, 1997). This weave of receptors intertwines with a weave of ligands, which similarly duplicate and mutate and adapt new shapes to better couple with new receptors. Given this scenario, the symbol for receptor–ligand coevolution is not an evolutionary tree, but an interweaving geometrical pattern, an evolutionary arabesque.

The enigma of animal receptors and plant ligands

The discovery of CB receptors led to an enigmatic question: why do animals have receptors for phytocannabinoids, which are compounds produced by plants? This question concerns not only the CB receptors and phytocannabinoids, but also the link between animal opioid receptors and plant morphine, animal VR1 receptors and plant capsicum, animal nicotinic receptors and plant nicotine, animal dopamine receptors and fungal ergot alkaloids, etc. Recent advances in molecular biology seem to link every newly elucidated animal neuroreceptor with a plant ligand. This series of seeming coincidences has several possible explanations: (1) the surreptitious mimic theory, (2) the theory of horizontal gene transfer, (3) the vestigial receptor hypothesis.

(1) The surreptitious mimic theory claims that plant ligands are surreptitious mimics of endogenous ligands produced by animals. The theory claims that THC simply imitates an endogenous ligand, termed 'anandamide', that exists in animal tissues (Devane *et al.*, 1992). As noted by McEno (1991), this concept is summarised by the pop-literature aphorism, 'humans surreptitiously evolved CB receptors that bind to cannabis compounds'. In reality, considering the relative ages of CB receptors and cannabis, the reverse may be true – cannabis surreptitiously evolved compounds that bind to CB receptors. The surreptitious mimic theory is undermined by the example of cannabis, where many compounds from the same plant work synergistically together. The probability of *many* synergistic mimics appearing simultaneously in one plant seems unlikely. Many medicinal plants follow this example.

(2) Horizontal gene transfer (HGT) has been evoked to explain the 'puzzling phenomena' of plant ligands coupling to animal neuroreceptors (Pirozynski, 1988). HGT is the direct non-sexual transmission of DNA between genomes of unrelated, reproductively isolated organisms. Over 200 human genes may have been obtained via HGT (International Human Genome Sequencing Consortium, 2001). McEno (1991) proposed that humans acquired CB genes from *C. sativa* via HGT. McEno conjectured that THC originally served as a ligand for CB receptors in the plant. HGT between these species could be vectored by parasites capable of bridging both hosts. For example, the bacterium *Agrobacterium tumefaciens* readily infects cannabis (McPartland *et al.*,

2000b) and humans (Hulse *et al.*, 1993), and is capable of vectoring DNA into mammalian nuclei (Ziemienowicz *et al.*, 1999). But *A. tumefaciens* is not known to infect germline cells (pollen and ova in plants, sperm and eggs in humans), so inheritance of HGT-vectored genes is unlikely. Furthermore, the CB-receptors-from-HGT hypothesis lost cachet after a search for CB genes in the genomes of *C. sativa*, *A. tumefaciens* and other potential plants and vectors proved unsuccessful (McPartland and Pruitt, 2002).

(3) The vestigial receptor hypothesis applies the evolutionary arabesque concept to the endocannabinoid system. We need to presume that the proto-CB receptor and its ligand evolved in primitive organisms that predated the divergence of animals and plants, shortly after GCPRs evolved 1.0 billion years ago. The proto-CB receptor survived in organisms that evolved into animals, whereas the organisms that evolved into plants lost the need for CB receptors. The CB ligands, however, persisted in plants; there is greater evolutionary pressure to conserve ligands than to conserve receptors (Hoyle, 1999). At present, organisms that produce cannabinoid-like ligands (in terms of structure or activity) scale the evolutionary ladder: algae (Soderstrom *et al.*, 1997), fungi (Quaghebeur *et al.*, 1994), liverworts (Toyota *et al.*, 2002), conifers (Nakane *et al.*, 2000) and angiosperms (Meschler and Howlett, 1999; Muhammad *et al.*, 2001). Cannabis may be the current flagship carrier of the phytocannabinoids, but far before its 34-million year history, previous organisms produced cannabinoid-like compounds – the earliest angiosperms evolved 140 million years ago, the conifers are twice as old, liverworts evolved 400 million years ago, and algae and fungi appeared a billion years ago (Benton and Ayala, 2003). Accordingly, when humans discovered cannabis – some time between 12 000 and 1.75 million years ago – this was not the first, but instead the *latest* linkage between an ancient ligand and an ancient receptor.

The vestigial receptor hypothesis proposes that pairs of receptors and ligands evolved among the earliest multicellular organisms, when membrane proteins became necessary for cell-to-cell signalling. Since then, the organisms that evolved into plants have lost CB receptors but retained the ligands, whereas organisms that evolved into animals retained CB receptors, which duplicated and mutated and paired with new ligands.

Deconstructing 'exogenous ligands'

Rather than a 'surreptitious coincidence' of 'exogenous ligands' that mimic 'endogenous ligands', we propose that the proto-CB receptor originally coupled with a ligand that resembled present-day phytocannabinoids. How and when did anandamide link with CB receptors? We know that anandamide serves as an endogenous ligand for CB receptors as well as VR1 receptors (reviewed by Szallasi and Di Marzo, 2000). VR1 regulates the sensation of pain, and may also modulate mood and memory. McPartland and Pruitt (2002) constructed a VR gene tree (Figure 4.3) and estimated the relative ages of the VR gene tree and the CB gene tree by comparing their respective divergences. This method is based on the neutrality theory of molecular evolution, which predicts that the rate of genetic divergence will be constant across time and across lineages. The VR tree exhibited deeper divergences than the CB gene tree at several levels. Since the degree of divergence correlates with evolutionary time, this analysis suggested that the ancestral VR receptor predated the ancestral CB receptor. It can be inferred that anandamide originally evolved as the ligand of the older receptor – VR1. As the proto-CB receptor morphed into a modern, recognisable structure, it evolved an affinity for the VR1 ligand, anandamide.

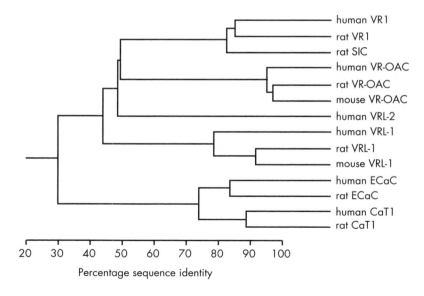

Figure 4.3 The vanilloid receptor gene tree, based on similarities between 14 cloned gene sequences.

Further along in evolutionary time, the proto-CB receptor duplicated and mutated into modern CB_1 and CB_2 – creating another bifurcation in the evolutionary arabesque. This duplication event may be the point where another ligand, 2-arachidonyl glycerol (2-AG), coupled with CB receptors, interweaving a new strand into the evolutionary arabesque. Subsequently, the CB_1 receptor again duplicated in at least one animal lineage, the teleost fishes, which express CB_{1a} and CB_{1b} receptors (Yamaguchi *et al.*, 1996). In other animal lineages, CB receptors have de-evolved and their genes completely degenerated, including insects (McPartland *et al.*, 2000b), nematodes (McPartland and Glass, 2001), and perhaps an entire clade of animals, the Ecdysozoa (McPartland *et al.*, 2001). Yet some of these animals without CB receptors (e.g. honey bees and fruit flies) continue to express 2-AG and perhaps even anandamide (McPartland *et al.*, 2001).

Although anandamide serves as a ligand for VR1, the receptor may be evolving away from anandamide and towards a temperature-gated mechanism. A splice variant of VR1 was recently described (Schumacher *et al.*, 2000), and it completely lost its ability to bind the ligand. For that matter, modern CB_1 may also be evolving away from anandamide. Shire *et al.* (1995) described a splice variant of CB_1 that translates into a truncated receptor which has lost some ability to bind anandamide (Rinaldi-Carmona *et al.*, 1996). CB_1 genes may also undergo a point mutation in their DNA sequences. These are known as single nucleotide polymorphisms (SNPs, pronounced 'snips'). Many CB_1 SNPs have been identified in the human population (SNP Consortium, http://snp.cshl.org). One CB_1 SNP may be associated with schizophrenia (Leroy *et al.*, 2001). Its ligand affinity has not been measured.

It is fascinating to note that the 'palaeontological' phytocannabinoid CBD (associated with the primeval biotype *C. ruderalis*) can bind to primeval VR1 with *greater* affinity than CBD can bind with CB receptors (see Chapter 5). The 'younger' phytocannabinoid, THC, can only bind with 'younger' CB receptors (THC cannot bind with 'older' VR1 receptors).

Plant ligands and 'the great leap forward'

Ligand–receptor coevolution is now generally accepted (Park *et al.*, 2002). Here we propose that a plant ligand may exert sufficient selection pressure to maintain the gene for a receptor in an animal. If the plant ligand improves the fitness of the receptor by serving as a 'proto-medicine' or a performance-enhancing substance, the ligand–receptor association could be evolutionarily conserved. In a hunter-gatherer society, the ability of phytocannabinoids to improve smell, night vision, discern edge and enhance the perception of colour would improve the evolutionary fitness of our species. Evolutionary fitness essentially mirrors reproductive success, and phytocannabinoids enhance the sensation of touch and the sense of rhythm, two sensual responses that may lead to increased replication rates.

Some authors have proposed that cannabis was the catalyst that synergised the emergence of syntactic language in Neolithic humans (McKenna, 1992). Language, in turn, probably caused what anthropologists call 'the great leap forward' in human behaviour, when humans suddenly crafted better tools out of new materials (e.g. fishhooks from bone, spear handles from wood, rope from hemp), developed art (e.g. painting, pottery, musical instruments), began using boats, and evolved intricate social (and religious) organisations. This rather abrupt transformation occurred about 50 000 years ago (Diamond, 1991). Some scientists hypothesise that the great leap forward was precipitated by a favorable mutation in *FOXP2*, a gene encoding a transcription factor that is associated with language development (reviewed by Marcus and Fisher, 2003). This hypothesis is impaired by the fact that *FOXP2* is not specific to our species. Furthermore, this recent burst of human evolution has been described as epigenetic (beyond our genes) – could it be due to the effects of plant ligands? *FOXP2* expression is greatest in the cerebral cortex, striatum, basal ganglia, cerebellum and thalamus – areas enriched with coexpressed CB_1. Conceivably, CB_1 activation by humans ingesting phytocannabinoids could enhance the expression pattern of *FOXP2*.

Evidence for coevolutionary adaptations in CB receptors

The pattern of CB_1 distribution and density in the rat brain (Herkenham *et al.*, 1991) differs subtly from the pattern of CB_1 in the human brain (Glass *et al.*, 1997). The rat cortex shows no lateralisation of CB_1 density, whereas human cortex shows greater CB_1 density in the left hemisphere (Glass *et al.*, 1997), known to be associated with verbal language development. An increased complexity and density of CB_1 patterns in the human forebrain probably mediate a THC 'high' in humans that is absent in rats. Similarly, CB_1 distribution in the human thalamus is more elaborate than the rat thalamus, with greatest density in the dorsomedial nucleus (Glass *et al.*, 1997), an area that mediates emotional tones from the amygdaloid complex, contributing to the formation of human personality. Do these shifts in CB_1 distribution represent simple mammalian evolution, or do they reflect *recent* coevolutionary adaptations from a thousand human generations exposed to phytocannabinoids? Certainly a small shift in receptor density or distribution yields significant changes in perception and behaviour. For example, THC produces aversive and anxiogenic effects in the Wistar strain of rats, whereas it produces rewarding effects in the Lewis strain (Arnold *et al.*, 2001). Wistar rats express higher densities of CB_1 in a part of the amygdala associated with cannabinoid-induced anxiety (Arnold *et al.*, 2001).

A 'gain-of-function' mutation (Lester and Karschin, 2000) of human CB_1 or CB_2, expressed as an increased affinity for phytocannabinoids, could be interpreted as a coevolutionary adaptation. Unfortunately no one has directly compared the affinity of THC for primary human brain tissue versus the affinity of THC for primary rodent brain tissue; nor has anyone done a head-to-head assessment of transfected human CB_1 versus transfected rodent CB_1. We do know that humans and rats respond differently to phytocannabinoids: humans are much more sensitive to phytocannabinoids. It takes 3 mg/kg of THC to affect a mouse (Varvel *et al.*, 2001), whereas only 0.06 mg/kg will work on a person (Ohlsson *et al.*, 1980).

Evidence for coevolutionary adaptations in plant ligands

Could human consumption of phytocannabinoids for thousands of years result in coevolutionary adaptations in cannabis plant phytochemistry? Good evidence shows that the wide array of compounds in cannabis synergistically enhance the beneficial effects of phytocannabinoids, while simultaneously decreasing the side-effects of phytocannabinoids (McPartland and Pruitt, 1999; McPartland and Russo, 2001). Each phytocannabinoid varies in its affinity for CB receptors (ability to bind with receptors), varies in its potency (efficacy at signal transduction), and varies in its activity, ranging from receptor agonists (e.g. Δ^9-THC) to receptor antagonists (e.g. CBD). Even the agonists vary in activity: Glass and Northup (1999) demonstrated that different cannabinoids cause CB receptors to couple with different G proteins (G_i, G_o or G_s), therefore stimulating different intracellular effectors.

These findings stretch the concept of ligand–receptor interactions beyond the classic key-in-lock metaphor. The results of Glass and Northup can be visualised as different keys (different cannabinoids) fitting the same lock (the CB_1 receptor), but opening the door into three different rooms (G_i, G_o or G_s).

Phytocannabinoids also exert non-CB receptor-mediated effects (reviewed by McPartland and Russo, 2001). CBD, for example, is not psychoactive like THC yet it possesses sedative properties. CBD provides neuroleptic benefits by functioning as an anticonvulsant, it increases dopamine activity, serves as a serotonin uptake inhibitor and enhances noradrenaline (norepinephrine) activity. CBD also protects neurons from glutamate toxicity by serving as an antioxidant. CBD is a potent anti-inflammatory agent – it inhibits the production of cyclooxygenase enzymes, lipoxygenase enzymes, tumour necrosis factor-alpha (TNFα) and inflammatory interleukins. It is also antifungal and antibacterial. Although CBD induces apoptosis in cancerous glioma cells, at the same time it protects normal but injured neurons from the same fate (Hampson *et al.*, 1998). Additionally, CBD modulates the pharmacodynamics and pharmacokinetics of THC: (1) it modulates THC signal transduction by perturbing the fluidity of membrane lipids surrounding the CB receptor and by remodelling G proteins and (2) it is a potent inhibitor of cytochrome P450 3A11 metabolism, thus blocking the hydroxylation of THC to its 11-hydroxy metabolite (Bornheim *et al.*, 1995). The 11-hydroxy metabolite is four times more psychoactive than unmetabolised THC (Browne and Weissman, 1981). This may be the reason why a clinical trial showed that CBD reduces anxiety and other unpleasant psychological side-effects provoked by pure THC (Zuardi *et al.*, 1982) – CBD partially blocks the conversion of THC to its more potently psychoactive metabolite. These complex pharmacokinetics are reviewed in Chapter 8.

The diverse qualities of the *Cannabis* biotypes may also be due to differences in terpenoid profiles, which vary by composition as well as concentration (Mediavilla and Steinemann, 1997). Many terpenoids vaporise near the same temperature as THC, they can be inhaled, and some are psychoactive by acting at CB receptors (Meschler and Howlett, 1999) or other receptors (Buchbauer *et al.*, 1993). Terpenoids can also alter the pharmacokinetics of the phytocannabinoids – they cause vasodilitation of alveolar capillaries (permitting more phytocannabinoids to be absorbed by the lung), and they increase blood–brain barrier permeability (Agrawal *et al.*, 1989), permitting more phytocannabinoids to enter the central nervous system.

It appears that our human interaction with cannabis has created a complex heterogeneous medicine that is optimally tolerated by *Homo sapiens*. The success of 12 000 or more years of human refinement with this botanical medication will be difficult to replicate in modern laboratories. Cannabis is but one example of why many of our best medicines come from ancient botanical sources.

Coevolution makes good medicine

The concept of coevolution between plant ligands and animal receptors is germane to any of our ancient medicinal plants. This concept also pertains to other conscious, plant-consuming primates, as well as the unconscious utilisation of medicinal plants by other animals, such as the documented coevolution of leaf-cutting ants and the antibiotic-producing fungi that they cultivate (Hinkle *et al.*, 1994).

Independent of our work, Sullivan and Hagen (2002) described plant alkaloids (such as nicotine and cocaine) serving an evolutionary role in animal survival during harsh environmental conditions. In a marginal environment, an animal's diet may be so poor that it cannot produce enough neurotransmitters of its own. The animal therefore consumes plant alkaloids to 'top up' its neurotransmitter levels during episodes of nutritional shortfalls. Sullivan and Hagen argued that this coevolutionary strategy dates to 'deep time', is deeply embedded in our behaviour, and explains our predilection for psychotropic substances.

The phytocannabinoids go an extra step beyond 'topping up' neurotransmitters during episodes of nutritional shortfalls – they also elicit 'the munchies' and promote appetite in animals. This is especially important during times of drought and famine, when the only foodstuffs available may not be very palatable. In newborns, the endocannabinoids in breast milk promote suckling and survival, and the administration of phytocannabinoids enhances this effect (Fride *et al.*, 2001). Moreover, phytocannabinoids increase the activity of osteoblasts (Bab *et al.*, 2003), so the extra food consumed under the influence of phytocannabinoids is converted into growth and development – an excellent survival mechanism.

Russo (2001) described 'endocannabinoid deficiency syndrome' (EDS), where the administration of phytocannabinoids corrected for deficiencies of either anandamide or CB receptors. EDS may arise from poor nutrition; in the case of anandamide, a deficit of dietary fatty acids may lead to decreased anandamide production. EDS may also arise from genetic dysfunctions. One CB_1 mutation may be associated with schizophrenia (Leroy *et al.*, 2001). The ligand affinity of this mutant receptor has not been measured, but if its affinity for endocannabinoids is decreased, this may explain why some schizophrenics successfully self-medicate their disease with phytocannabinoids (McPartland, unpublished data, 1999). These individuals treat their EDS by dosing their dysfunctional receptors with a surfeit of plant ligands.

In humans, the administration of exogenous phytocannabinoids appears to 'kick-start' our endocannabinoid system. For example, THC stimulates the release of anandamide (Burstein and Hunter, 1995), CBD stimulates the release of 2-AG, and CBD inhibits the breakdown of anandamide by fatty acid amide hydroxylase (FAAH) (Bisogno *et al.*, 2001). Acute administration of THC may increase the density of CB receptors in the central nervous system (Cichewicz *et al.*, 2001). On the other hand, chronic administration of high-dose THC leads to down-regulation and desensitisation of CB receptors, accompanied by tolerance to the drug (Breivogel *et al.*, 1999). Interestingly, CB receptors in different regions of the brain down-regulate at unequal rates and magnitudes, with greatest decrease in the hippocampus and little or no change in the nucleus accumbens and basolateral amygdala (Romero *et al.*, 1998). The evolutionary significance of this is open to conjecture.

Physiological tolerance to the phytocannabinoids is uncommon, partially because the ligands are partial agonists at CB receptors. Perhaps the best medicine (exogenous ligand) is a partial agonist – one that corrects the homeostatic decompensation but falls short of returning a person to total health. We are reminded of the 'sheep farmer' analogy: when the farmer finds a ewe on the wrong side of the fence, the farmer corrects the situation by placing the ewe on the other side of the fence, not by carrying the ewe over the fence and all the way to the centre of the paddock. Partial agonists produce more subtle effects than full agonists (especially in the presence of endogenous agonists), so they are less like to produce physiological tolerance.

Our tolerance to phytocannabinoids may also be due to the fact that CB_1 and CB_2 act as vestigial receptors. As receptors evolve into vestigial structures, their negative-feedback mechanisms may degenerate and become lost in the course of time. When vestigial receptors are activated, they go unopposed, at least for a while. If this activity is beneficial (and humans distinguished beneficial plants from base plants a long time ago), then the benefit is not opposed by biofeedback mechanisms. In contrast, non-vestigial receptors (those that regulate our physiology on a minute-by-minute basis, such as alpha- and beta-adrenergic receptors) are opposed by myriad mechanisms. When these receptors are stimulated, they are balanced by compensatory biofeedback systems, and these enzyme systems may be the source of physiological 'side-effects'.

Significantly, research suggests CB receptors are constituitively active – they constantly activate G proteins, even in the absence of agonist (Nie and Lewis, 2001). Consequently an 'endocannabinoid tone' must be maintained at an optimal magnitude; a decline from the proper magnitude results in a decline in health. The signals from tonically active receptors become amplified in the presence of agonists, and the administration of phytocannabinoids may recruit 'reserve' receptors (Gifford *et al.*, 1999). Conceivably, the phytocannabinoids could cause post-translational modifications in the structures of CB_1 and CB_2 that stabilise the receptors in a conformation that permits greater constituitive activity. This means that the administration of phytocannabinoids may enable CB receptors to remain constituitively active, even after the phytocannabinoids themselves have been metabolised by the body and excreted. This phenomenon happens to μ-opioid receptors after chronic exposure to opiates (Chavkin *et al.*, 2001).

Conclusions and future directions

We present a strong case for coevolution between *Cannabis* and *Homo sapiens*. Humans have certainly launched the evolution of cannabis into a new trajectory, transforming it from a modest weed restricted to Central Asia into one of the 'success stories' of the plant world. Cannabis now grows worldwide, from 0° (the equator) to approximately 63° latitude (McPartland *et al.*, 2000a). Humans, in turn, have benefited from the use of cannabis as a medicine. Over millennia, we have selected plants that provide maximal benefits and minimal side-effects. Furthermore, we develop tolerance to the side-effects of phytocannabinoids much faster than we develop tolerance to their benefits.

When molecular scientists sequence the genomes of organisms (or conduct ligand-binding studies), they cannot discern between the receptors involved in our daily lives and the vestigial receptors that remain in a relatively quiescent state. A method of mapping vestigial receptors and the mechanisms triggering their 'call-up' could be an ultimate diagnostic tool of the future. Are the triggers that up-regulate vestigial receptors what we currently call the 'prodrome' or the 'natural sequelae' of disease? Or does illness manifest a decompensation of vestigial systems? Experiments utilising cDNA microarray technology may ultimately answer these questions; Kittler *et al.* (2000) have already identified nearly 50 genes whose expression is altered by phytocannabinoid exposure in rats. The knowledge of how cannabis impacts gene expression in humans is just beginning.

Clinically, viewing CB_1 and CB_2 as vestigial receptors may explain why patients with identical diseases often respond differently to the same pharmaceutical intervention. As a disease progresses and a patient's homeostatic systems fail, the administration of phytocannabinoids permits a patient's system to recruit and activate some of its 'redundant' receptors back into service. Different patients may recruit different parts of the system and thus may respond very differently when exogenous ligands are introduced.

The therapeutic augmentation of vestigial receptors is vital for restoring homeostasis in an unbalanced animal. Cannabis has restored the health of humans for millennia. We look forward to restoring cannabis to the modern pharmacopoeia.

References

Abel E (1980). *Marijuana: The first 12,000 years.* New York: Plenum Press.

Agrawal A K, Kumar P, Gulati A, Seth P K (1989). Cannabis-induced neurotoxicity in mice: effects on cholinergic (muscarinic) receptors and blood brain barrier permeability. *Res Commun Substance Abuse* 10: 155–168.

Arnold J C, Topple A N, Mallet P E, Hunt G E, McGregor I S (2001). The distribution of cannabinoid-induced Fos expression in rat brain: differences between the Lewis and Wistar strain. *Brain Res* 921: 240–255.

Bab I, Ofek O, Fogel M, Attar-Namdar M, Shohami E, Mechoulam R (2003). Role of CB2 cannabinoid receptor in the regulation of bone remodeling. *Proceedings, 2003 Symposium on the Cannabinoids.* Burlington, VT: International Cannabinoid Research Society: 27.

Baker M E (1997). Steroid receptor phylogeny and vertebrate origins. *Mol Cell Endocrinol* 135: 101–107.

Bentham G, Hooker J D (1880). Urticaceae. *Genera Plantarum* 3: 341–395.

Benton M J, Ayala F J (2003). Dating the tree of life. *Science* 300: 1698–1700.

Beutler J A, Der Marderosian A H (1978). Chemotaxonomy of *Cannabis*. I. Crossbreeding between *Cannabis sativa* and *C. ruderalis*, with analysis of cannabinoid content. *Econ Bot* 32: 387–394.

Bisogno T, Hanus L, De Petrocellis L *et al.* (2001). Molecular targets for cannabidiol and its synthetic analogues: effect on vanilloid VR1 receptors and on the cellular uptake and enzymatic hydrolysis of anandamide. *Br J Pharmacol* 134: 845–852.

Bornheim L M, Kim K Y, Li J, Perotti B Y, Benet L Z (1995). Effect of cannabidiol pretreatment on the kinetics of tetrahydrocannabinol metabolites in mouse brain. *Drug Metab Disposition* 23: 825–831.

Breivogel C S, Childers S R, Deadwyler S A, Hampson R E, Vogt L J, Sim-Selley L J (1999). Chronic delta 9-tetrahydrocannabinol treatment produces a time-dependent loss of cannabinoid receptors and cannabinoid receptor-activated G proteins in rat brain. *J Neurochem* 73: 2447–2459.

Breivogel C S, Griffin G, Di Marzo V, Martin B R (2002). Evidence for a new G protein-coupled cannabinoid receptor in mouse brain. *Mol Pharmacol* 60: 155–163.

Browne R G, Weissman A (1981). Discriminative stimulus properties of delta 9-tetrahydrocannabinol: mechanistic studies. *J Clin Pharmacol* 21(8–9 Suppl): 227S–234S.

Buchbauer G, Jirovetz L, Jager W, Plank C, Dietrich H (1993). Fragrance compounds and essential oils with sedative effects upon inhalation. *J Pharm Sci* 82: 660–664.

Burstein S H, Hunter S A (1995). Stimulation of anandamide biosynthesis in N-18TG2 neuroblastoma cells by delta 9-tetrahydrocannabinol (THC). *Biochem Pharmacol* 49: 855–858.

Chavkin C, McLaughlin J P, Celver J P (2001). Regulation of opioid receptor function by chronic agonist exposure: constitutive activity and desensitization. *Mol Pharmacol* 60: 20–25.

Chiu J, DeSalle R, Lam H M, Meisel L, Coruzzi G (1999). Molecular evolution of glutamate receptors: a primitive signaling mechanism that existed before plants and animals diverged. *Mol Biol Evol* 16: 826–838.

Cichewicz D L, Haller V L, Welch S P (2001). Changes in opioid and cannabinoid receptor protein following short-term combination treatment with delta(9)-tetrahydrocannabinol and morphine. *J Pharmacol Exp Ther* 297: 121–127.

Clarke R C (1998). *Hashish!* Los Angeles, CA: Red Eye Press.

Collinson M E (1989). The fossil history of the Moraceae, Urticaceae (including Cecropiaceae) and Cannabaceae. In: Crane P R, Blackmore S, eds. *Evolution, Systematics and Fossil History of the Hamamelidae*, Vol 2: 'Higher' *Hamamelidae*. Systematics Association Special Volume. Oxford: Oxford University Press: 319–339.

DeCandolle A (1884). *Origin of Cultivated Plants*. New York: D Appleton and Co.

de Meijer E P M (1999). Cannabis germplasm resources. In: Ranalli P, ed. *Advances in Hemp Research*. New York: Haworth Press.

de Meijer E P M, Bagatta M, Carboni A *et al.* (2003). The inheritance of chemical phenotype in *Cannabis sativa* L. *Genetics* 163: 335–346.

de Meijer W J M, van der Kamp H J, van Eeuwijk F A (1992). Characterization of *Cannabis* accessions with regard to cannabinoid content in relation to other plant characters. *Euphytica* 62: 187–200.

Devane W A, Hanus L, Breuer A *et al.* (1992). Isolation and structure of a brain constituent that binds to the cannabinoid receptor. *Science* 258: 1946–1949.

Dewey L H (1914). Hemp. *U.S.D.A. Yearbook 1913*. Washington DC: United States Department of Agriculture: 283–347.

Diamond J (1991). *The Rise and Fall of the Third Chimpanzee*. London: Radius.

Di Marzo V, Fontana A (1995). Anandamide, an endogeonous cannabinomimetic eicosanoid: 'killing two birds with one stone'. *Prostaglandins Leukot Essent Fatty Acids* 53: 1–11.

DuToit B M (1980). *Cannabis in Africa*. Rotterdam: A A Balkema Press.

Ehrlich P R, Raven P H (1964). Butterflies and plants: a study in coevolution. *Evolution* 18: 586–608.

Elphick M R (1998). An invertebrate G-protein coupled receptor is a chimeric cannabinoid/melanocortin receptor. *Brain Res* 780: 170–173.

Endlicher S L (1837). Cannabaceae. *Genera Plantarum* 4: 286.

Engler A, Prantl K (1889). Moraceae. In: *Die natürlichen Pflanzenfamilien III*. Vol 1. Leipzig, Germany: Wilhelm Engelmann: 66–98.

Fellermeier M, Zenk M H (1998). Prenylation of olivetolate by a hemp transferase yields cannabigerolic acid, the precursor of tetrahydrocannabinol. *FEBS Lett* 427: 283–285.

Fredriksson R, Lagerström M C, Lundin L G, Schiöth H B (2003). The G-protein-coupled receptors in the human genome form five main families. Phylogenetic analysis, paralogon groups, and fingerprints. *Mol Pharmacol* 63: 1256–1272.

Fride E, Ginzburg Y, Breuer A, Bisogno T, Di Marzo V, Mechoulam R (2001). Critical role of the endogenous cannabinoid system in mouse pup suckling and growth. *Eur J Pharmacol* 419: 207–214.

Gaoni Y, Mechoulam R (1964). Isolation, structure and partial synthesis of an active constituent of hashish. *J Am Chem Soc* 86: 1646–1647.

Gifford A N, Bruneus M, Gatley S J, Lan R, Makriyannis A, Volkow ND (1999). Large receptor reserve for cannabinoid actions in the central nervous system. *J Pharmacol Exp Ther* 288: 478–483.

Glass M, Felder C C (1997). Concurrent stimulation of cannabinoid CB1 and dopamine D2 receptors augments cAMP accumulation in striatal neurons: evidence for a Gs linkage to the CB1 receptor. *J Neurosci* 17: 5327–5333.

Glass M, Northup J K (1999). Agonist selective regulation of G-proteins by cannabinoid CB1 and CB2 receptors. *Mol Pharmacol* 56: 1362–1369.

Glass M, Dragunow M, Faull R L (1997). Cannabinoid receptors in the human brain: a detailed anatomical and quantitative autoradiographic study in the fetal, neonatal and adult human brain. *Neuroscience* 77: 299–318.

Greuter W, Brummitt R K, Farr E, Kilian N, Kirk P M, Silva P C (1993). *Names in Current Use for Extant Plant Genera*. Königstein: Koeltz Scientific Books.

Hampson A J, Grimaldi M, Axelrod J, Wink D (1998). Cannabidiol and (–)delta9-tetrahydrocannabinol are neuroprotective antioxidants. *Proc Natl Acad Sci USA* 95: 8268–8273.

Herkenham M, Lynn A B, Johnson M R, Melvin L S, de Costa B R, Rice K C (1991). Characterization and localization of cannabinoid receptors in rat brain: a quantitative in vitro autoradiographic study. *J Neurosci* 11: 563–583.

Herodotus (1906) Reprint. *Herodotus IV (Melpomene)*. Cambridge: Cambridge University Press.

Hillig K W (2004a). Genetic evidence for speciation in *Cannabis (Cannabaceae)*. *Genet Res Crop Evol*, in press.

Hillig K W (2004b). Terpenoid variation in a *Cannabis* germplasm collection. *J Nat Prod*, in press.

Hillig K W, Mahlber P G (2004). A systematic analysis of cannabinoid variation in *Cannabis (Cannabaceae)*. *Am J Bot*, in press.

Hinkle G, Wetterer J K, Schultz T R, Sogin M L (1994). Phylogeny of the attine ant fungi based on analysis of small subunit ribosomal RNA gene sequences. *Science* 266: 1695–1697.

Hoyle C H V (1999). Neuropeptide families and their receptors: evolutionary perspectives. *Brain Res* 848: 1–25.

Hulse M, Johnson S, Ferrieri P (1993). *Agrobacterium* infections in humans: experience at one hospital and review. *Clin Infect Dis* 16: 112–127.

International Human Genome Sequencing Consortium (2001). Initial sequencing and analysis of the human genome. *Nature* 409: 860–920.

International Narcotics Control Board (1996). *Drug Report: West Asia*. United Nations INCB Regional Updates. www.un.org/ecosocdev/geninfo/drugs/regional.htm (accessed December 2003).

Jarai Z, Wagner J A, Varga K, Lake K D, Compton D R *et al.* (1999). Cannabinoid-induced mesenteric vasodilation through an endothelial site distinct from CB1 or CB2 receptors. *Proc Natl Acad Sci USA* 96: 14136–14141.

Kittler J T, Grigorenko E V, Clayton C *et al.* (2000). Large-scale analysis of gene expression changes during acute and chronic exposure to Δ9-THC in rats. *Physiol Genomics* 3: 175–185.

Leroy S, Griffon N, Bourdel M C, Olie J P, Poirier M F, Krebs M O (2001). Schizophrenia and the cannabinoid receptor type 1 (CB1): Association study using a single-base polymorphism in coding exon 1. *Am J Med Genet* 105: 749–752.

Lester H A, Karschin A (2000). Gain of function mutants: ion channels and G protein-coupled receptors. *Annu Rev Neurosci* 23: 89–125.

Li H L (1974). The origin and use of *Cannabis* in eastern Asia: linguistic-cultural implications. *Econ Bot* 28: 293–302.

Lynch M, Conery J S (2000). The evolutionary fate and consequences of duplicate genes. *Science* 290: 1151–1155.

McEno J (1991). *Cannabis,* radical agriculture, and the epistemology of plant pathology. In: McEno, ed. *Cannabis Ecology: A Compendium of Diseases and Pests*. Middlebury, Vermont: AMRITA Press: 106–122.

McKenna T (1992). *Food of the Gods*. New York: Bantam Books: 55.

McPartland J M (1984). Pathogenicity of *Phomopsis ganjae* on *Cannabis sativa* and the fungistatic effect of cannabinoids produced by the host. *Mycopathologia* 87: 149–153.

McPartland J M (1992). C.H. Persoon: a phanerogamic footnote. *Mycotaxon* 45: 257–258.

McPartland J M (1997). *Cannabis* as a repellent crop and botanical pesticide. *J Int Hemp Assoc* 4(2): 89–94.

McPartland J M, Glass M (2001). The nematocidal effects of *Cannabis* may not be mediated by cannabinoid receptors. *N Z J Crop Hort Sci* 29: 301–307.

McPartland J M, Mediavilla V (2001). Nichcannabinoide Inhaltsstoffe von *Cannabis*. In: Grotenhermen F, ed. *Cannabis und Cannabinoide*. Bern, Switzerland: Verlag Hans Huber: 429–436.

McPartland J M, Nicholson J (2003). Using parasite databases to identify potential nontarget hosts of biological control organisms. *N Z J Bot* 41(4): 699–706.

McPartland J M, Pruitt P L (1999). Side effects of pharmaceuticals not elicited by comparable herbal medicines: the case of tetrahydrocannabinol and marijuana. *Altern Ther Health Med* 5(4): 57–62.

McPartland J M, Pruitt P L (2002). Sourcing the code: searching for the evolutionary origins of cannabinoid receptors, vanilloid receptors, and anandamide. *J Cannabis Ther* 2(1): 73–103.

McPartland J M, Russo E B (2001). *Cannabis* and cannabis extracts: Greater than the sum of their parts? *J Cannabis Ther* 1(3–4): 103–132.

McPartland J M, Clarke R C, Watson D P (2000a). *Hemp Diseases and Pests: Management and Biological Control.* Wallingford, UK: CABI Publishing.

McPartland J M, Mercer A, Glass M (2000b). Agricultural applications of *Cannabis* and cannabinoids: are cannabinoid receptors involved? *Proceedings, 2000 Symposium on the Cannabinoids.* Burlington, VT: International Cannabinoid Research Society: 5.

McPartland J M, Di Marzo V, De Petrocellis L, Mercer A, Glass M (2001). Cannabinoid receptors are absent in insects. *J Comp Neurol* 436: 423–429.

Maddison W P (1997). Gene trees in species trees. *Syst Biol* 46: 523–536.

Marcus G F, Fisher S E (2003). FOXP2 in focus: what can genes tell us about speech and language? *Trends Cogn Sci* 7: 257–262.

Martin M, Ledent C, Parmentier M, Maldonado R, Valverde O (2002). Involvement of CB1 cannabinoid receptors in emotional behaviour. *Psychopharmacology* 159: 379–387.

Mechoulam R, Gaoni Y (1967). Recent advances in the chemistry of hashish. *Fortschritte der Chemie Organischer Naturstoffe* 25: 175–213.

Mechoulam R, Devane W A, Breuer A, Zahalka J (1991). A random walk through a cannabis field. *Pharmacol Biochem Behav* 40: 461–464.

Mechoulam R, Parker L A, Gallily R (2002). Cannabidiol: an overview of some pharmacological aspects. *J Clin Pharmacol* 42(11 Suppl): 11S–19S.

Mediavilla V, Steinemann S (1997). Essential oil of *Cannabis sativa* L. strains. *J Int Hemp Assoc* 4(2): 82–84.

Meschler J P, Howlett A C (1999). Thujone exhibits low affinity for cannabinoid receptors but fails to evoke cannabimimetic responses. *Pharmacol Biochem Behav* 62: 473–480.

Muhammad I, Li X C, Dunbar D C, ElSohly M A, Khan I A (2001). Antimalarial (+)-trans-hexahydrodibenzopyran derivatives from *Machaerium multiflorum*. *J Nat Prod* 64: 1322–1325.

Nakane S, Tanaka T, Satouchi K, Kobayashi Y, Waku K, Sugiura T (2000). Occurrence of a novel cannabimimetic molecule in the umbrella pine *Sciadopitys verticillata*. *Biol Pharm Bull* 23: 758–761.

Nie J, Lewis D L (2001). Structural domains of the CB1 cannabinoid receptor that contribute to constitutive activity and G-protein sequestration. *J Neurosci* 21: 8758–8764.

Ohlsson A, Lindgren J E, Wahlen A, Agurell S, Hollister L E, Gillespie H K (1980). Plasma delta-9 tetrahydrocannabinol concentrations and clinical effects after oral and intravenous administration and smoking. *Clin Pharmacol Ther* 28: 409–416.

Park Y, Kim Y J, Adams M E (2002). Identification of G protein-coupled receptors for *Drosophila* PRXamide peptides, CCAP, corazonin, and AKH supports a theory of ligand-receptor coevolution. *Proc Natl Acad Sci USA* 99: 11423–11428.

Pate D W (1999a). Hemp seed: a valuable food source. In: Ranalli P, ed. *Advances in Hemp Research*. New York: Haworth Press: 243–255.

Pate D W (1999b). Anandamide structure–activity relationships and mechanisms of action on intraocular pressure in the normotensive rabbit model. PhD thesis, University of Kuopio, Finland, 99 pp.

Peroutka S J, Howell T A (1994). The molecular evolution of G protein-coupled receptors: focus on 5-hydroxytryptamine receptors. *Neuropharmacology* 33: 319–324.

Pertwee R G, Ross R A, Craib S J, Thomas A (2002). Cannabidiol antagonizes receptor agonists and noradrenaline in the mouse vas deferens. *Eur J Pharmacol* 456: 99–106.

Pirozynski K A (1988). Coevolution by horizontal gene transfer: a speculation on the role of fungi. In: Pirozynski K A, Hawksworth D L, eds. *Coevolution of Fungi with Plants and Animals*. London: Academic Press: 247–268.

Pirozynski K A, Hawksworth D L (1988). Coevolution of fungi with plants and animals: introduction and overview. In: Pirozynski K A, Hawksworth D L, eds. *Coevolution of Fungi with Plants and Animals*. London: Academic Press: 1–29.

Pollan M (2001). *The Botany of Desire*. New York: Random House.

Quaghebeur K, Coosemans J, Toppet S, Compernolle F (1994). Cannabiorci- and 8-chlorocannabiorcichromenic acid as fungal antagonists from *Cylindrocarpon olidum*. *Phytochemistry* 37: 159–161.

Reininger W R (1946). Hashish. *Ciba Symp* 8: 374–404.

Renfrew J M (1973). *Palaeoethnobotany*. New York: Columbia University Press: 163.

Rinaldi-Carmona M, Calandra B, Shire D *et al.* (1996). Characterization of two cloned human CB1 cannabinoid receptor isoforms. *J Pharmacol Exp Ther* 278: 871–878.

Romero J, Berrendero F, Manzanares J *et al.* (1998). Time-course of the cannabinoid receptor down-regulation in the adult rat brain caused by repeated exposure to delta-9-tetrahydrocannabinol. *Synapse* 30: 298–308.

Ross S A, ElSohly M A (1996). The volatile oil composition of fresh and air-dried buds of *Cannabis sativa*. *J Nat Prod* 59: 49–51.

Rubin V (1975). *Cannabis and Culture*. The Hague: Mouton Publishers.

Rudenko S I (1970). *Frozen Tombs of Siberia* (English translation). Berkeley: University of California Press.

Russo E (2001). Hemp for headache. *J Cannabis Ther* 1(2): 21–92.

Schleiffer H (1979). *Narcotic Plants of the World*. Monticello, NY: Lubrecht & Cramer.

Schoenmakers N (1986). *The Seed Bank (1986)/1987 Catalogue*. Postbus 5, 6576 NZ, Ooy, the Netherlands.

Schultes R E (1970). Random thoughts and queries on the botany of *Cannabis*. In: Joyce C R B, Curry S H, eds. *The Botany and Chemistry of Cannabis*. London: J & A Churchill: 11–38.

Schultes R E, Klein W M, Plowman, T, Lockwood T E (1974). *Cannabis:* an example of taxonomic neglect. *Bot Mus Leaflet Harv Univ* 23: 337–367.

Schumacher, M A., Moff I, Sudanagunta S P, Levine J D (2000). Molecular cloning of an N-terminal splice variant of the capsaicin receptor. *J Biol Chem* 275: 2756–2762.

Shire D, Carillon C, Kaghad M *et al.* (1995). An amino-terminal variant of the central cannabinoid receptor resulting from alternative splicing. *J Biol Chem* 270: 3726–3731.

Shoyama Y, Taura F, Morimoto S (2001). Expression of tentrahydrocannabinoilic acid synthase in tobacco. *Proceedings, 2001 Symposium on the Cannabinoids.* Burlington, VT: International Cannabinoid Research Society: 9.

Small E, Beckstead H D (1973). Common cannabinoid phenotypes in 350 stocks of *Cannabis. Lloydia* 36: 144–165.

Small E, Cronquist A (1976). A practical and natural taxonomy for *Cannabis. Taxon* 25: 405–435.

Soderstrom K, Murray T F, Yoo H D *et al.* (1997). Discovery of novel cannabinoid receptor ligands from diverse marine organisms. *Adv Exp Med Biol* 433: 73–77.

Sullivan R J, Hagen E H (2002). Psychotropic substance-seeking: evolutionary pathology or adaptation? *Addiction* 97: 389–400.

Szallasi, A., Di Marzo V (2000). New perspectives on enigmatic vanilloid receptors. *Trends Neurosci* 23: 491–497.

Taura F, Morimoto S, Shoyama Y (1995). First direct evidence for the mechanism of tetrahydrocannabinolic acid biosynthesis. *J Am Chem Soc* 117: 9766–9767.

Thorne R F (1992). Classification and geography of the flowering plants. *Bot Rev* 58: 225–348.

Toyota M, Shimamura T, Ishii H, Renner M, Braggins J, Asakawa Y (2002). New bibenzyl cannabinoid from the New Zealand liverwort *Radula marginata. Chem Pharm Bull (Tokyo)* 50: 1390–1392.

Varvel S A, Hamm R J, Martin B R, Lichtman A H (2001). Differential effects of delta 9-THC on spatial reference and working memory in mice. *Psychopharmacology (Berlin)* 157: 142–50.

Vasquez C, Lewis D L (1999). The CB1 cannabinoid receptor can sequester G-proteins, making them unavailable to couple to other receptors. *J Neurosci* 19: 9271–9280.

Vavilov N I (1926). The origin of the cultivation of 'primary' crops, in particular of cultivated hemp. In: *Studies on the Origin of Cultivated Plants.* Leningrad: Institute of Applied Botany and Plant Breeding: 221–233.

Vavilov N I (1957). *Agroecological Survey of the Main Field Crops.* Moscow: Academy of Sciences of the USSR.

Vekua A, Lordkipanidze D, Rightmire G P *et al.* (2002). A new skull of early *Homo* from Dmanisi, Georgia. *Science* 297: 85–89.

Walton R P (1938). *Marihuana, America's New Drug Problem.* Philadelphia: J B Lippincott: 48–49.

Wirtshafter D (1997). Nutritional value of hemp seed and hemp seed oil. In: Mathre M L, ed. *Cannabis in Medical Practice.* Jefferson, NC: McFarland & Co.: 181–191.

Wood T B, Spivey W T, Easterfield T H (1899). Cannabinol. Part I. *J Chem Soc* 75: 20–36.

Yamaguchi F, Macrae A D, Brenner S (1996). Molecular cloning of two cannabinoid type 1-like receptor genes from the puffer fish *Fugu rubripes. Genomics* 35: 603–605.

Ziemienowicz A, Gorlich D, Lanka E, Hohn B, Rossi L (1999). Import of DNA into mammalian nuclei by proteins originating from a plant pathogenic bacterium. *Proc Natl Acad Sci USA* 96(7): 3729–3733.

Zimmer A, Zimmer A M, Hohmann A G, Herkenham M, Bonner T I (1999). Increased mortality, hypoactivity, and hypoalgesia in cannabinoid CB1 receptor knockout mice. *Proc Natl Acad Sci USA* 96: 5780–5785.

Zuardi A W, Shirakawa I, Finkelfarb E, Karniol I G (1982). Action of cannabidiol on the anxiety and other effects produced by Δ^9-THC in normal subjects. *Psychopharmacology* 76: 245–250.

5

Receptors and pharmacodynamics: natural and synthetic cannabinoids and endocannabinoids

Roger Pertwee

Development of medicines based on cannabis presupposes that the compounds present in the plant or extracts of the plant have pharmacological activity that is relevant to the proposed therapeutic use. Cannabis, and compounds isolated from it have been used in medicines from antiquity, but a rational explanation of the pharmacology and pharmacodynamics has only recently emerged. The discovery of specific receptors with a widespread distribution in the brain and the immune system helps to explain the effects of cannabis on behaviour and higher central nervous system (CNS) functions. However, receptor-mediated responses explain many, but not all of the effects of cannabis and cannabinoids. The discovery of an endocannabinoid system that is present in most phyla adds a new dimension to investigation of the physiological role of phytocannabinoids as therapeutic agents.

The plant *Cannabis sativa* is the unique source of a set of more than 60 oxygen-containing aromatic hydrocarbon compounds that are known collectively as cannabinoids and that include $(-)-\Delta^9$-tetrahydrocannabinol $((-)-\Delta^9$-THC), the compound that is largely responsible for the psychotropic properties of the plant (Pertwee, 1988). $(-)-\Delta^9$-THC and other cannabinoids have high lipid solubility and low water solubility and so were long thought to owe their pharmacological properties to an ability to perturb the phospholipid constituents of biological membranes. This changed in the 1980s with the discovery that $(-)-\Delta^9$-THC possesses highly selective modes of action that depend on the activation of specific cannabinoid receptors. Presently, there is firm evidence for the existence in mammalian tissues of just two types of cannabinoid receptor, CB_1 and CB_2. Mammalian tissues can also produce endogenous ligands for cannabinoid receptors, suggesting that these receptors have physiological as well as pharmacological significance.

Cannabinoid receptors and their endogenous ligands, the endocannabinoids, constitute the 'endocannabinoid system'; phytocannabinoids are derived from the plant kingdom.

Cannabinoid CB$_1$ and CB$_2$ receptors

CB$_1$ receptors, cloned in 1990 (Matsuda *et al.*, 1990), and CB$_2$ receptors, cloned in 1993 (Munro *et al.*, 1993), have been detected in several species including human, rat and mouse (Matsuda, 1997). As a result both CB$_1$ and CB$_2$ receptor knockout mice are now available (Ledent *et al.*, 1999; Zimmer *et al.*, 1999; Buckley *et al.*, 2000). The CB$_1$ receptor nucleotide sequence is well conserved across mammalian species, the sequences of human and rat being 90% identical, those of human and mouse 91% identical and those of rat and mouse 96% identical (Gérard *et al.*, 1990; Chakrabarti *et al.*, 1995). CB$_2$ receptors show greater interspecies differences. Thus, the predicted amino acid sequence of the mouse CB$_2$ receptor differs from that of the human CB$_2$ receptor in 60 residues (82% similarity) (Shire *et al.*, 1996). These differences are to be found mainly in the N-terminal extramembrane region. A spliced variant of CB$_1$ cDNA, CB$_{1a}$, has also been isolated (Shire *et al.*, 1995; Rinaldi-Carmona *et al.*, 1996). However, CB$_{1a}$ mRNA exists only as a minor transcript and there is no evidence for any important difference between the pharmacology of CB$_1$ and CB$_{1a}$ receptors.

CB$_1$ and CB$_2$ receptors are both members of the superfamily of G protein-coupled receptors and agonist stimulation of these receptors activates a number of signal transduction pathways (for references see Pertwee, 1997; Pertwee and Ross, 2002). For example, both receptor types are coupled through G$_{i/o}$ proteins, negatively to adenylate cyclase and positively to mitogen-activated protein kinase. In addition, mammalian CB$_1$ receptors are coupled through G$_{i/o}$ proteins to various ion channels. These include A-type and inwardly rectifying potassium channels, to which CB$_1$ receptors are positively coupled, and N-type and P/Q-type calcium channels and D-type potassium channels, to which CB$_1$ receptors are negatively coupled. There are also reports that CB$_1$ receptors are negatively coupled to postsynaptic M-type potassium channels in rat hippocampal CA1 pyramidal neurons and to voltage-gated L-type calcium channels in cat cerebral arterial smooth muscle cells. Other suggested effector mechanisms for CB$_1$ receptors involve closure of 5-HT$_3$ ion channels, modulation of nitric oxide production and mobilisation of arachidonic acid and of intracellular calcium stores.

CB$_1$ receptor activation can also initiate ceramide production through a non-G$_i$/G$_o$ mechanism and, under certain conditions, CB$_1$ receptors can activate adenylate cyclase and/or reduce outward potassium K current through G$_s$ proteins. Results from experiments with CB$_1$ and CB$_2$-transfected cells support the existence of even more signalling mechanisms for these receptors. However, since such cell lines tend to overexpress cannabinoid receptors, the physiological significance of these additional effector mechanisms remains to be established.

CB$_1$ receptors are present both in the central nervous system and in some peripheral tissues that include immune cells, reproductive and gastrointestinal tissues, sympathetic ganglia, adrenal and pituitary glands and heart, lung and urinary bladder (Pertwee, 1997). The distribution of CB$_1$ receptors within the brain is heterogeneous, areas that express this receptor type including the cerebral cortex, hippocampus, caudate-putamen, substantia nigra pars reticulata, globus pallidus, entopeduncular nucleus, cerebellum, periaqueductal grey, rostral ventromedial medulla, superior colliculus and certain nuclei of the thalamus and amygdala (Herkenham *et al.*, 1991; Pertwee, 1997, 2001). This distribution pattern accounts for several prominent pharmacological properties of CB$_1$ receptor agonists, for example their ability to impair cognition and memory, to affect the control of motor function and to produce signs of analgesia/antinociception both in humans and in animal models of acute pain and of tonic pain induced by nerve damage (neuropathic pain) or by the injection of an inflammatory agent. Thus, as detailed elsewhere (Pertwee, 2001; Salio *et al.*, 2001), CB$_1$ receptors are located on neurons associated with pain perception, both within the brain and outside it. These include neurons of the thalamus, periaqueductal grey and rostral ventromedial medulla, neurons that project from the brainstem to the spinal cord and intrinsic spinal neurons. CB$_1$ receptors have also been detected at the central and peripheral terminals of small-diameter C-fibres and larger diameter Aβ/Aδ-fibres of primary afferent neurons. This distribution pattern helps to explain the efficacy shown by CB$_1$ receptor agonists against signs of neuropathic pain as this kind of pain is thought to be elicited in part by abnormal spontaneous discharges of myelinated Aβ- and Aδ-fibres.

Many CB$_1$ receptors are expressed at the terminals of central and peripheral nerves, an important function of these presynaptic receptors being to reduce the release of a range of excitatory and inhibitory neurotransmitters (for references see Pertwee, 2001; Vizi *et al.*, 2001; Pertwee and Ross, 2002). Thus, results obtained from *in vitro* experiments with human, rat, mouse or guinea-pig brain tissue have indicated that pre-synaptic CB_1 receptors can mediate inhibition of the spontaneous or evoked neuronal release of acetylcholine, noradrenaline (norepineph-rine), 5-hydroxytryptamine (5-HT) and glutamate in cerebral cortex, of acetylcholine, noradrenaline, γ-aminobutyric acid (GABA), cholecys-tokinin and glutamate in hippocampus, of noradrenaline and 5-HT in hypothalamus, of dopamine, GABA and glutamate in striatum, of GABA and glutamate in nucleus accumbens, substantia nigra zona retic-ulata and periaqueductal grey, of GABA in rostral ventromedial medulla and of GABA, glutamate and D-aspartate in cerebellum.

Outside the brain, presynaptic CB_1 receptors appear to inhibit neu-ronal release of GABA, glutamate and glycine in the substantia gelati-nosa of spinal cord, of noradrenaline and dopamine release in retina, of noradrenaline release in heart, bronchus and vas deferens and of acetyl-choline in small intestine. Signs of CB_1-mediated inhibitory effects on acetylcholine release in cerebral cortex and hippocampus and of GABA release in striatum have also been detected *in vivo* in experiments with rats. The inhibitory effect of CB_1 receptor agonists on GABA, glutamate or glycine release in the periaqueductal grey, rostral ventromedial medulla and substantia gelatinosa most likely contributes to the ability of these agonists to modulate pain perception.

In some experiments with whole animals or with brain slices, CB_1 receptor agonists have been reported to enhance the central release of certain neurotransmitters. Examples include enhanced *in vivo* release of acetylcholine in prefrontal cortex and hippocampus (Acquas *et al.*, 2000, 2001) and enhanced dopamine release in nucleus accumbens, either *in vitro* (Cheer *et al.*, 2000) or *in vivo* (Chen *et al.*, 1990a,b, 1991; French, 1997; French *et al.*, 1997; Tanda *et al.*, 1997; Gessa *et al.*, 1998b; Melis *et al.*, 2000). However, it is possible that these effects also result from a CB_1 receptor-mediated inhibitory effect on neurotransmis-sion and that this is translated into a stimulatory effect on neurotrans-mitter release at some point downstream of the site at which the initial inhibitory effect is induced. For example, Robbe *et al.* (2001) have pos-tulated that stimulation of dopamine release in the nucleus accumbens by CB_1 receptor agonists may stem from a CB_1 receptor-mediated inhi-bition of glutamate release from extrinsic glutamatergic fibres onto GABAergic neurons that project from the nucleus accumbens to the ventral tegmental area to exert an inhibitory effect on dopaminergic meso-accumbens neurons (Figure 5.1). It is also possible that increased acetylcholine release in the prefrontal cortex induced by cannabinoids *in vivo* results from cannabinoid receptor-mediated disinhibition of

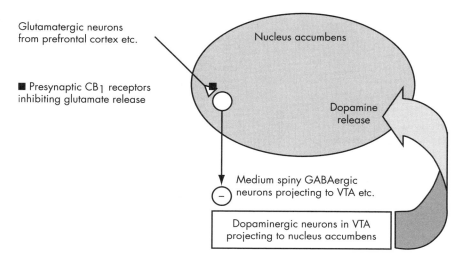

Glutamatergic neurons
from prefrontal cortex etc.

Nucleus accumbens

■ Presynaptic CB_1 receptors
inhibiting glutamate release

Dopamine
release

Medium spiny GABAergic
neurons projecting to VTA etc.

Dopaminergic neurons in VTA
projecting to nucleus accumbens

Figure 5.1 Schematic diagram illustrating how CB_1 receptor-mediated inhibition of glutamate release in the nucleus accumbens may indirectly enhance dopamine release in this brain area. VTA, ventral tegmental area.

dopamine release in the nucleus accumbens. Thus, dopamine released in this brain area is thought to disinhibit acetylcholine release in the pre-frontal cortex by acting on GABAergic neurons that project from the nucleus accumbens to the cortex (Moore *et al.*, 1999).

Turning now to the roles of CB_2 receptors, these may well include immunomodulation as this receptor type is expressed mainly by immune cells, particularly B cells and natural killer cells (Pertwee, 1997, 2001; Cabral, 2001). It is likely that CB_2 receptors regulate cytokine release in health and/or disease (Molina-Holgado *et al.*, 1999; Pertwee, 2001; Cabral, 2001). Consequently, since CB_1 receptors modulate neurotransmitter release, a common role of CB_1 and CB_2 receptors may be regulation of the release of chemical messengers. When activated by cannabinoids, CB_2 receptors (or possibly 'CB_2-like' receptors) also share the ability of CB_1 receptors to produce signs of analgesia/antinociception (Hanus *et al.*, 1999; Pertwee, 2001).

Endogenous ligands for CB_1 and CB_2 receptors

All endocannabinoids that have been identified so far are analogues of arachidonic acid. The most important of these 'eicosanoid' molecules (Figure 5.2) are arachidonoyl ethanolamide (anandamide), 2-arachidonoyl glycerol (2-AG) (Devane *et al.*, 1992; Di Marzo *et al.*, 1998;

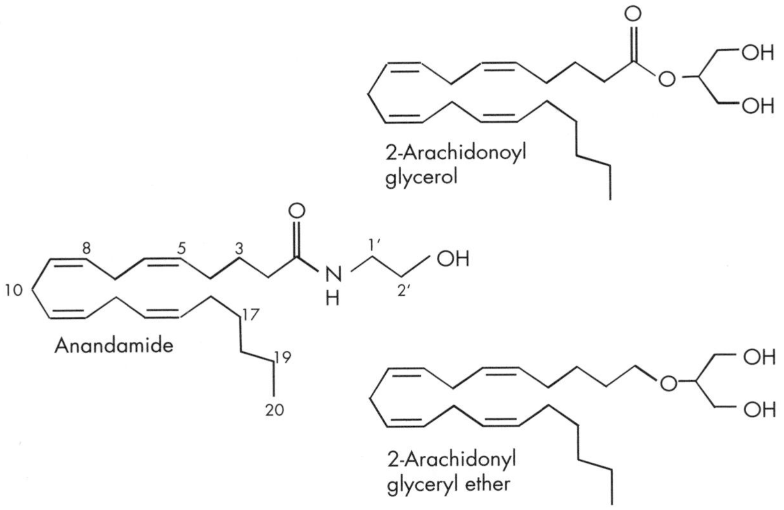

Figure 5.2 The structures of three endocannabinoids.

Mechoulam *et al.*, 1998; Sugiura and Waku, 2000) and probably also arachidonyl glyceryl ether (noladin ether) (Hanus *et al.*, 2001).

When protected from enzymic hydrolysis, anandamide exhibits a CB_1 affinity similar to that of (–)-Δ^9-THC (Table 5.1). It has marginally greater CB_1 than CB_2 affinity and behaves as a partial agonist at both these receptor types. Thus, in several CB_1 receptor-containing systems, the size of the maximal effect of anandamide has been found to fall well below that of higher efficacy cannabinoid receptor agonists such as CP55,940 and R-(+)-WIN55,212 (see next section) and its efficacy at CB_2 receptors is even less than at CB_1 receptors (Bayewitch *et al.*, 1995; Rinaldi-Carmona *et al.*, 1996; Griffin *et al.*, 1998; Pertwee, 1999). Indeed, in one set of experiments it has been found to attenuate CB_2 receptor-mediated responses to a higher efficacy agonist (2-AG) (Gonsiorek *et al.*, 2000), thus showing it to possess the mixed agonist–antagonist properties that are typical of a partial agonist.

As for 2-AG and noladin ether, the available data suggest that both are cannabinoid receptor agonists, that noladin ether has significantly higher affinity for CB_1 receptors than for CB_2 receptors (Table 5.1) whilst the affinity of 2-AG for CB_1 and CB_2 receptors is similar to that of anandamide, and that 2-AG exhibits higher efficacy than anandamide at both CB_1 and CB_2 receptors (Stella *et al.*, 1997; Sugiura *et al.*, 1997; Ben-Shabat *et al.*, 1998; Pertwee, 1999; Gonsiorek *et al.*, 2000; Hanus *et al.*, 2001; Savinainen *et al.*, 2001).

Table 5.1 K_i values of certain ligands for the *in vitro* displacement of [³H]CP55,940, [³H]R-(+)-WIN55,212 or [³H]HU-243 from CB_1- and CB_2-specific binding sites

Ligand	CB_1 K_i value (nM)	CB_2 K_i value (nM)	Reference
CB_1-selective ligands in order of decreasing CB_1/CB_2 selectivity			
ACEA	1.4[a,b]	>2000[a,b]	Hillard *et al.*, 1999
O–1812	3.4[b]	3870[b]	Di Marzo *et al.*, 2001
SR141716A	11.8	13 200	Felder *et al.*, 1998
	11.8	973	Felder *et al.*, 1995
	12.3	702	Showalter *et al.*, 1996
	5.6	>1000	Rinaldi-Carmona *et al.*, 1994
	1.98[b]	>1000[b]	Rinaldi-Carmona *et al.*, 1994
AM281	12[b]	4200[c]	Lan *et al.*, 1999
ACPA	2.2[a,b]	715[a,b]	Hillard *et al.*, 1999
2-Arachidonylglyceryl ether	21.2[b]	>3000	Hanus *et al.*, 2001
LY320135	141	14 900	Felder *et al.*, 1998
R-(+)-methanandamide	17.9[a,b]	868[a,c]	Lin *et al.*, 1998
	20[a,b]	815[c]	Khanolkar *et al.*, 1996
O-689	5.7[a]	132[a]	Showalter *et al.*, 1996
(+)-7-OH-4'-DMH-CBD	2.5[b]	44	Bisogno *et al.*, 2001
(+)-4'-DMH-CBD	17.4[b]	211	Bisogno *et al.*, 2001
Ligands without any marked CB_1/CB_2 selectivity			
Anandamide	61[a,b]	1930[a,c]	Lin *et al.*, 1998
	89[a]	371[a]	Showalter *et al.*, 1996
	543	1940	Felder *et al.*, 1995
	71.7[a,b]	279[a,b]	Hillard *et al.*, 1999
	252[b]	581	Mechoulam *et al.*, 1995
AM404	1760[a,b]	13 000[c]	Khanolkar *et al.*, 1996
Ajulemic acid (CT-3)	32.3[b]	170.5	Rhee *et al.*, 1997
2-Arachidonoylglycerol	472[b]	1400	Mechoulam *et al.*, 1995
	58.3[d]	145[d]	Ben-Shabat *et al.*, 1998
HU-210	0.0608	0.524	Felder *et al.*, 1995
	0.1[b]	0.17	Rhee *et al.*, 1997
	0.73	0.22	Showalter *et al.*, 1996
DMH-CBN	2[b]	1.5	Rhee *et al.*, 1997
CP55,940	5	1.8	Ross *et al.*, 1999a
	3.72	2.55	Felder *et al.*, 1995
	1.37[b]	1.37[b]	Rinaldi-Carmona *et al.*, 1994
	0.58	0.69	Showalter *et al.*, 1996
	0.50[a,b]	2.80[a,b]	Hillard *et al.*, 1999

(*continued*)

Table 5.1 *Continued*

Ligand	CB_1 K_i value (nM)	CB_2 K_i value (nM)	Reference
Δ^9-THC	53.3	75.3	Felder *et al.*, 1995
	39.5[b]	40	Bayewitch *et al.*, 1996
	40.7	36.4	Showalter *et al.*, 1996
	80.3[b]	32.2	Rhee *et al.*, 1997
	35.3[b]	3.9[b]	Rinaldi-Camona *et al.*, 1994
Δ^8-THC	47.6[b]	39.3[c]	Busch-Petersen *et al.*, 1996
O-1238	3.5	7.8	Ross *et al.*, 1999b
O-1184	5.2	7.4	Ross *et al.*, 1999b
(−)-CBD	4350	2860	Showalter *et al.*, 1996
	>10 000[b]	>10 000	Bisogno *et al.*, 2001
CBN	211.2[b]	126.4	Rhee *et al.*, 1997
	308	96.3	Showalter *et al.*, 1996
	1130	301	Felder *et al.*, 1995
(+)-CBD	842[b]	203	Bisogno *et al.*, 2001
R-(+)-WIN55,212	9.94[b]	16.2[b]	Rinaldi-Carmona *et al.*, 1994
	4.4[a,b]	1.2[a,b]	Hillard *et al.*, 1999
	1.89	0.28	Showalter *et al.*, 1996
	62.3	3.3	Felder *et al.*, 1995
	123	4.1	Shire *et al.*, 1996

CB_2-selective ligands in order of increasing CB_2/CB_1 selectivity

AM630	5152	31.2	Ross *et al.*, 1999a
JWH-133	677[b]	3.4	Huffman *et al.*, 1999
L-759633	1043	6.4	Ross *et al.*, 1999a
	15 850	20	Gareau *et al.*, 1996
L-759656	4888	11.8	Ross *et al.*, 1999a
	>20 000	19.4	Gareau *et al.*, 1996
HU-308	>10 000[b]	22.7	Hanus *et al.*, 1999
SR144528	437	0.60	Rinaldi-Carmona *et al.*, 1998
	305[b]	0.30[b]	Rinaldi-Carmona *et al.*, 1998
	>10 000	5.6	Ross *et al.*, 1999a

[a]With phenylmethylsulphonyl fluoride (PMSF).
[b]Binding to rat cannabinoid receptors on transfected cells or on brain (CB_1) or spleen tissue (CB_2).
[c]Binding to mouse spleen cannabinoid receptors.
[d]Species unspecified. All other data from experiments with human cannabinoid receptors.
CBD, cannabidiol; CBN, cannabinol; DMH, dimethylheptyl; THC, tetrahydrocannabinol.
See text for other definitions and figures for the structures of compounds.

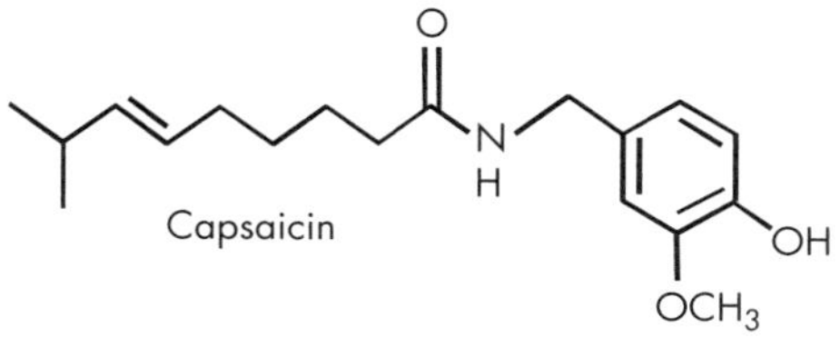

Figure 5.3 The structure of capsaicin.

There is firm evidence that as well as being a cannabinoid receptor agonist, anandamide shares the ability of capsaicin (Figure 5.3), a pungent constituent of hot chilli peppers, to activate vanilloid receptors (VR1) (Zygmunt *et al.*, 1999; Smart *et al.*, 2000). In contrast, neither 2-AG nor established non-eicosanoid CB$_1$ or CB$_2$ receptor agonists act on these receptors. Vanilloid receptors form Ca^{2+}-permeable ion channels that can be gated by acid pH and high temperature and their presence on a subset of primary afferent neurons suggests that they may well play a part in nociception. Interestingly, results from recent experiments with rat hippocampal slices suggest that, whereas 2-AG reduces paired-pulse depression of population spikes by acting through hippocampal CB$_1$ receptors, anandamide acts selectively on hippocampal vanilloid receptors to increase paired-pulse depression (Al-Hayani *et al.*, 2001). The potency and efficacy of anandamide at vanilloid receptors is rather low (Ross *et al.*, 2001), casting doubt on the possibility that it serves as an endogenous ligand for these receptors. It is possible, however, that metabolites of anandamide have such a role (see Pertwee and Ross, 2002; Ross *et al.*, 2002). Thus, for example, data obtained in experiments with guinea-pig isolated bronchus suggest that anandamide can be converted by lipoxygenase to metabolites that exhibit higher efficacy than their parent compound at vanilloid receptors (Craib *et al.*, 2001).

Anandamide and 2-AG probably both serve as neurotransmitters or neuromodulators. Thus, there is evidence that they can undergo depolarisation-induced release from neurons, in which they appear to be synthesised on demand, and that after their release they are rapidly removed from the extracellular space by a membrane transport process that has still to be fully characterised (Di Marzo *et al.*, 1998; Maccarrone *et al.*, 1998; Di Marzo, 1999; Piomelli *et al.*, 1999; Hillard and Jarrahian, 2000). Recent data also indicate that endocannabinoid molecules may function as retrograde synaptic messengers (see Pertwee and Ross, 2002 and Figure 5.4). Once it has been transported into the cell, anandamide is most probably hydrolysed to arachidonic acid and ethanolamine by the microsomal enzyme fatty acid amide hydrolase

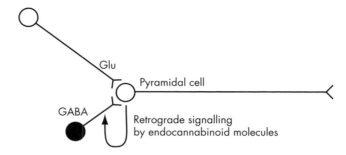

Figure 5.4 Schematic diagram illustrating endocannabinoid-mediated retrograde feedback inhibition in the hippocampus. Increases in intracellular calcium caused by strong depolarisation of postsynaptic hippocampal pyramidal cells rapidly trigger the biosynthesis and non-vesicular release from these cells of endocannabinoid molecules. These molecules are then thought to act through presynaptic CB$_1$ receptors to inhibit the presynaptic release of the inhibitory transmitter γ-aminobutyric acid (GABA) from hippocampal neurons, thereby augmenting synaptic transmission (depolarisation-induced suppression of inhibition) (Ohno-Shosaku et al., 2001; Wilson and Nicoll, 2001). Evidence also exists for endocannabinoid-mediated retrograde feedback inhibition of both glutamate (Glu) and GABA release in the cerebellum (Kreitzer and Regehr, 2001a,b; Maejima et al., 2001; Diana et al., 2002).

(FAAH) (Di Marzo et al., 1998; Maccarrone et al., 1998; Ueda et al., 2000) or converted to other metabolites by lipoxygenase or cyclooxygenase (see Pertwee and Ross, 2002). 2-AG can also be hydrolysed enzymically both by FAAH and by intracellular lipases (Di Marzo et al., 1998; Khanolkar and Makriyannis, 1999). Mechanisms underlying the production and fate of noladin ether have still to be identified.

The finding that anandamide and 2-AG undergo membrane transport and intracellular enzymic hydrolysis has prompted the development of inhibitors of these processes. The first uptake inhibitor to be developed was N-(4-hydroxyphenyl) arachidonylamide (AM404) (Figure 5.5 and Table 5.1). This has been shown not only to inhibit anandamide uptake by rat cultured cortical neurons (EC$_{50}$ = 1 μM) and astrocytes (EC$_{50}$ = 5 μM) (Beltramo et al., 1997) but also to increase plasma levels of anandamide in rats (Giuffrida et al., 2000) and to potentiate anandamide in certain in vitro and in vivo assays (Beltramo et al., 1997). AM404 also shares the ability of direct CB$_1$ receptor agonists to decrease locomotor activity in rats in an SR141716A-sensitive manner (González et al., 1999; Beltramo et al., 2000; Giuffrida et al., 2000).

However, it does not produce two other typical effects of CB$_1$ receptor agonists in rats: antinociception in the hot plate test and catalepsy (Beltramo et al., 2000). At concentrations at which it inhibits

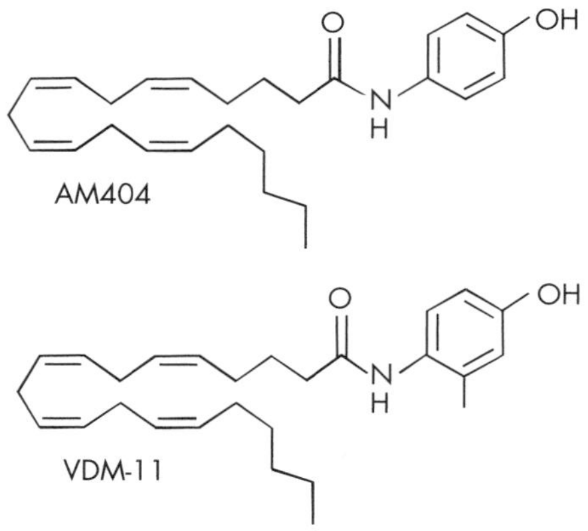

Figure 5.5 The structures of the endocannabinoid uptake inhibitors, AM404 and VDM-11.

the membrane transport of endocannabinoids, AM404 activates vanilloid VR1 receptors (Jerman *et al.*, 2000; Zygmunt *et al.*, 2000) and binds to CB$_1$ receptors (Khanolkar *et al.*, 1996). However, there are no reports as yet that AM404 behaves as a CB$_1$ receptor agonist or antagonist. VDM-11 (Figure 5.5), a structural analogue of AM404, is also an inhibitor of endocannabinoid membrane transport (De Petrocellis *et al.*, 2000). Like AM404, VDM-11 binds to CB$_1$ receptors at concentrations at which it inhibits membrane transport. However, it shows markedly less efficacy than AM404 as a vanilloid receptor agonist. Other arachidonic acid derivatives with the ability to inhibit anandamide membrane transport have been designed and synthesised by Piomelli *et al.* (1999) and by López-Rodríguez *et al.* (2001).

One compound frequently used to inhibit the enzymic hydrolysis of anandamide is the non-specific irreversible serine protease inhibitor, phenylmethylsulfonyl fluoride (PMSF) (see Pertwee, 1997). More recently developed inhibitors of anandamide metabolism include palmitylsulphonyl fluoride (AM374) and stearylsulphonyl fluoride (AM381) (Figure 5.6), both of which inhibit FAAH irreversibly. These two agents are markedly more potent than PMSF and are also much more potent as FAAH inhibitors than as CB$_1$ receptor ligands (Deutsch *et al.*, 1997). In line with its ability to inhibit FAAH, AM374 has been reported to potentiate the ability of anandamide both to inhibit evoked [³H]acetylcholine release in rat hippocampal slices (Gifford *et al.*, 1999) and to suppress rat operant lever pressing and open field locomotor activity (Cervone *et al.*, 1999). Certain members of a recently developed series

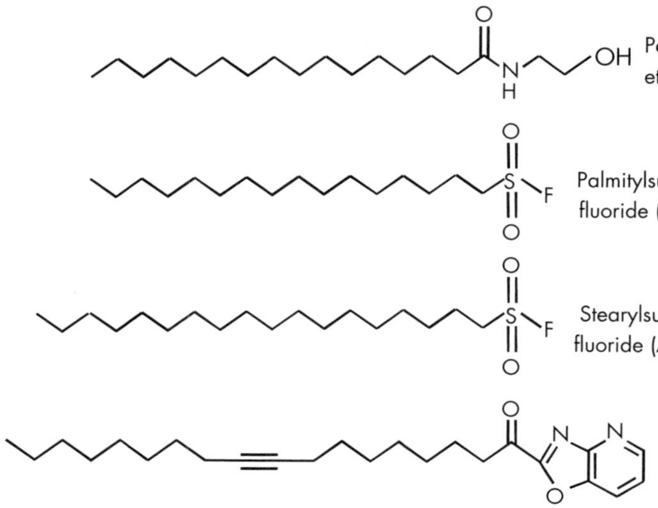

Figure 5.6 The structures of palmitoylethanolamide and of the FAAH inhibitors, AM374, AM381 and compound 59.

of α-keto bicyclic heterocycles with alkyl or phenylalkyl side-chains (e.g. compound 59 in Figure 5.6) are even more potent than AM374 and AM381 as FAAH inhibitors, showing inhibitory activity in the picomolar range (Boger *et al.*, 2000). These agents inhibit FAAH competitively and reversibly. Their ability to interact with cannabinoid receptors or to potentiate endocannabinoids has still to be reported.

There are several reports that endogenous substrates for FAAH such as linoleoylethanolamide, oleoylethanolamide and oleamide serve as reversible inhibitors of this enzyme (Desarnaud *et al.*, 1995; Maurelli *et al.*, 1995; Mechoulam *et al.*, 1997; Maccarone *et al.*, 1998). This has prompted the hypothesis that anandamide may be protected from enzymic hydrolysis by endogenously produced FAAH inhibitors in what has been termed an 'entourage' effect (Mechoulam *et al.*, 1998). A similar entourage effect may well extend to 2-AG which can be protected from the esterase action of FAAH by the endogenous fatty acid derivatives, 2-linoleylglycerol and 2-palmitylglycerol (Ben-Shabat *et al.*, 1998; Mechoulam *et al.*, 1998; Gallily *et al.*, 2000).

Other agonists for CB₁ and CB₂ receptors

Cannabinoid receptor agonists can be divided into four chemical groups that are often referred to as classical, non-classical, aminoalkylindole and eicosanoid (see Pertwee, 1999). Classical cannabinoids are tricyclic dibenzopyran derivatives, important examples including the psychotropic plant cannabinoids, (–)-Δ^9-THC, (–)-Δ^8-THC and cannabinol (Figure 5.7), and the synthetic cannabinoids, (–)-11-hydroxy-Δ^8-THC-dimethylheptyl (HU-210) and L-nantradol (CP50,556) (Figure 5.8). Pate (1999) has proposed that Δ^9-THC and other cannabinoids produced by cannabis are referred to as 'phytocannabinoids' in order to distinguish them from synthetic classical cannabinoids such as HU-210. Non-classical cannabinoids are bicyclic or tricyclic analogues of (–)-Δ^9-THC with no pyran ring, for example CP55,940 (Figure 5.8). This group of compounds was developed by a Pfizer research team (Johnson and Melvin, 1986). The aminoalkylindole group, developed by a Sterling Winthrop research team (Martin *et al.*, 1991; Pacheco *et al.*, 1991), contains compounds such as *R*-(+)-WIN55,212 (Figure 5.9) that are structurally quite different from classical or non-classical cannabinoids. In line with this structural difference is evidence that *R*-(+)-WIN55,212 binds differently to the CB_1 receptor than classical or non-classical cannabinoids, albeit it in a manner that still permits mutual displacement between *R*-(+)-WIN55,212 and non-aminoalkylindole cannabinoids at CB_1 binding sites (see Pertwee, 1999). The prototypic member of the eicosanoid group of cannabinoid receptor agonists is the endocannabinoid anandamide (see above).

(–)-Δ^9-THC undergoes significant binding to cannabinoid receptors at submicromolar concentrations, with similar affinities for CB_1

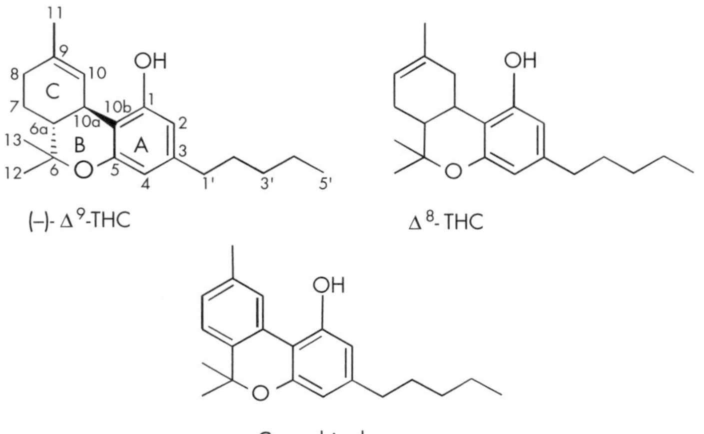

(–)-Δ^9-THC Δ^8-THC

Cannabinol

Figure 5.7 The structures of three phytocannabinoids: (–)-Δ^9-THC, Δ^8-THC and cannabinol.

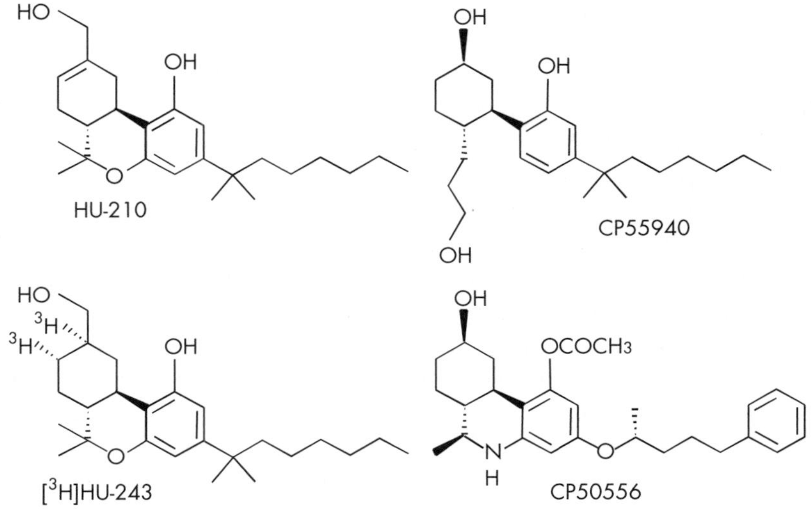

Figure 5.8 The structures of the synthetic classical cannabinoids, HU-210, HU-243 and L-nantradol (CP50,556) and of the non-classical cannabinoid, CP55,940.

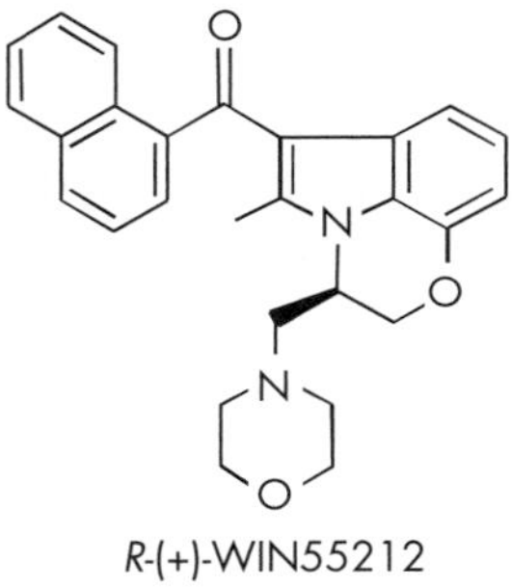

R-(+)-WIN55212

Figure 5.9 The structure of the aminoalkylindole cannabinoid receptor agonist, *R*-(+)-WIN55,212.

and CB_2 receptors (Table 5.1). It resembles anandamide in behaving as a partial agonist at CB_1 receptors (Gérard *et al.*, 1991; Breivogel *et al.*, 1998; Griffin *et al.*, 1998; Pertwee, 1999) and in exhibiting less CB_2 than CB_1 efficacy (Bayewitch *et al.*, 1996; Pertwee, 1999). In line with its classification as a CB_2 receptor partial agonist, (−)-Δ^9-THC shares the ability of anandamide to behave as an antagonist at CB_2 receptors under at least some experimental conditions (Bayewitch *et al.*, 1996) and can also attenuate responses mediated by CB_1 receptors (Sim *et al.*, 1996;

Griffin *et al.*, 1998; Shen and Thayer, 1999). As for (–)-Δ^8-THC, this resembles (–)-Δ^9-THC both in its affinities for CB_1 and CB_2 receptors (Table 5.1) and in its CB_1 receptor efficacy (Matsuda *et al.*, 1990; Gérard *et al.*, 1991). Another phytocannabinoid in the classical group that is known to bind to CB_1 and CB_2 receptors, albeit with less affinity than (–)-Δ^9-THC, is cannabinol (see Pertwee, 1999 and Table 5.1). At CB_1 receptors, this behaves as a partial agonist with even less efficacy than Δ^9-THC. However, at CB_2 receptors, it has been found to behave as an agonist in one bioassay system but as an inverse agonist in another, producing an effect opposite in direction to that of established CB_2 agonists. HU-210, CP55,940 and *R*-(+)-WIN55,212 all have high affinities for CB_1 and CB_2 receptors (Table 5.1) and exhibit relatively high efficacy at both these receptor types (see Pertwee, 1999). While HU-210 and CP55,940 bind more or less equally well to CB_1 and CB_2 receptors, *R*-(+)-WIN55,212 has slightly greater affinity for CB_2 than for CB_1 receptors. HU-210 is a particularly potent cannabinoid receptor agonist as it has even higher affinity than CP55,940 or *R*-(+)-WIN55,212 for cannabinoid receptors. Its pharmacological effects *in vivo* are also exceptionally long lasting. The enhanced affinity and efficacy shown by HU-210 at cannabinoid receptors can be attributed largely to the replacement of the pentyl side-chain of Δ^8-THC with a dimethylheptyl group. The same structural modification also markedly increases the affinity of cannabinol for CB_1 and CB_2 receptors (see dimethylheptyl cannabinol in Table 5.1). As for HU-210, these increases in affinity are not accompanied by any marked changes in relative affinity for CB_1 and CB_2 receptors. Less lipophilic than classical cannabinoids, ^{3}H-labelled CP55,940 and *R*-(+)-WIN55,212 are often used to characterise the binding properties of other cannabinoid receptor ligands and to map out the tissue distribution of CB_1 and CB_2 receptors. Because of its remarkably high affinity for CB_1 and CB_2 receptors, the structural analogue of HU-210, [^{3}H]HU-243 (Figure 5.8), has also been developed as a probe for these receptors. Typical K_d values for [^{3}H]CP55,940, [^{3}H]*R*-(+)-WIN55,212 and [^{3}H]HU-243 are 0.07–4 nM, 1.9–16.2 nM and 0.045 nM respectively at CB_1 receptors and 0.2–7.4 nM, 2.1–3.8 nM and 0.061 nM respectively at CB_2 receptors (see Pertwee, 1999).

Chirality of cannabinoids

Cannabinoid receptor agonists usually contain chiral centres, the resulting stereoisomers often exhibiting marked potency differences (see

Pertwee, 1997, 1999). Thus, classical and non-classical cannabinoids with the same absolute stereochemistry as $(-)$-Δ^9-THC at 6a and 10a (6aR, 10aR) show the greater activity at cannabinoid receptors, whilst R-$(+)$-WIN55,212 is much more potent than S-$(-)$-WIN55,212. Although anandamide does not contain any chiral centres, some of its synthetic analogues do. One example is methanandamide, the R-$(+)$-isomer of which has nine times greater affinity for CB_1 receptors than the S-$(-)$-isomer (Abadji et al., 1994).

Several cannabinoid receptor agonists with significant selectivity for CB_1 receptors have been developed (Table 5.1). The most important of these are all structurally related to anandamide (Figure 5.10). They include arachidonyl-2′-chloroethylamide (ACEA) and arachidonylcyclopropylamide (ACPA), which share the susceptibility of anandamide to enzymic hydrolysis (Hillard et al., 1999; Pertwee, 1999), and methanandamide, O-689 and O-1812, which are protected from enzymic hydrolysis by the presence of a methyl substituent on the 1′ or 2 carbon (Pertwee, 1999; Di Marzo et al., 2001). O-1812 has much higher affinity than anandamide for the CB_1 receptor (Table 5.1) and exhibits greater in vivo potency as a CB_1 receptor agonist.

Among the best CB_2-selective agonists to have been developed so far (Figure 5.11) are L-759633, L-759656, JWH-133 and HU-308

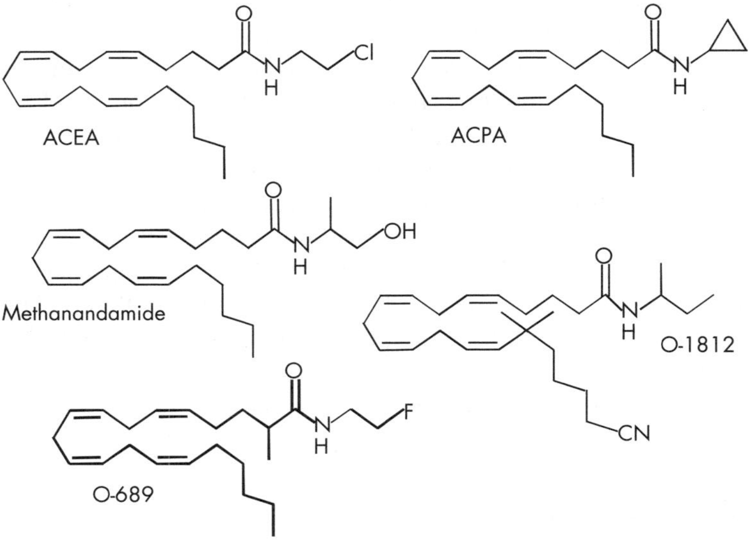

Figure 5.10 The structures of the CB_1-selective synthetic cannabinoid receptor agonists ACEA, ACPA, methanandamide, O-1812 and O-689.

(Hanus *et al.*, 1999; Ross *et al.*, 1999a; Pertwee, 2000), all of which bind to CB_2 receptors at concentrations in the low nanomolar range (Table 5.1). Each of these agonists is a structural analogue of THC in which the phenolic OH group has been replaced by a methoxy group or removed altogether. L-759633 and L-759656 have similar potencies and efficacies to CP55,940, as measured by inhibition of forskolin-stimulated cyclic AMP accumulation in Chinese hamster ovary (CHO) cells expressing recombinant CB_2 receptors (Ross *et al.*, 1999a). L-759656 (10 µM) is inactive at CB_1 receptors, while L-759633 behaves as a weak CB_1 receptor agonist with an EC_{50} of about 10 µM (Ross *et al.*, 1999a). Similarly, HU-308 and JWH-133 have been reported to be much more potent as inhibitors of forskolin-stimulated cyclic AMP production by CB_2- than by CB_1-transfected CHO cells (Hanus *et al.*, 1999; Pertwee, 2000).

One phytocannabinoid that does not appear to have any significant affinity for CB_1 or CB_2 receptors is (–)-cannabidiol (Figure 5.12 and Table 5.1). In contrast, its (+)-enantiomer does have significant affinity for both these receptor types, as do the (+)-enantiomers of 4'-dimethylheptyl-CBD and 7-OH-4'-dimethylheptyl-cannabidiol (Figure 5.12 and Table 5.1), each of which also has significantly greater affinity for CB_1 and CB_2 receptors than its corresponding (–)-enantiomer (Bisogno *et al.*, 2001). Thus, unlike classical cannabinoids such as THC (see above), it is the (+) (3*S*,4*S*) enantiomers of cannabidiol and its structural analogues that show the greater affinity for CB_1 and CB_2 receptors. Both (+)- and (–)-cannabidiol have also been reported to

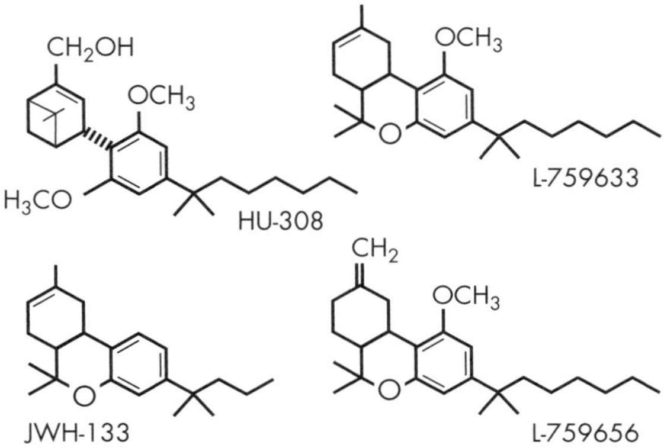

Figure 5.11 The structures of the CB_2-selective cannabinoid receptor agonists HU-308, L-759633, L-759656 and JWH-133.

behave as vanilloid receptor agonists (Bisogno *et al.*, 2001). They are equipotent with EC_{50} values in the low micromolar range. Also of interest are reports that (–)-cannabidiol can attenuate at least two types of response to CP55,940 or *R*-(+)-WIN55,212 that are thought to be CB_1 receptor mediated. Thus, it has been found, firstly, that at 10 μM, (–)-cannabidiol reduces the ability of CP55,940 to enhance $[^{35}S]GTP\gamma S$ binding to rat cerebellar membranes (Petitet *et al.*, 1998) and secondly, that at concentrations of 316 nM and above (–)-cannabidiol significantly attenuates *R*-(+)-WIN55,212-induced inhibition of electrically evoked contractions of the mouse isolated vas deferens (Craib *et al.*, 2002). It remains possible that (–)-cannabidiol was acting as a competitive antagonist of CP55,940 in the first of these studies as there is one report that its K_i for displacing $[^3H]CP55,940$ from CB_1 binding sites is 4.35 μM (Table 5.1). However, the potency it displayed as an antagonist in the second investigation ($K_B = 0.12$ μM) makes it unlikely that (–)-cannabidiol was attenuating responses of the vas deferens to *R*-(+)-WIN55,212 by competing with this agonist for CB_1 receptors.

CB_1 and CB_2 receptor antagonists

The discovery of cannabinoid receptors has also led to the development of selective CB_1 and CB_2 receptor antagonists, the most notable of

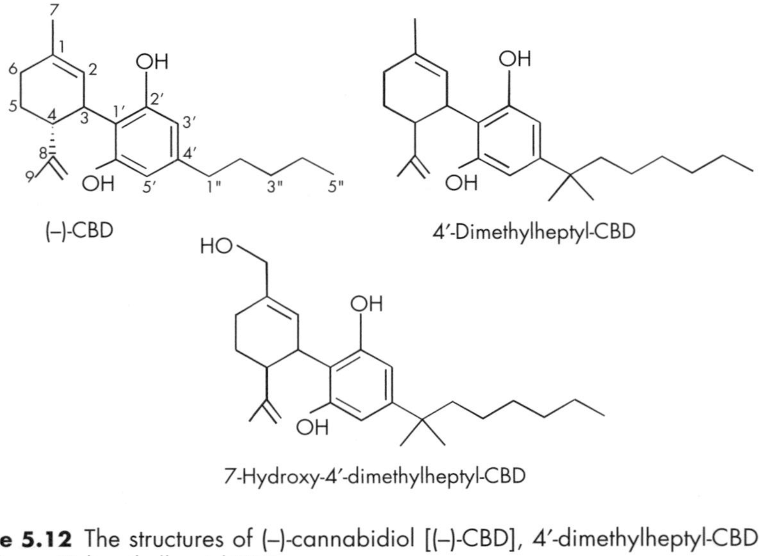

Figure 5.12 The structures of (–)-cannabidiol [(–)-CBD], 4′-dimethylheptyl-CBD and 7-hydroxy-4′-dimethylheptyl-CBD.

which are two diarylpyrazoles that were developed by Sanofi: the CB$_1$-selective SR141716A (Figures 5.13 and 5.14) and the CB$_2$-selective SR144528 (Figure 5.13) (Rinaldi-Carmona *et al.*, 1994, 1998; Pertwee, 1999). Although SR141716A is CB$_1$-selective it is not CB$_1$-specific (Table 5.1). Thus, whilst it is safe to assume that in tissues containing both CB$_1$ and CB$_2$ receptors, concentrations of SR141716 in the low or mid-nanomolar range will interact mainly with CB$_1$ receptors, this assumption should not be made for higher concentrations of SR141716A. Similarly, SR144528 is not CB$_2$-specific (Table 5.1) and there is evidence that at concentrations in the high nanomolar and micromolar range it can block

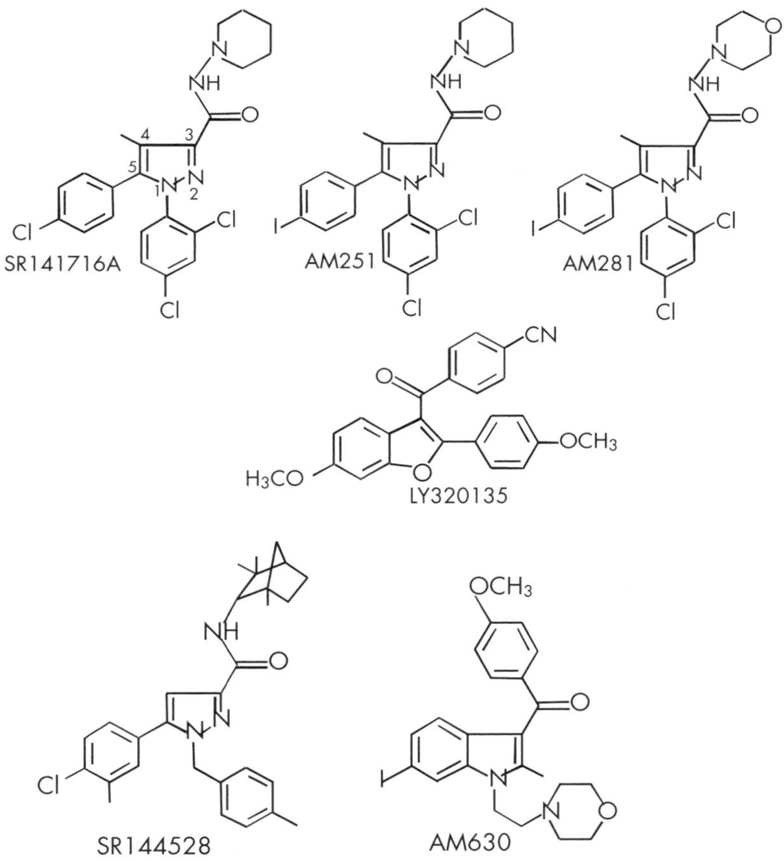

Figure 5.13 The structures of cannabinoid receptor antagonists/inverse agonists with CB$_1$ selectivity (SR141716A, AM251, AM281 and LY320135) or CB$_2$ selectivity (SR144528 and AM630).

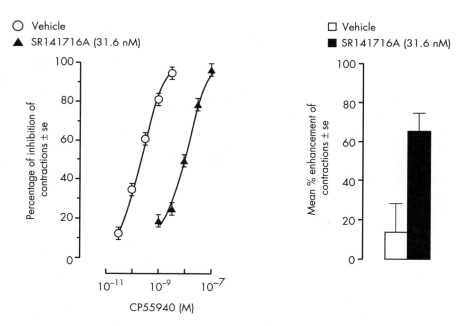

○ Vehicle
▲ SR141716A (31.6 nM)

□ Vehicle
■ SR141716A (31.6 nM)

CP55940 (M)

Figure 5.14 Data from experiments with the mouse isolated vas deferens, a tissue in which presynaptic CB_1 receptors mediate inhibition of electrically evoked contractions by suppressing the release of contractile transmitters (n = 6–8). The left panel shows that SR141716A behaves as a potent competitive, surmountable antagonist of the CB_1 agonist CP55,940 in this bioassay system (data from Pertwee *et al.*, 1995b). The right panel shows that when administered by itself, SR141716A enhances the amplitude of electrically evoked contractions, an indication of its inverse agonist activity and/or that there is on-going endocannabinoid release (Pertwee and Stevenson, unpublished).

CB_1 receptor-mediated effects (Rinaldi-Carmona *et al.*, 1998). There is also evidence that at 10 μM (but not 1 μM), SR141716A can inhibit potassium channels and L-type voltage-operated calcium channels (White and Hiley, 1998). By themselves, SR141716A and SR144528 can both produce effects in some bioassay systems that are opposite in direction from those elicited by CB_1 or CB_2 receptor agonists (Pertwee, 1999) (see also Figure 5.14).

These 'inverse' effects may sometimes be attributable to antagonism of endogenously produced endocannabinoid(s). However, there is also evidence that CB_1 and CB_2 receptors can exhibit signal transduction activity (constitutive activity) in the absence of endogenous or exogenous agonists and that SR141716A and SR144528 can reduce the constitutive activity of these signal transduction pathways, thereby acting as 'inverse agonists' rather than as 'silent' or 'neutral' antagonists (Bouaboula *et al.*, 1997; MacLennan *et al.*, 1998; Pan *et al.*, 1998; Rinaldi-Carmona *et al.*, 1998; Portier *et al.*, 1999; Ross *et al.*, 1999a; Coutts *et al.*, 2000; Sim-Selley *et al.*, 2001). In some investigations, SR141716A has proved to be more potent in blocking responses to CB$_1$ receptor agonists than in producing inverse cannabimimetic effect by itself (Gessa *et al.*, 1997, 1998a; Schlicker *et al.*, 1997; Acquas *et al.*, 2000; Sim-Selley *et al.*, 2001). Possibly SR141716A binds to two sites on the CB$_1$ receptor, the agonist binding site for which it has high affinity and another site for which it has lower affinity, and that it is the lower affinity site that is responsible for the inverse agonist properties of SR141716A (Sim-Selley *et al.*, 2001).

Two other diarylpyrazoles capable of blocking CB$_1$ receptor-mediated effects are AM251 and AM281 (Figure 5.13) (Gifford *et al.*, 1997; Al-Hayani and Davies, 2000; Cosenza *et al.*, 2000; Izzo *et al.*, 2000; Al-Hayani *et al.*, 2001; Huang *et al.*, 2001; Maejima *et al.*, 2001; Simoneau *et al.*, 2001; Wilson and Nicoll, 2001). Like SR141716A, AM281 binds much more readily to CB$_1$ than CB$_2$ receptors (Table 5.1). It also shares the ability of SR141716A to behave as an inverse agonist when administered alone (Gifford *et al.*, 1997; Cosenza *et al.*, 2000; Izzo *et al.*, 2000). [^{3}H]SR141716A (CB$_1$ K_d = 0.19–1.24 nM) has been synthesised for use as a CB$_1$-selective probe. So too have the ^{123}I-labelled analogues of AM251 (CB$_1$ K_d = 0.23–0.62 nM) (Lan *et al.*, 1996; Gatley *et al.*, 1997) and AM281 (Gatley *et al.*, 1998) and the ^{18}F-labelled analogue of SR141716A (SR144385) (Barth, 1998), all of which were developed as potential probes for single photon emission computed tomography (SPECT) or positron emission tomography (PET) experiments. Results obtained from animal experiments with [^{123}I]AM281 have been particularly promising (Gatley *et al.*, 1998).

Other notable cannabinoid receptor antagonists/inverse agonists are the CB$_1$-selective substituted benzofuran LY320135 and the CB$_2$-selective aminoalkylindole 6-iodopravadoline (AM630) (Figure 5.13 and Table 5.1). LY320135, developed by Eli Lilly, shares the ability of SR141716A not only to block effects of CB$_1$ receptor agonists (Felder *et al.*, 1998; Coruzzi *et al.*, 1999; Holland *et al.*, 1999; Molderings *et al.*, 1999; Christopoulos *et al.*, 2001) but also to behave as an inverse agonist (Felder *et al.*, 1998; Christopoulos *et al.*, 2001). It has less affinity than SR141716A for CB$_1$ receptors and, at concentrations in the low micromolar range, also binds to muscarinic and 5-HT$_2$ receptors (Felder *et al.*, 1998). The ability of AM630 to behave as a cannabinoid receptor antagonist was first noted in experiments with the mouse isolated vas deferens, which yielded dissociation constant (K_B) values for AM630 against Δ^9-THC and CP55,940 of 14.0 and 17.3 nM respectively (Pertwee *et al.*, 1995a). More recently, experiments with human CB_2-transfected CHO cell preparations showed that AM630 could potently reverse CP55,940-induced inhibition of forskolin-stimulated cyclic AMP production (EC_{50} = 128.6 nM) and that when administered by itself, it could enhance forskolin-stimulated cyclic AMP production (EC_{50} = 230.4 nM) and inhibit [^{35}S]GTPγS binding (EC_{50} = 76.6 nM) (Ross *et al.*, 1999a). This inverse agonist activity at CB_2 receptors appears to be less than that of SR144528 (Ross *et al.*, 1999b). As for the ability of AM630 to interact with CB_1 receptors, there are some reports that it behaves as a low-affinity partial agonist, exhibiting mixed agonist–antagonist properties (Pertwee *et al.*, 1996; Hosohata *et al.*, 1997a,b; Pertwee, 1999; Ross *et al.*, 1999a). However, there is also one report that it can behave as a low-potency inverse agonist at CB_1 receptors (Landsman *et al.*, 1998).

Other cannabinoid receptor ligands

Two of these that merit special mention are the classical cannabinoids, 6′-azidohex-2′-yne-Δ^8-THC (O-1184) and 6′-azidohex-*cis*-2′-ene-Δ^8-THC (O-1238) (Figure 5.15 and Table 5.1). Thus, these ligands are

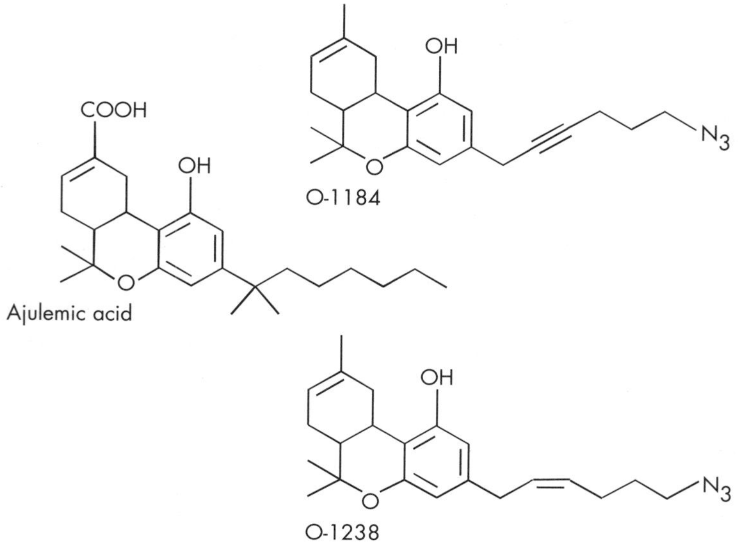

Figure 5.15 The structures of ajulemic acid, O-1184 and O-1238.

close to being silent cannabinoid receptor antagonists, albeit at both CB_1 and CB_2 receptors. In addition to a terminal N_3 group, the alkyl side-chain of O-1184 contains a carbon–carbon triple bond, and this structural modification reduces the CB_1 and CB_2 efficacy of O-1184 but not its CB_1 or CB_2 affinity. As a result, this cannabinoid behaves as a high-affinity low-efficacy agonist at CB_1 receptors and as a high-affinity low-efficacy inverse agonist at CB_2 receptors (Ross *et al.*, 1998, 1999b). O-1238, in which the carbon–carbon triple bond of O-1184 is replaced by a carbon–carbon double bond, has higher efficacy than O-1184 at CB_1 receptors and behaves as a high-affinity low-efficacy partial agonist at CB_2 receptors (Ross *et al.*, 1999b).

Other cannabinoid receptors?

Data obtained from experiments with the endogenous fatty acid amide palmitoylethanolamide (Figure 5.6) have prompted Calignano *et al.* (1998, 2001) to postulate the existence of a 'CB$_2$-like' receptor. They found that even though palmitoylethanolamide lacks significant affinity for CB_2 (or CB_1) receptors (Devane *et al.*, 1992; Felder *et al.*, 1993; Showalter *et al.*, 1996; Sheskin *et al.*, 1997; Lambert *et al.*, 1999), it could induce antinociceptive effects that are attenuated by the CB$_2$-selective antagonist SR144528, although not by the CB$_1$-selective antagonist SR141716A. These results were obtained in the mouse formalin paw test after intraplantar injection of palmitoylethanolamide and in the mouse abdominal stretch test after intraperitoneal injection of this compound. In the same bioassays, anandamide was found to be antagonised by SR141716A but not SR144528, and palmitoylethanolamide and anandamide were found to act synergistically (Calignano *et al.*, 1998, 2001). The proposed 'CB$_2$-like' receptor is unlikely to be a vanilloid receptor as palmitoylethanolamide does not share the ability of anandamide or of the vanilloid receptor antagonist capsazepine to suppress paw-licking behaviour when coadministered with capsaicin into mouse hind-paw (Calignano *et al.*, 2001). Evidence also exists for the presence of CB$_2$-like receptors in the mouse vas deferens (Griffin *et al.*, 1997).

Another compound that may induce anti-inflammatory/analgesic effects by acting through CB_2 or CB$_2$-like receptors is 1′,1′-dimethyl-heptyl-Δ^8-THC-11-oic acid (ajulemic acid or CT-3) (Figure 5.15). As detailed elsewhere (Pertwee, 2001), this agent has been reported to reduce signs of inflammation in rodent models after both single and repeated oral administration at doses as low as 0.01 or 0.1 mg/kg

(Burstein *et al.*, 1992; Zurier *et al.*, 1998). It has also been found to be active as an antinociceptive agent in the mouse hot plate test, mouse formalin paw test and phenylbenzoquinone abdominal stretch test (Burstein *et al.*, 1992, 1998). Whether any of the *in vitro* or *in vivo* effects of ajulemic acid can be antagonised by SR144528 (or SR141716A) has yet to be established. Even so, it has been proposed that at least some of these effects are mediated by CB_2 (or CB_2-like) receptors rather than CB_1 receptors. This hypothesis has been prompted by evidence from *in vitro* experiments that ajulemic acid is more potent as an agonist for CB_2 receptors than for CB_1 receptors (Rhee *et al.*, 1997) (even though it does have 5 times more affinity for CB_1 receptors than for CB_2 receptors (Table 5.1)). Moreover, ajulemic acid has been found not to induce any sign of CB_1 receptor agonism (catalepsy) in mice at anti-inflammatory/antinociceptive doses (Burstein *et al.*, 1992; Burstein, 1999). It is also noteworthy that whilst ajulemic acid shows activity in the mouse hot plate test, palmitoylethanolamide (Calignano *et al.*, 2001) and the CB_2-selective agonist HU-308 (Hanus *et al.*, 1999) do not. Another possibility is that ajulemic acid produces its anti-inflammatory effects by suppressing eicosanoid synthesis in inflamed tissue. Thus, Burstein *et al.* (1992) and Zurier *et al.* (1998) have reported that ajulemic acid is an inhibitor of cyclooxygenase-2 (COX-2), an enzyme that seems to be activated during inflammation and to catalyse the production of inflammatory eicosanoids. Zurier *et al.* (1998) also found that ajulemic acid can inhibit COX-2 at concentrations having no effect on COX-1 activity, raising the possibility that it may be able to relieve inflammation without producing unwanted effects such as gastrointestinal and kidney toxicity that limit the clinical usefulness of less selective non-steroidal anti-inflammatory agents (Burstein *et al.*, 1998; Burstein, 1999).

Recently, experiments with brain tissue from CB_1 knockout mice ($CB_1^{-/-}$ mice) in which the measured response was cannabinoid-induced activation of $[^{35}S]GTP\gamma S$ binding, have provided evidence for the existence of a novel G protein-coupled, SR141716A-insensitive, non-CB_1, non-CB_2 cannabinoid receptor (Di Marzo *et al.*, 2000; Breivogel *et al.*, 2001). Data from these experiments suggest that this putative receptor can be activated by anandamide and *R*-(+)-WIN55,212 but not by three other established CB_1/CB_2 agonists, Δ^9-THC, HU-210 and CP55,940. Since it was also found that membranes from $CB_1^{-/-}$ cerebral cortex, hippocampus and brainstem contained specific binding sites for $[^3H]R$-(+)-WIN55,212 but not for $[^3H]CP55,940$ (Breivogel *et al.*, 2001), it is unlikely that the proposed new cannabinoid receptor is a CB_2 receptor.

Nor is it likely to be a vanilloid receptor, as this receptor type is not G protein coupled and is not activated by R-(+)-WIN55,212 (Zygmunt *et al.*, 1999). The results obtained by Breivogel *et al.* (2001) in the [^{35}S]GTPγS binding assay point to the presence of the novel cannabinoid receptor in $CB_1^{-/-}$ cerebral cortex, midbrain, hippocampus, diencephalon and brainstem and to its absence from $CB_1^{-/-}$ caudate-putamen/ globus pallidus and cerebellum, two brain areas that are well-populated with CB_1 receptors in wild-type ($CB_1^{+/+}$) animals. Evidence that there are R-(+)-WIN55,212-sensitive receptors in $CB_1^{-/-}$ mouse brain has also been obtained by Hájos *et al.* (2001) from electrophysiological experiments with hippocampal slices. The results from this investigation suggest that these are presynaptic neuronal non-CB_1 cannabinoid receptors that mediate inhibition of evoked glutamate release when activated by R-(+)-WIN55,212.

Finally, Kunos and his colleagues have obtained evidence for the presence of SR141716A-sensitive non-CB_1, non-CB_2 cannabinoid receptors on mesenteric arteries (Járai *et al.*, 1999; Wagner *et al.*, 1999). They found that anandamide, methanandamide and the cannabidiol analogues, abnormal cannabidiol and O-1602 (Figure 5.16) could all induce concentration-related relaxations of rat or mouse precontracted mesenteric arteries. It is unlikely that this effect was mediated by CB_1 or CB_2 receptors as Δ^9-THC, HU-210, R-(+)-WIN55,212 and 2-arachidonoyl glycerol were not vasorelaxant in these experiments and as abnormal cannabidiol and O-1602 lack significant affinity for rat brain CB_1 receptors (Járai *et al.*, 1999).

Moreover, anandamide, methanandamide and abnormal cannabidiol also evoke relaxant responses in precontracted mesenteric arteries obtained from $CB_1^{-/-}$ knockout mice or from $CB_1^{-/-}/CB_2^{-/-}$ double-knockout mice (Járai *et al.*, 1999). It is also unlikely that the proposed new receptors are vanilloid receptors because the relaxant effect of abnormal cannabidiol in rat precontracted mesenteric arteries was unaffected by a concentration of capsazepine (5 µM) that did attenuate the

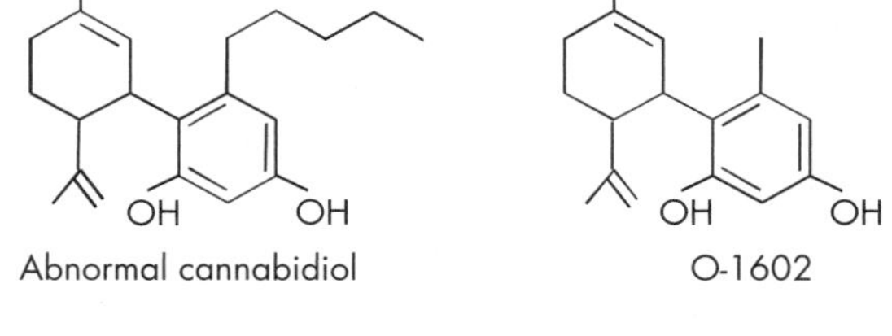

Figure 5.16 The structures of abnormal cannabidiol and O-1602.

relaxant effect of capsaicin (Járai *et al.*, 1999). The relaxant effects of anandamide, abnormal cannabidiol or O-1602 on precontracted mesenteric arteries from rats or from $CB_1^{+/+}$ or $CB_1^{-/-}$ mice were attenuated by SR141716A at 0.5, 1 or 5 µM and by (–)-cannabidiol at 10 µM (Járai *et al.*, 1999; Wagner *et al.*, 1999). Cannabidiol exhibited some degree of selectivity as an antagonist in these experiments as the same concentration of this non-psychotropic phytocannabinoid did not attenuate vasorelaxant responses to acetylcholine, bradykinin or sodium nitroprusside (Járai *et al.*, 1999). The relaxant effects of abnormal cannabidiol and O-1602 in rat precontracted mesenteric arteries seem to be largely endothelium dependent, as is the ability of SR141716A to attenuate the vasorelaxant effect of anandamide (Járai *et al.*, 1999). Hence, the SR141716A-sensitive, non-CB_1, non-CB_2 cannabinoid receptors proposed by Kunos and his colleagues are most probably present on the endothelium and absent from mesenteric smooth muscle. Interestingly, anandamide-induced relaxation is detectable in endothelium-denuded as well as in endothelium-intact precontracted rat mesenteric arteries (Wagner *et al.*, 1999; Kunos *et al.*, 2000), pointing to the existence of a second mechanism by which this endocannabinoid can relax precontracted mesenteric arteries.

Conclusions

Although considerable progress has been made in the pharmacological and physiological characterisation of cannabinoid receptors and their ligands, a number of important questions remain to be addressed. In particular, it will be important:

- to develop cannabinoid receptor antagonists that lack inverse agonist properties
- to investigate the possibility of developing CB_1 receptor agonists that do not cross the blood–brain barrier but retain the ability to relieve pain by activating CB_1 receptors located outside the central nervous system, for example on the peripheral terminals of primary afferent sensory neurons
- to establish the physiological and pathophysiological importance and the pharmacological properties both of CB_2 receptors and of novel cannabinoid receptor types that have already been proposed or that remain to be discovered
- to develop selective and potent agonists and antagonists for any novel cannabinoid receptor type that proves to exist

- to seek out pharmacological actions of cannabinoids that are not mediated by known or unknown cannabinoid receptors
- to characterise the pharmacological properties of phytocannabinoids singly and in combination, focusing particularly on those cannabinoids or combinations that have been subjected to little or no investigation in the past
- to gain a more complete understanding of the physiological/pathophysiological roles and pharmacological properties of all known endocannabinoids and their metabolites and to look for additional endocannabinoids
- to explore the therapeutic potential of inhibitors of endocannabinoid membrane transport or metabolism (indirect cannabinoid receptor agonists).

With regard to the therapeutic potential of indirect cannabinoid receptor agonists, recent data from animal experiments suggest that such agents may have applications in the clinic, for example for the relief of inflammatory pain or the management of the spasticity and pain of multiple sclerosis. Some of these data come from experiments performed with Biozzi ABH mice with chronic relapsing experimental allergic encephalomyelitis (CREAE), induced by injecting the animals subcutaneously with an emulsion of mouse spinal cord homogenate in Freund's complete adjuvant (Baker *et al.*, 2001). These experiments showed that inhibitors of endocannabinoid membrane transport (AM404) or of fatty acid amide hydrolase (AM374) share the ability of direct cannabinoid receptor agonists to ameliorate spasticity in CREAE mice and that spastic CREAE mice have elevated concentrations of the endocannabinoids, anandamide and 2-arachidonoyl glycerol, in their brains and spinal cords. As to inflammatory pain, there is evidence from rat experiments that peripheral inflammatory pain triggers increased release of anandamide in at least one area of the brain at which CB_1 receptors can mediate signs of analgesia, the periaqueductal grey area of the midbrain (Walker *et al.*, 1999).

References

Abadji V, Lin S, Taha G *et al.* (1994). (R)-methanandamide: a chiral novel anandamide possessing higher potency and metabolic stability. *J Med Chem* 37: 1889–1893.

Acquas E, Pisanu A, Marrocu P *et al.* (2000). Cannabinoid CB_1 receptor agonists increase rat cortical and hippocampal acetylcholine release in vivo. *Eur J Pharmacol* 401: 179–185.

Acquas E, Pisanu A, Marrocu P *et al.* (2001). Δ^9-Tetrahydrocannabinol enhances cortical and hippocampal acetylcholine release in vivo: a microdialysis study. *Eur J Pharmacol* 419: 155–161.

Al-Hayani A, Davies S N (2000). Cannabinoid receptor mediated inhibition of excitatory synaptic transmission in the rat hippocampal slice is developmentally regulated. *Br J Pharmacol* 131: 663–665.

Al-Hayani A, Wease K N, Ross R A *et al.* (2001). The endogenous cannabinoid anandamide activates vanilloid receptors in the rat hippocampal slice. *Neuropharmacology* 41: 1000–1005.

Baker D, Pryce G, Croxford J L *et al.* (2001). Endocannabinoids control spasticity in a multiple sclerosis model. *FASEB J* 15: 300–302.

Barth F (1998). Cannabinoid receptor agonists and antagonists. *Exp Opin Ther Patents* 8: 301–313.

Bayewitch M, Avidor-Reiss T, Levy R *et al.* (1995). The peripheral cannabinoid receptor: adenylate cyclase inhibition and G protein coupling. *FEBS Lett* 375: 143–147.

Bayewitch M, Rhee M-H, Avidor-Reiss T *et al.* (1996). (–)-Δ^9-tetrahydrocannabinol antagonizes the peripheral cannabinoid receptor-mediated inhibition of adenylyl cyclase. *J Biol Chem* 271: 9902–9905.

Beltramo M, Stella N, Calignano A *et al.* (1997). Functional role of high-affinity anandamide transport, as revealed by selective inhibition. *Science* 277: 1094–1097.

Beltramo M, Rodríguez de Fonseca F, Navarro M *et al.* (2000). Reversal of dopamine D_2 receptor responses by an anandamide transport inhibitor. *J Neurosci* 20: 3401–3407.

Ben-Shabat S, Fride E, Sheskin T *et al.* (1998). An entourage effect: inactive endogenous fatty acid glycerol esters enhance 2-arachidonoyl-glycerol cannabinoid activity. *Eur J Pharmacol* 353: 23–31.

Bisogno T, Hanus L, De Petrocellis L *et al.* (2001). Molecular targets for cannabidiol and its synthetic analogues: effect on vanilloid VR1 receptors and on the cellular uptake and enzymatic hydrolysis of anandamide. *Br J Pharmacol* 134: 845–852.

Boger D L, Sato H, Lerner A E *et al.* (2000). Exceptionally potent inhibitors of fatty acid amide hydrolase: the enzyme responsible for degradation of endogenous oleamide and anandamide. *Proc Natl Acad Sci USA* 97: 5044–5049.

Bouaboula M, Perrachon S, Milligan L *et al.* (1997). A selective inverse agonist for central cannabinoid receptor inhibits mitogen-activated protein kinase activation stimulated by insulin or insulin-like growth factor 1. Evidence for a new model of receptor/ligand interactions. *J Biol Chem* 272: 22330–22339.

Breivogel C S, Selley D E, Childers S R (1998). Cannabinoid receptor agonist efficacy for stimulating [^{35}S]GTPγS binding to rat cerebellar membranes correlates with agonist-induced decreases in GDP affinity. *J Biol Chem* 273: 16865–16873.

Breivogel C S, Griffin G, Di Marzo V *et al.* (2001). Evidence for a new G protein-coupled cannabinoid receptor in mouse brain. *Mol Pharmacol* 60: 155–163.

Buckley N E, McCoy K L, Mezey É *et al.* (2000). Immunomodulation by cannabinoids is absent in mice deficient for the cannabinoid CB_2 receptor. *Eur J Pharmacol* 396: 141–149.

Burstein S H (1999). The cannabinoid acids: nonpsychoactive derivatives with therapeutic potential. *Pharmacol Ther* 82: 87–96.

Burstein S H, Audette C A, Breuer A *et al.* (1992). Synthetic nonpsychotropic cannabinoids with potent antiinflammatory, analgesic, and leukocyte antiadhesion activities. *J Med Chem* 35: 3135–3141.

Burstein S H, Friderichs E, Kögel B *et al.* (1998). Analgesic effects of 1′,1′dimethyl-heptyl-Δ^8-THC-11-oic acid (CT3) in mice. *Life Sci* 63: 161–168.

Busch-Petersen J, Hill W A, Fan P *et al.* (1996). Unsaturated side chain beta-11-hydroxyhexahydrocannabinol analogs. *J Med Chem* 39: 3790–3796.

Cabral G A (2001). Marijuana and cannabinoids: effects on infections, immunity, and AIDS. *J Cannabis Ther* 1: 61–85.

Calignano A, La Rana G, Giuffrida A *et al.* (1998). Control of pain initiation by endogenous cannabinoids. *Nature* 394: 277–281.

Calignano A, La Rana G, Piomelli D (2001). Antinociceptive activity of the endogenous fatty acid amide, palmitylethanolamide. *Eur J Pharmacol* 419: 191–198.

Cervone K, Keene A, Lin S *et al.* (1999). Behavioral investigation of the interactions between amidase inhibitors and the cannabinoid agonist anandamide. *Proc Soc Neurosci* 25: 2077.

Chakrabarti A, Onaivi E S, Chaudhuri G (1995). Cloning and sequencing of a cDNA encoding the mouse brain-type cannabinoid receptor protein. *DNA Sequence* 5: 385–388.

Cheer J F, Marsden C A, Kendall D A *et al.* (2000). Lack of response suppression follows repeated ventral tegmental cannabinoid administration: an *in vitro* electrophysiological study. *Neuroscience* 99: 661–667.

Chen J, Paredes W, Lowinson J H *et al.* (1990a). Δ^9-Tetrahydrocannabinol enhances presynaptic dopamine efflux in medial prefrontal cortex. *Eur J Pharmacol* 190: 259–262.

Chen J, Paredes W, Li J *et al.* (1990b). Δ^9-Tetrahydrocannabinol produces naloxone-blockable enhancement of presynaptic basal dopamine efflux in nucleus accumbens of conscious, freely-moving rats as measured by intracerebral microdialysis. *Psychopharmacology* 102: 156–162.

Chen J, Paredes W, Lowinson J H *et al.* (1991). Strain-specific facilitation of dopamine efflux by Δ^9-tetrahydrocannabinol in the nucleus accumbens of rat: an *in vivo* microdialysis study. *Neurosci Lett* 129: 136–140.

Christopoulos A, Coles P, Lay L *et al.* (2001). Pharmacological analysis of cannabinoid receptor activity in the rat vas deferens. *Br J Pharmacol* 132: 1281–1291.

Coruzzi G, Adami M, Coppelli G *et al.* (1999). Inhibitory effect of the cannabinoid receptor agonist WIN 55,212-2 on pentagastrin-induced gastric acid secretion in the anaesthetized rat. *Naunyn-Schmiedeberg's Arch Pharmacol* 360: 715–718.

Cosenza M, Gifford A N, Gatley S J *et al.* (2000). Locomotor activity and occupancy of brain cannabinoid CB1 receptors by the antagonist/inverse agonist AM281. *Synapse* 38: 477–482.

Coutts A A, Brewster N, Ingram T *et al.* (2000). Comparison of novel cannabinoid partial agonists and SR141716A in the guinea-pig small intestine. *Br J Pharmacol* 129: 645–652.

Craib S J, Ellington H C, Pertwee R G *et al.* (2001). A possible role of lipoxygenase in the activation of vanilloid receptors by anandamide in the guinea-pig bronchus. *Br J Pharmacol* 134: 30–37.

Craib S J, Thomas A, Ross R A *et al.* (2002). Cannabidiol attenuates responses of the mouse isolated vas deferens to WIN55212-2 and noradrenaline. *Br J Pharmacol* 136: 53.

De Petrocellis L, Bisogno T, Davis J B *et al.* (2000). Overlap between the ligand recognition properties of the anandamide transporter and the VR1 vanilloid receptor: inhibitors of anandamide uptake with negligible capsaicin-like activity. *FEBS Lett* 483: 52–56.

Desarnaud F, Cadas H, Piomelli D (1995). Anandamide amidohydrolase activity in rat brain microsomes. Identification and partial characterization. *J Biol Chem* 270: 6030–6035.

Deutsch D G, Lin S, Hill W A G *et al.* (1997). Fatty acid sulfonyl fluorides inhibit anandamide metabolism and bind to the cannabinoid receptor. *Biochem Biophys Res Commun* 231: 217–221.

Devane W A, Hanus L, Breuer A *et al.* (1992). Isolation and structure of a brain constituent that binds to the cannabinoid receptor. *Science* 258: 1946–1949.

Diana M A, Levenes C, Mackie K *et al.* (2002). Short-term retrograde inhibition of GABAergic synaptic currents in rat Purkinje cells is mediated by endogenous cannabinoids. *J Neurosci* 22: 200–208.

Di Marzo V (1999). Biosynthesis and inactivation of endocannabinoids: relevance to their proposed role as neuromodulators. *Life Sci* 65: 645–655.

Di Marzo V, Melck D, Bisogno T *et al.* (1998). Endocannabinoids: endogenous cannabinoid receptor ligands with neuromodulatory action. *Trends Neurosci* 21: 521–528.

Di Marzo V, Breivogel C S, Tao Q *et al.* (2000). Levels, metabolism, and pharmacological activity of anandamide in CB_1 cannabinoid receptor knockout mice: evidence for non-CB_1, non-CB_2 receptor-mediated actions of anandamide in mouse brain. *J Neurochem* 75: 2434–2444.

Di Marzo V, Bisogno T, De Petrocellis L *et al.* (2001). Highly selective CB_1 cannabinoid receptor ligands and novel CB_1/VR1 vanilloid receptor 'hybrid' ligands. *Biochem Biophys Res Commun* 281: 444–451.

Felder C C, Briley E M, Axelrod J *et al.* (1993). Anandamide, an endogenous cannabimimetic eicosanoid, binds to the cloned human cannabinoid receptor and stimulates receptor-mediated signal transduction. *Proc Natl Acad Sci USA* 90: 7656–7660.

Felder C C, Joyce K E, Briley E M *et al.* (1995). Comparison of the pharmacology and signal transduction of the human cannabinoid CB_1 and CB_2 receptors. *Mol Pharmacol* 48: 443–450.

Felder C C, Joyce K E, Briley E M *et al.* (1998). LY320135, a novel cannabinoid CB1 receptor antagonist, unmasks coupling of the CB1 receptor to stimulation of cAMP accumulation. *J Pharmacol Exp Ther* 284: 291–297.

French E D (1997). Δ^9-Tetrahydrocannabinol excites rat VTA dopamine neurons through activation of cannabinoid CB1 but not opioid receptors. *Neurosci Lett* 226: 159–162.

French E D, Dillon K, Wu X (1997). Cannabinoids excite dopamine neurons in the ventral tegmentum and substantia nigra. *Neuroreport* 8: 649–652.

Gallily R, Breuer A, Mechoulam R (2000). 2-Arachidonylglycerol, an endogenous cannabinoid, inhibits tumor necrosis factor-α production in murine macrophages, and in mice. *Eur J Pharmacol* 406: R5–R7.

Gareau Y, Dufresne C, Gallant M *et al.* (1996). Structure activity relationships of tetrahydrocannabinol analogues on human cannabinoid receptors. *Bioorg Med Chem Lett* 6: 189–194.

Gatley S J, Lan R, Pyatt B *et al.* (1997). Binding of the non-classical cannabinoid CP 55,940, and the diarylpyrazole AM251 to rodent brain cannabinoid receptors. *Life Sci* 61: PL191–197.

Gatley S J, Lan R, Volkow N D *et al.* (1998). Imaging the brain marijuana receptor: development of a radioligand that binds to cannabinoid CB1 receptors in vivo. *J Neurochem* 70: 417–423.

Gérard C, Mollereau C, Vassart G *et al.* (1990). Nucleotide sequence of a human cannabinoid receptor cDNA. *Nucleic Acids Res* 18: 7142.

Gérard C M, Mollereau C, Vassart G *et al.* (1991). Molecular cloning of a human cannabinoid receptor which is also expressed in testis. *Biochem J* 279: 129–134.

Gessa G L, Mascia M S, Casu M A *et al.* (1997). Inhibition of hippocampal acetylcholine release by cannabinoids: reversal by SR141716A. *Eur J Pharmacol* 327: R1–R2.

Gessa G L, Casu M A, Carta G *et al.* (1998a). Cannabinoids decrease acetylcholine release in the medial-prefrontal cortex and hippocampus, reversal by SR 141716A. *Eur J Pharmacol* 355: 119–124.

Gessa G L, Melis M, Muntoni A *et al.* (1998b). Cannabinoids activate mesolimbic dopamine neurons by an action on cannabinoid CB_1 receptors. *Eur J Pharmacol* 341: 39–44.

Gifford A N, Tang Y, Gatley S J *et al.* (1997). Effect of the cannabinoid receptor SPECT agent, AM 281, on hippocampal acetylcholine release from rat brain slices. *Neurosci Lett* 238: 84–86.

Gifford A N, Bruneus M, Lin S *et al.* (1999). Potentiation of the action of anandamide on hippocampal slices by the fatty acid amide hydrolase inhibitor, palmitylsulphonyl fluoride (AM 374). *Eur J Pharmacol* 383: 9–14.

Giuffrida A, Rodríguez de Fonseca F, Nava F *et al.* (2000). Elevated circulating levels of anandamide after administration of the transport inhibitor, AM404. *Eur J Pharmacol* 408: 161–168.

Gonsiorek W, Lunn C, Fan X *et al.* (2000). Endocannabinoid 2-arachidonyl glycerol is a full agonist through human type 2 cannabinoid receptor: antagonism by anandamide. *Mol Pharmacol* 57: 1045–1050.

González S, Romero J, de Miguel R *et al.* (1999). Extrapyramidal and neuroendocrine effects of AM404, an inhibitor of the carrier-mediated transport of anandamide. *Life Sci* 65: 327–336.

Griffin G, Fernando S R, Rors R A *et al.* (1997). Evidence for the presence of CB_2-like cannabinoid receptors on peripheral nerve terminals. *Eur J Pharmacol* 339: 53–61.

Griffin G, Atkinson P J, Showalter V M *et al.* (1998). Evaluation of cannabinoid receptor agonists and antagonists using the guanosine-5′-O-(3-[^{35}S]thio)-triphosphate binding assay in rat cerebellar membranes. *J Pharmacol Exp Ther* 285: 553–560.

Hájos N, Ledent C, Freund T F (2001). Novel cannabinoid-sensitive receptor mediates inhibition of glutamatergic synaptic transmission in the hippocampus. *Neuroscience* 106: 1–4.

Hanus L, Breuer A, Tchilibon S *et al.* (1999). HU-308: a specific agonist for CB_2, a peripheral cannabinoid receptor. *Proc Natl Acad Sci USA* 96: 14228–14233.

Hanus L, Abu-Lafi S, Fride E *et al.* (2001). 2-arachidonyl glyceryl ether, an endogenous agonist of the cannabinoid CB_1 receptor. *Proc Natl Acad Sci USA* 98: 3662–3665.

Herkenham M, Lynn A B, Johnson M R *et al.* (1991). Characterization and localization of cannabinoid receptors in rat brain: a quantitative *in vitro* autoradiographic study. *J Neurosci* 11: 563–583.

Hillard C J, Jarrahian A (2000). The movement of N-arachidonoylethanolamine (anandamide) across cellular membranes. *Chem Phys Lipids* 108: 123–134.

Hillard C J, Manna S, Greenberg M J *et al.* (1999). Synthesis and characterization of potent and selective agonists of the neuronal cannabinoid receptor (CB1). *J Pharmacol Exp Ther* 289: 1427–1433.

Holland M, Challiss R A J, Standen N B *et al.* (1999). Cannabinoid CB_1 receptors fail to cause relaxation, but couple via G_i/G_o to the inhibition of adenylyl cyclase in carotid artery smooth muscle. *Br J Pharmacol* 128: 597–604.

Hosohata K, Quock R M, Hosohata Y *et al.* (1997a). AM630 is a competitive cannabinoid receptor antagonist in the guinea pig brain. *Life Sci* 61: PL115–118.

Hosohata Y, Quock R M, Hosohata K *et al.* (1997b). AM630 antagonism of cannabinoid-stimulated [^{35}S]GTPγS binding in the mouse brain. *Eur J Pharmacol* 321: R1–R3.

Huang C-C, Lo S-W, Hsu K-S (2001). Presynaptic mechanisms underlying cannabinoid inhibition of excitatory synaptic transmission in rat striatal neurons. *J Physiol* 532: 731–748.

Huffman J W, Liddle J, Yu S *et al.* (1999). 3-(1′,1′-dimethylbutyl)-1-deoxy-Δ^8-THC and related compounds: synthesis of selective ligands for the CB_2 receptor. *Bioorg Med Chem* 7: 2905–2914.

Izzo A A, Mascolo N, Tonini M *et al.* (2000). Modulation of peristalsis by cannabinoid CB_1 ligands in the isolated guinea-pig ileum. *Br J Pharmacol* 129: 984–990.

Járai Z, Wagner J A, Varga K *et al.* (1999). Cannabinoid-induced mesenteric vasodilation through an endothelial site distinct from CB1 or CB2 receptors. *Proc Natl Acad Sci USA* 96: 14136–14141.

Jerman J C, Brough S J, Davis J B *et al.* (2000). The anandamide transport inhibitor AM404 is an agonist at the rat vanilloid receptor (VR1). *Br J Pharmacol (Proc Suppl)* 129: 73P.

Johnson M R, Melvin L S (1986). The discovery of nonclassical cannabinoid analgetics. In: Mechoulam R, ed. *Cannabinoids as Therapeutic Agents*. Boca Raton: CRC Press: 121–145.

Khanolkar A D, Makriyannis A (1999). Structure-activity relationships of anandamide, an endogenous cannabinoid ligand. *Life Sci* 65: 607–616.

Khanolkar A D, Abadji V, Lin S *et al.* (1996). Head group analogs of arachidonylethanolamide, the endogenous cannabinoid ligand. *J Med Chem* 39: 4515–4519.

Kreitzer A C, Regehr W G (2001a). Retrograde inhibition of presynaptic calcium influx by endogenous cannabinoids at excitatory synapses onto Purkinje cells. *Neuron* 29: 717–727.

Kreitzer A C, Regehr W G (2001b). Cerebellar depolarization-induced suppression of inhibition is mediated by endogenous cannabinoids. *J Neurosci* 21 (RC174): 1–5.

Kunos G, Járai Z, Bátkai S *et al.* (2000). Endocannabinoids as cardiovascular modulators. *Chem Phys Lipids* 108: 159–168.

Lambert D M, DiPaolo F G, Sonveaux P *et al.* (1999). Analogues and homologues of *N*-palmitoylethanolamide, a putative endogenous CB_2 cannabinoid, as potential ligands for the cannabinoid receptors. *Biochim Biophys Acta* 1440: 266–274.

Lan R, Gatley S J, Makriyannis A (1996). Preparation of iodine-123 labeled AM251: a potential SPECT radioligand for the brain cannabinoid CB1 receptor. *J Lab Comp Radiopharm* 38: 875–881.

Lan R, Gatley J, Lu Q *et al.* (1999). Design and synthesis of the CB1 selective cannabinoid antagonist AM281: a potential human SPECT ligand. *AAPS Pharmsci* 1: U13–U24, article 4, http://www.pharmsci.org/

Landsman R S, Makriyannis A, Deng H *et al.* (1998). AM630 is an inverse agonist at the human cannabinoid CB_1 receptor. *Life Sci* 62: PL109–113.

Ledent C, Valverde O, Cossu G *et al.* (1999). Unresponsiveness to cannabinoids and reduced addictive effects of opiates in CB_1 receptor knockout mice. *Science* 283: 401–404.

Lin S, Khanolkar A D, Fan P *et al.* (1998). Novel analogues of arachidonyl-ethanolamide (anandamide): affinities for the CB1 and CB2 cannabinoid receptors and metabolic stability. *J Med Chem* 41: 5353–5361.

López-Rodríguez M L, Viso A, Ortega-Gutiérrez S *et al.* (2001). Design, synthesis and biological evaluation of novel arachidonic acid derivatives as highly potent and selective endocannabinoid transporter inhibitors. *J Med Chem* 44: 4505–4508.

Maccarrone M, van der Stelt M, Rossi A *et al.* (1998). Anandamide hydrolysis by human cells in culture and brain. *J Biol Chem* 273: 32332–32339.

Maclennan S J, Reynen P H, Kwan J *et al.* (1998). Evidence for inverse agonism of SR141716A at human recombinant cannabinoid CB_1 and CB_2 receptors. *Br J Pharmacol* 124: 619–622.

Maejima T, Hashimoto K, Yoshida T *et al.* (2001). Presynaptic inhibition caused by retrograde signal from metabotropic glutamate to cannabinoid receptors. *Neuron* 31: 463–475.

Martin B R, Compton D R, Thomas B F *et al.* (1991). Behavioral, biochemical, and molecular modeling evaluations of cannabinoid analogs. *Pharmacol Biochem Behav* 40: 471–478.

Matsuda L A (1997). Molecular aspects of cannabinoid receptors. *Crit Rev Neurobiol* 11: 143–166.

Matsuda L A, Lolait S J, Brownstein M J *et al.* (1990). Structure of a cannabinoid receptor and functional expression of the cloned cDNA. *Nature* 346: 561–564.

Maurelli S, Bisogno T, De Petrocellis L *et al.* (1995). Two novel classes of neuroactive fatty acid amides are substrates for mouse neuroblastoma 'anandamide amidohydrolase'. *FEBS Lett* 377: 82–86.

Mechoulam R, Ben-Shabat S, Hanus L *et al.* (1995). Identification of an endogenous 2-monoglyceride, present in canine gut, that binds to cannabinoid receptors. *Biochem Pharmacol* 50: 83–90.

Mechoulam R, Fride E, Hanus L et al. (1997). Anandamide may mediate sleep induction. *Nature* 389: 25–26.

Mechoulam R, Fride E, Di Marzo V (1998). Endocannabinoids. *Eur J Pharmacol* 359: 1–18.

Melis M, Gessa G L, Diana M (2000). Different mechanisms for dopaminergic excitation induced by opiates and cannabinoids in the rat midbrain. *Prog Neuro-Psychopharmacol Biol Psychiat* 24: 993–1006.

Molderings G J, Likungu J, Göthert M (1999). Presynaptic cannabinoid and imidazoline receptors in the human heart and their potential relationship. *Naunyn-Schmiedeberg's Arch Pharmacol* 360: 157–164.

Molina-Holgado E, Guaza C, Borrell J et al. (1999). Effects of cannabinoids on the immune system and central nervous system. Therapeutic implications. *Biodrugs* 12: 317–326.

Moore H, Fadel J, Sarter M et al. (1999). Role of accumbens and cortical dopamine receptors in the regulation of cortical acetylcholine release. *Neuroscience* 88: 811–822.

Munro S, Thomas K L, Abu-Shaar M (1993). Molecular characterization of a peripheral receptor for cannabinoids. *Nature* 365: 61–65.

Ohno-Shosaku T, Maejima T, Kano M (2001). Endogenous cannabinoids mediate retrograde signals from depolarized postsynaptic neurons to presynaptic terminals. *Neuron* 29: 729–738.

Pacheco M, Childers S R, Arnold R et al. (1991). Aminoalkylindoles: actions on specific G-protein-linked receptors. *J Pharmacol Exp Ther* 257: 170–183.

Pan X, Ikeda S R, Lewis D L (1998). SR 141716A acts as an inverse agonist to increase neuronal voltage-dependent Ca^{2+} currents by reversal of tonic CB1 cannabinoid receptor activity. *Mol Pharmacol* 54: 1064–1072.

Pate D W (1999). Anandamide structure-activity relationships and mechanisms of action on intraocular pressure in the normotensive rabbit model. PhD thesis, University of Kuopio, Finland.

Pertwee R G (1988). The central neuropharmacology of psychotropic cannabinoids. *Pharmacol Ther* 36: 189–261.

Pertwee R G (1997). Pharmacology of cannabinoid CB_1 and CB_2 receptors. *Pharmacol Ther* 74: 129–180.

Pertwee R G (1999). Pharmacology of cannabinoid receptor ligands. *Curr Med Chem* 6: 635–664.

Pertwee R G (2000). Cannabinoid receptor ligands: clinical and neuropharmacological considerations, relevant to future drug discovery and development. *Expert Opin Invest Drugs* 9: 1553–1571.

Pertwee R G (2001). Cannabinoid receptors and pain. *Prog Neurobiol* 63: 569–611.

Pertwee R G, Ross R A (2002). Cannabinoid receptors and their ligands. *Prostaglandins Leukot Essent Fatty Acids* 66: 101–121.

Pertwee R, Griffin G, Fernando S et al. (1995a). AM630, a competitive cannabinoid receptor antagonist. *Life Sci* 56: 1949–1955.

Pertwee R G, Griffin G, Lainton J A H et al. (1995b). Pharmacological characterization of three novel cannabinoid receptor agonists in the mouse isolated vas deferens. *Eur J Pharmacol* 284: 241–247.

Pertwee R G, Fernando S R, Nash J E et al. (1996). Further evidence for the presence of cannabinoid CB_1 receptors in guinea-pig small intestine. Br J Pharmacol 118: 2199–2205.

Petitet F, Jeantaud B, Reibaud M et al. (1998). Complex pharmacology of natural cannabinoids: evidence for partial agonist activity of Δ^9-tetrahydrocannabinol and antagonist activity of cannabidiol on rat brain cannabinoid receptors. Life Sci 63: PL1–PL6.

Piomelli D, Beltramo M, Glasnapp S et al. (1999). Structural determinants for recognition and translocation by the anandamide transporter. Proc Natl Acad Sci USA 96: 5802–5807.

Portier M, Rinaldi-Carmona M, Pecceu F et al. (1999). SR 144528, an antagonist for the peripheral cannabinoid receptor that behaves as an inverse agonist. J Pharmacol Exp Ther 288: 582–589.

Rhee M-H, Vogel Z, Barg J et al. (1997). Cannabinol derivatives: binding to cannabinoid receptors and inhibition of adenylylcyclase. J Med Chem 40: 3228–3233.

Rinaldi-Carmona M, Barth F, Héaulme M et al. (1994). SR141716A, a potent and selective antagonist of the brain cannabinoid receptor. FEBS Lett 350: 240–244.

Rinaldi-Carmona M, Calandra B, Shire D et al. (1996). Characterization of two cloned human CB1 cannabinoid receptor isoforms. J Pharmacol Exp Ther 278: 871–878.

Rinaldi-Carmona M, Barth F, Millan J et al. (1998). SR 144528, the first potent and selective antagonist of the CB2 cannabinoid receptor. J Pharmacol Exp Ther 284: 644–650.

Robbe D, Alonso G, Duchamp F et al. (2001). Localization and mechanisms of action of cannabinoid receptors at the glutamatergic synapses of the mouse nucleus accumbens. J Neurosci 21: 109–116.

Ross R A, Brockie H C, Fernando S R et al. (1998). Comparison of cannabinoid binding sites in guinea-pig forebrain and small intestine. Br J Pharmacol 125: 1345–1351.

Ross R A, Brockie H C, Stevenson L A et al. (1999a) Agonist-inverse agonist characterization at CB_1 and CB_2 cannabinoid receptors of L759633, L759656 and AM630. Br J Pharmacol 126: 665–672.

Ross R A, Gibson T M, Stevenson L A et al. (1999b) Structural determinants of the partial agonist-inverse agonist properties of 6'-azidohex-2'-yne-Δ^8-tetrahydrocannabinol at cannabinoid receptors. Br J Pharmacol 128: 735–743.

Ross R A, Gibson T M, Brockie H C et al. (2001). Structure-activity relationship for the endogenous cannabinoid, anandamide, and certain of its analogues at vanilloid receptors in transfected cells and vas deferens. Br J Pharmacol 132: 631–640.

Ross R A, Craib S J, Stevenson L A et al. (2002). Pharmacological characterization of the anandamide cycloxygenase metabolite: PGE_2 ethanolamide. J Pharmacol Exp Ther 301: 900–907.

Salio C, Fischer J, Franzoni M F et al. (2001). CB1-cannabinoid and μ-opioid receptor co-localization on postsynaptic target in the rat dorsal horn. Neuroreport 12: 3689–3692.

Savinainen J R, Järvinen T, Laine K *et al.* (2001). Despite substantial degradation, 2-arachidonoylglycerol is a potent full efficacy agonist mediating CB_1 receptor-dependent G-protein activation in rat cerebellar membranes. *Br J Pharmacol* 134: 664–672.

Schlicker E, Timm J, Zentner J *et al.* (1997). Cannabinoid CB_1 receptor-mediated inhibition of noradrenaline release in the human and guinea-pig hippocampus. *Naunyn-Schmiedeberg's Arch Pharmacol* 356: 583–589.

Shen M, Thayer S A (1999). Δ^9-Tetrahydrocannabinol acts as a partial agonist to modulate glutamatergic synaptic transmission between rat hippocampal neurons in culture. *Mol Pharmacol* 55: 8–13.

Sheskin T, Hanus L, Slager J *et al.* (1997). Structural requirements for binding of anandamide-type compounds to the brain cannabinoid receptor. *J Med Chem* 40: 659–667.

Shire D, Carillon C, Kaghad M *et al.* (1995). An amino-terminal variant of the central cannabinoid receptor resulting from alternative splicing. *J Biol Chem* 270: 3726–3731.

Shire D, Calandra B, Rinaldi-Carmona M *et al.* (1996). Molecular cloning, expression and function of the murine CB2 peripheral cannabinoid receptor. *Biochim Biophys Acta* 1307: 132–136.

Showalter V M, Compton D R, Martin B R *et al.* (1996). Evaluation of binding in a transfected cell line expressing a peripheral cannabinoid receptor (CB2): identification of cannabinoid receptor subtype selective ligands. *J Pharmacol Exp Ther* 278: 989–999.

Sim L J, Hampson R E, Deadwyler S A *et al.* (1996). Effects of chronic treatment with Δ^9-tetrahydrocannabinol on cannabinoid-stimulated [^{35}S]GTPγS autoradiography in rat brain. *J Neurosci* 16: 8057–8066.

Sim-Selley L J, Brunk L K, Selley D E (2001). Inhibitory effects of SR141716A on G-protein activation in rat brain. *Eur J Pharmacol* 414: 135–143.

Simoneau, I. I., Hamza M S, Mata H P *et al.* (2001). The cannabinoid agonist WIN55,212-2 suppresses opioid-induced emesis in ferrets. *Anesthesiology* 94: 882–887.

Smart D, Gunthorpe M J, Jerman J C *et al.* (2000). The endogenous lipid anandamide is a full agonist at the human vanilloid receptor (hVR1). *Br J Pharmacol* 129: 227–230.

Stella N, Schweitzer P, Piomelli D (1997). A second endogenous cannabinoid that modulates long-term potentiation. *Nature* 388: 773–778.

Sugiura T, Waku K (2000). 2-Arachidonoylglycerol and the cannabinoid receptors. *Chem Phys Lipids* 108: 89–106.

Sugiura T, Kodaka T, Kondo S *et al.* (1997). Inhibition by 2-arachidonoylglycerol, a novel type of possible neuromodulator, of the depolarization-induced increase in intracellular free calcium in neuroblastoma × glioma hybrid NG108-15 cells. *Biochem Biophys Res Commun* 233: 207–210.

Tanda G, Pontieri F E, Di Chiara G (1997). Cannabinoid and heroin activation of mesolimbic dopamine transmission by a common μ_1 opioid receptor mechanism. *Science* 276: 2048–2050.

Ueda N, Puffenbarger R A, Yamamoto S *et al.* (2000). The fatty acid amide hydrolase (FAAH). *Chem Phys Lipids* 108: 107–121.

Vizi E S, Katona I, Freund T F (2001). Evidence for presynaptic cannabinoid CB_1 receptor-mediated inhibition of noradrenaline release in the guinea pig lung. *Eur J Pharmacol* 431: 237–244.

Wagner J A, Varga K, Járai Z *et al.* (1999). Mesenteric vasodilation mediated by endothelial anandamide receptors. *Hypertension* 33: 429–434.

Walker J M, Huang S M, Strangman N M *et al.* (1999). Pain modulation by release of the endogenous cannabinoid anandamide. *Proc Natl Acad Sci USA* 96: 12198–12203.

White R, Hiley C R (1998). The actions of the cannabinoid receptor antagonist, SR 141716A, in the rat isolated mesenteric artery. *Br J Pharmacol* 125: 689–696.

Wilson R I, Nicoll R A (2001). Endogenous cannabinoids mediate retrograde signalling at hippocampal synapses. *Nature* 410: 588–592.

Zimmer A, Zimmer A M, Hohmann A G *et al.* (1999). Increased mortality, hypoactivity, and hypoalgesia in cannabinoid CB1 receptor knockout mice. *Proc Natl Acad Sci USA* 96: 5780–5785.

Zurier R B, Rossetti R G, Lane J H *et al.* (1998). Dimethylheptyl-THC-11-oic acid. A nonpsychoactive antiinflammatory agent with a cannabinoid template structure. *Arthritis Rheum* 41: 163–170.

Zygmunt P M, Petersson J, Andersson D A *et al.* (1999). Vanilloid receptors on sensory nerves mediate the vasodilator action of anandamide. *Nature* 400: 452–457.

Zygmunt P M, Chuang H, Movahed P *et al.* (2000). The anandamide transport inhibitor AM404 activates vanilloid receptors. *Eur J Pharmacol* 396: 39–42.

6

Therapeutic potential of cannabis and cannabinoids in experimental models of multiple sclerosis

David Baker

Multiple sclerosis (MS) is the major demyelinating disease of the central nervous system (CNS). Although the precise aetiology of MS is unknown, it appears that an environmental factor acts on an individual with a susceptible genetic background to trigger an inflammatory cascade that is associated with: repeated episodes of blood–brain barrier dysfunction and mononuclear cells entry into the CNS; paralytic clinical episodes; demyelinated lesions and axonal destruction that slowly accumulates over a number of years to leave the affected individual with progressively increasing disability and the development of troublesome symptoms that greatly affect 'quality of life' (Compston and Coles, 2002). The clinical course can be very varied, from a benign 'self-limiting' form of MS, to acute MS that is rapidly fatal, primary progressive disease with accumulating disability from onset, or the more common relapsing-remitting MS, where some recovery occurs between episodes of active clinical disease that often evolves into secondary progressive disease with accumulating disability (Compston and Coles, 2002). Whatever the cause, there is accumulating evidence that the disease involves an immune-mediated component that can be modified by agents affecting the immune system (Coles *et al.*, 1999; SPECTRIMS Study Group, 2001; Wiendl and Hohlfeld, 2002; Miller *et al.*, 2003) and this element has been modelled in experimental animal models. Whilst no non-human animal spontaneously develops a disease identical to MS, many animal species can be induced to develop disease with features that occur in MS. The majority of studies have focused on rodents, which provide a more useful medium for experimentation (t'Hart and Amor, 2003).

Some believe that MS is caused by an infectious agent and there are a number of pathogens that can induce demyelinating disease in animals, but within the context of cannabinoid research in MS, the

Theiler's mouse encephalomyelitis virus (TMEV) model is the only system so far investigated (Arévalo-Martin *et al.*, 2003; Croxford and Miller, 2003). TMEV is a natural pathogen of mice that upon infection of the CNS induces an immune-mediated demyelination and slow accumulation of paresis in susceptible animals strains (Dal Canto *et al.*, 1996). Despite many potential pathogens found in MS tissues, no single agent has been found in all cases or shown to have a causal relationship to MS.

Another school of thought believes that MS represents an organ-specific autoimmune disease, and many of the pathological features of MS can be modelled in experimental allergic encephalomyelitis (EAE). This is an autoimmune disease induced by autoimmunity to CNS components, in particular to CNS myelin (t'Hart and Amor, 2003). EAE can be induced in many species, including humans (e.g. acute disseminated encephalomyelitis following vaccination with rabies virus contaminated with brain tissues). The clinico/histopathological features vary greatly depending on the species and the strain being investigated, the nature of the inducing antigen and, importantly, the length of duration of the study (t'Hart and Amor, 2003).

The autoimmune and infectious aetiologies are not mutually exclusive and environmental agents can trigger autoimmunity, as occurs in TMEV infection (Croxford *et al.*, 2002), via a number of experimentally supported mechanisms (Van Noort *et al.*, 2000; Croxford *et al.*, 2002; Wekerle and Holmfeld, 2003). These MS models have largely been used to investigate the therapeutic use of anti-inflammatory and immunosuppressive agents in disease control. However, despite the thousands of agents that prevent the development of EAE, very few have been translated into clinical use (Watson *et al.*, 1991; Wiendl and Hohlfeld, 2002; Miller *et al.*, 2003). These many clinical failures underscore the realisation that MS is a neurodegenerative process (Coles *et al.*, 1999; SPECTRIMS Study Group, 2001; Bjartmar *et al.*, 2003), probably triggered by the microenvironment created following immune attack.

Clinically, monotherapies have so far had limited success (Wiendl and Hohlfeld, 2002) and therefore one needs multiple solutions for multiple problems. Cannabis may offer potential for the treatment of multiple pathways in the disease process in MS.

Cannabis as a therapeutic in MS

Although it is recognised that Δ^9-tetrahydrocannabinol (Δ^9-THC) is the major psychoactive cannabinoid in marijuana (Mechoulam and Gaoni,

1967), cannabis contains many different compounds that may interact to give the therapeutic effect. It is important that any therapeutic effect is understood so that it can be improved. However, from a scientific perspective, few people work with a cocktail of agents in experimental systems relevant to MS. The focus has been on the use of single agents with a relatively specific activity. The development of specific and highly active cannabinoid compounds was a forerunner to the discovery of cannabinoid receptors (CB_1 receptors expressed in the brain and CB_2 receptors on leukocytes). Subsequently, endogenous endocannabinoid ligands such as anandamide and 2-arachidonoyl glycerol (2-AG) and a homeostatic endocannabinoid degradation system have been described (Pertwee 1999; Howlett *et al.*, 2002; Maccarrone and Finazzi-Agro, 2002; Sugiura *et al.*, 2002). This has revolutionised cannabinoid biology and now allows us to underpin the mechanisms and biology of the many anecdotal observations of millennia of human use.

Whatever cannabis does, it works because it is affecting biological systems. We are only recently beginning to unravel these. Unlike the typical pharmaceutical approach of targeting a novel agent to a disease condition in the hope that it works, the widespread use of cannabis means that people with diseases are already giving us the indications for clinical use, particularly in relation to symptom management, and there are many people who claim that cannabis gives symptom relief in MS (Consroe *et al.*, 1997; House of Lords Select Committee on Science and Technology, 1998; Schnelle *et al.*, 1999). It is well established that cannabis has mind-altering potential, and while this may be part of the therapeutic effect (Howlett *et al.*, 2002; Pertwee, 2002), it is not a complete explanation.

Until recently, objective scientific evidence for the value of cannabis in symptom control in MS was lacking, apart from some small-scale clinical studies (Pertwee, 2002). While animals lack the cognitive capacities of humans, they provide a tool to obtain objective evidence and, importantly, to dissect out mechanisms of activity using recently available tools such as specific, synthetic receptor agonists, antagonists and gene knockout animals (Howlett *et al.*, 2002). The claims for the therapeutic activities of cannabis are varied; science is now beginning to underpin these.

Symptom control

Many people with MS claim that cannabis gives symptom benefit for spasticity and spasms, pain, tremor and bladder function (Consroe *et al.*, 1997; House of Lords Select Committee on Science and Technology, 1998; Schnelle *et al.*, 1999; Pertwee, 2002). The symptoms that develop as a consequence of MS are very varied and depend on the location of the lesions and the efficacy of the compensation mechanisms within the neural circuit controlling the behaviour (Compston and Coles, 2002). However, on a simplistic level these are all problems associated with impaired neural transmission. It is well recognised that demyelination is a pathological hallmark of MS and that demyelinated axons have aberrant conduction patterns and are particularly sensitive to agents that cause conduction block (Smith *et al.*, 2001; Waxman, 2002). Furthermore, inflammation also induces many axonal transections and axonal loss, which contributes further to loss of fine control of excitory and inhibitory neural circuits (Trapp *et al.*, 1998; Bjartmar *et al.*, 2003).

Recently it has been shown that one of the important functions of the cannabinoid system is in the control of synaptic neurotransmission (Kreitzer and Regehr, 2001; Wilson and Nicoll, 2001, 2002; Freund *et al.*, 2003). In these studies it was shown that postsynaptic endocannabinoids, released in response to neurotransmitter activity, deliver retrograde synaptic signals via presynaptic CB_1 to limit further neurotransmission (Wilson and Nicoll, 2002), but postsynaptic inhibitory effects have also been observed (Nogueron *et al.*, 2001; Pryce *et al.*, 2003a). It is therefore not surprising that cannabis can mediate control of many effects, the location of the receptor determining whether the outcome is positive or negative, as it can affect both excitory and inhibitory neural circuits (Kreitzer and Regehr, 2001; Wilson and Nicoll, 2001, 2002).

Pain and bladder function

Many people with MS have claimed relief of pain following use of cannabis (Consroe *et al.*, 1997). Unfortunately, as most experimental pain systems rely on movement behaviours away from painful stimuli and in EAE movement is known to be adversely affected, pain in experimental MS has yet to be analysed effectively. However, cannabinoids have been shown to be very effective at controlling pain (acute, chronic and neuropathic pain) in every experimental paradigm (Walker and Huang, 2002).

Cannabinoid receptors are highly expressed in dorsal root ganglia (Bridges *et al.*, 2003), which are the gateways of afferent sensory pathways between the peripheral and central nervous system. Control of pain can be found in peripheral, spinal and supraspinal sites which are controlled by CB_1 and also by a putative CB_2-like receptor and can be controlled by cannabinoids without significant psychoactive potential (Walker and Huang, 2002).

Although incontinence of the bladder and bowel is a feature of EAE, the role of cannabinoids in the control of these signs has not yet been investigated. However, using experimental models of bladder hyperreactivity CB_1-mediated control of bladder hyperactivity has been found (Martin *et al.*, 2000). Recent studies with sublingual medical cannabis extract appear to demonstrate some efficacy at treating bladder dysfunction (Brady *et al.*, 2002).

Tremor

Tremor is a common occurrence in MS and is difficult to treat (Alusi *et al.*, 2001). Both fore and hindlimb tremor occur in mice during chronic EAE, but with a relatively low frequency which makes it difficult to study. However, it is clear that CB_1 antagonism can worsen EAE-induced tremor, and likewise CB_1 agonism (such as with Δ^9-THC) could ameliorate tremor (Baker *et al.*, 2000). Tremor present in the rodent autoimmune CNS disease is substantially more aggressive than that typical of humans (40 Hz in mice compared with a maximum of 5–8 Hz in humans). It is difficult to treat, as doses that inhibit spasticity may not always adequately control the tremor. It is most effectively treated using potent CB_1 agonists (Baker *et al.*, 2000, unpublished).

Examination of mutant animals with tremors may provide an alternative way to investigate the actions of cannabinoids on tremors. *Rumpshaker* (proteolipid protein mutation) and *Shiverer* (myelin basic protein mutation) mice both exhibit body tremors (12–25 Hz), which can be inhibited by CB agonism (WIN55,212-2). These are, however, typically intention tremors initiated during movement. Here, inhibition of body tremor was particularly associated with the development of hypomotility and control of tremor may therefore be secondary to the induction of hypomotility (unpublished observations). Likewise, cannabinoids could affect the limb tremor associated with the 'startle' response in glycine receptor *spastic* mutant mice, however doses which inhibited tremor in EAE were found to actually exacerbate tremor in these mutant mice (Baker and Pryce, 2004). This CB_1-mediated tremor-inducing potential of WIN55,212-2 was absent in CB_1-deficient *Spastic* mutant mice (unpublished observations).

Cannabinoids therefore can have paradoxical effects on symptoms, as has been noted with the effects of cannabis in humans (House of Lords Select Committee on Science and Technology, 1998). This further argues that the outcome of effects will be dependent on the location of the receptor within the neural circuit. Although tremor is a common occurrence in MS (Alusi *et al.*, 2001), its pathophysiology will undoubtedly be varied. Some tremors, such as seen with nystagmus of the eye, may respond (Schon *et al.*, 1999), whereas other tremors may not. As the pathophysiology of experimental and clinical tremors is better understood it may be possible to target therapeutic agents to this condition with more accuracy.

Spasticity

Spasticity (uncontrolled limb stiffness) is a common occurrence in MS (Barnes *et al.*, 2003) and occurs frequently in EAE after significant neurological deficit and nerve loss has occurred (Baker *et al.*, 2000). This represents a neurological deficit that is left as a consequence of damage accumulated during repeated episodes of paralytic attack (Baker *et al.*, 2000; Barnes *et al.*, 2003). While CB_1 agonists can rapidly inhibit spasticity (Baker *et al.*, 2000, 2001), most important was the observation that CB_1 antagonists transiently worsened spasticity and tremor, whereas they did not affect non-spastic animals (Baker *et al.*, 2000). This suggests that the cannabinoid system becomes particularly active once normal homeostatic control is lost and is involved in the control of this sign. Mice that are deficient in CB_1 develop spasticity more rapidly following the development of EAE (Pryce *et al.*, 2003a) and can be used to definitively demonstrate that CB_1 agonists such as CP55,940 are mediating their activity by a CB_1-dependent mechanism (unpublished observations).

Although some CB_2 agonists were also antispastic agents (Baker *et al.*, 2000, unpublished), this effect was lost in EAE-induced spastic CB_1-deficient mice. This suggests that the antispastic effect was due to CB_1 cross-reactivity, which is a problem with all currently available CB_2 agonists (Pertwee, 1999; Howlett *et al.*, 2002). However, importantly, this indicates that agents with weak CB_1-stimulating potential may be useful and indeed may be preferable to strong agonists. There may be a small therapeutic window between effect, side-effect or no effect. Potent full agonists can rapidly and strongly stimulate CB_1 and have a great potential for psychoactivity and the induction of receptor tolerance, which will limit efficacy (Howlett *et al.*, 2002; Sim-Selley and Martin, 2002). However, weak agonists may allow more effective dose-titration and probably give better bio-distribution of agent as they allow more to be administered.

In comparison with some synthetic cannabinoids such as CP55,940 (K_i at CB_1 ~0.5 nM), THC is significantly less active at CB_1 receptor agonism (K_i at CB_1 ~40 nM), however, endocannabinoids have an even lower affinity (K_i at CB_1 ~100–500 nM) (Pertwee, 1999) and offer potential for therapy whilst minimising psychoactive effects (Baker et al., 2001, 2003).

Experimentally, many of the adverse effects and positive effects such as pain relief by cannabis can be attributed to the action of Δ^9-THC on the CB_1 receptor. However, marijuana smoke has also been shown to exhibit some biologically active, non-CB_1 receptor-mediated effects (Lichtman et al., 2001). While Δ^9-THC could be shown to inhibit tremor and spasticity in EAE, cannabidiol failed to demonstrate inhibition of experimental spasticity (Baker et al., 2000). Furthermore, removal of THC from a cannabis extract inhibited the capacity of the extract to inhibit spasticity (Wilkinson et al., 2003). This indicates that the main and important antispastic agent in cannabis is THC and therefore it is unlikely that it will be possible to truly dissociate the psychoactive from the therapeutic effects.

However, in direct comparisons of cannabis and THC, while they were found to be equally effective at inhibiting signs, cannabis appeared to be more rapidly active. This suggests that it contains other elements that contribute to the effects of THC (Williamson, 2001; Wilkinson et al., 2003). It is possible that components of cannabis harbour chemicals that stimulate or alter other receptors that are in a homeostatic feedback with the cannabinoid system (Giuffrida et al., 1999; Maejima et al., 2001; Kim et al., 2002; Fowler, 2003). Alternatively, other components of marijuana may contribute to enhanced pharmacokinetics, CNS permeability or alter the tolerability of THC. Cannabidiol (CBD) can ameliorate clinical anxiety provoked by pure Δ^9-THC (Zuardi et al., 1982) and increases levels of Δ^9-THC in the brain of mice after administration of both drugs (Bornheim et al., 1995). It also blocks CYP450 3A11, the enzyme responsible for hydroxylation of Δ^9-THC to the 11-hydroxy metabolite, a more potent CB_1 agonist (Bornheim et al., 1995; Pertwee, 1999).

The plant may also contain other cannabinoids with some modest CB_1 affinity such as Δ^8-THC, which may be insufficient to mediate therapeutic or psychoactive effect in itself but can augment the effects of THC (Pertwee, 1999). While cannabinol (CBN), which is a breakdown product of THC, may not be present in significant quantities within the plant, it can appear when THC is degraded during storage. It has weak CB_1 affinity and may account for some of the enhanced effects seen experimentally (Lichtman et al., 2001; Wilkinson et al., 2003).

There may be many more cannabinoid components in cannabis that have not been sufficiently purified to allow examination of their *in vitro* and *in vivo* biological effects. In addition there may be components in cannabis that can affect endocannabinoid degradation by acting as a substrate for fatty acid amide hydrolase (FAAH). FAAH degrades anandamide (Cravatt and Lichtman, 2002; Deutsch *et al.*, 2002; Lichtman *et al.*, 2002) and monoglycerol lipase (MGL) degrades 2-arachidonoyl glycerol (Dinh *et al.*, 2002; Lichtman *et al.*, 2002). Inhibition of these enzymes thus provides additional CB_1 stimulation by indirect mechanisms. CBD has been reported to block anandamide re-uptake (Bisogno *et al.*, 2001; Jacobsson and Fowler, 2001), and thus may contribute to an antispastic effect. However, while CBD has this activity at a level similar to that of prototype synthetic re-uptake inhibitors *in vitro* (Bisogno *et al.*, 2001; Jacobsson and Fowler, 2001), it was relatively inactive at inhibiting spasticity in comparison with the synthetic drugs, such as AM404 and VDM11 (Baker *et al.*, 2001; Baker and Pryce, 2004).

Recently, the existence of an anandamide-specific transporter, thought to represent a diffusion-facilitated transporter (Hillard and Jarrahian, 2000), has been questioned (Glaser *et al.*, 2003). The re-uptake activity of compounds is usually active in the micromolar range, compared with the nanomolar effects on the receptors, and is not truly dependent on the level of anandamide being inhibited. Furthermore, in contrast to the expression of CB_1 receptor and FAAH (Howlett *et al.*, 2002; Romero *et al.*, 2002; Egertova *et al.*, 2003), the transporter activity is essentially ubiquitous in virtually every cell type (Hillard and Jarrahian, 2000) and even so-called negative cell lines such as Cos7 and HeLa cells (Hillard and Jarrahian, 2000; Deutsch *et al.*, 2001).

Most transport inhibitor compounds have additional activities that may account for their *in vivo* activity. These include weak CB_1 affinity, vanilloid receptor 1 (VR1) affinity and particularly FAAH activity (Beltramo *et al.*, 1997; De Petrocellis *et al.*, 2000; Jarrahian *et al.*, 2000; Lopez-Rodriguez *et al.*, 2001; Ralevic *et al.*, 2001; Ortar *et al.*, 2003), all of which may contribute to their biological activity as anti-spastic agents (Baker *et al.*, 2000, 2001; Brooks *et al.*, 2002). In particular it has been suggested that enzymes such as FAAH simply drive a diffusion gradient through the cell (Day *et al.*, 2001; Deutsch *et al.*, 2001). Nevertheless, the *in vitro* re-uptake activity of anandamide is selectively inhibited by certain cannabinoids but not by others, such as palmitoethanolamide (Beltramo *et al.*, 1997; Rakhshan *et al.*, 2000; Jacobsson and Fowler, 2001). It is possible that such compounds compete for diffusion sites dictated by the physiochemical properties of the compound through the plasma membrane of the cell, but until such a molecule is cloned, the therapeutic value of such agents must be interpreted with caution. However, transport inhibitors have been reported to increase anandamide levels *in vivo* in biological fluids (Giuffrida *et al.*, 2000) and to inhibit experimental spasticity (Baker *et al.*, 2001, unpublished). Inhibition of degradation of endocannabinoid inhibition may prove to be a new avenue towards therapy in MS (Baker *et al.*, 2003).

An important observation was that SR141617A transiently worsened spasticity, indicating that an endocannabinoid tone was involved in the limitation of these signs and therefore exogenous CB_1 agonism should have the potential to augment this and control signs (Baker *et al.*, 2000, 2001). These observations underpinned the rationale for clinical trials and indeed there appears to be clinical translation of our observations in some studies (Fox *et al.*, 2001; Brady *et al.*, 2002; GW Pharmaceuticals, 2002; Notcutt *et al.*, 2002; Vaney *et al.*, 2002; Wade *et al.*, 2003). While CB antagonists may actually exhibit inverse agonism *in vitro* (Pertwee, 1999; Hurst *et al.*, 2002), the observation that elevated levels of endocannabinoids were being produced in the spastic lesions are more consistent with antagonism of tonic control by the endocannabinoid system (Baker *et al.*, 2001).

While changes in endocannabinoids have been detected in other experimental neuropathies (Di Marzo *et al.*, 2000; Lastres-Becker *et al.*, 2001), it is difficult to determine whether this occurs in human disease, although microdialysis of a stroke patient indicated that disease was associated with increases in endocannabinoid levels (Schabitz *et al.*, 2002). However post-mortem increases in endocannabinoids (Felder *et al.*, 1996) means that it is unlikely that these observations can be replicated in MS, but analysis of cerebrospinal fluid (CSF) from severely spastic MS patients showed no significant differences in the levels of anandamide or palmitoyethanolamide compared with non-spastic neurological disease controls (unpublished). However, the endocannabinoid levels in spastic MS were comparable to levels previously detectable in people with schizophrenia, who had significantly elevated anandamide levels compared with their respective controls (Leweke *et al.*, 1999).

Since CSF lacks 2-AG, which is abundant in tissues (Leweke *et al.*, 1999; Schabitz *et al.*, 2002), it probably is not indicative of tissue events. However, local alterations of the endocannabinoid system observed in animal models suggests that it may be possible to get some selectivity of action of CB_1 in lesional areas. This will limit psychoactive potential controlled by different brain centres, particularly as endo-cannabinoids have lower CB_1 receptor affinities than THC (Pertwee, 1999; Baker *et al.*, 2001, 2003). CB_1 agonism may be achieved through stimulation of endocannabinoid release or through inhibition of endo-cannabinoid degradation. Inhibitors of FAAH have been found to exhibit antispastic activity (Boger *et al.*, 2000; Baker *et al.*, 2001). This may be a novel route to therapy that utilises the therapeutic benefits of the cannabinoid system while limiting the known adverse side-effects. Although CB_1 is the major mediator of cannabinoid-induced control of spasticity, other systems can inhibit spasticity independently of the CB_1 receptor (Brooks *et al.*, 2002). As we understand more about the biology of MS and the full extent of the cannabinoid system, such as novel receptors and ligands (Howlett *et al.*, 2002), there is even more scope for cannabinoids in the therapeutic control of MS.

Immunomodulation

Although some people believe that cannabis may affect the course of the disease (Consroe *et al.*, 1997), as yet objective scientific data are lacking, and the clinical course of MS is notoriously variable and difficult to predict (Compston and Coles, 2002). Although CB_1 is highly expressed through the neural compartments, particularly within the CNS (Howlett *et al.*, 2002; Egertova *et al.*, 2003), it is also expressed on leukocytes, which also can express CB_2 receptors (Parolaro, 1999; Noe *et al.*, 2001; Howlett *et al.*, 2002). Although present on T cells, CB_1 and CB_2 receptors are expressed particularly on B cells and macrophages, which can also produce endocannabinoids (Parolaro *et al.*, 2002). Cannabinoids, including THC, CBD and CBN, have been shown to influence the nature and level of cytokine production and function and cell fate (Herring and Kaminski, 1999; Berdyshev, 2000; Buckley *et al.*, 2000; Sacerdote *et al.*, 2000; Zhu *et al.*, 2000; Herring *et al.*, 2001; Klein *et al.*, 2001; McKallip *et al.*, 2002; Yuan *et al.*, 2002). Both cannabinoids and cytokines have been shown to inhibit the generation of autoimmunity (Malfait *et al.*, 2000; Li *et al.*, 2001), including the development of EAE (Lyman *et al.*, 1989; Wirguin *et al.*, 1994).

In EAE, treatment was performed prior to initial disease develop-ment. Inhibition of the development of paralysis was associated with prevention of events leading to leukocyte accumulation and possibly at the level of initial sensitisation, which has minor therapeutic relevance (Lyman *et al.*, 1989; Wirguin *et al.*, 1994). Indeed naïve T cells were found to be more sensitive to the effects of cannabinoid than primed T cells (Croxford and Miller, 2003). Synthetic cannabinoid receptor agonists have been shown to influence disease course in a viral model of MS (Arévalo-Martin *et al.*, 2003; Croxford and Miller, 2003). These effects were largely CB_1-mediated, although a CB_2 agonist, which also has some affinity for CB_1, could also mediate disease-ameliorating effects that were prolonged (about a month) after cessation of a short course of treatment (Arévalo-Martin *et al.*, 2003; Croxford and Miller, 2003).

Disease inhibition was associated with inhibition of microglial activation and anti-inflammatory cytokine production (Arévalo-Martin *et al.*, 2003; Croxford and Miller 2003). However, in one study (Croxford and Miller, 2003) disease-modifying effects were only seen with very high doses of a CB_1/CB_2 full agonist (WIN55,212-2) that can induce significant adverse (catelepsy, hypomotility) effects and are probably too high to be relevant for the human condition. Cannabinoid-mediated immunosuppression may also be independent of direct stimulation of CB receptors on leukocytes. It could be due to CNS-expressed CB receptors in areas controlling neuropeptide release to lymphoid organs, or the release or activity of immunosuppressive hormonal agents such as leptin (Di Marzo *et al.*, 2001; Sanna *et al.*, 2003) or glucocorticosteroids (Bolton *et al.*, 1997; Di *et al.*, 2003; Pryce *et al.*, 2003b).

Disease-modifying effects could also be due to effects on vascular biology, which may not even be CB receptor mediated (Hogestatt and Zygmunt, 2002; Offertaler *et al.*, 2003; Sancho *et al.*, 2003). Some non-CB binding cannabinoids can mediate their effects through inhibition of *N*-methyl D-aspartate (NMDA) receptor-induced vascular permeability that prevents leukocyte accumulation in EAE (Bolton and Paul, 1997; Achiron *et al.*, 2000).

Cannabidiol (CBD) can exhibit anti-inflammatory properties and exhibits inhibitory effects in autoimmune arthritis (Malfait *et al.*, 2000). While Δ^9-THC does have the potential to inhibit the generation of EAE by a CB_1-dependent mechanism (Lyman *et al.*, 1989; Baker *et al.*, 2000, unpublished), as yet we have been unable to find any evidence showing that CBD has any immunosuppressive potential in mouse EAE when treatment was initiated during sensitisation or shortly before the onset of clinical signs, in contrast to that seen in experimental arthritis (unpublished observations). Furthermore, immunosuppression occurred at relatively high doses of THC that can induce a glucocorticosteroid response (Pertwee, 1974; Lyman *et al.*, 1989; Wirguin *et al.*, 1994; Bolton *et al.*, 1997). In a clinical context, such dose levels may not be achieved and chronic cannabis smokers are not hugely immunosuppressed, although they may exhibit some immune perturbations (Bredt *et al.*, 2002; Pacifici *et al.*, 2003).

People with human immunodeficiency virus (HIV) regularly use cannabis for symptom control (Schnelle *et al.*, 1999) and THC is licensed for the treatment of wasting disease associated with HIV infection. It would therefore be surprising if therapeutic doses of THC caused marked immunosuppression; this would be a contraindication for use in HIV, as it would contribute to the problems associated with acquired immune deficiency syndrome (AIDS). Recent studies following trials of smoked marijuana in people with HIV have shown few changes in immunological parameters (Bredt *et al.*, 2002). Other clinical studies in MS indicate that oral doses of THC that are not therapeutic but are capable of inducing some adverse physiological effects, such as dry mouth (Killestein *et al.*, 2002), fail to demonstrate significant immunomodulation (Killestein *et al.*, 2003).

Although perhaps marginal, any immunosuppressive activity could be beneficial as, at least initially, acute EAE is T cell mediated, whereas cannabinoid receptors are predominantly expressed by B lymphocytes and macrophages and microglia (Howlett *et al.*, 2002; Zhang *et al.*, 2003). These are important in the demyelinating processes that occur in chronic relapsing EAE (t'Hart and Amor, 2003) and have yet to be treated with cannabinoids in an experimental context. The effects of cannabis on immune function is being analysed in ongoing clinical trials, however, more importantly, the biology of the cannabinoid system indicates that cannabinoids may be neuroprotective.

Neuroprotection

The major cause of permanent disability in MS is the underlying neurodegeneration, which has so far evaded any satisfactory treatment. This leads to the development of the troublesome symptoms that greatly reduce 'quality of life' (Compston and Coles 2002; Bjartmar *et al.*, 2003). There is increasing evidence that cannabinoids, including endocannabinoid tone, can limit acute neurodegeneration in ischaemia/stroke, head trauma and associated excitotoxicity (Nagayama *et al.*, 1999; Panikashvilli *et al.*, 2001; van der Stelt *et al.*, 2001; Hansen *et al.*, 2002; Parmentier-Batteur *et al.*, 2002; Pryce *et al.*, 2003a). Although the pathological causes of chronic neurodegeneration such as in Alzheimer's disease, Huntington's disease, motor neuron diseases and MS are varied, there appears to be some commonality with nerve death effector pathways in both acute and chronic neurodegeneration. These appear to involve oxidative attack and glutamate exocitoxicity, which eventually lead to toxic (Ca^{2+}) ion imbalances and metabolic failure (Choi and Rothman, 1990; Koprowski *et al.*, 1993; Rosen *et al.*, 1993; Rossi *et al.*, 2000; Smith *et al.*, 2000, 2001; Werner *et al.*, 2001; Knoller *et al.*, 2002; Kalkers *et al.*, 2003; Kapoor *et al.*, 2003; Reisberg *et al.*, 2003). In contrast to stroke and trauma, where these elements are rapid and often catastrophic, in chronic neurodegeneration they accumulate more slowly and less aggressively and thus there is a greater window for therapeutic modulation.

During MS and EAE, inflammatory events rapidly generate a damaging microenviroment in which inflammation induces axonal transections and Wallerian degeneration in addition to demyelination (Trapp *et al.*, 1998; Compston and Coles, 2002; Bjartmar *et al.*, 2003; Filippi *et al.*, 2003). This creates an increasing burden on the neuronal circuitry through chronic demyelination and associated impaired neural transmission, loss of trophic support and nerve loss. Hyperexcited demyelinated axons are particularly vulnerable to damage and death (Smith *et al.*, 2001; Waxman, 2002, 2003). This may lead to a slow death cascade that accelerates as a 'slow burn-out', where nerves die and neural plasticity is exhausted, ultimately leading to progressive neurological dysfunction (Compston and Coles, 1999). Once set in motion, degeneration may progress independently of significant inflammation and occurs despite immunotherapy (Coles *et al.*, 1999; SPECTRIMS Study Group, 2001). It progresses at a remarkably steady rate in both primary and secondary MS once a certain level of disability is achieved (Confavreux *et al.*, 2000).

The cannabinoid system can regulate potential degenerative events at multiple levels within the vasculature and CNS, including antioxidant activity, inhibition of glutamate release and signalling, and in addition is negatively coupled with a number of calcium channels (Twitchell *et al.*, 1997; Hampson *et al.*, 1998, 2000; Parmentier-Battuer *et al.*, 2002; Pryce *et al.*, 2003a). Furthermore, cannabinoids can inhibit microglial migration and activation, which may be central to the maintenance of the neurodegenerative microenvironment (Waksman *et al.*, 1999; Sacerdote *et al.*, 2000; Arévalo-Martin *et al.*, 2003). While not all neuroprotective elements of cannabis and the endocannabinoids may be mediated by CB_1 stimulation, the actions of this receptor can act at many levels within the death cascade that leads to toxic ion influxes, cell metabolic failure and activation of death effector molecules. This would be consistent with the rapid neurodegeneration that occurs in CB_1-deficient mice after both excitotoxicity and, importantly, in an inflammatory model of MS (Parmentier-Battuer et al., 2002; Pryce et al., 2003a). Here CB_1-deficient animals demonstrate poor recovery from the effects of inflammatory attack and accumulate significant axonal loss. This also implicates a role for endocannabinoids in neuroprotection.

The nature of the endogenous neuroprotective endocannabinoid has yet to be definitively resolved and may involve more than one CB_1-mediated pathway, possibly dependent on the neural circuit involved. While in head trauma it has been suggested that 2-AG may mediate neuroprotection (Panikashvili et al., 2001), in other studies anandamide, which is elevated in stroke (Schabitz et al., 2002), was shown to be active (Sinor et al., 2000; Hansen et al., 2001; Milton, 2002). However, as both anandamide and 2-AG are elevated in chronic lesions during EAE (Baker et al., 2001), it may be that both participate in endogenous neuroprotective mechanisms.

Consistent with the increased neurodegeneration during EAE that was associated with the lack of CB_1 expression, exogenous CB_1 agonism was also neuroprotective against inflammation-induced neurodegeneration (Pryce et al., 2003a, unpublished observations). This was evident in autoimmune uveitis in the eye (Pryce et al., 2003a) and during chronic relapsing EAE, using doses of cannabinoids that were not overtly immunosuppressive and therefore did not prevent the development of relapsing disease but significantly slowed the accumulation of deficits due to inflammatory attack (unpublished observations). As CB_1 receptor stimulation mediates these effects it is not surprising that THC can be shown to exhibit neuroprotective effects during experimental autoimmune disease (Pryce et al., 2003a).

Additional elements within cannabis offer a degree of neuroprotection. Notably, CBD exhibits antioxidant effects that are CB_1 independent and has shown neuroprotection against glutamate excitoxicity (Hampson et al., 1998, 2000).

The above indicates that in addition to symptom management, cannabis may offer the potential to slow disease progression. The fact that cannabis contains multiple compounds may exhibit advantages over a mononeuroprotective therapeutic agent. However, the capacity of cannabis or other cannabinoids to give benefit in MS will be dependent on sufficient neural circuitry being intact and the ability of the individual to tolerate neuroprotective levels of cannabinoids. Nevertheless, as not all these will be psychoactive it offers great potential.

As cannabinoids can regulate both excitory and inhibitory neural pathways, the outcome will be dependent on the location of CB_1 within that circuitry and could even enhance symptoms or neuronal effects (Clement *et al.*, 2003). At least in experimental MS models, studies indicate that cannabis may be beneficial at multiple levels of the disease process. Time will tell how this translates in human studies.

Acknowledgements

D Baker is a Senior Research Fellow of the Multiple Sclerosis Society of Great Britain and Northern Ireland.

References

Achiron A, Miron S, Lavie V, Margalit R, Biegon A (2000). Dexanabinol (HU-211) effect on experimental autoimmune encephalomyelitis: implications for the treatment of acute relapses of multiple sclerosis. *J Neuroimmunol* 102: 26–31.

Alusi S H, Worthington J, Glickman S, Bain P G (2001). A study of tremor in multiple sclerosis. *Brain* 124: 720–730.

Arévalo-Martin A, Vela J M, Molina-Holgado E, Borrell J, Guaza C (2003). Therapeutic action of cannabinoids in a murine model of multiple sclerosis. *J Neurosci* 23: 2511–2516.

Baker D, Pryce G (2004). The potential role of the endocannabinoid system in the control of multiple sclerosis. Medicinal Chemistry-Central Nervous System Agents (CMC-CNSA). Therapeutic implications of the endogenous cannabinoid system in the central nervous system, in press.

Baker D, Pryce G, Croxford J L *et al.* (2000). Cannabinoids control spasticity and tremor in a multiple sclerosis model. *Nature* 404: 84–87.

Baker D, Pryce G, Croxford J L *et al.* (2001). Endocannabinoids control spasticity in a multiple sclerosis model. *FASEB J* 15: 300–302.

Baker D, Pryce G, Giovannoni G, Thompson A J (2003). Therapeutic potential of cannabis. *Lancet Neurol* 2: 291–298.

Barnes M P, Kent R M, Semlyen J K, McMullen K M (2003). Spasticity in multiple sclerosis. *Neurorehabil Neural Repair* 17: 66–70.

Beltramo M, Stella N, Calignano A, Lin S Y, Makriyannis A, Piomelli D (1997). Functional role of high-affinity anandamide transport, as revealed by selective inhibition. *Science* 277: 1094–1097.

Berdyshev E V (2000). Cannabinoid receptors and the regulation of immune response. *Chem Phys Lipids* 108: 169–190.

Bisogno T, Hanus L, De Petrocellis L *et al.* (2001). Molecular targets for cannabidiol and its synthetic analogues: effect on vanilloid VR1 receptors and on the cellular uptake and enzymatic hydrolysis of anandamide. *Br J Pharmacol* 134: 845–852.

Bjartmar C, Wujek J R, Trapp B D (2003). Axonal loss in the pathology of MS: consequences for understanding the progressive phase of the disease. *J Neurol Sci* 206: 165–171.

Boger D L, Sato H, Lerner A E *et al.* (2000). Exceptionally potent inhibitors of fatty acid amide hydrolase: the enzyme responsible for degradation of endogenous oleamide and anandamide. *Proc Natl Acad Sci USA* 97: 5044–5049.

Bolton C, Paul C (1997). MK-801 limits neurovascular dysfunction during experimental allergic encephalomyelitis. *J Pharmacol Exp Ther* 282: 397–402.

Bolton C, O'Neill J K, Allen S J, Baker D (1997). Regulation of chronic relapsing experimental allergic encephalomyelitis by endogenous and exogenous glucocorticoids. *Int Arch Allergy Immunol* 114: 74–80.

Bornheim L M, Kim K Y, Li J, Perotti B Y, Benet L Z (1995). Effect of cannabidiol pretreatment on the kinetics of tetrahydrocannabinol metabolites in mouse brain. *Drug Metab Dispos* 23: 825–831.

Brady C M, Das Gupta R, Wiseman O J, Dalton C M, Berkley K J, Fowler C J (2002). The effects of cannabis based medicinal extracts on lower urinary tract dysfunction in advanced multiple sclerosis: preliminary results. *J Neurol Neurosurg Psychiatry* 72: 139.

Bredt B M, Higuera-Alhino D, Shade S B, Hebert S J, McCune J M, Abrams D I (2002). Short-term effects of cannabinoids on immune phenotype and function in HIV-1-infected patients. *J Clin Pharmacol* 42 (Suppl): 82S–89S.

Bridges D, Rice A S, Egertova M, Elphick M R, Winter J, Michael G J (2003). Localisation of cannabinoid receptor 1 in rat dorsal root ganglion using in situ hybridisation and immunohistochemistry. *Neuroscience* 119: 803–812.

Brooks J W, Pryce G, Bisogno T *et al.* (2002). Arvanil-induced inhibition of spasticity and persistent pain: evidence for therapeutic sites of action different from the vanilloid VR1 receptor and cannabinoid CB(1)/CB(2) receptors. *Eur J Pharmacol* 439: 83–92.

Buckley N E, McCoy K L, Mezey E *et al.* (2000). Immunomodulation by cannabinoids is absent in mice deficient for the cannabinoid CB(2) receptor. *Eur J Pharmacol* 396: 141–149.

Choi D, Rothman S M (1990). The role of glutamate neurotoxicity in hypoxic-ischemic neuronal death. *Annu Rev Neurosci* 13: 171–182.

Clement A B, Hawkins E G, Lichtman A H, Cravatt B F (2003). Increased seizure susceptibility and proconvulsant activity of anandamide in mice lacking fatty acid amide hydrolase. *J Neurosci* 23: 3916–3923.

Coles A J, Wing M G, Molyneux P *et al.* (1999). Monoclonal antibody treatment exposes three mechanisms underlying the clinical course of multiple sclerosis. *Ann Neurol* 46: 296–304.

Compston A, Coles A (2002). Multiple sclerosis. *Lancet* 359: 1221–1231.

Confavreux C, Vukusic S, Moreau T, Adeleine, P (2000). Relapses and progression of disability in multiple sclerosis. *N Engl J Med* 343: 1430–1438.

Consroe P, Musty R, Rein J, Tillery W, Pertwee R (1997). The perceived effects of smoked cannabis on patients with multiple sclerosis. *Eur Neurol* 38: 44–48.

Cravatt B F, Lichtman A H (2002). The enzymatic inactivation of the fatty acid amide class of signaling lipids. *Chem Phys Lipids* 121: 135–148.

Croxford J L, Miller S D (2003). Immunoregulation of a viral model of multiple sclerosis using the synthetic cannabinoid R(+)WIN55,212. *J Clin Invest* 111: 1231–1240.

Croxford J L, Olson J K, Miller S D (2002). Epitope spreading and molecular mimicry as triggers of autoimmunity in the Theiler's virus-induced demyelinating disease model of multiple sclerosis. *Autoimmunol Rev* 1: 251–260.

Dal Canto M C, Kim B S, Miller S D, Melvold R W (1996). Theiler's murine encephalomyelitis virus (TMEV)-induced demyelination: a model for human multiple sclerosis. *Methods* 10: 453–461.

Day T A, Rakhshan F, Deutsch D G, Barker E L (2001). Role of fatty acid amide hydrolase in the transport of the endogenous cannabinoid anandamide. *Mol Pharmacol* 59: 1369–1375.

De Petrocellis L, Bisogno T, Davis J B, Pertwee R G, Di Marzo V (2000). Overlap between the ligand recognition properties of the anandamide transporter and the VR1 vanilloid receptor: inhibitors of anandamide uptake with negligible capsaicin-like activity. *FEBS Lett* 483: 52–56.

Deutsch D G, Glaser S T, Howell J M *et al.* (2001). The cellular uptake of anandamide is coupled to its breakdown by fatty-acid amide hydrolase. *J Biol Chem* 276: 6967–6973.

Deutsch D G, Ueda N, Yamamoto S (2002). The fatty acid amide hydrolase (FAAH). *Prostaglandins Leukot Essent Fatty Acids* 66: 201–210.

Di S, Malcher-Lopes R, Halmos K C, Tasker J G (2003). Nongenomic glucocorticoid inhibition via endocannabinoid release in the hypothalamus: a fast feedback mechanism. *J Neurosci* 23: 4850–4857.

Di Marzo V, Hill M P, Bisogno T, Crossman A R, Brotchie J M (2000). Enhanced levels of endogenous cannabinoids in the globus pallidus are associated with a reduction in movement in an animal model of Parkinson's disease. *FASEB J* 14: 1432–1438.

Di Marzo V, Goparaju S K, Wang L *et al.* (2001). Leptin-regulated endocannabinoids are involved in maintaining food intake. *Nature* 410: 822–825.

Dinh T P, Freund T F, Piomelli D (2002). A role for monoglyceride lipase in 2-arachidonoylglycerol inactivation. *Chem Phys Lipids* 121: 149–158.

Egertova M, Cravatt B F, Elphick M R (2003). Comparative analysis of fatty acid amide hydrolase and cb(1) cannabinoid receptor expression in the mouse brain: evidence of a widespread role for fatty acid amide hydrolase in regulation of endocannabinoid signaling. *Neuroscience* 119: 481–496.

Felder C C, Nielsen A, Briley E M *et al.* (1996). Isolation and measurement of the endogenous cannabinoid receptor agonist, anandamide, in brain and peripheral tissues of human and rat. *FEBS Lett* 16(393): 231–235.

Filippi M, Bozzali M, Rovaris M *et al.* (2003). Evidence for widespread axonal damage at the earliest clinical stage of multiple sclerosis. *Brain* 126: 433–437.

Fowler C J (2003). Plant-derived, synthetic and endogenous cannabinoids as neuroprotective agents. Non-psychoactive cannabinoids, 'entourage' compounds and inhibitors of N-acyl ethanolamine breakdown as therapeutic strategies to avoid pyschotropic effects. *Brain Res Brain Res Rev* 41: 26–43.

Fox P, Thompson A, Zajicek J (2001). A multicentre randomised controlled trial of cannabinoids in multiple sclerosis. *J Neurol Sci* 187: S453.

Freund T F, Katona I, Piomelli D (2003). Role of endogenous cannabinoids in synaptic signaling. *Physiol Rev* 83: 1017–1066.

Giuffrida A, Parsons L H, Kerr T M, Rodriguez de Fonseca F, Navarro M, Piomelli D (1999). Dopamine activation of endogenous cannabinoid signaling in dorsal striatum. *Nat Neurosci* 2: 358–363.

Giuffrida A, Rodriguez de Fonseca F, Nava F, Loubet-Lescoulie P, Piomelli D (2000). Elevated circulating levels of anandamide after administration of the transport inhibitor, AM404. *Eur J Pharmacol* 408: 161–168.

Glaser S T, Abumrad N A, Fatade F, Kaczocha M, Studholme K M, Deutsch D G (2003). Evidence against the presence of an anandamide transporter. *Proc Natl Acad Sci USA* 100: 4269–4274.

GW Pharmaceuticals (2002). GW announces positive results from each of four phase three clinical trials. http://www.gwpharm.com/news_pres_05_nov_02.htm (accessed 5 November 2002).

Hampson A J, Grimaldi M, Axelrod J, Wink D (1998). Cannabidiol and (–)Δ^9-tetrahydrocannabinol are neuroprotective antioxidants. *Proc Natl Acad Sci USA* 95: 8268–8273.

Hampson A J, Grimaldi M, Lolic M, Wink D, Rosenthal R, Axelrod J (2000). Neuroprotective antioxidants from marijuana. *Ann N Y Acad Sci* 899: 274–282.

Hansen H H, Schmid P C, Bittigau P *et al.* (2001). Anandamide, but not 2-arachidonoylglycerol accumulates during in vivo neurodegeneration. *J Neurochem* 78: 1415–1427.

Hansen H H, Azcoitia I, Pons S *et al.* (2002). Blockade of cannabinoid CB(1) receptor function protects against in vivo disseminating brain damage following NMDA-induced excitotoxicity. *J Neurochem* 82: 154–158.

Herring A C, Kaminski N E (1999). Cannabinol-mediated inhibition of nuclear factor-kappaB, cAMP response element-binding protein, and interleukin-2 secretion by activated thymocytes. *J Pharmacol Exp Ther* 291: 1156–1163.

Herring A C, Faubert Kaplan B L, Kaminski N E (2001). Modulation of CREB and NF-kappaB signal transduction by cannabinol in activated thymocytes. *Cell Signal* 13: 241–250.

Hillard C J, Jarrahian A (2000). The movement of N-arachidonoylethanolamine (anandamide) across cellular membranes. *Chem Phys Lipids* 108: 123–134.

Hogestatt E D, Zygmunt P M (2002). Cardiovascular pharmacology of anandamide. *Prostaglandins Leukot Essent Fatty Acids* 66: 343–351.

House of Lords Select Committee on Science and Technology (1998) *Cannabis: The Scientific and Medical Evidence*. The House of Lords Session 1997–8, 9th report. London: Stationery Office.

Howlett A C, Barth F, Bonner T I *et al.* (2002). International Union of Pharmacology. XXVII. Classification of cannabinoid receptors. *Pharmacol Rev* 54: 161–202.

Hurst D P, Lynch D L, Barnett-Norris J *et al.* (2002). N-(Piperidin-1-yl)-5-(4-chlorophenyl)-1-(2,4-dichlorophenyl)-4-methyl-1H-pyrazole-3-carboxamide (SR141716A) interaction with LYS 3.28(192) is crucial for its inverse agonism at the cannabinoid CB1 receptor. *Mol Pharmacol* 62: 1274–1287.

Jacobsson S O, Fowler C J (2001). Characterization of palmitoylethanolamide transport in mouse neuro-2a neuroblastoma and rat RBL-2H3 basophilic leukaemia cells: comparison with anandamide. *Br J Pharmacol* 132: 1743–1754.

Jarrahian A, Manna S, Edgemond W S, Campbell W B, Hillard C J (2000). Structure-activity relationships among N-arachidonylethanolamine (anandamide) head group analogues for the anandamide transporter. *J Neurochem* 74: 2597–2606.

Kalkers N F, Barkhof F, Bergers E, van Schijndel R, Polman C H (2002). The effect of the neuroprotective agent riluzole on MRI parameters in primary progressive multiple sclerosis: a pilot study. *Multiple Sclerosis* 8: 532–533.

Kapoor R, Davies M, Blaker P A, Hall S M, Smith K J (2003). Blockers of sodium and calcium entry protect axons from nitric oxide-mediated degeneration. *Ann Neurol* 53: 174–180.

Killestein J, Hoogervorst E L, Reif M *et al.* (2002). Safety, tolerability, and efficacy of orally administered cannabinoids in MS. *Neurology* 58: 1404–1407.

Killestein J, Hoogervorst E L, Reif M *et al.* (2003) Immunomodulatory effects of orally administered cannabinoids in multiple sclerosis. *J Neuroimmunol* 137: 140–143.

Kim J, Isokawa M, Ledent C, Alger B E (2002). Activation of muscarinic acetylcholine receptors enhances the release of endogenous cannabinoids in the hippocampus. *J Neurosci* 22: 10182–10191.

Klein T W, Newton C A, Friedman H (2001). Cannabinoids and the immune system. *Pain Res Manag* 6: 95–101.

Knoller N, Levi L, Shoshan I *et al.* (2002). Dexanabinol (HU-211) in the treatment of severe closed head injury: a randomized, placebo-controlled, phase II clinical trial. *Crit Care Med* 30: 548–554.

Koprowski H, Zheng Y M, Heber-Katz E *et al.* In vivo expression of inducible nitric oxide synthase in experimentally induced neurologic diseases. *Proc Natl Acad Sci USA* 90: 3024–3027.

Kreitzer A C, Regehr W G (2001). Retrograde inhibition of presynaptic calcium influx by endogenous cannabinoids at excitatory synapses onto Purkinje cells. *Neuron* 29: 717–727.

Lastres-Becker I, Fezza F, Cebeira M *et al.* (2001). Changes in endocannabinoid transmission in the basal ganglia in a rat model of Huntington's disease. *Neuroreport* 12: 2125–2129.

Leweke F M, Giuffrida A, Wurster U, Emrich H M, Piomelli D (1999). Elevated endogenous cannabinoids in schizophrenia. *Neuroreport* 10: 1665–1669.

Li X, Kaminski N E, Fischer L J (2001). Examination of the immunosuppressive effect of delta9-tetrahydrocannabinol in streptozotocin-induced autoimmune diabetes. *Int Immunopharmacol* 1: 699–712.

Lichtman A H, Poklis J L, Poklis A, Wilson D M, Martin B R (2001). The pharmacological activity of inhalation exposure to marijuana smoke in mice. *Drug Alcohol Depend* 63: 107–116.

Lichtman A H, Hawkins E G, Griffin G, Cravatt B F (2002). Pharmacological activity of fatty acid amides is regulated, but not mediated, by fatty acid amide hydrolase in vivo. *J Pharmacol Exp Ther* 302: 73–79.

Lopez-Rodriguez M L, Viso A, Ortega-Gutierrez S *et al.* (2001). Design, synthesis and biological evaluation of novel arachidonic acid derivatives as highly potent and selective endocannabinoid transporter inhibitors. *Med Chem* 44: 4505–4508.

Lyman W D, Sonett J R, Brosnan C F, Elkin R, Bornstein, M B (1989). Delta 9-tetrahydrocannabinol: a novel treatment for experimental autoimmune encephalomyelitis. *J Neuroimmunol* 23: 73–81.

Maccarrone M, Finazzi-Agro A (2002). Endocannabinoids and their actions. *Vitam Horm* 65: 225–255.

McKallip R J, Lombard C, Martin B R, Nagarkatti M, Nagarkatti P S (2002). Delta(9)-tetrahydrocannabinol-induced apoptosis in the thymus and spleen as a mechanism of immunosuppression in vitro and in vivo. *J Pharmacol Exp Ther* 302: 451–465.

Maejima T, Hashimoto K, Yoshida T, Aiba A, Kano M (2001). Presynaptic inhibition caused by retrograde signal from metabotropic glutamate to cannabinoid receptors. *Neuron* 31: 463–475.

Malfait A M, Gallily R, Sumariwalla P F *et al.* (2000). The nonpsychoactive cannabis constituent cannabidiol is an oral anti-arthritic therapeutic in murine collagen-induced arthritis. *Proc Natl Acad Sci USA* 97: 9561–9566.

Martin R S, Luong L A, Welsh N J, Eglen R M, Martin G R, MacLennan S J (2000). Effects of cannabinoid receptor agonists on neuronally-evoked contractions of urinary bladder tissues isolated from rat, mouse, pig, dog, monkey and human. *Br J Pharmacol* 129: 1707–1715.

Mechoulam R, Gaoni Y (1967). The absolute configuration of delta-1-tetrahydrocannabinol, the major active constituent of hashish. *Tetrahedron Lett* 12: 1109–1111.

Miller D H, Khan O A, Sheremata W A *et al.* (2003) A controlled trial of natalizumab for relapsing multiple sclerosis. *N Engl J Med* 348: 15–23.

Milton N G (2002). Anandamide and noladin ether prevent neurotoxicity of the human amyloid-beta peptide. *Neurosci Lett* 332: 127–130.

Nagayama T, Sinor A D, Simon R P *et al.* (1999). Cannabinoids and neuroprotection in global and focal cerebral ischemia and in neuronal cultures. *J Neurosci* 19: 2987–2995.

Noe S N, Newton C, Widen R, Friedman H, Klein T W (2001). Modulation of CB1 mRNA upon activation of murine splenocytes. *Adv Exp Med Biol* 493: 215–221.

Nogueron M I, Porgilsson B, Schneider W E, Stucky C L, Hillard C J (2001). Cannabinoid receptor agonists inhibit depolarization-induced calcium influx in cerebellar granule neurons. *J Neurochem* 79: 371–381.

Notcutt W, Price M, Sansom C, Simmons S, Phillips C (2002). Medicinal cannabis extract in chronic pain: overall results of 29 "N of 1" studies (CBME-1). *Proceedings, 2002 Symposium on the Cannabinoids.* Burlington, VT: International Cannabinoid Research Society: 55. (http://www.cannabinoidsociety.org/progab2.pdf)

Offertaler L, Mo F M, Batkai S *et al.* (2003). Selective ligands and cellular effectors of a G protein-coupled endothelial cannabinoid receptor. *Mol Pharmacol* 63: 699–705.

Ortar G, Ligresti A, De Petrocellis L, Morera E, Di Marzo V (2003). Novel selective and metabolically stable inhibitors of anandamide cellular uptake. *Biochem Pharmacol* 65: 1473–1481.

Pacifici R, Zuccaro P, Pichini S *et al.* (2003). Modulation of the immune system in cannabis users. *JAMA* 289: 1929–1931.

Panikashvili D, Simeonidou C, Ben-Shabat S *et al.* (2001). An endogenous cannabinoid (2-AG) is neuroprotective after brain injury. *Nature* 413: 527–531.

Parmentier-Batteur S, Jin K, Mao X O, Xie L, Greenberg D A (2002). Increased severity of stroke in CB1 cannabinoid receptor knock-out mice. *J Neurosci* 22: 9771–9775.

Parolaro D (1999). Presence and functional regulation of cannabinoid receptors in immune cells. *Life Sci* 65: 637–644.

Parolaro D, Massi P, Rubino T, Monti E (2002). Endocannabinoids in the immune system and cancer. *Prostaglandins Leukot Essent Fatty Acids* 66: 319–332.

Pertwee R G (1974). Tolerance to the effect of delta1-tetrahydrocannabinol on corticosterone levels in mouse plasma produced by repeated administration of cannabis extract or delta1-tetrahydrocannabinol. *Br J Pharmacol* 51: 391–397

Pertwee R G (1999). Pharmacology of cannabinoid receptor ligands. *Curr Med Chem* 6: 635–664.

Pertwee R G (2002). Cannabinoids and multiple sclerosis. *Pharmacol Ther* 95: 165–174.

Pryce G, Ahmed Z, Hankey D J R *et al.* (2003a). Cannabinoids inhibit neurodegeneration in models of multiple sclerosis. *Brain* 126: 2191–2202.

Pryce G, Giovannoni G, Baker D (2003b). Mifepristone or inhibition of 11beta-hydroxylase activity potentiates the sedating effects of the cannabinoid receptor-1 agonist delta(9)-tetrahydrocannabinol in mice. *Neurosci Lett* 341: 164–166.

Rakhshan F, Day T A, Blakely R D, Barker E L (2000). Carrier-mediated uptake of the endogenous cannabinoid anandamide in RBL-2H3 cells. *J Pharmacol Exp Ther* 292: 960–967.

Ralevic V, Kendall D A, Jerman J C, Middlemiss D N, Smart D (2001). Cannabinoid activation of recombinant and endogenous vanilloid receptors. *Eur J Pharmacol* 424: 211–219.

Reisberg B, Doody R, Stoffler A *et al.* (2003). Memantine in moderate-to-severe Alzheimer's disease. *N Engl J Med* 348: 1333–1341.

Romero J, Hillard C J, Calero M, Rabano A (2002). Fatty acid amide hydrolase localization in the human central nervous system: an immunohistochemical study. *Brain Res Mol Brain Res* 30(100): 85–93.

Rosen D, Siddique T, Patterson D *et al.* (1993). Mutations in Cu/Zn superoxide dismutase gene are associated with familial amyotrophic lateral sclerosis. *Nature* 362: 59–62.

Rossi D J, Oshima T, Attwell D (2000). Glutamate release in severe brain ischaemia is mainly by reversed uptake. *Nature* 403: 316–321.

Sacerdote P, Massi P, Panerai A E, Parolaro D (2000). In vivo and in vitro treatment with the synthetic cannabinoid CP55,940 decreases the in vitro migration of macrophages in the rat: involvement of both CB1 and CB2 receptors. *J Neuroimmunol* 109: 155–163.

Sancho R, Calzado M A, Di Marzo V, Appendino G, Munoz E (2003). Anandamide inhibits nuclear factor-kappaB activation through a cannabinoid receptor-independent pathway. *Mol Pharmacol* 63: 429–438.

Sanna V, Di Giacomo A, La Cava A *et al.* (2003). Leptin surge precedes onset of autoimmune encephalomyelitis and correlates with development of pathogenic T cell responses. *J Clin Invest* 111: 241–250.

Schabitz W R, Giuffrida A, Berger C *et al.* (2002). Release of fatty acid amides in a patient with hemispheric stroke: a microdialysis study. *Stroke* 33: 2112–2114.

Schnelle M, Grotenhermen F, Reif M, Gorter R W (1999). Results of a standardized survey on the medical use of cannabis products in the German-speaking area. *Forsch Komplementärmed* 6 (Suppl 3): 28–36.

Schon F, Hart P, Hodgson T R, Williamson E M, Kennard C, Ruprah M (1999). Suppression of pendular nystagmus by cannabis in a patient with multiple sclerosis. *Neurology* 53: 2209–2210.

Sim-Selley L J, Martin B R (2002). Effect of chronic administration of R-(+)-[2,3-Dihydro-5-methyl-3-[(morpholinyl)methyl]pyrrolo[1,2,3-de]-1,4-benzoxazinyl]-(1-naphthalenyl) methanonemesylate (WIN55,212-2) or delta(9)-tetrahydrocannabinol on cannabinoid receptor adaptation in mice. *J Pharmacol Exp Ther* 303: 36–44.

Sinor AD, Irvin S M, Greenberg D A (2000). Endocannabinoids protect cerebral cortical neurons from in vitro ischemia in rats. *Neurosci Lett* 278: 157–160.

Smith K J, Kapoor R, Hall S M, Davies M (2001). Electrically active axons degenerate when exposed to nitric oxide. *Ann Neurol* 49: 470–476.

Smith T, Groom A, Zhu B. Turski L (2000). Autoimmune encephalomyelitis ameliorated by AMPA antagonists. *Nat Med* 6: 62–66.

SPECTRIMS Study Group (2001). Secondary progressive efficacy clinical trial of recombinant interferon-beta-1a in MS. *Neurology* 56: 1496–1504.

Sugiura T, Kobayashi Y, Oka S, Waku K (2002). Biosynthesis and degradation of anandamide and 2-arachidonoylglycerol and their possible physiological significance. *Prostaglandins Leukot Essent Fatty Acids* 66: 173–192.

t'Hart B, Amor S (2003). The use of animal models to investigate the pathogenesis of neuroinflammatory disorders of the central nervous system. *Curr Opin Neurol* 16: 375–384.

Trapp B D, Peterson J, Ransohoff R M, Rudick R, Mork S, Bo L (1998). Axonal transection in the lesions of multiple sclerosis. *N Engl J Med* 338: 278–285.

Twitchell W, Brown S, Mackie K (1997). Cannabinoids inhibit N- and P/Q-type calcium channels in cultured rat hippocampal neurons. *J Neurophysiol* 78: 43–50.

van der Stelt M, Veldhuis W B, van Haaften G W *et al.* (2001) Exogenous anandamide protects rat brain against acute neuronal injury in vivo. *J Neurosci* 21: 8765–8771.

Vaney C, Jobin P, Tscopp F, Heinzel M, Schnelle M (2002). Efficacy, safety and tolerability of an orally administered cannabis extract in the treatment of spasticity in patients with multiple sclerosis. *Proceedings, 2002 Symposium on the Cannabinoids*. Burlington, VT: International Cannabinoid Research Society: 57. (http://www.cannabinoidsociety.org/progab2.pdf)

van Noort J M, Bajramovic J J, Plomp A C, van Stipdonk M J (2000). Mistaken self, a novel model that links microbial infections with myelin-directed autoimmunity in multiple sclerosis. *J Neuroimmunol* 105: 46–57.

Wade D T, Robson P, House H, Makela P, Aram J (2003). A preliminary controlled study to determine whether whole-plant cannabis extracts can improve intractable neurogenic symptoms. *Clin Rehabil* 17: 21–29.

Waksman Y, Olson J M, Carlisle S J, Cabral G A (1999). The central cannabinoid receptor (CB1) mediates inhibition of nitric oxide production by rat microglial cells. *J Pharmacol Exp Ther* 288: 1357–1366.

Walker J, Huang S (2002). Cannabinoid analgesia. *Pharmacol Ther* 95: 127–135.

Watson C M, Davison A N, Baker D, O'Neill J K, Turk J L (1991). Suppression of demyelination by mitoxantrone. *Int J Immunopharmacol* 13: 923–930.

Waxman S G (2002). Ion channels and neuronal dysfunction in multiple sclerosis. *Arch Neurol* 59: 1377–1380.

Waxman S G (2003). Nitric oxide and the axonal death cascade. *Ann Neurol* 53: 150–153.

Wekerle H, Hohlfeld R (2003). Molecular mimicry in multiple sclerosis. *N Engl J Med* 349: 185–186.

Werner P, Pitt D, Raine C S. Multiple sclerosis: altered glutamate homeostasis in lesions correlates with oligodendrocyte and axonal damage. *Ann Neurol* 50: 169–180.

Wiendl H, Hohlfeld R (2002). Therapeutic approaches in multiple sclerosis: lessons from failed and interrupted treatment trials. *BioDrugs* 16: 183–200.

Wilkinson J, Whalley B J, Baker D *et al.* (2003). Medicinal cannabis: the whole plant extract, or isolated delta^9-tetrahydrocannabinol? *J Pharm Pharmacol* 55: 1687–1694.

Williamson E M (2001). Synergy and other interactions in phytomedicines. *Phytomedicine* 8: 401–440

Wilson R I, Nicoll R A (2001). Endogenous cannabinoids mediate retrograde signalling at hippocampal synapses. *Nature* 410: 588–592.

Wilson R I, Nicoll R A (2002). Endocannabinoid signaling in the brain. *Science* 296: 678–682.

Wirguin I, Mechoulam R, Breuer A, Schezen E, Weidenfeld J, Brenner T (1994). Suppression of experimental autoimmune encephalomyelitis by cannabinoids. *Immunopharmacology* 28: 209–214.

Yuan M, Kiertscher S M, Cheng Q, Zoumalan R, Tashkin D P, Roth M D (2002). Delta 9-tetrahydrocannabinol regulates Th1/Th2 cytokine balance in activated human T cells. *J Neuroimmunol* 133: 124–131.

Zhang J, Hoffert C, Vu H K, Groblewski T, Ahmad S, O'Donnell D (2003). Induction of CB2 receptor expression in the rat spinal cord of neuropathic but not inflammatory chronic pain models. *Eur J Neurosci* 17: 2750–2754.

Zhu L X, Sharma S, Stolina M *et al.* (2000). Delta-9-tetrahydrocannabinol inhibits antitumor immunity by a CB2 receptor-mediated, cytokine-dependent pathway. *J Immunol* 165: 373–380.

Zuardi A W, Shirakawa I, Finkelfarb E, Karniol I G (1982). Action of cannabidiol on the anxiety and other effects produced by delta-9-THC in normal subjects. *Psychopharmacology* 76: 245–250.

7

Natural cannabinoids: interactions and effects

Richard E Musty

The distribution of naturally occurring cannabinoids is known to vary according to geographical source and derivation from different landraces. Within this range, most New World varieties contain predominantly THC as the principal cannabinoid. The proportions of delta^9-tetrahydrocannabinol (Δ^9-THC) and cannabidiol (CBD) are the most important variables that determine the activity of different strains of cannabis. In an analysis of samples, Turner (1985) reported differences in the THC:CBD ratio ranging from 211:1 to 22.3:1. These large variations have been shown to produce different pharmacological effects, thus the ratio of THC:CBD is a very important factor to consider when attempting to understand the potential therapeutic effects of cannabis, as well as potential adverse or side-effects that may occur. In addition to these two principal cannabinoids, there are several others present in the plant, usually at lower concentrations. These include cannabinol (CBN), cannabichromene (CBC), cannabigerol (CBG) and tetrahydrocannabivarin (THCV). Early experiments demonstrated that when CBD was combined with THC there were interactive effects as reported by Carlini *et al.* (1973).

In addition to the cannabinoid compounds present in the plant, there are also other non-cannabinoid compounds (e.g. flavonoids and terpenoids), which may enhance cannabinoid activity by acting with beneficial synergy or by mitigating the side-effects of dominant active ingredients (McPartland and Russo, 2001). Some of these compounds and their interactions with cannabinoid receptors are discussed in this chapter; for further information see Chapters 2, 4 and 9. In an overview, Meschler and Howlett (1999) discussed mechanisms by which terpenoids could modulate THC activity. Theories put forward were that they might:

• bind to cannabinoid receptors
• modulate the affinity of THC for its own receptor by sequestering THC

- act by perturbing annular lipids surrounding the receptor
- act by increasing the fluidity of neuronal membranes.

It was also postulated that terpenoids may:

- alter the signalling cascade by remodelling G proteins
- alter THC pharmacokinetics by altering the blood–brain barrier (BBB)
- act on other receptors and neurotransmitters
- act as serotonin uptake inhibitors
- enhance norepinephrine activity
- increase dopamine activity
- augment GABA.

The concept of an 'entourage effect', that is, the ability of non-receptor-binding endocannabinoid precursors to influence clinical effects (Ben-Shabat *et al.*, 1998; Mechoulam and Ben-Shabat, 1999), seems to apply equally well to phytocannabinoids beyond THC and CBD, as well as to their terpenoid cousins.

Monoterpenes, some of which are abundant in cannabis resin, have been suggested to:

- inhibit cholesterol synthesis
- promote hepatic enzyme activity to detoxify carcinogens
- stimulate apoptosis in cells with damaged DNA
- inhibit protein phosphorylation implicated in malignant deterioration (Jones, 1999).

Cannabis produces approximately 20 flavonoid-type compounds (Turner *et al.*, 1980) and up to 1% of the leaf mass is attributed to their content (Paris *et al.*, 1976). Flavonoids may modulate the pharmacokinetic activity of THC via a mechanism that is shared by CBD, which is the inhibition of P450 3A11 and P450 3A4 enzymes. P450-suppressing compounds serve as chemoprotective agents by shielding healthy cells from the activation of benzo[α]pyrene and aflatoxin B1 (Offord *et al.*, 1997), which are two procarcinogens potentially located in cannabis smoke (McPartland and Pruitt, 1997). Other terpenoids present to a greater or lesser extent in cannabis are limonene, pulegone, 1,8-cineole, α-terpineol (plus terpinen-4-ol and 4-terpineol) and *p*-cymene. These are cited as having immunomodulating effects, CNS effects relevant to Alzheimer's disease, antifungal effects, antibacterial effects and antioxidant properties respectively (Carson and Tiley, 1995; Komori *et al.*, 1995; Raman *et al.*, 1995; Miyazawa *et al.*, 1997). These terpenoids may also interact and/or synergise with the cannabinoids, although not as much is known about their pharmacological interactions as is known about those of the terpenoids myrcene, β-caryophyllene, linalool and α-pinene and the flavonoids apigenin and quercetin.

Background references

The pharmacological interactions between CBD and THC have been studied in rabbits, rats and mice by administering mixtures containing varying amounts of both substances. THC suppressed the nictitating membrane corneal reflex (Gayer Test) in rabbits, whereas CBD had no effect, even at high doses (Karniol and Carlini, 1973). When THC and CBD were combined in a ratio of 1:1, the dose of THC required to block the reflex to pressure was increased by approximately 30%, and by approximately 60% when the ratio was 1:4. It appeared from these results that increasing the amount of CBD in the combined material increased the effect of THC.

In a second test, THC alone induced catatonia in mice in a dose-dependent manner. CBD also produced catatonia, but the durations were very brief. When THC and CBD were administered simultaneously (2.5, 5.0 and 10.0 mg/kg) in a 1:1 ratio, the percentage decreases in catatonia were approximately 66%, 76% and 66% for each dose, respectively. These results suggested that the decrease in catatonia varied little across a range of combined doses.

In the hot plate test, 3-month-old mice were administered drugs (i.p.) in the following doses: THC (5 and 10 mg/kg), CBD (20 mg/kg), THC (5 mg/kg) + CBD (10 mg/kg), or THC (5 mg/kg) + CBD (20 mg/kg). THC produced significant analgesia at both 5 and 10 mg/kg, when compared with controls. Interestingly, at 5 mg/kg, analgesia occurred only at 30 minutes post injection, but at 10 mg/kg, analgesia was significant at 30, 60, 90 and 120 minutes post injection (all compared with controls). Irrespective of the combined doses of THC and CBD, CBD significantly potentiated the analgesic effects of THC. Although the effect was greater with the THC + CBD combination at the THC (5 mg/kg) plus CBD (20 mg/kg) dose level, these data suggested that the lower the THC:CBD ratio the greater the potentiation of analgesia (see the section on Pain below). Other models studied by this group were the 'climbing rope method', the rapid eye movement (REM) sleep deprivation and aggressiveness models, and the 'open field method'.

In the climbing rope test, a dose of 10 mg/kg Δ^9-THC impaired climbing performance; however CBD, although inactive *per se*, did potentiate Δ^9-THC effects. It was observed that doses of 10, 20 and 40 mg/kg CBD potentiated nearly 100% the impairing effects of 10 mg/kg Δ^9-THC on the climbing rope performance of the rats.

In the REM sleep deprivation/aggressiveness test a first dose of 10 mg/kg of Δ^9-THC induced strong aggressive behaviour in rats that had been stressed by REM sleep deprivation. Aggressive behaviour was still present after doubling the dose to 20 mg/kg. Twenty or 40 mg/kg doses of CBD or control solution were still inactive. Again, although inactive *per se*, CBD blocked aggressiveness-inducing properties of Δ^9-THC, and the authors concluded that CBD partially blocked Δ^9-THC-induced aggressiveness. In the 'open-field method' the researchers found that CBD did not alter acute Δ^9-THC-mediated defecation or ambulation, however it did block the chronic effects of Δ^9-THC.

In a drug discrimination task, rats were trained to run to one arm of a T-maze when administered THC and to the other arm when administered placebo (Zuardi *et al.*, 1981). When given CBD, the rats ran to the placebo arm, indicating that they could not discriminate CBD from placebo. When THC and CBD were administered together, rats ran to the placebo arm, indicating that the addition of CBD blocked the feeling of intoxication produced by THC alone, i.e. the ability to discriminate THC+CBD from a control injection (Zuardi *et al.*, 1981).

In normal volunteers Karniol *et al.* (1974) administered THC alone or THC and CBD in ratios of 2:1, 1:1 and 1:2 (p.o.). Heart rate was elevated with THC alone, but decreased as the ratios decreased. This same result was found in a time estimation study by estimating the passage of a minute and the rated degree of intoxication over it. Dalton *et al.* (1976), using smoked cannabis, found that the self-rated degree of intoxication or 'high' was decreased by the addition of CBD to the smoked material. These studies supported the view that CBD antagonised several of the pharmacological effects of THC, including the 'high' that is perceived as pleasant by some patients and dysphoric by others.

Some of the symptoms of dysphoria are dizziness, perceptions that one's heart is pounding and occasional feelings of panic. With regard to CBD alone, it is clear that this compound does not produce feelings of intoxication, nor does it have any degree of negative effect(s) in the studies reported above.

Finally, there is evidence that CBD effects are attributable to antagonism of CB_1 receptors *in vitro*. Petitet *et al.* (1998) in rat cerebellar homogenate and Thomas *et al.* (1998) in rat brain membrane assays both reported that CBD was an antagonist of the receptor in the micromolar range, suggesting that CBD had pharmacological effects and was an antagonist at the CB_1 receptor. The significance of these findings *in vivo* or with respect to natural phytocannabinoid extracts is unclear.

Another critical factor to consider is the ability of CBD to stimulate vanilloid receptors (VR1) with similar affinity to capsaicin, to inhibit uptake of the endocannabinoid anandamide (AEA) and to inhibit its hydrolysis weakly (Bisogno *et al.*, 2001).

Pain

Reports of cannabis-induced analgesia date back several millennia (Hall *et al.*, 1994; Russo, 2002). Studying the antinociceptive and anti-hyperalgesic roles of cannabinoids previously has been difficult due to the lack of identification and characterisation of receptors, and selective agonists and antagonists (Richardson *et al.*, 1998a). This situation changed in the early 1990s when the CB_1 and CB_2 receptor subtypes were cloned and found to be members of the seven-transmembrane (7-TM) G protein-coupled receptor family (Matsuda *et al.*, 1990; Munro *et al.*, 1993). Selective synthetic cannabinoids have been developed and endogenous ones have been discovered previous to and since then (Lemberger and Rowe, 1975; D'Ambra *et al.*, 1992; Hanus *et al.*, 1993; Mechoulam *et al.*, 1995; Sugiura *et al.*, 1995). These developments have resulted in the determination that activation of central CBD receptors produces antinociception (Yaksh, 1981; Herkenham *et al.*, 1991; Lichtman and Martin, 1991; Martin *et al.*, 1993, 1995, 1996; Hohmann *et al.*, 1995; Hohmann and Herkenham 1997; Richardson 1998b).

Tetrahydrocannabivarin (THCV) is a phytocannabinoid that may attain significant proportions in certain South African and South-East Asian cannabis strains. It is said to produce a faster and clearer 'high' than THC, with about 25% of the subjective psychoactivity (Hollister, 1974). This may prove to be a useful component in conditions such as breakthrough pain or spasm, and is undergoing additional investigation by GW Pharmaceuticals.

A terpenoid that has been cited as having analgesic activity is myrcene, specifically β-myrcene. This is the most abundant terpenoid produced by cannabis (Ross and ElSohly, 1996). It has been shown to have potent analgesic activity, acting at central sites antagonised by naloxone (Rao *et al.*, 1990), suggesting an opioid mechanism of action. This compound also works via a peripheral mechanism shared by CBD,

CBG and CBC, which is that of blocking inflammatory activity of prostaglandin E_2 (PGE_2) (Lorenzetti *et al.*, 1991).

Animal models

Few studies have examined the effects of extracts with a low THC:CBD ratio or experimentally varied pure THC and CBD mixtures. In an early study by Sofia and colleagues (1975), a comparison of the pain-relieving effects of Δ^9-THC were compared with those of a crude cannabis extract, cannabinol (CBN), cannabidiol (CBD), morphine sulfate and aspirin (all p.o.). The rat acetic acid-induced abdominal constriction test, the hot plate test and the Randall–Selitto paw pressure tests were used to determine potential analgesic effects.

Δ^9-THC and morphine were equipotent in all tests except for the 'elevating pain threshold' test in the uninflamed rat hind-paw, where morphine was significantly more potent. In terms of Δ^9-THC content, crude marijuana extract (CME) was approximately equipotent in the hot plate and the Randall–Selitto tests, but was three times more potent in the acetic acid abdominal constriction test. Conversely, CBN, like aspirin, was only effective in reducing abdominal constriction frequency in mice (being three times more potent than aspirin) and in raising the pain threshold of the inflamed hind-paw in the rat model (wherein it was shown to be equipotent with aspirin). CBD did not display a significant analgesic effect in any of the test systems used. The results of this investigation suggested that both Δ^9-THC and CME possess analgesic activity similar to that produced by morphine, while CBN appears to be non-analgesic at the doses used.

Bicher and Mechoulam (1968) found that Δ^9-THC and Δ^8-THC (i.p.) were approximately half as effective as morphine (s.c.) in three tests of analgesia used, those being the hot plate test, the abdominal constriction test and the rat tail flick test.

Human studies

In a recent review of the cannabinoid literature on pain, Walker *et al.* (2002) concluded that cannabinoids suppressed nociceptive neurotransmission, that synthetic agonists were as potent as morphine, and that there were direct effects on the spinal cord, the periphery and the brain. Particularly important is the finding that the pain-modulating mechanisms in the periqueductal grey matter of the brainstem are under endocannabinoid control (Walker *et al.*, 1999).

In a review of both human anecdotal and controlled studies by Musty (2002), pain relief was reported. Two double blind placebo-controlled studies were reviewed where THC was administered for cancer pain. THC was effective orally at doses of 15 and 20 mg in one study (Noyes *et al.*, 1975b), and in the second study, THC (20 mg) taken orally was equal in analgesia to 120 mg of codeine (Noyes *et al.*, 1975a). In a study of pain following extraction of unpacked molar teeth (Raft *et al.*, 1977), diazepam was more effective than placebo and intravenous THC at doses of 0.22 mg/kg or 0.44 mg/kg. Levonantradol (a synthetic analogue of THC) was effective in postoperative pain at doses of 1.5–3 mg i.m. (Jain *et al.*, 1981).

In a questionnaire study, Dunn and Davis (1974) reported that patients who smoked cannabis found relief from phantom limb pain, and in a single case report, Finnegan-Ling and Musty (1995) reported that THC administered orally was more effective than conventional pain medications, including opiates and non-steroidal anti-inflammatory drugs (NSAIDs).

Only one human case study, which used an extract containing known amounts of THC, CBD and CBN, has been published (Holdcroft *et al.*, 1997) prior to recent reports with sublingually administered extracts (see Chapters 9 and 10). The extract contained THC (5.75%), CBD (4.73%) and CBN (2.42%) and was administered orally to a volunteer patient with chronic abdominal pain associated with familial Mediterranean fever in a six-week randomised placebo-controlled study. Both normal use of morphine and escape use (dosing when an acute attack of pain occurs) were significantly reduced. A self-report on a visual analogue scale also demonstrated significant reductions in perception of pain following the use of this characterised extract.

Another study with known THC intake and very low CBD provided information on musculoskeletal pain relief in two patients with hereditary connective tissue diseases (Russo *et al.*, 2002). Both utilised National Insititute on Drug Abuse (NIDA) cannabis in the US Compassionate Use Investigational New Drug Program for many years with good pain control and no dose escalation. One male with nail–patella syndrome used 7 g of 3.75% THC daily, and another with multiple congenital cartilaginous exostoses required 9 g of 2.75% cannabis per day. Interestingly, neither noted any subjective associated intoxication, and neither ever experienced withdrawal symptoms (other than increased pain burden) during periods of inadequate supplies.

Anxiety

Linalool is a non-cyclic monoterpenoid that constitutes 5% or less of cannabis essential oil (Ross and ElSohly, 1996). Buchbauer *et al.* (1993) assayed the sedative effects of over 40 terpenoids upon inhalation by mice and found that linalool was the most powerful, reducing mouse motility by 37% after 1 hour's inhalation. Citronellol and α-terpineol, also present in cannabis, were also deeply sedating at low concentrations. Combinations of effects were found to be synergistic in their sedative effects, suggesting that these terpenoids might mitigate the anxiety produced by pure THC. It was also found that inhalation of the terpenoids, particularly limonene, with which cannabis essential oil is well endowed, provided antidepressant and immune-stimulating effects (Komori *et al.*, 1995).

Animal models

In a study by Musty (1984), mice (type C57Bl6J) were trained to avoid receiving shocks in a running wheel. Drugs administered were CBD, THC, diazepam (DZP) or saline control (SAL). As shown in Figure 7.1, CBD produced a dose-related decrease in the number of shocks received, which compared well with THC and DZP. Musty *et al.* (1985) also found that CBD increased 'licking for water' behaviour in the 'lick suppression test' in a concentration-dependent manner. This model involves rats being trained to lick from a water tube after 23 hours of water deprivation for 7 days. On test days each rat was placed in the test chamber for 20 minutes following an injection of either vehicle, CBD or DZP (i.p.), at varying doses. Each rat was allowed to drink water freely for 1 minute, after which the water spout was electrified to deliver a small shock to the tongue. For 9 minutes the number of punished licks were recorded. Significant reductions in punished licks were found for both drugs (Musty, 1984) (Figure 7.2), and equivalent effects were found with the classic anxiolytic drug DZP. To test the potential for greater potency, two analogues were also used: 2-pinyl-5-dimethylheptyl resorcinol (PR-DMH) and monomethyl cannabidiol (ME-CBD-2). ME-CBD-2 had anxiolytic activity but was less potent than CBD; PR-DMH had no anxiolytic properties and both were less potent than DZP.

For a different indication, it was also found that CBD produced a dose-dependent inhibition of the development of stress-induced ulcers in rats when compared with DZP (Musty, 1984), which produced an equivalent reduction in the number of stress-induced ulcers (Figure 7.3).

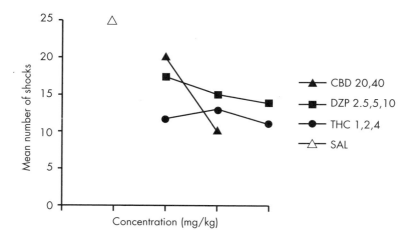

Figure 7.1 Mice (C57Bl6J) were trained to run in a running wheel which delivered a shock of 0.25 mA until the mouse ran and the wheel turned at least one-half revolution. Once this occurred, the shock was terminated for 20 s. If the mouse continued to run, each half revolution delayed the shock for 20 s. If the mouse remained motionless for 20 s the shock reoccurred. Separate groups of mice were injected i.p. with either the vehicle comprising Tween 80 (0.6%) + saline (SAL) or 1, 2 and 4 mg/kg Δ^9-tetrahydrocannabinol (THC). Cannabidiol (CBD) was administered at doses of 20 and 40 mg/kg. The comparison drug used was diazepam (DZP), which was administered to separate groups of mice at doses of 2.5, 5 and 10 mg/kg. Significant reductions in shocks received were found for each of the three drugs. Adapted from Musty (1984).

Guimaraes *et al.* (1990) tested rats in the elevated plus maze model of anxiety. In the first test, rats were placed in a 'plus'-shaped maze, which was elevated from the floor. Two of the maze arms were enclosed with walls and two were not. Time spent in the enclosed arms was taken as a measure of anxiety or fear. Both CBD and DZP decreased the amount of time spent by the rats in the enclosed arms at all doses tested.

Human studies

In normal healthy volunteers, Zuardi *et al.* (1982) tested the hypothesis that CBD would antagonise anxiety induced by THC. Subjects were tested in a double-blind crossover procedure with doses of 0.5 mg/kg of THC, 1.0 mg/kg CBD, a mixture of 0.5 mg/kg Δ^9-THC plus 1 mg/kg CBD, placebo and DZP (10 mg) as controls. Each volunteer received treatments in a different sequence, and the doses exceeded the

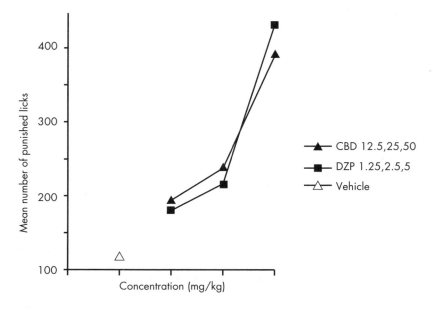

Figure 7.2 Hooded rats were trained for 7 days to lick from a water tube after 23 h of water deprivation. On test days each rat was placed in the test chamber for 20 min following injection of either vehicle, cannabidiol (CBD) or diazepam (DZP), i.p. at doses shown in the key (mg/kg). Each rat was allowed to drink water freely for 1 min, after which the water spout was electrified to deliver a 0.016 mA shock to the tongue. For 9 min the number of punished licks were recorded. Significant reductions in punished licks were found for both drugs. Adapted from Musty (1984).

concentration a person would need to take to induce the intoxicating effect of the drug and that would make them feel anxious.

Subjects reported a pleasant high at a THC concentration of 0.25 mg/kg using the same oral route of administration as that which did not produce anxiety. CBD (1.0 mg/kg) was shown to block anxiety produced by Δ^9-THC but the effect also extended to cannabis-like effects and to other subjective alterations induced by Δ^9-THC. This antagonism was not thought to be due to general blocking of Δ^9-THC, as no change was reported in pulse-rate measurements. Several other effects were observed that were typical of CBD and were of an opposite nature to those produced by Δ^9-THC, suggesting that the effects of CBD, as opposed to those of THC, might be involved in the antagonism of effects between the two cannabinoids.

In a second study, Zuardi *et al.* (1993a) induced anxiety in healthy normal subjects by having them prepare a 4-minute speech

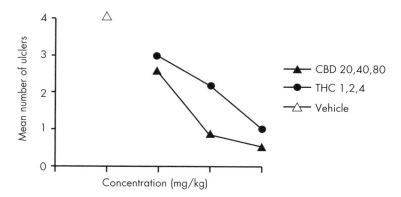

Figure 7.3 Mice (CD-1) were administered either vehicle, cannabidiol (CBD) or diazepam (DZP), i.p. at doses shown in the key (mg/kg) and placed in a cylindrical chamber 2 cm in diameter and 10 cm long. An electrode was attached to the tail and shocks (0.24 mA) were delivered to the feet of the mouse on a variable-interval 60-s schedule for 18 h. The mice were then returned to their home cage without food or water being available for 6 h. After this, the mice were sacrificed under ether anaesthesia, stomachs were removed, washed and examined under a dissecting microscope. Photographs were taken and observers, blind to the experimental condition, counted the number of ulcers. Significant reductions in ulcers were found at all doses of both drugs. Adapted from Musty (1984).

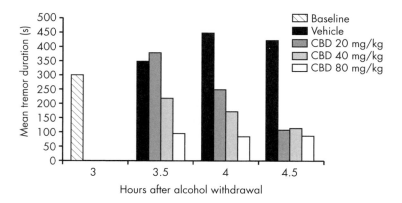

Figure 7.4 The effects of CBD on tremor in mice fed an alcohol diet of Sustacal, water and alcohol until they reached a phase in which they showed grossly impaired gait. Drugs were injected after the 3-h baseline period which reflects the beginning of withdrawal. Doses are shown in the key. CBD produced a significant decrease in mean tremor duration (s) at the 4 and 4.5 h points. Redrawn from Musty (1984).

about a topic from an educational course they had taken earlier during the year, and they were told that a psychologist would videotape the speech for later analysis. The subject began the speech while viewing his or her image on a video monitor. Anxiety measures were recorded using a visual analogue scale of mood, including anxiety, physical sedation, mental sedation and other feelings (e.g. degree of interest). Measurements were recorded at five time points: (1) baseline, (2) immediately prior to instructions, (3) immediately prior to speech, (4) in the middle of the speech, and (5) after the speech. The heart rate and blood pressure of the volunteers were also recorded.

Subjects were randomly assigned to one of the four treatments, which were either CBD (300 mg), isapirone (5 mg), diazepam (10 mg) or placebo. Following analysis of the data it was observed that anxiety and systolic blood pressure were decreased by CBD, diazepam and isapirone. Physical and mental sedation were not affected by CBD. Diazepam did not produce feelings of physical sedation.

Cortisol levels are associated with stress and anxiety; for example, cortisol levels have been shown to decrease in anxious HIV patients who were given relaxation training and this correlated with a decrease in anxiety (Cruess et al., 2000). Cortisol levels have been found to be elevated in patients with mixed anxiety-depressive disorder (Karra et al., 2000) and in graduate students undergoing oral exams (Lacey et al., 2000).

Zuardi et al. (1993b) measured the effects of CBD on plasma prolactin, growth hormone and cortisol in 11 normal healthy volunteers who were administered placebo or CBD (300 mg (n = 7) or 600 mg (n = 4), p.o.), in a double-blind study in two experimental sessions that were at least one week apart. Measurements were performed using radioimmunoassay. Basal prolactin (and growth hormone) levels were not affected by placebo or CBD. In contrast, plasma cortisol levels were significantly decreased during the placebo session (basal measurement = 11.0 ± 3.7 µg/dL; at 120 minutes placebo = 7.1 ± 3.9 µg/dL) in agreement with the normal circadian rhythm of the hormone. The decrease in cortisol levels was significantly attenuated after CBD, the basal measurement being 10.5 ± 4.9 µg/dL; 120 minutes after 300 mg CBD the level was 9.9 ± 6.2 µg/dl; and 120 minutes after dosing with 600 mg CBD the level was 11.6 ± 11.6 µg/dL. CBD was thus observed to interfere with cortisol secretion and it had a sedative effect as determined by the self-evaluation scales.

Thus it seemed there was good correlation between the anxiolytic properties of CBD and lowered cortisol levels in humans. Furthermore,

CBD could antagonise the anxiogenic effects of THC, which have been reported to occur in some cases. In addition, CBD alone seemed to have anxiolytic properties.

Depression

Animal models

The tail suspension test in mice is an animal model that has been developed to test for potentially antidepressive effects of drugs. In this model Musty *et al.* (2002b) reported that a cannabis-derived extract produced by GW Pharmaceuticals, containing high levels of CBD and no significant levels of other cannabinoids, reduced immobility when mice were suspended by the tail. In this model, whereas struggling is a measure of resisting, giving up is a primary symptom of depression. The extract produced an increase in struggling movements at 20 and 40 mg/kg of CBD. The results were virtually the same (at a concentration of 30 mg/kg) as those of imipramine. When using the GW Pharmaceuticals extract containing high levels of THC (drugs were administered i.p. 30 minutes prior to testing for effects), a decrease in struggling was observed at doses of 4 and 8 mg/kg THC. It was proposed that when THC reduced the distress produced in the tail suspension test the motivation to struggle or attempt to escape was reduced. This conclusion was supported by the observation that grooming in the open field (a measure of emotionality and distress) was significantly reduced in THC-treated animals. This pattern of behavioural responses thus suggested that THC extracts may have potential as anxiolytic agents.

When THC and CBD were combined at doses that produced significant effects, the struggling behaviour was similar to vehicle controls, suggesting that the cannabinoids had opposite effects. While these data were certainly not conclusive with regard to the antidepressive effects of CBD, they were strongly suggestive of efficacy, and future behavioural tests should focus on models of anxiety (e.g. the mouse emergence model or the chick separation test).

Following on from this work, a GW Pharmaceuticals cannabichromene (CBC) extract was tested in a similar fashion (Deyo and Musty, 2003) with escalating doses versus imipramine. Higher doses of CBC were comparable to imipramine in the tail suspension test, affirming significant antidepressant properties.

Human studies

In a recent review on the potential effects of cannabinoids on depression (see Musty, 2002), a study carried out with human volunteers observed that there was a positive correlation on the depression scale of the Minnesota Multiphasic Personality Inventory (MMPI) which was associated with feelings of euphoria after smoking cannabis, and which at the same time showed no correlation between anxiety on the hysteria scale and somatic concerns on the hypochondriasis scale. This suggested an antidepressive effect from the use of marijuana.

In a survey of 128 patients in Germany, Schnelle *et al.* (1999) reported that 12% of subjects used marijuana for the relief of depression. Consroe *et al.* (1997) found that depression was reduced in patients with multiple sclerosis (MS) in a self-report questionnaire. In another self-report study, Consroe *et al.* (1998) observed that patients with spinal cord injuries who used cannabis reported similar reductions in depression.

In cancer patients Regelson *et al.* (1976) found that THC relieved depression in advanced cancer patients and, in addition, Warner *et al.* (1994) reported relief from depression in a survey of 79 mentally ill patients. Russo *et al.* (2002) found unexpectedly low Beck Depression Inventory values in a cohort of four seriously ill subjects with high chronic daily intake of THC-predominant cannabis supplied through the US Compassionate Use Investigational New Drug Program.

At present there has been very little formal data reported supporting the hypothesis that cannabinoids might relieve depression, but tests of both agonists and antagonists against the CB_1 receptor are clearly necessary to test this hypothesis.

Whether or not CBD produces a primary effect on depressive symptoms is presently open to question and requires further investigation. In addition, it is possible that both CBD and THC may play some role in the diminution of depressive symptoms due to anxiolytic properties. This seems possible, since in control experiments, THC-and CBD-treated mice showed decreased emotional behaviour in the open field test. At present, it seems important to continue investigations at the level of the animal models in human patients and normal healthy subjects in order to evaluate the potential of these compounds as antidepressive therapeutic agents.

Alcohol dependence

Animal models

Alcoholism causes neurological disorders in humans and animals including memory and cognitive dysfunction, and binge drinking is a wide-

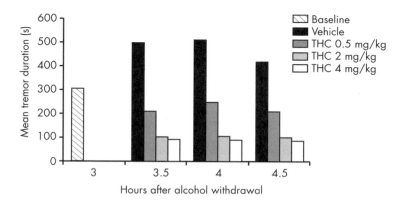

Figure 7.5 The effects of THC on tremor in mice fed an alcohol diet (as in Figure 7.4). Injection procedure as in Figure 7.4. Doses are shown in the key. THC at 2 and 4 mg/kg produced a significant decrease in mean tremor duration (s) at the 4 and 4.5 h points. Redrawn from Musty (1984).

spread form of alcoholism in society today. A study carried out by Musty *et al.* (1984) used mice (type C57Bl6J), which were fed a diet of liquid food and alcohol for 4 days. Healthy mice that had grossly impaired bodily movements or that were comatose were withdrawn from the diet. Mice were given THC, CBD or clonidine and the effects in this model were monitored. Tremors during withdrawal were video-taped and the durations scored. Results for these drugs are shown in Figures 7.4 and 7.5 (THC versus control).

All of these drugs significantly reduced body tremor during alcohol withdrawal, and in addition CBD, Δ^9-THC and clonidine reduced audiogenic seizures during alcohol withdrawal. Equivalent reductions in tremors and seizures were found with clonidine. Both human and animal studies suggested that cannabinoids may be useful for the treatment of opiate and alcohol withdrawal and, since CBD is not psycho-active, this drug seems to be the best candidate for future human clinical trials.

Spasticity

Animal models

Cannabidiol attenuates dystonia and torticollis in mutant rats (Consroe *et al.*, 1988). In an experiment, mutant dystonic (dt) rats at 16–20 days old were studied. Characteristic behaviour of animals with this disorder includes displaying torticollis (characterised as a perpetual twist in the neck with the muscles spasmodically and involuntarily pulling in one direction causing pain), clasping of the forepaws, rigidity, behaviour and jerky uncontrolled running. The rats were administered 0 (vehicle), 20, 40 and 80 mg/kg of CBD in a counterbalanced, crossover design with 7 days separating each test dose. Rats were videotaped in an open field for 3 minutes at 0, 15, 30, 45 and 60 minutes following injection. Raters, who were blind to the experimental conditions, recorded the duration of each of the aforementioned dystonic behaviours with an inter-rate reliability greater than 90%. Torticollis, forepaw clasping and rigidity were significantly decreased at the 20 mg/kg dose to a total decrease of at least 50% at the 80 mg/kg dose for each of the symptoms recorded. Spasmodic running and rolling behaviour were significantly decreased at the 20 and 40 mg/kg doses respectively, and this activity dropped to virtually zero at the 80 mg/kg dose.

In a second experiment, the investigators studied tetrabenazine (TBZ)-induced parkinsonian symptoms in rats. Groups of 10 rats were injected with TBZ (4 mg/kg, s.c.) and 45 minutes later were injected with 0 (vehicle), 10, 15, 20 or 30 mg/kg (i.v.) of CBD. During the subsequent 15-minute period, the duration of the hypokinesic (catatonic) state was measured. When either catatonia ceased or 15 minutes had passed, tremor, ptosis, hunchback posture and tail rigidity were measured. CBD augmented the duration of hypokinesia, but had no effect on the other symptoms.

In a third study, apomorphine-induced turning movements in rats with unilateral nigrostriatal lesions and aggressive behaviour in an L-pyroglutamate-induced model of Huntington's disease were studied (Conti et al., 1988). In the first experiment, 6-hydroxydopamine was injected unilaterally into the caudate-putamen. Following recovery from surgery, apomorphine was administered at 0.5 mg/g i.p., which induced the rat to turn in a circular motion. The animals were then injected with 10, 20 or 40 mg/kg of CBD (i.v.). CBD reduced the number of rotations observed in this model.

In the second experiment carried out by this group, dyskinetic symptoms were induced by bilateral injections of L-pyroglutamate into the caudate nucleus. The symptoms resembled those in Huntington's disease (HD) (e.g. aggressive outbursts). After bilateral injections of L-pyroglutamate, rats were allowed to recover from surgery. These rats were then placed in an observation chamber with a normal demonstrator rat. L-Pyroglutamate-treated rats were given injections of 5, 10 or 20 mg/kg (i.v.) of CBD and then placed in the chamber with the demonstrator animal. Attack, threats and aggressive posturing behaviour between animals was measured. All three doses of CBD reduced aggressive behaviours to near zero. Taken together, these experiments appeared to demonstrate that CBD selectively reduced dystonia, dyskinesia and aggressive behaviour in rats at the concentrations tested.

More recently, studies in the rodent chronic relapsing allergic encephalomyelitis (CRAE) model of multiple sclerosis have demonstrated that resulting spasticity and tremor are under the control of endocannabinoid mechanisms (Baker *et al.*, 2001).

Human studies

Sandyk *et al.* (1988) conducted a preliminary trial with four human patients suffering with Huntington's disease (HD). The patient's behaviour was recorded on videotape for a one-week period prior to drug administration. In the first week, patients were administered 300 mg of CBD in the morning, followed by neurological and clinical assessments at the end of the experimental week. For the following three weeks patients were administered 300 mg of CBD at 8:00 a.m. and 300 mg at 2:00 p.m. for a 3- to 4-week period. Assessments were made one week after cessation of CBD treatment. A reduction in choreic symptoms was observed in three patients during CBD treatment. In addition, an improvement in mood and sociability was observed. In the fourth patient, who had advanced HD, marginal improvements were also observed, but these were not as marked as in the other patients.

Consroe and Snider (1986) reported results on five patients with various dystonias in an open trial in which patients received 100–600 mg of CBD for six weeks. Twenty to fifty per cent reductions in dystonias were reported in all cases, but tremor and hypokinesia still occurred in patients with coexisting Parkinson's disease. (*Note*: This correlates well with the animal research reported above.)

Consroe *et al.* (1991) conducted a double-blind crossover study with 15 human Huntington's disease patients and administered 10 mg/kg/day of CBD orally in sesame oil capsules for six weeks, however there were no beneficial effects observed. One of the reasons for this observation could be the low bioavailability of orally administered CBD.

If one considers the results of the animal studies cited above, it can be seen that lower doses of CBD (e.g. 5 mg/kg) produced marked reductions in experimental dystonias. Furthermore, when CBD was delivered to normal healthy human volunteers in a minute amount of alcohol plus orange juice (Karniol and Carlini, 1973), or in smoked form (Dalton *et al.*, 1976), it appeared to be rapidly absorbed.

Schizophrenia

Antipsychotic drugs are also referred to as neuroleptics and generally tranquillise without impairing consciousness and without causing para-doxical excitement. For conditions such as schizophrenia the tranquillising effect is of secondary importance and this class of drugs is used to relieve florid psychotic symptoms (e.g. thought disorder, hallucinations and delusions), and to prevent relapse. Antipsychotic drugs are considered to act by interfering with dopaminergic transmission in the brain, principally by blocking dopamine receptors; they may also affect cholinergic, α-adrenergic, histaminergic and serotonergic receptors.

Animal models

Expression of c-fos is induced by both the typical (e.g. chlorpromazine, haloperidol and flupenthixol) and atypical (e.g. clozapine, amisulpride and risperidone) antipsychotic drug therapies. Haloperidol produces expression of c-fos in the dorsal striatum and the nucleus accumbens and clozapine produces expression in the prefrontal cortex and the nucleus accumbens (Zuardi *et al.*, 2002).

Various events such as stress, seizures, pain, visual stimuli, olfactory stimuli and drugs cause expression of the proto-oncogene c-fos in many brain regions (Morgan and Curran, 1995). The presence of this 55 000 molecular weight phosphoprotein has been linked to the patho-physiology of schizophrenia and several studies have investigated this (Sebens *et al.*, 1995; Klarner *et al.*, 1998; Abdel-Naby Sayed *et al.*, 2001; Todorova *et al.*, 2003).

Abdel-Naby Sayed *et al.* (2001) carried out immunohistochemistry studies on c-fos protein in order to study changes in neuronal activity in discrete brain areas of mice repeatedly treated with phencyclidine (PCP), which were showing enhancement of immobility in the forced swimming test. This behavioural change is considered as avolition, which is one of the negative symptoms of schizophrenia. Repeated treatment with PCP significantly prolonged immobility time in the forced swimming test, compared with saline treatment. The c-fos protein expression of mice showing PCP-induced enhancement of immobility was increased in certain brain regions, such as the retrosplenial cortex, pyriform cortices, pontine nuclei, cingulate, frontal cortex and the thalamus, compared with that of PCP-treated, non-swimming and saline-treated, swimming groups. These results suggested that increased c-fos protein was involved in the expression of PCP-induced enhancement of immobility, and c-fos expression played a role in negative symptom-like behavioural changes associated with schizophrenia.

Todorova *et al.* (2003) have found that in the cerebellar vermis of schizophrenic patients, studies have revealed alterations in the mitogen-activated protein (MAP) kinase signalling cascade and downstream transcription factors within the c-fos promoter. Since the proteins of the Fos and Jun families of immediate-early genes dimerise to form activating protein (AP)-1, they examined the expression of Jun transcription factors in schizophrenic and control subjects.

Protein levels of c-Jun, Jun B and Jun D were determined, as well as the levels of c-Jun mRNA by relative reverse transcription-polymerase chain reaction (RT-PCR) in post-mortem samples from cerebellar vermis. The expression of c-Jun protein and c-Jun mRNA were significantly increased in the cerebellar vermis of patients with schizophrenia, whereas no significant differences were found in the expression of Jun B or Jun D proteins. Studies in rats indicated that the abnormal expression of c-Jun transcription factor observed in schizophrenic patients was not related to post-mortem intervals or chronic treatment with antipsychotic medications. These studies provided new insights into the cerebellar abnormalities of schizophrenia.

Recently, Zuardi *et al.* (2002) examined c-fos expression after the administration of CBD. They found that the number of immunoreactive neurons in the lateral septal nucleus and the prefrontal cortex were significantly different from that of vehicle administration. Haloperidol produced significant neuroleptic effects in the lateral septum and the dorsal striatum, and after treatment with clozapine, significant effects were found in the lateral septum and the prefrontal cortex. The CBD dose was similar to that used in an animal model of psychosis (Zuardi *et al.*, 1995). In addition, Musty *et al.* (2000a) demonstrated that the inverse CB1 antagonist, SR141716, attenuated symptoms of schizophrenia in rats following administration of ketamine in a prepulse inhibition task. Alonso *et al.* (1999) found that SR141716 induced c-fos expression in the ventrolateral septum, the nucleus accumbens and the dorsomedial caudate-putamen. Taken together, these data suggested that CBD and SR141716 acted in areas of the brain like the atypical antipsychotics. The results lend further support to their potential use as antipsychotic therapies.

Zuardi *et al.* (1991) tested the effects of CBD and haloperidol in an animal model that was used to predict antipsychotic activity in rats. The effects of CBD were compared with those produced by haloperidol. Several doses of CBD (15–480 mg/kg) and haloperidol (0.062–1.0 mg/kg) were tested in each model. CBD increased the effective doses (50%) (or ED_{50} value) of apomorphine necessary for inducing the sniffing and biting behaviours induced by the drug at a concentration of 6.4 mg/kg, increased plasma prolactin levels and produced palpebral ptosis when compared with control solutions. Both drugs (CBD and haloperidol) decreased the frequency of these behaviours. CBD did not induce catalepsy even at very high doses, although haloperidol did. The authors concluded that CBD had a pharmacological profile similar to that of the atypical antipsychotic drugs though the mechanism of action was uncertain and it was postulated that it could be different to that of the dopamine antagonists.

Human studies

Zuardi *et al.* (1995) reported an experiment with a single case in which a patient was being treated for psychosis with haloperidol at a mean dose of 4 mg/kg a day. The medication was terminated due to side effects (amenorrhoea, galactorrhoea and weight gain), and was followed by a return of symptoms, which led to hospitalisation. At this point the patient was given placebo medication for 4 days, after which she was administered CBD (two doses per day) on an increasing dose schedule up to 750 mg twice daily until the 26th day. This was followed by 4 days of placebo and finally by a return to haloperidol for four weeks. Interviews were conducted with the patient and videotaped, and were followed by rating of interviews using the Brief Psychiatric Rating Scale (BPRS) and the Interactive Observation Scale for Psychiatric Patients (IOSPP). A psychiatrist who was blind to treatment conditions rated the patient on the BPRS, and in addition, nursing assistants who were blind to treatment and conditions independently rated the patient on the IOSPP scale. When comparing placebo with the CBD condition, hostility-suspiciousness dropped by 50% of the BPRS maximum scale score (mss), thought-disturbance decreased by 37.5% of the mss, anxiety-depression by 43.7%, activation by 41.6%, and anergia decreased by 31.3% of the mss. During the following 4-day period of placebo, all five scale scores increased somewhat. The patient was returned to haloperidol treatment and the subsequent scores were close to those with CBD treatment. This 'n of 1' (*n*=1) experiment demonstrated that CBD is a candidate for testing in, and a potential therapy for, human schizophrenia. At present, the mechanism of action of CBD in the case remains unknown.

Considerable controversy has recently surrounded allegations that cannabis, particularly THC, may cause or precipitate psychosis in humans. These data have been recently reviewed (Fride and Russo, 2004; Grinspoon and Russo, 2004). In the opinion of these authors, there has been little convincing evidence for an aetiological role of cannabis in schizophrenia, nor epidemiological studies supporting an increase in baseline rates of psychosis in any population based on increases in its utilisation.

Epilepsy

Epilepsy is caused by abnormal electric impulses in groups of neurons in the brain. For diagnostic purposes, epilepsy is divided into the two main groups: idiopathic and symptomatic epilepsy. In idiopathic epilepsy (from Greek *idos*, for 'self') the cause is unknown. However, it is believed that attacks are caused by the lack of a particular group of neurotransmitters used to regulate the electric impulses in the brain. There may be a hereditary (genetic) background, as epilepsy of the same type is often seen among relatives. Moreover, EEG irregularities similar to those of the patient are often seen among family members, even if they do not suffer from epilepsy themselves. New research has shown that certain cases of idiopathic epilepsy are clearly hereditary, and are caused by chromosomal abnormality. A patient will not have any other signs of neurological illness or mental defects and computerised tomography (CT) and magnetic resonance imaging (MRI) scans will be normal.

Symptomatic epilepsy is caused by a known illness in the brain. Numerous illnesses or types of brain damage can cause epilepsy:

- Developmental anomalies, where damage occurs to the brain as it develops during the first three months of pregnancy. This can be revealed by modern MRI scans and causes many of the difficult-to-control cases in children. On the other hand, damage inflicted during delivery (cerebral palsy) is fairly uncommon.
- Trauma to the skull. Whereas the incidence of post-traumatic epilepsy is under 2% in closed head injuries, it may attain 50% following a depressed skull fracture, where the brain tissue has been partly damaged, or a gunshot wound to the head.

- Blood clots (infarcts) and haemorrhages in the brain. Approximately 10% of all brain infarcts cause epilepsy.
- Brain tumours, in particular slow-growing superficial tumours.
- Encephalitis, when prolonged seizures and fever convulsions can induce brain damage.
- Alcohol abuse. Epilepsy may occur as a result of the alcohol withdrawal associated with delirium tremens. In certain cases, an MRI scan reveals abnormalities in the brain, but no evidence of neurological illness. Such cases are called cryptogenic (from Greek *kryptos*, for 'hidden').

Animal models

CBD has been found to raise electroshock-induced seizure thresholds in mice (Consroe and Snider, 1986) and to have a protective index (PI) (toxic dose$_{50}$/effective dose$_{50}$) comparable in animal models to that of the classic antiepileptic drugs (e.g. phenytoin, phenobarbital and carbamazepine), which are effective against grand mal and partial seizures. Seizures are commonly induced in mice chemically by pentylenetetrazol (PTZ).

In genetically susceptible animals, however, conclusions from the literature are mixed. CBD has been shown to be 'generally effective' more often than not. Cannabidiol has been shown to decrease convulsions in mice and, in addition, cannabinoids have been shown to have antiseizure and anticonvulsant effects in a variety of species and paradigms (Consroe and Snider, 1986). Leite *et al.* (1982) have also demonstrated antiseizure effects of (+) and (–) isomers of CBD and THC and their dimethylheptyl homologues. All cannabinoids were anticonvulsant and potentiated pentobarbitone sleeping time. The (+) isomer was more active than the (–) isomer.

More recent studies have greatly contributed to our understanding of cannabinoids and seizures. Wallace *et al.* (2002) demonstrated in mice that seizure threshold was mediated by cannabinoid mechanisms via CB_1, and that this effect was antagonised by SR141716A. In a subsequent study (Wallace *et al.*, 2003), a pilocarpine-induced seizure model in rats was employed that mimics drug-resistant complex partial seizure disorders in humans, the most common source of patients who fail conventional approaches. THC produced a 100% reduction in seizures, whereas phenobarbital and diphenylhydantoin did not. The animals demonstrated both acute increases in endocannabinoid production and a long-term up-regulation of CB_1 production as apparent compensatory effects counteracting glutamate excitotoxicity.

Human studies

Of the three controlled studies carried out (Karniol and Carlini, 1973; Karniol *et al.*, 1974; Cunha *et al.*, 1980), mixed results were obtained but it seemed that CBD had some potential to control epilepsy.

One study in particular warrants a detailed discussion. Cunha *et al.* (1980) studied 15 patients with secondary generalised epilepsy with temporal lobe foci who were tested in a double-blind two-group procedure with CBD. Patients remained on the antiepileptic drug which they were receiving for the duration of the study. Doses (200–300 mg per day of CBD in gelatin capsules) were given to patients in the study which took place over a minimum 6- to 18-week period.

One week prior to beginning administration, the placebo group had a median value of 4.5 focal convulsions and a median value of 1 (range 1–3) generalised convulsion(s) per week. The CBD group had a median value of 6.5 focal convulsions and a median value of 2.5 (range 1–4) generalised convulsion(s) per week. Each week patients were rated on a clinical efficacy scale, where 0 = total absence of convulsions and self-reported improvement; 2 = subjective self-reported improvement; and 3 = no reduction in convulsions and no self-reported improvement. Over the total drug phase for each subject the placebo group had a median rating of 3 (6 rated 3 and 1 rated 0) and the CBD-treated group had a median rating of 1.6 (4 rated 0, 2 rated 2 and 1 rated 3). No side-effects occurred in any of the patients. These data at least supported the hypothesis that CBD could be used as an adjunctive drug to current drug therapy for the treatment of epilepsy. Due to the small sample size, however, further clinical trials are warranted. Another possibility is that mixtures of agonists and antagonists might be useful for treating epilepsy since it has been demonstrated that CBD attenuates the psycho-activity of THC (Karniol and Carlini, 1973; Karniol, *et al.*, 1974). The data of Wallace *et al.* (2002, 2003) certainly argue for a therapeutic role of THC in epilepsy, which is quite contrary to the current perceived wisdom.

Antioxidant effects

The term 'oxidative associated diseases' refers to pathological conditions that result at least in part from the production of or exposure to free radicals, particularly oxyradicals, or reactive oxygen species (ROS). Free radicals are unstable atom groups in the body linked to tissue damage in a wide array of diseases, including those of pain, inflammation (peripheral and CNS, general and localised to particular areas of the body, e.g. rheumatoid arthritis (RA)), ischaemia, coronary heart disease (CHD) and debilitating neurodegenerative conditions including Alzheimer's and Parkinson's diseases and multiple sclerosis (MS). The number of studies investigating potential antioxidant effects of cannabinoids is increasing and their potential use for a variety of diseases is being investigated where relevant models are available; the areas relevant to neurodegeneration are under particular scrutiny. Antioxidants are substances that, when present in a mixture containing an oxidisable substrate, the biological molecule, significantly delay or prevent its oxidation. Antioxidants can act by scavenging biologically important free radicals or other ROS (e.g. $\cdot O_2^-$, H_2O_2, $\cdot OH$, HOCl, ferryl, peroxyl, peroxynitrile), or by preventing their formation, or by catalytically converting the free radical or other ROS to a less reactive species.

Most pathological conditions are multifactorial, and assigning or identifying the predominant causal factors for any particular condition is frequently difficult. For these reasons, the term 'free radical-associated disease' encompasses pathological states that are recognised as conditions in which free radicals or ROS contribute to the pathology of the disease, or wherein administration of a free radical inhibitor (e.g. desferrioxamine), scavenger (e.g. tocopherol or glutathione) or catalyst (e.g. SOD), is shown to produce detectable benefit by decreasing symptoms, increasing survival or providing other detectable clinical benefits in treating or preventing pathological states.

Different mechanisms have been proposed to explain how free radicals might specifically mediate CNS damage, including the theory that decreased levels of antioxidants may promote increased sensitivity to enzymes (e.g. lipoxygenase), which then stimulates the production of leukotrienes thereby increasing the immuno-inflammatory processes in peripheral and CNS tissues and cells (Hutter, 1993). With particular relevance to MS, it is thought that excessive concentrations of free radicals might trigger heightened T cell activity via the arachidonic acid cascade, or that direct damage to myelin or myelin sheaths that protect the neurons is caused directly by these molecules (Cooper, 1997) and thus contributes to the pathophysiology of the disease.

Two studies have found evidence linking low antioxidant levels to MS: superoxide dismutase (SOD) and glutathione peroxidase were both found to be present at low levels in the red blood cells (RBCs) of patients with MS (Zagorski et al., 1991; Dudek et al.,

1992). The researchers concluded that the RBCs in these patients were more vulnerable to oxidative stress than those of healthy human controls.

In a comparative study, an examination of the cerebrospinal fluid (CSF) of patients with MS found that glutathione reductase activity (which guards against free radical production) was reduced by approximately one half (Calabrese *et al.*, 1994). In addition, direct examination of MS plaque revealed increased free radical activity together with decreased levels of α-tocopherol (vitamin E) and glutathione (Langermann *et al.*, 1992). Thus, in the small number of studies carried out to date researching the link between antioxidants and MS, there is significant evidence to warrant further investigation of antioxidants as a therapy for this disease, with these studies extending to the inclusion of CBD or other cannabis-derived compounds or extracts.

When Hampson *et al.* (1998) exposed rat cortical neuronal cell cultures that had been previously treated with the excitatory neurotransmitter glutamate, it was found that CBD protected against neurotoxic effects. Using cyclic voltametry they also demonstrated that CBD had antioxidant effects. In both a chemical (Fenton reaction) system and in neuronal cell cultures, cannabidiol was shown to prevent hydroperoxide-induced oxidative damage as well as, or better than, the antioxidants α-tocopherol and ascorbate. Cannabidiol was more protective against glutamate neurotoxicity than either ascorbate or α-tocopherol, indicating its potential as an antioxidant. The authors also concluded that the data suggested that the naturally occurring non-psychotropic cannabinoid cannabidiol might be a potentially useful therapeutic agent for the treatment of oxidative neurological disorders such as cerebral ischaemia.

Neuroprotective effects have been described for many cannabinoids in several neurotoxicity models (Marsicano *et al.*, 2002); however, the exact mechanisms and how they relate to cannabinoid structures are not clearly understood yet. Antioxidant neuroprotective effects of cannabinoids, and their involvement with the cannabinoid receptors, have been analysed using cell-free biochemical assays and cellular assays using mouse hippocampal HT22 cells and also rat primary cerebellar cell cultures.

The HT22 cell line contained a stably transfected CB_1 receptor and the protective potentials of compounds were compared against the HT22 control cells. Oxidative stress experiments were performed in cultured cerebellar granule cells that were derived from CB_1 knockout mice or control wild-type littermates.

The results suggested that CB_1 was not involved in the cellular antioxidant neuroprotective effects of cannabinoids after comparing structure–activity relationships (SARs) of compounds that were either phenolic and did not bind to the CB_1 receptor, non-phenolic and bound to the CB_1 receptor or were phenolic and bound to the CB_1 receptor.

Chen and Buck (2000) also found that cannabinoids could protect cells from oxidative cell death by receptor-independent mechanisms. They observed that submicromolar concentrations of THC, Δ^9-THC, cannabidiol and cannabinol but not WIN55,212-2, prevented β-lymphoblastoid cells and fibroblasts from dying in serum-depleted media after 2 days. Normally serum is required for the maintenance and growth of most animal cells. It was also found that THC synergised with platelet-derived growth factor in activating resting NIH-3T3 fibroblasts.

This growth supportive effect did not correlate with the ability of the cannabinoid compounds to bind to known CBD receptors and, in addition, showed no stereoselectivity that would indicate a non-receptor-mediated pathway/mode of action. Direct measurement of oxidative stress revealed that the cannabinoids prevented serum-deprived cell death by antioxidation. This was confirmed by their ability to antagonise oxidative stress and the consequent cell death induced by the retinoid antihydroretinol. Thus in their model it was demonstrated that cannabinoids acted as antioxidants to modulate cell survival and to stimulate growth of β-lymphocytes and fibroblasts.

4-Terpineol, an essential oil component of cannabis, demonstrated 'respectable' radical scavenging and antioxidant effects (Burits and Bucar, 2000).

Quercetin, a flavonoid in cannabis, is able to act as an antioxidant and its importance as an inhibitor of nuclear transcription factor kappa (NF-κB) has been of interest for over a decade (Greenspan, 1993; Musonda and Chipman, 1998; Herring and Kaminski, 1999). Downstream products of NF-κB activation include inflammatory cytokines important for leukocyte activation and recruitment, tumour necrosis factor (TNF), nitric oxide synthase (NOS), and thus regulation of vascular tone, cell adhesion molecule expression involved in inflammatory responses, and viral activation such as in HIV. Free radicals activate NF-κB and quercetin has been shown to arrest the formation of this molecule by blocking the protein kinase C (PKC)-induced phosphorylation of an inhibitory subunit of NF-κB termed IκB (Musonda and Chipman, 1998). The results of this are that quercetin may actively inhibit carcinogenesis and stimulation/development of some inflammatory diseases. Greenspan (1993) has shown that NF-κB has a role in activating HIV-1 and thus quercetin may also play an active role in inhibiting replication of this virus. CBN has also been shown to down-regulate NF-κB, thus together, CBN and quercetin may synergise to down-regulate THC-induced NF-κB (Herring and Kaminski, 1999).

Anti-inflammatory effects

In vitro models

While the role of peripheral cannabinoid receptors in nociceptive modulation is not quite as well understood as that of the central cannabinoid receptors, peripheral CB_2 receptors have been reported to modulate inflammation in *in vitro* models (Richardson *et al.*, 1998c).

The mouse macrophage nitric oxide synthetase (NOS) gene is maximally activated by a combination of lipopolysaccharide (LPS) and interferon-γ (IFNγ) (Ding *et al.*, 1988). Nitric oxide (NO) is converted within seconds to nitrite, which is then slowly oxidised to nitrate in biological systems. Preliminary experiments by Coffey *et al.* (1996) demonstrated that THC did not affect the kinetics of nitrite appearance or the ratio of nitrite:nitrate. The researchers administered Δ^9-THC (i.p.) to thioglycollate-treated mice and, after an 18-hour period, the peritoneal macrophages were harvested and NO production was induced by LPS and IFNγ at concentrations of 1 μg/mL and 0.1–10 U/mL respectively. Macrophages from the THC-treated mice produced approximately half as much NO as those from the controls. When THC (1 μg/mL) was added *in vitro*, further inhibition of the inflammatory mediator was observed with the greatest inhibition being produced at the lower concentration of IFNγ used in the assay. Thus THC was demonstrated to have inhibitory activity against this inflammatory mediator.

Following on from these findings, the effects of two cannabinoid receptor agonists, WIN55,212-2 and cannabinol (CBN), were investigated for their ability to inhibit the production of NO and inducible nitric oxide synthase (iNOS) expression in the C6 rat glioma cell line (Esposito *et al.*, 2001). Glioma cells were stimulated with the chemical agents LPS and IFNγ which would produce an inflammatory reaction. Twenty-four hours following treatment with LPS (at 1 μg/mL) and IFNγ (at 300 U/mL), a significant increase in NO production was produced in the culture medium surrounding the glioma cells, which was evaluated as nitrite.

The compounds WIN55,212-2 and CBN were shown to dose-dependently inhibit the production of nitrite and had different EC_{50} values, with WIN55,212-2 being the more potent (WIN55,212-2, EC_{50} = 4.2 nm, CBN EC_{50} = 700 nm). WIN55,212-2 also inhibited iNOS expression when incubated at the same time as LPS and IFN, but it had no effect when it was added to the cells 2 hours following LPS/IFNγ treatment, indicating a possible interference at the protein synthesis level or at an earlier step such as gene transcription.

The cannabinoid CB_1 receptor antagonist SR141716A was shown to decrease, in a dose-related manner, the CBN-induced inhibition of nitrite production, and this compound also reversed the WIN55,212-2-induced inhibition of iNOS expression. The data suggested that some cannabinoid compounds acting selectively through cannabinoid CB_1 receptor activation, which in turn inhibits iNOS expression and NO overproduction in glioma cells, might be potential therapies for inhibiting NO-mediated inflammation, which may lead to neurodegeneration.

THC has 20 times the anti-inflammatory activity of acetylsalicylic acid, and twice that of hydrocortisone (Evans, 1991). Numerous other phytocannabinoids are anti-inflammatory, notably cannabigerol (CBG), which exceeds the antierythemic, analgesic and lipoxygenase-blocking effects of THC (Evans, 1991).

With reference to the non-cannabinoid compounds present in cannabis with anti-inflammatory activity, β-caryophyllene, which is the most common sesquiterpenoid produced by cannabis (Mediavilla and Steinman, 1997), demonstrated anti-inflammatory effects of the oleoresin in rats comparable to phenylbutazone in reduction of granuloma formation. A decreased vascular permeability to injected histamine was also observed. α-Pinene, a bicyclic monoterpenoid, was shown to be effective in preventing acute inflammation in a carrageenan-induced plantar oedema model (Gill *et al.*, 1970). It was also shown to have bronchodilatory effects.

TNFα, a cytokine expressed by monocytes and macrophages (Gerritsen *et al.*, 1995), induces and maintains inflammation and is associated with rheumatoid arthritis and multiple sclerosis. THC decreased TNFα production, possibly by a non-receptor-mediated mechanism (Burnette-Curley and Cabral, 1995). Conversely, a second study by Shivers *et al.* (1994) suggested that THC might induce TNFα. The flavonoid apigenin has been shown to inhibit the production of TNFα, thus apigenin facilitates beneficial suppression of TNFα, either in parallel or by counteracting THC effects.

Cannflavin A is a prenylated flavone which so far is unique to cannabis (Barrett *et al.*, 1986). This compound has been shown to be an inhibitor of PGE_2 in human rheumatoid synovial cells with an IC_{50} value 30 times more potent than aspirin in the same model. It has also been shown to inhibit cyclooxygenase (COX) and lipoxygenase (LO) more potently than THC (Evans *et al.*, 1987) but repeat experiments are necessary to ensure that the solvent (ethanol) in which the compound was dissolved did not adversely affect the results.

Animal models

The endocannabinoid palmitoylethanolamide (PMEA), a selective CB_2 cannabinoid receptor agonist, has been shown to attenuate mechanical hyperalgesia by carrageenan. A potential mechanism for the antihyper-algesic effect of PMEA is the inhibition of mast cell degranulation (Mazzari *et al.*, 1996), which would modulate the release of histamine and serotonin. These compounds are capable of producing the inflam-matory effects of vasodilatation, increased vascular permeability (plas-ma extravasation) and nociceptor activation, potentially contributing to the observed effects of hyperthermia, oedema and hyperalgesia (which are all characteristic of carrageenan-induced hyperalgesia) (Vinegar *et al.*, 1976; Hargreaves *et al.*, 1988; Rang *et al.*, 1994). Clayton *et al.* (2002) have shown that CB_1 and CB_2 receptors are implicated in inflammatory hypersensitivity using the carrageenan-induced acute hypersensitivity test, the (nociceptive) mechanical paw withdrawal threshold test, weight bearing dual channel weight averager (a measure of hypersensitivity to pain) and the oedema (increase in paw volume) tests using the agonist compounds HU-210 and GW405833 and the antagonists AM281 and SR144528.

The results showed that HU-210 was anti-inflammatory and anti-nociceptive, with these effects being antagonised by the CB_1 antagonist AM281 but not SR144528. This suggested the antinociceptive actions were mediated primarily through the CB_1 receptor. AM281 had a minor inhibitory effect on the antihypersensitive effects of HU-210. GW405833 is a potent CB_2 receptor agonist as demonstrated when used in conjunction with the selective CB_2 antagonist SR144528. Experiments with SR144528 confirmed that a major component of the inflammatory hypersensitivity response was mediated via the CB_2 receptor; thus GW405833 decreased the hypersensitivity and paw oedema induced by carrageenan and the effect was reversed by SR144528. The authors concluded that both CB_1 and CB_2 receptors had anti-inflammatory hypersensitivity activity. Activation of the CB_2 receptor alone was sufficient to produce a substantial anti-inflammatory (and analgesic) effect in the carrageenan model used in their studies.

Smith *et al.* (2001) evaluated cannabinoid receptor ligands in mice for effects on the development of peritoneal inflammation elicited in mice using thioglycollate broth or *Staphylococcus* enterotoxin A. The compounds studied were the cannabinoid receptor agonists HU-210, WIN55,212-2 and SR144528.

Both HU-210 and WIN55,212-2 blocked the migration of neutrophils into the peritoneal cavity in response to the inflammatory stimuli. The effect was caused by a delay in the production of neutrophil chemoattractants and macrophage inflammatory protein 2.

HU-210 and WIN55,212-2 blocked neutrophil chemokines and neutrophil administered s.c. or i.c.v. These effects were antagonised by SR141716A (centrally administered), the selective CB_1 receptor antagonist. The ability of the cannabinoid receptor agonists to suppress peritoneal inflammation at low doses compared to when administered i.c.v. indicated a role for central cannabinoid receptors in the anti-inflammatory activities of HU-210 and WIN55,212-2. The agonists had no effect on monocyte migration elicited by thioglycollate despite the ability to suppress monocyte chemotactic protein 1 levels in lavage fluids. SR144528 inhibited peritoneal inflammation in a manner analogous to that of HU-210 and WIN55,212-2 when administered i.c.v. but did not appear to act through central CB_1 receptors. These observations increase the knowledge of the diverse interactions the CB agonist and antagonists have with the inflammatory cascade and highlight diverse anti-inflammatory properties.

Richardson *et al.* (1998b) have demonstrated activation of spinal CB_1 receptors that can result in both antihyperalgesia and the inhibition of neuropeptide release from central termination of capsaicin-sensitive primary efferent nociceptive fibres and that cannabinoid binding sites can be measured in sensory neurons.

Tchilibon *et al.* (2000) used an ear-swelling assay to test the anti-inflammatory effects of CBD compared with the activity of the pharmacological compound indometacin. The results showed that the CBD metabolites, as well as the dimethylheptyl homologues, were anti-inflammatory, and the acids were more potent than the hydroxy derivatives. CBD, when compared with aspirin, had anti-inflammatory efficacy at doses lower than that of aspirin.

Malfait *et al.* (2000) conducted an experiment in which collagen-induced arthritis (CIA) was produced in mice and was followed by CBD treatment. They found that CBD reduced clinical signs of arthritic symptoms and resulted in histological evidence of improvement in the hind-feet joints of the mice. In order to induce CIA, DBA/1 mice were immunised with type II collagen in complete Freund's adjuvent by intradermal injection of 100 μg of bovine collagen II. After day 15, mice were evaluated daily for the onset of clinical arthritis using clinical scores as follows: 1 = slight swelling and erythema, 2 = pronounced oedema and 3 = joint rigidity. Each limb was graded on this scale for a maximum possible score of 12. Arthritis was monitored over 12 days, at which point the animals were killed and histology of the hind limbs was conducted.

When the first clinical signs of CIA were observed, CBD was administered in the order of 0 (vehicle), 2.5, 5, 10 or 20 mg/kg (i.p.) or oral administration of 0 (in olive oil), 10, 25 or 50 mg/kg (p.o.). In chronic rather than acute experiments, mice were treated for five weeks with CBD at 5 or 10 mg/kg (i.p.) or CBD at 25 mg/kg orally using the same vehicle controls.

With regard to clinical signs, using the i.p. route, a concentration of 5 mg/kg had the optimal effect of suppressing the disease, or eliminating all signs of the disease. In the chronic model (i.p. injection) the same dose was found to be the most effective in suppressing the symptoms with orally administered doses of 10, 25 and 50 mg/kg. The drugs were shown to be virtually 100% effective in suppressing the clinical symptoms, while the 25 mg/kg dose was found to be the most effective treatment for the chronic progression of the disease over the four-week treatment period. With reference to joint damage from histological examination, both the 5 mg/kg dose delivered i.p. and the 25 mg/kg delivered orally resulted in ratings of joint changes as shown in Table 7.1. Amelioration of CIA occurred at medium doses in both the emerging disease (acute) and the chronic relapsing model. These data suggested that CBD could have clinical utility in the treatment of arthritis, but also demonstrated that in order to optimise successful therapeutic concentrations for therapy, dose ranging experiments would be of utmost importance in early clinical evaluations.

Conclusions

Based on the research to date, it seems clear that CBD can antagonise many of the pharmacological and/or 'negative' effects of THC. These include cardiovascular acceleration, distortion of time perception and the anxiogenic effects of THC, e.g. tachycardia and the perception of the

Table 7.1 Effect of CBD on histological ratings of hyperplasia and joint destruction in mice with collagen-induced arthritis (CIA)

	i.p.		p.o.		
	Control (%)	CBD (5 mg/kg) (%)	Control (%)	CBD (25 mg/kg) (%)	CBD (50 mg/kg) (%)
Acute CIA					
Normal	0	34.0	0	0	0
Mild	31.0	26.0	20.0	41.0	34.0
Moderate	31.0	20.0	5.0	34.0	16.0
Severe	38.0	20.0	75.0	25.0	50.0
Chronic CIA					
Normal	0	30.0	0	36.0	
Mild	25.0	50.0	20.0	28.0	
Moderate	65.0	10.0	80.0	36.0	
Severe	10.0	10.0	0	0	

'high' (which is not necessarily considered a negative issue by all patients and/or users). It is known that if a patient takes CBD prior to THC the potential adverse effects may not be experienced, however, the reverse scenario does not apply. It is also known that synthetic cannabinergic compounds have efficacies different to those of naturally derived cannabinoid compounds. The fact that CBD and THC have additive and/or synergistic effects justifies their use as a co-therapy for multifactorial diseases. This interaction between CBD and THC may explain why patients obtain a better or smoother effect with a combined product rather than when using them singly. However, until recently the evidence of efficacy was mostly anecdotal. Thus far, THC and CBD ratios have been administered to a maximum 1:1 ratio (see Chapters 9 and 10), yet the studies cited above suggest that alternative ratios of CBD:THC should be tested for their pharmacological and clinical effects.

CBD alone seems to have pharmacological actions independent of interactions with THC and, since CBD is a weak antagonist, this may account for its unique pharmacological actions. Potentially, CBD may have antiepileptic, antipsychotic, anxiolytic, antidepressive, antioxidant and anti-inflammatory effects. These putative effects should be studied both in animals and humans in order to further elucidate the potential of these cannabinoids for a variety of diseases that have unmet clinical needs.

The roles of other phytocannabinoids such as cannabichromene, cannabigerol and tetrahydrocannabivarin, and cannabis terpenoid essential oil and flavonoid components have only recently been considered. Their future contributions to cannabinoid therapeutics may prove to be considerable.

References

Abdel-Naby Sayed M, Noda Y, Hamdy M *et al.* (2001). Enhancement of immobility induced by repeated phencyclidine injection: association with c-Fos protein in the mouse brain. *Behav Brain Res* 124: 71–76.

Alonso R, Voutinos B, Labie C *et al.* (1999). Blockade of cannabinoid receptors by SR141716 selectively increases Fos expression in rat mesocorticolimbic areas via reduced dopamine D2 function. *Neuro* 91: 607–620

Baker D, Pryce G, Croxford J L *et al.* (2001). Endocannabinoids control spasticity in a multiple sclerosis model *FASEB J* 15(2): 300–302.

Barrett M L, Scutt A M, Evans F J (1986). Cannflavin A and B, prenylated flavones from *Cannabis sativa* L. *Experientia* 42: 452–453.

Ben-Shabat S, Fride E, Sheskin T *et al.* (1998). An entourage effect: inactive endogenous fatty acid glycerol esters enhance 2-arachidonoyl-glycerol cannabinoid activity. *Eur J Pharmacol* 353(1): 23–31.

Bicher H I, Mechoulam R (1968). Pharmacolgical effects of two active constituents of marihuana. *Arch Int Pharmacodyn Ther* 172: 24–31.

Bisogno T, Hanus L, De Petrocellis L *et al.* (2001). Molecular targets for cannabidiol and its synthetic analogues: effect on vanilloid VR1 receptors and on the cellular uptake and enzymatic hydrolysis of anandamide. *Br J Pharmacol* 134: 845–852.

Buchbauer G, Jirovetz L, Jager W *et al.* (1993). Fragrance compounds and essential oils with sedative effects upon inhalation. *J Pharm Sci* 82: 660–664.

Burits M, Bucar F (2000). Antioxidant activity of *Nigella sativa* essential oil. *Phytother Res* 14: 323–328.

Burnette-Curley D, Cabral G A (1995). Differential inhibition of RAW-264.7 macrophage tumoricidal activity by Δ^9-tetrahydrocannabinol. *Proc Soc Exp Biol Med* 210: 64–76.

Calabrese V, Raggaele R, Cosentino E *et al.* (1994). Changes in cerebrospinal fluid levels of malonaldehyde and glutathione reductase activity in multiple sclerosis. *Int J Clin Pharmacol Res* 14: 119–123.

Carlini E A, Santos M, Claussen V *et al.* (1973). Structure activity relationship of four tetrahydrocannabinols and the pharmacological activity of five semipurified extracts of *Cannabis sativa*. *Psychopharmacology* 18: 82–93.

Carson C F, Tiley T V (1995). Antimicrobial activity of the major components of the essential oil of *Melaleuca alternifolia*. *J Appl Bacter* 78: 264–269.

Chen Y, Buck J (2000). Cannabinoids protect cells from oxidative cell death: a receptor-independent mechanism. *J Pharmacol Exp Ther* 293: 807–812.

Clayton N, Marshall F H, Bountra C, O'Shaughnessy C T (2002). CB1 and CB2 cannabinoid receptors are implicated in inflammatory pain. *Pain* 96: 253–260.

Coffey R G, Snella E, Johnson K, Pross S (1996). Inhibition of macrophage nitric oxide production by tetrahydrocannabinol *in vivo* and *in vitro*. *Int J Immunopharmacol* 18: 749–752.

Consroe P, Snider S R (1986). Therapeutic potential of cannabinoids in neurological disorders. In: Mechoulam R, ed. *Cannabinoids as Therapeutic Agents*. Boca Raton, FL: CRC Press: 21–49.

Consroe P, Musty R E, Conti L H (1988). Effects of cannabidiol in animal models of neurologic dysfunction. In: Chesher G, Consroe P, Musty R E, eds. *Marihuana: An International Research Report*. Canberra: Australian Government Publishing Service: 141–146.

Consroe P, Laguna J, Allender J *et al.* (1991). Controlled clinical trial of cannabidiol in Huntington's disease. *Pharmac Biochem Behav* 40: 701–708.

Consroe P, Musty R E, Tillery W, Pertwee R (1997). Perceived effects of cannabis smoking in patients with multiple sclerosis. *Eur Neurol* 38: 44–48.

Consroe P, Tillery W, Rein J, Musty R E (1998). Reported marijuana effects in patients with spinal cord injury. *Proceedings, 1998 Symposium on the Cannabinoids*. Burlington, VT: International Cannabinoid Research Society: 64.

Conti L H, Johanessen J, Musty R E, Consroe P (1988). Anti-dyskinetic effects of cannabidiol. In: Chesher G, Consroe P, Musty R E, eds. *Marihuana: An International Research Report*. Canberra: Australian Government Publishing Service: 153–156.

Cooper R J (1997). Multiple sclerosis: an immune legacy? *Med Hypotheses* 49: 307–311.

Cruess D G, Antoni M H, Schneiderman N *et al.* (2000). Cognitive-behavioral stress management increases free testosterone and decreases psychological distress in HIV-seropositive men. *Health Psychol* 19: 12–20.

Cunha J M, Carlini E A, Pereira A E *et al.* (1980). Chronic administration of cannabidiol to healthy volunteers and epileptic patients. *Pharmacology* 21: 175–185.

Dalton W S, Martz R, Lemberger L (1976). Influence of cannabidiol on delta-9-tetrahydrocannabinol effects. *Clin Pharmacol Ther* 19: 300–309.

D'Ambra W A, Hanus L, Breuer A *et al.* (1992). Conformationally restrained analogues of pravadoline: nanomolar potent, enantioselective (aminoalkyl)indole agonists of the cannabinoid receptor. *J Med Chem* 35: 124–135.

Deyo R A, Musty R E (2003). A cannabichromene (CBC) extract alters behavioral despair on the mouse tail suspension test of depression. In: *Proceedings, 2003 Symposium on the Cannabinoids*. Cornwall, ON, Canada: International Cannabinoid Research Society: 146.

Ding A H, Nathan C F, Stuehr D J (1988). Release of reactive nitrogen intermediates and reactive oxygen intermediates from mouse peritoneal macrophages. Comparison of activating cytokines and evidence for independent production. *J Immunol* 141: 2407–2412.

Dudek I, Zagorski T, Liskiewicz J, Kedziora J, Chmielewski H (1992). Effect of gamma radiation on selected indicators of oxygen metabolism in erythrocytes of patients with multiple sclerosis. *Neurol Neurochir* 26: 34–39.

Dunn M, Davis R (1974). The perceived effects of marijuana on spinal cord injured males. *Paraplegia* 12: 175.

Esposito G, Izzo A, Di Rosa M, Iuvone T (2001). Selective cannabinoid CB1 receptor-mediated inhibition of inducible nitric oxide synthase protein expression in C6 rat glioma cells. *J Neurochem* 78: 835–841.

Evans A T, Formukong E A, Evans F J (1987). Actions of cannabis constituents on enzymes of arachidonate metabolism: anti-inflammatory potential. *Biochem Pharmacol* 36: 2035–2037.

Evans F J (1991). Cannabinoids: The separation of central from peripheral effects on a structural basis. *Planta Med* 57: S60–67.

Finnegan-Ling D, Musty R E (1995). Marinol and phantom limb pain: a case study. Paper presented at the International Cannabis Research Society, 21–23 July. L'Esterel, Quebec, Canada.

Fride E, Russo E B (2004). Neuropsychiatry: Schizophrenia, depression, and anxiety. In: Onaivi E, Sugiura T, Di Marzo V, eds. *Endocannabinoids: The Brain and Body's Marijuana and Beyond*. London: Taylor and Francis, in press.

Gerritsen M E, Carley W W, Ranges G E *et al.* (1995). Flavonoids inhibit cytokine-induced endothelial cell adhesion protein gene expression. *Am J Pathol* 147: 278–292.

Gill E W, Paton W D M, Pertwee R G (1970). Preliminary experiments on the chemistry and pharmacology of cannabis. *Nature* 228: 134–136.

Greenspan H C (1993). The role of reactive oxygen species, antioxidants and phytopharmaceuticals in human immunodeficiency virus activity. *Med Hypotheses* 40: 85–92.

Grinspoon L, Russo E (2004). Marihuana. In: Lowinson J H, Ruiz L, Millman R B, Langrod J G, eds. *Substance Abuse: a Comprehensive Textbook*. New York: Lippincott, Williams and Wilkins, in press.

Guimaraes F S, Chiaretti T M, Graeff F G, Zuardi A W (1990). Anti-anxiety effect of cannabidiol in the elevated plus-maze. *Psychopharmacology* 100: 558–559.

Hall W, Solowij N, Lemon J (1994). The therapeutic effects of cannabinoids. In: *The Health and Psychological Consequences of Cannabis Use*. National Drug Strategy Monograph Series No. 25. Canberra: Australian Government Publishing Service: 185–202.

Hampson A J, Grimaldi M, Axelrod J, Wink D (1998). Cannabidiol and (–)9-tetrahydrocannabinol are neuroprotective antioxidants. *Proc Natl Acad Sci USA* 95: 8268–8273.

Hanus L, Gopher A, Almog S *et al.* (1993). Two new unsaturated fatty acid ethanolamides in brain that bind to the cannabinoid receptor. *J Med Chem* 36: 3032–3034.

Hargreaves K, Dubner R, Brown F *et al.* (1988). A new and sensitive method for measuring thermal nociception in cutaneous hyperalgesia. *Pain* 32: 77–88.

Herkenham M, Lynn A B, Little M D *et al.* (1991). Characterisation of cannabinoid receptors in rat brain: a quantitative *in vitro* autoradiographic study. *J Neurosci* 11: 563–583.

Herring A C, Kaminski N E (1999). Cannabinol-mediated inhibition of nuclear factor-kB, cAMP response element-binding protein, and interleukin-2 secretion by activated thymocytes. *J Pharmacol Exp Ther* 291: 1156–1163.

Hohmann A G, Herkenham M (1997). Localization of cannabinoid receptor (CB1). mRNA in neuronal subpopulations of rat spinal cord and dorsal root ganglia. *Abstr Soc Neurosci* 23: 1954.

Hohmann A G, Martin W J, Tsou K *et al.* (1995). Inhibition of noxious stimulus-evoked activity of spinal cord dorsal horn neurons by the cannabinoid WIN55,212-2. *Life Sci* 56: 2111–2118.

Holdcroft A, Smith A, Jacklin A *et al.* (1997). Pain relief with oral cannabinoids in familial Mediterranean fever. *Anaesthesia* 52: 483–486.

Hollister L E (1974). Structure-activity relationships in man of cannabis constituents, and homologs and metabolites of delta9-tetrahydrocannabinol *Pharmacology* 11: 3–11.

Hutter C (1993). On the causes of multiple sclerosis. *Med Hypotheses* 41: 93–96.

Jain A K, Ryan J R, McMahon F G, Smith G (1981). Evaluation of intramuscular levonantradol and placebo in acute postoperative pain. *J Clin Pharmacol* 21(8–9 Suppl): 320S–326S.

Jones C L A (1999). Monoterpenes: essence of a cancer cure. *Nutr Sci News* 4: 190.

Karniol I G, Carlini E A (1973). Pharmacological interaction between cannabidiol and delta 9-tetrahydrocannabinol. *Psychopharmacology* 33: 53–70.

Karniol I G, Shirakawa I, Kasinski N *et al.* (1974). Cannabidiol interferes with the effects of delta-9-tetrahydrocannabinol in man. *Eur J Pharmacol* 28: 172–177.

Karra S, Yazici K M, Gulec C, Unsal I (2000). Mixed anxiety-depressive disorder and major depressive disorder: comparison of the severity of illness and biological variables. *Psychiatry Res* 94: 59–66.

Klarner A, Koch M, Schnitzler H U (1998). Induction of Fos-protein in the forebrain and disruption of sensorimotor gating following N-methyl-D-aspartate infusion into the ventral hippocampus of the rat. *Neuroscience* 84: 443–452.

Komori T R, Fujiwara M, Tanida, M *et al.* (1995). Effects of citrus fragrance on immune function and depressive states. *Neuroimmunomodulation* 2: 174–180.

Lacey K, Zaharia M D, Griffiths J *et al.* (2000). A prospective study of neuroendocrine and immune alterations associated with the stress of an oral academic examination among graduate students. *Psychoneuroendocrinology* 25: 339–356.

Langermann H, Kabiersch A, Newcombe J (1992). Measurement of low-molecular weight antioxidants, uric acid, tyrosine and tryptophan in plagues and white matter from patients with multiple sclerosis. *Eur Neurol* 32: 248–252.

Leite J R, Carlini E A, Lander N, Mechoulam R (1982). Anti-convulsant effects of the (-) and + isomers of cannabdiol and their dimethylheptyl homologs. *Pharmacology* 24: 141–146.

Lemberger L, Rowe H (1975). Clinical pharmacology of nabilone, a cannabinoid derivative. *Clin Pharmacol Ther* 18: 720–726.

Lichtman A H, Martin B R (1991). Spinal and supraspinal components of cannabinoid-induced antinociception. *J Pharmacol Exp Ther* 258: 517–523.

Lorenzetti B B, Souza G E P, Sarti S J *et al.* (1991). Myrecene mimics the peripheral analgesic activity of lemongrass tea. *J Ethnopharmacol* 34: 43–48.

McPartland J M, Pruitt P P (1997). Medical marijuana and its use by the immunocompromised. *Altern Ther* 3: 39–45.

McPartland J M, Russo E B (2001). Cannabis and cannabis extracts: greater than the sum of their parts?. *J Cannabis Ther* 1: 103–132.

Malfait A M, Gallily R, Sumariwalla P F *et al*. (2000). The nonpsychoactive cannabis constituent cannabidiol is an oral anti-arthritic therapeutic in murine collagen-induced arthritis. *Proc Natl Acad Sci USA* 97: 9561–9566.

Marsicano G, Moosmann B, Hermann H (2002). Neuroprotective properties of cannabinoids against oxidative stress: role of the cannabinoid receptor CB1. *J Neurochem* 80: 448–456.

Martin W J, Lai N K, Patrick S L *et al*. (1993). Antinociceptive actions of cannabinoids following intraventricular administration in rats. *Brain Res* 629: 300–304.

Martin W J, Patrick S L, Coffin P O *et al*. (1995). An examination of the central sites of action of cannabinoid-induced antinociception in the rat. *Life Sci* 56: 2103–2109.

Martin W J, Hohmann A G, Walker J M (1996). Suppression of noxious stimulus-evoked activity in the ventral posterolateral nucleus of the thalamus by a cannabinoid agonist: correlation between electrophysiological and antinociceptive effects. *J Neursci* 16: 6601–6611.

Matsuda L A, Lolait S J, Brownstein M J *et al*. (1990). Structure of a cannabinoid receptor and functional expression of the cloned cDNA. *Nature* 346: 561–564.

Mazzari S, Canella R, Petrelli L (1996). N-(2-hydroxyethyl) hexadecanamide is orally active in reducing edema formation and inflammatory hyperalgesia by down-modulating mast cell activation. *Eur J Pharmacol* 300: 227–236.

Mechoulam R, Ben-Shabat S (1999). From gan-zi-gun-nu to anandamide and 2-arachidonoylglycerol: The ongoing story of cannabis. *Nat Prod Rep* 16: 131–143.

Mechoulam R, Ben-Shabat S, Hanus L *et al*. (1995). Identification of an endogenous 2-monoglyceride present in canine gut that binds to cannabinoid receptors. *Biochem Pharmacol* 50: 83–90.

Mediavilla V, Steinman S (1997). Essential oil of *Cannabis sativa* L. strains. *J Int Hemp Assoc* 4: 82–84.

Meschler J P, Howlett A C (1999). Thujone exhibits low affinity for cannabinoid receptors but fails to evoke cannabimimetic responses. *Pharmacol Biochem Behav* 62: 473–480.

Miyazawa M, Watanbe H, Kameoka H (1997). Inhibition of acetylcholinesterase activity by monoterpenoids with a *p*-methane skeleton. *J Agric Food Chem* 45: 677–679.

Morgan J I, Curran T (1995). Proto-oncogenes: Beyond second messengers. In: Bloom F E, Kupfer D J, eds. *The Fourth Generation of Progress. Psychopharmacology* 55: 263–265.

Munro S, Thomas K L, Abu-Shaar M (1993). Molecular characterization of a peripheral receptor for cannabinoids. *Nature* 365: 61–65.

Musonda C A, Chipman, J K (1998). Quercetin inhibits hydrogen peroxide-induced NF-kB DNA binding activity and DNA damage in HepG2 cells. *Carcinogen* 19: 1583–1589.

Musty R E (1984). Possible anxiolytic effects of cannabidiol. In: Agurell S, Dewey W, Willette R, eds. *The Cannabinoids*. New York: Academic Press: 829–844.

Musty R E (2002). Cannabinoid therapeutic potential in motivational processes, psychological disorders and central nervous system disorders. In: Onaivi E, ed. *Biology of Marijuana*. New York: Taylor and Francis: 45–74.

Musty R E, Conti L H, Mechoulam R (1985). Anxiolytic properties of cannabidiol. In: Harvey D, ed. *Marihuana '84*. Oxford: IRL Press: 713–719.

Musty R E, Deyo R A, Baer J L *et al.* (2000a). Effects of SR141716 on animal models of schizophrenia. *Proceedings, 2001 Symposium on the Cannabinoids*. Burlington, VT: International Cannabinoid Research Society.

Musty R E, Bouldin M J, Erickson J R, Deyo R (2002b). CBD and THC extracts after behavioral despair on the mouse tail suspension test. *Proceedings, 2001 Symposium on the Cannabinoids*. Burlington, VT: International Cannabinoid Research Society: 140.

Noyes R, Jr, Brunk S F, Avery D A H, Canter A C (1975a). The analgesic properties of delta-9-tetrahydrocannabinol and codeine. *Clin Pharmacol Ther* 18: 84–89.

Noyes R, Jr, Brunk S F, Baram D A, Canter A (1975b). Analgesic effect of delta-9-tetrahydrocannabinol. *J Clin Pharmacol* 15: 139–143.

Offord E A, Mace K, Avanti O (1997). Mechanisms involved in the chemoprotective effects of rosemary extracts studied in human liver and bronchial cells. *Cancer Lett* 114: 275–281.

Paris R R, Henri E, Paris M (1976). Sur les c-flavonoides du *Cannabis sativa* L. *Plantes Med Phytother* 10: 144–154.

Petitet F, Jeantaud B, Reibaud M *et al.* (1998). Complex pharmacology of natural cannabinoids: evidence for partial agonist activity of delta-9-tetrahydrocannabinol and antagonist activity of cannabidiol on rat brain cannabinoid receptors. *Life Sci* 63: 1–6.

Raft D, Gregg J, Ghia J, Harris L (1977). Effects of intravenous tetrahydrocannabinol on experimental and surgical pain. Psychological correlates of the analgesic response *Clin Pharmacol Ther* 21: 26–33.

Raman A, Weir U, Bloomfield S F (1995). Antimicrobial effects of tea-tree oil and its major components on *Staphylococcus aureus*, *Staph. epidermidis* and *Propionibacterium acnes*. *Lett Appl Microbiol* 21: 242–245.

Rang H P, Bevan S, Dray A (1994). Inflammatory pain. In: Wall P D, Melzack R, eds. *Textbook of Pain*, 3rd edn. New York: Churchill Livingstone: 57–78.

Rao V S N, Menezes A M S, Viana G S B (1990). Effects of myrecene on nociception in mice. *J Pharm Pharmacol* 42: 877–878.

Regelson W, Butler J R, Schultz J *et al.* (1976). D9-tetrahydrocannabinol as an effective antidepressant and appetite stimulating agent in advanced cancer patients. In: Braude M C, Lszara S, eds. *Pharmacology of Marijuana*. New York: Raven Press: 763–776.

Richardson J D, Aanonsen L, Hargreaves K M (1998a). Antihyperalgesic effects of spinal cannabinoids. *Eur J Pharmacol* 345: 145–153.

Richardson J D, Aanonsen L, Hargreaves K M (1998b). Hypoactivity of the spinal cannabinoid system results in NMDA-dependent hyperalgesia. *J Neurosci* 18: 451–457.

Richardson J D, Kilo S, Hargreaves K M (1998c). Cannabinoids reduce hyperalgesia and inflammation via interaction with peripheral CB1 receptors. *Pain* 75: 111–119.

Ross S A, ElSohly M A (1996). The volatile oil composition of fresh and air-dried buds of *Cannabis sativa*. *J Nat Prod* 59: 49–51.

Russo E B (2002). Role of cannabis and cannabinoids in pain management. In: Weiner R S, ed. *Pain Management: A Practical Guide for Clinicians*. Boca Raton, FL: CRC Press: 357–375.

Russo E B, Mathre M L, Byrne A *et al.* (2002). Chronic cannabis use in the Compassionate Investigational New Drug Program: An examination of benefits and adverse effects of legal clinical cannabis. *J Cannabis Ther* 2: 3–57.

Sandyk R, Consroe P, Stern L *et al.* (1988). Preliminary trial of cannabidiol in Huntington's disease. In: Chesher G, Consroe P, Musty R E, eds. *Marihuana: An International Research Report*. Canberra: Australian Government Publishing Service: 157–162.

Schnelle M, Grotenhermen F, Reif M, Gorter R W (1999). Ergebnisse einer standardisierten Umfrage zur medizinischen Verwendung von Cannabisprodukten im deutschen Sprachraum [Results of a standardized survey on the medical use of cannabis products in the German-speaking area]. *Forsch Komplementarmed Suppl* 3: 28–36.

Sebens J B, Koch T, Ter Horst G J, Korf J (1995). Differential Fos-protein induction in rat forebrain regions after acute and long-term haloperidol and clozapine treatment. *Eur J Pharmacol* 273: 175–182.

Shivers S C, Newton C, Friedman H *et al.* (1994). Δ^9-Tetrahydrocannabinol (THC) modulates IL-1 bioactivity in human monocyte/macrophage cell lines. *Life Sci* 54: 1281–1289.

Smith S, Denhardt G, Terminelli C (2001). The anti-inflammatory activities of cannabinoid receptor ligands in mouse peritonitis models. *Eur J Pharmacol* 432: 107–119.

Sofia R D, Vassar H B, Knobloch L C (1975). Comparative analgesic activity of various naturally occurring cannabinoids in mice and rats. *Psychopharmacology* 40: 285–295.

Sugiura T, Kondo S, Sukagawa A (1995). 2-Arachidonylglycerol: a possible endogenous cannabinoid receptor ligand in brain. *Biochem Biophys Res Commun* 215: 89–97.

Tchilibon S, Mechoulam R, Fride E, Hanus L (2000). Cannabidiol metabolites and analogues: synthesis and their anti-inflammatory effect. *Proceedings, 2000 Symposium on the Cannabinoids*. Burlington, VT: International Cannabinoid Research Society: 118.

Thomas B F, Gilliam A F, Burcj D F *et al.* (1998). Comparative receptor binding analyses of cannabinoid agonists and antagonists. *J Pharmacol Exp Ther* 285: 285–292.

Todorova V K, Elbein A D, Kyosseva S V (2003). Increased expression of c-Jun transcription factor in cerebellar vermis of patients with schizophrenia. *Neuropsychopharmacology* 28(8): 1506–1514.

Turner C E (1985). Marijuana and cannabis: research why the conflict. In: Harvey D, ed. *Marihuana '87*. Oxford: IRL Press: 31–36

Turner C E, ElSohly M A, Boeren E G (1980). Constituents of *Cannabis sativa* L. XVII. A review of the natural constituents. *J Nat Prod* 43: 169–304.

Vinegar R, Truax J F, Selph J J (1976). Quantitative studies of the pathway to acute carrageenan inflammation. *Fedn Proc* 35: 2447–2456.

Walker J M, Huang S M, Strangman N M, Tsou K, Sanudo-Pena M C (1999). Pain modulation by the release of the endogenous cannabinoid anandamide *Proc Natl Acad Sci USA* 96: 12198–12203.

Walker J M, Strangman N M, Huang S M (2002). Cannabinoids as analgesics. In: Onaivi E, ed. *Biology of Marijuana*. New York: Taylor and Francis: 573–590.

Wallace M J, Martin B R, DeLorenzo R J (2002). Evidence for a physiological role of endocannabinoids in the modulation of seizure threshold and severity. *Eur J Pharmacol* 452: 295–301.

Wallace M J, Blair R E, Falenski K W *et al.* (2003). The endogenous cannabinoid system regulates seizure frequency and duration in a model of temporal lobe epilepsy. *J Pharmacol Exp Ther* 307: 129–137.

Warner R, Taylor D, Wright J *et al.* (1994). Substance use among the mentally ill: Prevalence, reasons for use, and effects on illness. *Am J Orthopsychiatry* 64: 30–39.

Yaksh T L (1981). The antinociceptive effects of intrathecally administered levonantradol and desacetyllevonantradol in the rat. *J Clin Pharmacol* 21: 3345–3405.

Zagorski T, Dudek I, Berkan L *et al.* (1991). Superoxide dismutase (SOD-1) activity in erythrocytes of patients with multiple sclerosis. *Neurol Neurochir Pol* 25: 725–730.

Zuardi A W, Finkelfarb E, Bueno O F A *et al.* (1981). Characteristics of the stimulus produced by the mixture of cannabidiol with Δ^9-tetrahydrocannabinol. *Arch Int Pharmacod Ther* 249: 137–146.

Zuardi A W, Shirakawa I, Finkelfarb E, Karniol I G (1982). Action of cannabidiol on the anxiety and other effects produced by delta 9-THC in normal subjects. *Psychopharmacology* 76: 245–250.

Zuardi A W, Rodrigues J A, Cunha J M (1991). Effects of cannabidiol in animal models predictive of antipsychotic activity. *Psychopharmacology* 104: 260–264.

Zuardi A W, Cosme R A, Graeff F G, Guimaraes F S (1993a). Effects of ipsapirone and cannabidiol on human experimental anxiety. *J Psychopharmacol* 7: 82–88.

Zuardi A W, Guimaraes F S, Moreira A C (1993b). Effect of cannabidiol on plasma prolactin, growth hormone and cortisol in human volunteers. *Braz J Med Biol Res* 26: 213–217.

Zuardi A W, Morais S L, Guimaraes F S, Mechoulam R (1995). Antipsychotic effect of cannabidiol. *J Clin Psychiatry* 56: 485–486.

Zuardi A W, Guimares V M C, Del Bel E A (2002). Cannabidiol: possible therapeutic actions. In: Grotenhermen F, Russo E, eds. *Cannabis and Cannabinoids. Pharmacology, Toxicology, and Therapeutic Potential*. Binghampton, NY: Haworth Press: 359–369.

8

Metabolism and pharmacokinetics of cannabinoids

Gabrielle Hawksworth and Karen McArdle

Pharmacokinetics is a means of describing all the processes that affect the disposition of a drug in the body over time (Clarke and Smith, 1993; McLeod, 1999). The pharmacokinetics of a drug depend on a number of factors, including the route of administration, the lipophilicity of the drug, metabolism, drug–drug interactions and elimination. The cannabinoids are no exception and numerous studies have been conducted over the last 30 years to investigate the factors that influence the pharmacokinetics of these plant-derived compounds. The main focus of these studies has been on Δ^9-tetrahydrocannabinol (Δ^9-THC), not just because it is the most potent psychoactive component of marijuana, but because it also has a number of therapeutic applications (Pertwee 1999a; Darmani, 2001a,b; Kumar *et al.*, 2001).

The term cannabinoid is given to the C_{21} compounds (and their metabolites) found in extracts of *Cannabis sativa* L. (Turner *et al.*, 1980; Harvey and Paton, 1984; Harvey, 1992). Classical cannabinoids have a dibenzopyran-type structure, with a hydroxyl group at the C-1 aromatic position and an alkyl group at the C-3 aromatic position (Figure 8.1). Most of the major cannabinoids possess a pentyl side-chain at C-3, however lower homologues also exist, as in the case of Δ^9-tetrahydrocannabivarin (THCV), which has a propyl side-chain (Figure 8.1). The most abundant cannabinoids found in a typical cannabis extract are, Δ^9-THC, its precursor cannabidiol (CBD), and cannabinol, which is spontaneously formed from Δ^9-THC (Figure 8.1). Δ^8-Tetrahydrocannabinol (Δ^8-THC), although not an abundant cannabinoid (Hively *et al.*, 1966), is of interest because it displays similar pharmacological activity to Δ^9-THC (Hollister and Gillespie, 1973; Mechoulam *et al.*, 1999). Two numbering schemes exist for cannabinoids: the monoterpene system (Δ^1) and the dibenzopyran (Δ^9) system. The dibenzopyran system is more popular in recent literature, however the monoterpene system is still adopted for CBD (Figure 8.1).

Δ⁹-Tetrahydrocannabinol

Δ⁸-Tetrahydrocannabinol

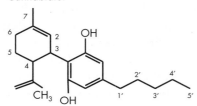

Cannabidiol

Cannabinol

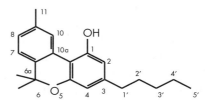

Δ⁹-Tetrahydrocannabivarin

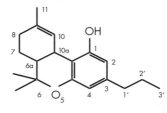

Figure 8.1 Structures of the major cannabinoids: Δ⁹-tetrahydrocannabinol, Δ⁸-tetrahydrocannabinol, cannabidiol, cannabinol and Δ⁹-tetrahydrocannabivarin.

Molecular modelling and structure–activity studies have found that there are three regions of the classical cannabinoid structure that are important for cannabimimetic activity: the phenolic hydroxyl (C-1), the side-chain and the substitution at C-9 (Burstein, 1999; Pertwee, 2001; Martin *et al.*, 2002). Modifications to any one of these regions can lead to changes in pharmacological activity. Substitution of the C-1 hydroxyl group with fluorine caused a substantial decrease in CB₁ receptor affinity and cannabimimetic potency (Martin *et al.*, 2002). This study also showed that the hydroxyl group on C-1 donated electrons for hydrogen bonding to the CB₁ receptor. Hydroxymethyl substitution at

C-9 increases the cannabimimetic potency of the resulting derivative. For example, 11-hydroxy-Δ^9-THC (11-OH-THC) and 11-hydroxy-Δ^8-THC are more potent than their parent compounds. However, conversion of the hydroxymethyl group to a carboxylated analogue leads to a reduction in the cannabimimetic activity. Δ^9-THC-11-oic-acid (THCCOOH), an abundant Δ^9-THC metabolite, is not psychoactive. On the other hand, carboxylated derivatives possess analgesic and anti-inflammatory properties equivalent to those of the parent molecules, indicating that these effects are mediated via a different pathway from the cannabimimetic effects (Burstein *et al.*, 1986, 1988, 1989). The length and the conformational mobility of the cannabinoid side-chain are important determinants of the pharmacological activity (Keimowitz *et al.*, 2000). Alterations to the side-chain can often lead to elevated activity. When the pentyl side-chain of the non-psychoactive THCCOOH was substituted with a dimethylheptyl side-chain, the outcome was an active analogue equipotent to Δ^9-THC. Additionally, cannabinoids with the same absolute configuration as $(-)\Delta^9$-THC at C-6a and C-10a *(R,R)* have greater cannabimimetic activity than the (+) enantiomers (Burstein, 1999; Pertwee, 1999b, 2001).

Cannabinoids are highly lipophilic compounds with log K_{ow} values >5 (Table 8.1). They are rapidly distributed to various tissues such as the brain, liver, kidney and fat, from where they are slowly released back into the bloodstream. A steady state volume of distribution for Δ^9-THC ranging from 500 to 800 L has been reported (Hunt and Jones 1980; Busto *et al.*, 1989), which is indicative of highly lipophilic compounds. Protein binding studies have shown that almost 90% of Δ^9-THC and some of its metabolites are bound to blood plasma proteins. Approximately 10% is bound to red blood cells (Wahlqvist *et al.*, 1970;

Table 8.1 Octanol–water (K_{ow}) coefficient for the major cannabinoids and their metabolites

Compound	Log K_{ow}	
	HPLC	*Calculated*
Δ^9-THC	6.97	7.18
11-OH-Δ^9-THC	5.33	5.19
Δ^8-THC	7.41	7.18
Cannabidiol	5.79	6.92
Cannabinol	6.20	7.40

From Thomas *et al.* (1990).

Widman *et al.*, 1973, 1974; Garrett and Hunt 1974; Giroud *et al.*, 2001). The accumulation of cannabinoids in fatty tissue and their slow release are responsible for the protracted elimination of cannabinoids from the body and hence the prolonged pharmacological effect.

Metabolism of Δ^9-THC, cannabidiol, cannabinol and Δ^9-tetrahydrocannabivarin in humans

The metabolism of Δ^9-THC is complex and has been extensively studied in a number of species (Harvey *et al.*, 1978; Harvey and Paton, 1984; Agurell *et al.*, 1986; Harvey, 1992). Although the metabolic profile is similar across species, there are quantitative differences in the formation of metabolites. Over 100 metabolites of Δ^9-THC have been identified (Harvey, 1985, 1992). The primary metabolite is 11-OH-THC, which is further metabolised to the 11-oic acid (THCCOOH). Both of these metabolites are excreted in the urine as glucuronides, as are the side-chain hydroxylated metabolites (Williams and Moffat, 1980; Harvey and Paton, 1984; Agurell *et al.*, 1986). The other main oxidative metabolites are 8α- and 8β-hydroxy-Δ^9-THC (8-OH-THC), with the 8β-metabolite predominating in humans. The pentyl side-chain of Δ^9-THC can be hydroxylated in several positions and several dihydroxy metabolites are formed, following oxidation at allylic positions and on the side-chain (Harvey *et al.*, 1980; Halldin *et al.*, 1982a,b).

Δ^9-THC and the 11-OH-THC metabolite are equipotent in their psychotropic effects, whereas the 8β-OH metabolite is about one-third as potent and the 8α-OH metabolite is less potent than the 8β-OH metabolite (Hollister, 1973; Wall and Perez-Reyes, 1981; Agurell *et al.*, 1986). Interactions leading to altered formation of the metabolites at the 11 or 8 allylic position may result in altered pharmacological effects. During intravenous (i.v.) infusion Δ^9-THC remains in the blood at higher levels than 11-OH-THC, but this ratio is altered after oral administration, due to the extensive first pass elimination (Ohlsson *et al.*, 1980; Wall *et al.*, 1983; Law *et al.*, 1984; Agurell *et al.*, 1986). The ratio of 11-OH-THC to Δ^9-THC after i.v. infusion is 1:15, whereas after oral administration, the ratio is approximately 0.75:1 (Wall *et al.*, 1983). In animal studies 11-OH-THC crosses the blood–brain barrier more efficiently than the parent compound. This correlates with behavioural effects where the speed of onset is faster after injecting 11-OH-THC than parent compound. About a third of the dose of parent compound and metabolites is excreted in the urine, with 15% being excreted over the first 72 hours. The major urinary metabolite is Δ^9-THC-11-oic acid, followed by 4'OH-Δ^9-THC-11-oic acid (Halldin *et al.*, 1982a,b).

Cannabidiol (CBD), a non-psychoactive cannabinoid of therapeutic interest, undergoes monohydroxylation at C-7, with the formation of 7-OH-CBD and the 7-oic acid (Agurell *et al.*, 1981, 1985). The 7-oic acid is abundant in both urine and plasma. There is also hydroxylation at each of the carbons on the pentyl side-chain. Side-chain hydroxylated derivatives of CBD-7-oic acid are particularly abundant in human urine (Harvey, 1992). Dihydroxylated metabolites have also been identified and about 90% are present as 7-OH metabolites (Martin *et al.*, 1976). The excretion rate of metabolites in human urine is similar to the excretion of Δ^9-THC in humans (Wall *et al.*, 1976).

Cannabinol (CBN) is mainly metabolised to monohydroxy CBN with the 7-OH metabolite being the predominant metabolite (Wall *et al.*, 1976; Agurell *et al.*, 1981, 1985). The levels in plasma are about 10% of the CBN levels after i.v. administration. The metabolic profile is less diverse than that seen following Δ^9-THC administration, due to one more ring being aromatic in nature. Only 8% of a CBN dose was excreted in urine within 72 hours (Agurell *et al.*, 1986).

In general, side-chain hydroxylations are minor pathways in humans. Long-chain fatty acid conjugates of hydroxylated metabolites of these cannabinoids have been reported in the rat (Yisak *et al.*, 1978).

Δ^9-Tetrahydrocannabivarin (9-THCV) is a natural component of the cannabis plant, with a propyl instead of a pentyl side-chain as in Δ^9-THC. The major urinary metabolite, similar to the other cannabinoids described above, is 11-nor-Δ^9-THCV-9-COOH. The presence of this metabolite in a urine specimen indicates prior ingestion of 9-THCV, which exists only in cannabis preparations and is not a component of Marinol (ElSohly *et al.*, 2001).

Metabolism *in vitro* in humans

Only limited data are available on the *in vitro* metabolism of cannabinoids in humans. These mainly focus on the major cannabinoids, Δ^9-THC, CBD and CBN (Wall *et al.*, 1976; Wall and Perez-Reyes, 1981; Halldin *et al.*, 1982c; Yamamoto *et al.*, 1983; Harvey and Paton 1984; Harvey and Brown, 1990). The *in vitro* systems used (e.g. hepatic microsomes and hepatocytes) have been useful in elucidating the phase I and II metabolites. Other cannabinoids such as cannabichromene and cannabielsoin have also been investigated in several species (Yamamoto *et al.*, 1988; Brown and Harvey, 1990).

Phase I metabolism of cannabinoids is catalysed by the cytochrome P450 (CYP) mixed function oxidase system (Bornheim *et al.*, 1992; McArdle *et al.*, 2001). The CYPs are a superfamily of haem-containing enzymes that are found mainly in the liver but also in small intestine and kidney. These enzymes are responsible for the oxidation of about 90% of drugs administered to humans (Shimada *et al.*, 1994; Bertz and Granneman, 1997). The elucidation of the CYP isoforms involved in phase I metabolism is important in highlighting any potential drug–drug interactions. Such interactions could alter the pharmacokinetic profile of coadministered drugs (Spatzenegger and Jaeger, 1995). The hepatic CYPs involved in phase I metabolism in humans and their relative abundance are shown in Figure 8.2.

The primary route of metabolism for the cannabinoids *in vitro* (Figure 8.3) is hydroxylation at C-11 to give 11-OH-Δ^9-THC, -Δ^8-THC and -CBN (Halldin *et al.*, 1982c; Harvey and Paton, 1984; Agurell *et al.*, 1986; Bornheim *et al.*, 1992). CBD is also hydroxylated at this position and the metabolite is designated 7-OH-CBD (see Fig. 8.1). Δ^9-THC and CBD also undergo allylic hydroxylation at C-8 (C-6 for CBD) to yield 8α- and 8β-OH-Δ^9-THC or 6α- and 6β-OH-CBD. Δ^8-THC undergoes hydroxylation at C-7 to yield 7α- and 7β-OH-Δ^8-THC. The 11-OH metabolite undergoes further oxidation to its corresponding aldehyde (e.g. 11-oxo-Δ^9-THC). The C-11 aldehyde is then further oxidised to its carboxylic acid, THCCOOH. Likewise the 8-OH metabo-

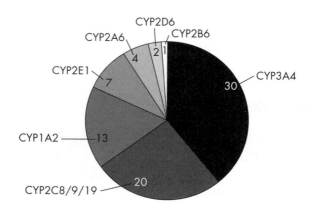

Figure 8.2 The major hepatic cytochrome P450 isoforms involved in human metabolism and their relative abundance (%). Adapted from Shimada *et al.* (1994).

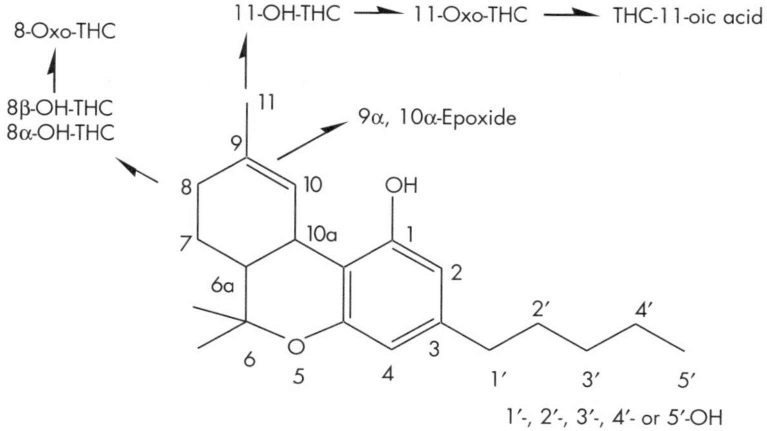

Figure 8.3 Δ^9-Tetrahydrocannabinol Phase I hepatic metabolism. Adapted from Narimatsu *et al.* (1991).

lites are oxidised to their corresponding ketones. Epoxidation and side-chain hydroxylation are minor routes of metabolism in human *in vitro* systems (Yamamoto *et al.*, 1984; Agurell *et al.*, 1986; Bornheim *et al.*, 1992).

Hepatic cytochrome P450s (CYPs) responsible for phase 1 metabolism of cannabinoids

The CYP isoforms responsible for the oxidative metabolism of Δ^9-THC have been identified in several species, including rat (Narimatsu *et al.*, 1990a, 1991), mouse (Bornheim and Correia, 1990, 1991), guinea-pig (Narimatsu *et al.*, 1990b) and human (Bornheim *et al.*, 1992; McArdle *et al.*, 2001). All of these studies implicate the 2C and 3A subfamilies in the formation of the phase I metabolites. A summary of the major CYP isoforms involved in the oxidative metabolism of Δ^9-THC in a number of species is given in Table 8.2.

In humans, the formation of 11-OH-THC is primarily catalysed by CYP2C9, CYP2C19 and CYP2D6 (Bornheim *et al.*, 1992; McArdle *et al.*, 2001). CYP2C19 is also the key isoform involved in the formation of 7-OH-CBD, with contributions from CYP2C9 and CYP3A4/5. The oxidation of the 11-oxo-metabolite to the 11-oic acid (Figure 8.3) for both Δ^9-THC and Δ^8-THC is catalysed by microsomal aldehyde oxygenase (MALDO) (Watanabe *et al.*, 1991, 1993, 1995).

Table 8.2 Summary of major cytochrome P450 isoforms involved in metabolism of Δ⁹-tetrahydrocannabinol

	11-OH-THC	*8β-OH-THC*	*8α-OH-THC*	*3'-OH-THC*	*Minor metabolites*
Human	CYP2C9 CYP2C19 CYP2C8[a] CYP2D6	CYP3A4	CYP2C19 CYP3A4	–	CYP3A4/5
Rat (male)	CYP2C11 CYP2C13[a] CYP2A2[a]	CYP2A2		CYP2C11	
Rat (female)	CYP2C6				
Mouse	CYP2C29	CYP3A11	CYP2C29	–	
Guinea-pig	CYP2B	CYP3A		–	

[a]Slight activity.

Watanabe *et al.* (1995) suggest that the MALDO activity is catalysed by a member of the CYP2C subfamily. Hydroxylation at C-8 is catalysed by CYP3A4/5 and CYP2C19 for Δ⁹-THC, with CYP2C19 displaying stereoselectivity in the formation of 8α-OH-THC but not the 8β-OH metabolite (McArdle *et al.*, 2001). The isoform(s) responsible for the oxidation of 8-OH-THC to 8-oxo-Δ⁹ metabolites has not been identified in humans. It is probable that CYP3A4/5 is responsible since the oxidation of 7-OH-Δ⁸-THC to 7-oxo-Δ⁸-THC is catalysed by CYP3A4 (Narimatsu *et al.*, 1988; Matsunaga *et al.*, 1998, 2000, 2001).

Inhibition and induction of oxidative metabolism in the liver by cannabinoids

Many drugs have the ability to modify the metabolism of other drugs. These drug–drug interactions may lead to an alteration in the therapeutic effect of many drugs (Spatzenegger and Jaeger, 1995). Concomitant administration of drugs increases the possibility of drug–drug interactions through the induction or inhibition of drug-metabolising enzymes. Table 8.3 lists some key features of CYP induction and inhibition.

Induction results in increased enzyme activity, which is brought about by an increase in enzyme synthesis. The mechanism of induction is complex and involves the activation of nuclear receptors, which bind

Table 8.3 Key features of cytochrome P450 induction and inhibition

Induction	*Inhibition*
↑ mRNA	Competitive, non-competitive or mechanism based inhibition
↑ Enzyme activity	↓ Enzyme activity
↓ Parent drug	↑ Parent drug
↓ Pharmacological effect when parent drug is the active form	↑ Toxicity when the parent drug is the active form

to DNA response elements and stimulate the transcription of a CYP gene. Certain inducers display selectivity towards CYP isoforms in humans (e.g. rifampicin selectively induces CYP3A4).

Inhibition can occur when two drugs compete for the same isoform of a drug-metabolising enzyme, resulting in a decreased rate of metabolism for one or both drugs. Toxicity may occur due to inhibition of metabolism. Inhibitors differ in their selectivity for CYP isoforms (e.g. sulfaphenazole selectively inhibits CYP2C9) and are classified according to their mode of inhibition.

Inhibition

CBD affects the metabolism of several drugs *in vitro* and *in vivo*, including Δ^9-THC, by selectively inhibiting or inactivating isozymes belonging to the CYP2C and CYP3A subfamilies (Bornheim *et al.*, 1981, 1993; Watanabe *et al.*, 1987; Bornheim and Correia, 1989, 1990, 1991; McArdle *et al.*, 2001). A recent study by Mathews *et al.* (2000) on the inhibitory effects of CBD on a range of CYPs showed that CBD also inhibits CYP2D6 activity *in vitro* in humans and CYP2D1 activity *in vivo* in the rat.

CBD differentially inhibits the oxidative metabolism of Δ^9-THC in human hepatic microsomal samples (Jaeger *et al.*, 1996; McArdle *et al.*, 2001). CBD has no inhibitory effect on the formation of the 11-OH metabolite when preincubated with an NADPH-generating system. McArdle *et al.* (2001) have shown that CBD coincubated with Δ^9-THC and an NADPH-generating system results in a decrease in 11-OH-THC formation. One possible mode of inhibition is that CBD is competing with Δ^9-THC for the CYP2C9 and/or CYP2C19 active sites. A time-dependent decrease in 8β-OH-THC production after pretreatment with CBD and an NADPH-generating system *in vitro* suggests that CBD and/or a CBD metabolite is responsible for the inhibition of CYP3A4/5 activity. Bornheim and Grillo (1998) suggest that a CBD-hydroxyquinone intermediate formed at the CYP3A11 active site in the mouse covalently binds to specific amino acid residues on CYP3A11, rendering the isoform inactive. CBD attenuates the psychotropic effects of Δ^9-THC when both are coadministered to humans (Hollister, 1973; Karniol *et al.*, 1974). Since CBD does not significantly modulate the pharmacokinetics of Δ^9-THC (Agurell *et al.*, 1981; Hunt *et al.*, 1981), this reduction in Δ^9-THC effects could be attributed to interactions at the receptor level.

Δ^9-THC displays weak inhibitory effects on the metabolism of antipyrine, pentobarbital and ethanol in humans (Benowitz and Jones, 1977). Prolonged ingestion of Δ^9-THC increased the plasma half-lives of antipyrine and pentobarbital, delayed the absorption of pentobarbital and ethanol and delayed the disappearance of ethanol from blood. Benowitz and Jones attribute these effects to increased distribution volume and decreased metabolism.

Mechanisms of Δ^9-THC inhibition of drug-metabolising enzymes have been investigated in the rat. Gosh and Poddar (1992) showed that Δ^9-THC competitively inhibited *N*- and *O*-demethylase activity under *in vitro* conditions. In contrast, aniline hydroxylase displayed non-competitive and mixed-type inhibition. Similar results were obtained for these enzymes by Mitra *et al.* (1976), who proposed that Δ^9-THC elicits its inhibitory effect by either specific or non-specific interaction of Δ^9-THC with the active site of the CYPs or perturbations of the microsomal membrane by Δ^9-THC.

Induction

Evaluation of the inducing effects of cannabinoids has mainly focused on the potent CYP inhibitor CBD (Watanabe *et al.*, 1987; Bornheim and Correia 1989, 1990; Deutsch *et al.*, 1991; Bornheim *et al.*, 1994; Roth *et al.*, 2001). Drugs that inhibit or inactivate CYPs can also induce this family of enzymes after prolonged exposure. Bornheim *et al.* (1994) demonstrated that repetitive administration of CBD results in a >10-fold increase in mouse CYP2B10 mRNA. The mRNA levels correlate with increased CYP2B protein content and enzyme activity. Previous experiments by Bornheim and Correia (1989) support the induction of a CYP displaying similarities to the phenobarbital-induced CYP2B. A twofold increase in CYP3A and CYP2C mRNA levels was also obtained (Bornheim *et al.*, 1994). As expected, this small increase in mRNA level did not increase the enzymatic activity of either CYP.

Marked induction of CYP2B1 (phenobarbital-inducible rat isoform) by CBD was shown by McArdle *et al.* (2003). Rats treated repetitively with 150 mg/kg CBD showed a 140-fold increase in CYP2B1 mRNA, which correlated well with the induction of CYP2B1/2 protein. A similar study by Bornheim *et al.* (1994) showed a ninefold induction in CYP2B1/2 protein coupled with a sevenfold increase in CYP2B enzyme activity. In contrast, Deutsch *et al.* (1991) reported that CBD did not induce CYP2B1/2 mRNA levels when administered alone, but had the ability to potentiate the inducing effect of phenobarbital. Bornheim *et al.* (1994) suggest that the discrepancy between the two studies may be related to species differences or that the CBD dose (30 mg/kg) used in the Deutsch study was insufficient to induce CYP2B1/2 by itself. A more modest induction of rat CYP3A23 mRNA (threefold) and protein was also observed by McArdle *et al.* The induction of CYP2B1 and CYP3A23 by CBD appears to be transcriptionally regulated and is probably mediated through activation of the nuclear receptors, constitutive androstane receptor (CAR) and pregnane X receptor (PXR), respectively (Muangmoonchai *et al.*, 2000; Kliewer and Wilson, 2002). CBD also displays post-transcriptional regulation of CYP induction in rat, possibly through protein stabilisation. CYP1A2 was markedly induced at the protein level but no increase in mRNA was observed (McArdle *et al.*, 2003). These rat studies show that CBD is a complex compound with both transcriptional and post-transcriptional modes of CYP induction. They also highlight the potential for CBD to induce the human equivalents of these rat CYPs, mainly CYP2B6 and CYP3A4, following extended periods of administration.

Extracts of a marijuana cigarette induced higher levels of CYP1A1 mRNA than extracts from a tobacco cigarette when both were compared *in vitro* using a murine hepatoma cell line (Roth *et al.*, 2001). This difference was attributed to Δ^9-THC, which was shown to induce CYP1A1 via the aryl hydrocarbon receptor. Δ^9-THC also competitively inhibited the CYP1A1-dependent ethoxyresorufin dealkylation. Since CYP1A1 is responsible for the activation of procarcinogens found in marijuana and tobacco smoke (polycyclic aromatic hydrocarbons), the induction of this enzyme by Δ^9-THC in marijuana could increase the risk of cancer in marijuana smokers. However, the ability of Δ^9-THC to competitively inhibit CYP1A1 activity may counteract these harmful effects and hence the risk would depend on the relative levels of induction and inhibition.

Pharmacokinetics by different routes of administration

In drug development, the route of administration is an important consideration as it will influence the bioavailability (systemic availability) of a drug and hence the efficacy. Currently Δ^9-THC is prescribed as an antiemetic (Marinol) and is administered orally in an oil formulation. This therapy displays poor efficacy due to the low bioavailability of active Δ^9-THC when administered orally. Administration via smoking or intravenous infusion, two routes known to elevate the bioavailability of Δ^9-THC, is neither feasible nor acceptable. This section of the chapter gives a brief outline of three routes of administration. In addition, rectal administration, a practical alternative to oral administration, is mentioned.

Administration of Δ^9-THC by smoking

The amount of Δ^9-THC in a marijuana cigarette is typically in the range 5–30 mg (Busto *et al.*, 1989). Inhalation of Δ^9-THC in the form of a marijuana cigarette is characterised by rapid absorption from the lungs into the bloodstream, then immediate distribution to various organs such as the brain and deep tissue compartments (e.g. fatty tissue). Therefore, the reintroduction of Δ^9-THC into the bloodstream is the rate-limiting step in the formation and elimination of Δ^9-THC metabolites. The plasma versus time profile for smoked Δ^9-THC is very similar to the profile following i.v. administration, except that the plasma levels are approximately half those found after i.v. infusion (Lemberger *et al.*, 1972; Ohlsson *et al.*, 1980; Chiang and Barnett, 1984; Busto *et al.*, 1989). Δ^9-THC peak plasma levels are reached within 3–8 minutes from the start of smoking (Perez-Reyes *et al.*, 1981, 1982; Barnett *et al.*, 1982; Huestis *et al.*, 1992a,b,c). Huestis *et al.* (1992b) also noted that Δ^9-THC can be detected in plasma following the first inhalation of a marijuana cigarette, with a mean concentration of 7 ng/mL and 18 ng/mL for a 15.8 mg and 33.8 mg Δ^9-THC content respectively. Mean peak Δ^9-THC levels after smoking a single cigarette often exceed 100 ng/mL. However, the decline is rapid and at 2 hours from the start of smoking the level drops to <10 ng/mL (Ohlsson *et al.*, 1980;

Perez-Reyes *et al.*, 1981, 1982; Barnett *et al.*, 1982; Lindgren *et al.*, 1982; Reeve *et al.*, 1983; Chiang and Barnett, 1984; Law *et al.*, 1984; Huestis *et al.*, 1992b,c). Despite this sudden decrease, Δ^9-THC is still detectable in plasma after 12 hours (Huestis *et al.*, 1992b,c). A mean Δ^9-THC plasma half-life between 1 and 4 days has been shown (Barnett *et al.*, 1982; Ohlsson *et al.*, 1982; Wall *et al.*, 1983; Johansson *et al.*, 1987, 1988, 1989; Johansson and Halldin, 1989). There is some conflict in the suggestion that differences in plasma half-life exist between heavy and light marijuana smokers. Lemberger *et al.* (1972) found the half-life for Δ^9-THC in heavy smokers (28 hours) was half as long as in light users (57 hours), intimating that induction of metabolism in chronic users is responsible. In contrast, Hunt and Jones and Ohlsson found no differences in the pharmacokinetics of either group following prolonged exposure to Δ^9-THC (Hunt and Jones, 1980; Ohlsson *et al.*, 1982). A direct correlation between plasma Δ^9-THC levels and the Δ^9-THC content of a cigarette have been found (Perez-Reyes *et al.*, 1982).

The active Δ^9-THC metabolite 11-OH-THC appears rapidly after the first or second inhalation of a Δ^9-THC cigarette (Huestis *et al.*, 1992b,c). The plasma levels remain low relative to Δ^9-THC, typically 6–10% of the Δ^9-THC concentration up to 45 minutes after initiation of smoking (McBurney *et al.*, 1986; Huestis *et al.*, 1992b,c; Cone, 1998). 11-OH-THC declines gradually and is detectable for up to 12 hours (McBurney *et al.*, 1986; Huestis *et al.*, 1992b,c). Similar to Δ^9-THC, the AUC for 11-OH-THC demonstrates a dose–response relationship (Huestis *et al.*, 1992b,c).

The acid metabolite, THCCOOH, appears gradually in plasma and plateaus after 1 hour for an extended period of time – 2–4 hours (Huestis *et al.*, 1992b,c; Cone and Huestis, 1993). Typically, the mean peak plasma and serum concentrations for THCCOOH are lower than those for Δ^9-THC but higher than those for 11-OH-THC (Law *et al.*, 1984; Huestis *et al.*, 1992b,c; Reiter *et al.*, 2001). A cigarette containing 30 mg Δ^9-THC will produce a peak THCCOOH level of 50 ng/mL (Perez-Reyes *et al.*, 1982; Huestis *et al.*, 1992b,c). Plasma half-lives of 22 hours for THCCOOH and 21 hours for THCCOOH acid glucuronide are reported by Law *et al.* (1984). The slow reintroduction of Δ^9-THC into the bloodstream leads to extended elimination of Δ^9-THC and its metabolites from the body. A urinary excretion half-life between 2 and 5 days is typical for THCCOOH, although half-lives of 10 days and greater are possible (Crindland *et al.*, 1983; Law *et al.*, 1984; Ellis *et al.*, 1985; Johansson and Halldin, 1989; Johansson *et al.*, 1989, 1990; Kelly and Jones, 1992; Heustis and Cone, 1998).

The bioavailability of Δ^9-THC during smoking is usually in the range of 10–27% and is influenced by a number of factors such as loss in sidestream smoke, pyrolysis and perhaps some metabolism by the lungs (Lindgren et al., 1981; Wall et al., 1983; Cone and Huestis, 1993). Heavy users tend to have greater bioavailability compared with light smokers, probably due to more efficient inhalation by the experienced users.

Oral administration of Δ^9-THC

Following oral ingestion, the cannabinoid plasma levels are much lower than those produced after intravenous infusion and smoking (Lemberger et al., 1972; Ohlsson et al., 1980; Hollister et al., 1981; Perez-Reyes et al., 1982; Mattes et al., 1993; Brenneisen et al., 1996). This is most likely due to degradation by gastric acids and first pass metabolism in the liver (Ohlsson et al., 1980; Wall et al., 1983; Agurell et al., 1986). The plasma profiles post oral administration are highly variable when compared with the other two forms of administration. This can probably be attributed to first pass metabolism by CYPs in the small intestine, e.g. CYP3A5 (Busto et al., 1989; Mattes et al., 1993). Peak plasma levels for Δ^9-THC rise slowly (1–6 hours) and are usually in the range 1–17 ng/mL (Ohlsson et al., 1980; Law et al., 1984; Brenneisen et al., 1996).

After oral administration of Δ^9-THC the metabolites are often detectable in plasma before and persist longer than Δ^9-THC itself (Ohlsson et al., 1980; Wall et al., 1983; Law et al., 1984; Agurell et al., 1986). It is not uncommon to observe plasma levels equal to Δ^9-THC for 11-OH-Δ^9-THC and these can persist up to 6 hours after dosing (Wall and Perez-Reyes, 1981; Wall et al., 1983; Law et al., 1984). Indeed, Wall et al. (1983) found levels of the 11-OH metabolite twice as high as the parent drug. It is therefore reasonable to assume that following oral administration of Δ^9-THC, the 11-OH metabolite contributes greatly to the psychotropic effects of Δ^9-THC. Plasma levels as high as 250 ng/mL for THCCOOH (occurring between 2 and 8 hours) are reported (Law et al., 1984; Brenneisen et al., 1996). Often the plasma level of the acid can be 35 times greater then that of Δ^9-THC. This is in contrast to smoking, where the Δ^9-THC plasma level is approximately 3 times higher than THCCOOH (Huestis et al., 1992b,c; Cone, 1998).

In common with the other main routes of administration, THCCOOH glucuronide is the predominant metabolite excreted in urine after oral dosing (Lemberger et al., 1972; Halldin et al., 1982b;

Law *et al.*, 1984; Johansson *et al.*, 1990). Peak urinary cannabinoid levels after an oral dose of Δ^9-THC (20 mg) range from 190 ng/mL to 2900 ng/mL (Law *et al.*, 1984; Johannson *et al.*, 1990). A urinary half-life for Δ^9-THC metabolites between 16 and 25 hours has been reported after an oral dose of 20 mg Δ^9-THC, with positive results recorded for 12 days after ingestion (Law *et al.*, 1984; Johansson *et al.*, 1990).

On average the systemic availability of Δ^9-THC is 6% due to degradation in the gut and first pass metabolism (Ohlsson *et al.*, 1980; Wall *et al.*, 1983). Brenneisen *et al.* (1996) showed that the bioavailability after oral dosing is 45–55% of that achieved by the rectal route. The vehicle used to deliver the oral dose has an influence on systemic availability, for example an oil suspension of Δ^9-THC will increase bioavailability to 20% (Brenneisen *et al.*, 1996).

Intravenous administration of Δ^9-THC

The plasma profile for Δ^9-THC after i.v. administration parallels that of smoking except that the plasma concentrations are approximately twice as high post i.v. infusion. Peak plasma levels for Δ^9-THC are in the range 200–400 ng/mL after i.v. infusion of 5 mg of Δ^9-THC (Lemberger *et al.*, 1972; Hunt and Jones, 1980; Ohlsson *et al.*, 1980; Hollister *et al.*, 1981; Lindgren *et al.*, 1981; Hollister, 1988; Kelly and Jones, 1992). The time to reach peak plasma levels is short, approximately 3 minutes. Δ^9-THC has a short plasma half-life of 1–2 hours, which is probably due to rapid distribution.

The 11-OH metabolite is present at the low nanogram per millilitre level in plasma after i.v. administration. Wall *et al.* (1983) found that only 10% of infused Δ^9-THC is in the form of 11-OH-THC. Peak plasma level for the acid metabolite THCCOOH is reached between 20 and 45 minutes after administration and the ratio of THCCOOH to Δ^9-THC is less than 1 only before 45 minutes. THCCOOH has a plasma half-life between 4 and 6 days (Kelly and Jones, 1992). A mean urinary half-life of 2 days for THCCOOH was also found in this study.

Rectal administration of Δ^9-THC

As a means of bypassing the first pass elimination associated with oral administration, rectal administration of Δ^9-THC has been proposed (ElSohly *et al.*, 1991a,b; Mattes *et al.*, 1993; Brenneisen *et al.*, 1996). Administration of Δ^9-THC hemisuccinate ester via a rectal suppository to dogs yielded a bioavailability of 67% (ElSohly *et al.*, 1991a). In humans, a comparison between oral (sesame oil formulation) and rectal (hemisuccinate ester) administration of Δ^9-THC showed a marked and sustained increase in Δ^9-THC plasma levels after rectal administration (Mattes *et al.*, 1993). This study also found that the AUC for Δ^9-THC was 30-fold greater than after oral administration.

Routes of administration for CBD and CBN

Human studies following the pharmacokinetic profile of CBD and CBN by different routes of administration are few (Wall *et al.*, 1976; Agurell *et al.*, 1981, 1986; Ohlsson *et al.*, 1984, 1986; Johansson *et al.*, 1987; Consroe *et al.*, 1991). Oral administration of CBD results in low peak plasma levels in the region of 5 ng/mL (Agurell *et al.*, 1981). Even repetitive oral administration of CBD (700 mg daily over six weeks) gave a low, narrow range of plasma CBD levels (6–12 ng/mL after one week) (Consoe *et al.*, 1991). The bioavailability of oral CBD in humans is estimated at 6%, compared with 31% after smoking. Again, first pass metabolism in the liver is the most likely explanation for poor bioavailability following oral administration, although the isomerisation of CBD to Δ^9-THC may play a small part (Ohlsson *et al.*, 1986). A pharmacokinetic study of CBD in the dog confirmed that first pass elimination is responsible for the low bioavailability (Samara *et al.*, 1988). Consroe *et al.* (1991) found that CBD was eliminated over 2–3 weeks after oral ingestion and estimated a half-life of 2–5 days. Ohlsson *et al.* (1986) estimated terminal half-lives for CBD of 24 hours after i.v. infusion and 31 hours after smoking.

   Peak plasma levels for CBN after i.v. infusion and smoking of 20 mg CBN were 434 ng/mL and 126 ng/mL respectively (Johansson *et al.*, 1987). This study also found a mean systemic availability of 39% for CBD after smoking. Again the infrequent users had lower bioavailability of CBN (7%) when compared with frequent users (55%). Like Δ^9-THC, CBD and CBN rapidly disappear from plasma once peak plasma levels have been reached, after smoking and i.v. administration (Agurell *et al.*, 1986; Johansson *et al.*, 1987; Consroe *et al.*, 1991).

Conclusion

To maximise the bioavailability of the cannabinoids, rectal or sublingual administrations are the routes of choice. The major primary metabolites of Δ^9-THC and CBD are the 11-OH and 8α and 8β metabolites. The ratio of metabolite to parent compound levels in plasma depends on the route of administration.

Interactions between Δ^9-THC and CBD or THC/CBD and coadministered drugs could lead to altered therapeutic effect, although detailed extrapolations from *in vitro* to *in vivo* effects have not yet been carried out. The CYPs that are implicated in these interactions are CYP3A4/5, CYP2C9 and CYP2C19. The relevance for *in vivo* kinetics will depend on the relative plasma levels of Δ^9-THC, CBD and the coadministered drugs. An additional factor to consider is the relative inhibitory or inducing effects of CBD on the metabolism of coadministered drugs and the effects of potent CYP3A4 inducers on 8β- and 8α-OH-THC formation.

References

Agurell S, Carlsson S, Lindgren J E, Ohlsson, A, Gillespie H, Hollister L (1981). Interactions of delta-1-tetrahydrocannabinol with cannabinol and cannabidiol following oral administration in man. Assay of cannabinol and cannabidiol by mass fragmentography. *Experientia* 37: 1090–1092.

Agurell S, Gillespie H, Halldin M *et al.* (1985). A review of recent studies on the pharmacokinetics and metabolism of Δ^1-tetrahydrocannabinol, cannabidiol and cannabinol in man. In: Harvey D J, ed. *Marihuana' 84*. Oxford: IRL Press: 49–62.

Agurell S, Halldin M, Lindgren J E *et al.* (1986). Pharmacokinetics and metabolism of Δ^1-tetrahydrocannabidiol and other cannabinoids with emphasis on man. *Pharmacol Rev* 38: 21–43.

Barnett G, Chiang C W N, Perez-Reyes M, Owens S M (1982). Kinetic study of smoking marijuana. *J Pharmacokinet Biopharm* 10: 495–506.

Benowitz N L, Jones R T (1977). Effects of delta-9-tetrahydrocannabinol on drug distribution and metabolism, antipyrine, pentobarbital and ethanol. *Clin Pharmacol Ther* 22: 259–268.

Bertz R J, Granneman G R (1997). Use of *in vitro* and *in vivo* data to estimate the likelihood of metabolic pharmacokinetic interactions. *Clin Pharmacokinet* 32: 210–258.

Bornheim L M, Correia M A (1989). Effect of cannabidiol on cytochrome P-450 isozymes. *Biochem Pharmacol* 38: 2789–2794.

Bornheim L M, Correia M A (1990). Selective inactivation of mouse liver cytochrome P450IIIA by cannabidiol. *Mol Pharmacol* 38: 319–326.

Bornheim L M, Correia M A (1991). Purification and characterisation of the major hepatic cannabinoid hydroxylase in the mouse: a possible member of the cytochrome P-450IIC subfamily. *Mol Pharmacol* 40: 228–234.

Bornheim L M, Grillo M P (1998). Characterization of cytochrome P450 3A inactivation by cannabidiol: possible involvement of cannabidiol-hydroxyquinone as a P450 inactivator. *Chem Res Toxicol* 11: 1209–1216.

Bornheim L M, Borys H K, Karler R (1981). Effect of cannabidiol on cytochrome P-450 and hexobarbital sleep time. *Biochem Pharmacol* 30: 503–507.

Bornheim L M, Lasker M J, Raucy J L (1992). Human hepatic microsomal metabolism of Δ^1-tetrahydrocannabidiol. *Drug Metab Dispos* 20: 241–246.

Bornheim L M, Everhart E T, Jianmin L, Correia M A (1993). Characterization of cannabidiol-mediated cytochrome P450 inactivation. *Biochem Pharmacol* 45: 1323–1331.

Bornheim L M, Everhart E T, Jianmin L, Correia M A (1994). Induction and genetic regulation of mouse hepatic cytochrome P450 by cannabidiol. *Biochem Pharmacol* 48: 161–171.

Brenneisen R, Egli A, ElSohly M A, Henn V, Spiess Y (1996). The effect of orally and rectally administered Δ^9-tetrahydrocannabinol on spasticity: a pilot study with 2 patients. *Int J Clin Pharmacol Ther* 34: 446–452.

Brown N K, Harvey D J (1990). *In vitro* metabolism of cannabicromene in seven common laboratory animals. *Drug Metab Dispos* 18: 1065–1070.

Burstein S H (1999). The cannabinoid acids: nonpsychoactive derivatives with therapeutic potential. *Pharmacol Ther* 82: 87–96.

Burstein S, Hunter S A, Latham V, Renzulli L (1986). Prostaglandins and cannabis. XVI. Antagonism of Δ^1-THC action by its metabolites. *Biochem Pharmacol* 35: 2553–2558.

Burstein S H, Hull K, Hunter S A, Latham V (1988). Cannabinoids and pain responses: a possible role for prostaglandins. *FASEB J* 2: 3022–3026.

Burstein S H, Audette C A, Doyle S A, Hull K, Hunter S A, Latham V (1989). Antagonism to the actions of PAF by a nonpsychoactive cannabinoid. *J. Pharmacol Exp Ther* 251: 531–535.

Busto U, Bendayan R, Sellers E M (1989). Pharmacokinetics of non-opiate abused drugs. *Clin Pharmacokinet* 16: 1–26.

Chiang C W N, Barnett G (1984). Marijuana effect and delta-9-tetrahydrocannabinol plasma level. *Clin Pharmacol Ther* 36: 234–238.

Clark B, Smith D S (1993). *An Introduction to Pharmacokinetics*, 2nd edn. Oxford: Blackwell Scientific.

Cone E J (1998). Recent discoveries in pharmacokinetics of drugs of abuse. *Toxicol Lett* 102–103: 97–101.

Cone E J, Huestis M A (1993). Relating blood concentrations of tetrahydrocannabinol and metabolites to pharmacologic effects and time of marijuana usage. *Ther Drug Monitor* 15: 527–532.

Consoe P, Kennedy K, Schram K (1991). Assay of plasma cannabidiol by capillary gas chromatography/ion trap mass spectrometry following high dose repeated daily oral administration to humans. *Pharmacol Biochem Behav* 40: 517–522.

Crindland J S, Rottanburg D, Robins A H (1983). Apparent half-life of excretion of cannabinoids in man. *Hum Toxicol* 2: 641–644.

Darmani N A (2001a). Δ^9-Tetrahydrocannabinol and synthetic cannabinoids prevent emesis produced by the cannabinoid CB$_1$ receptor antagonist/inverse agonist SR141716A. *Neuropsychopharmacology* 24: 198–203.

Darmani N A (2001b). Δ^9-Tetrahydrocannabinol differentially suppresses cisplatin-induced emesis and indices of motor function via cannabinoid CB$_1$ receptors in the least shrew. *Pharmacol Biochem Behav* 69: 239–249.

Deutsch D G, Tombler E R, March J E, Lo S H C, Adesinik M (1991). Potentiation of the inductive effect of phenobarbital on cytochrome P450 mRNAs by cannabidiol. *Biochem Pharmacol* 42: 2048–2063.

Ellis G M Jnr, Mann M A, Judson B E, Schramm N T, Tashehian A (1985). Excretion patterns of cannabinoid metabolites after last use in a group of chronic users. *Clin Pharmacol Ther* 38: 562–578.

ElSohly M A, Little T L, Hikal A, Harland E, Stanford D F, Walker L (1991a). Rectal bioavailability of delta-9-tetrahydrocannabinol from various esters. *Pharmacol Biochem Behav* 40: 497–502.

ElSohly M A, Stanford D F, Harland E C *et al.* (1991b). Rectal bioavailability of delta-9-tetrahydrocannabinol from the hemmisuccinate ester in monkeys. *J Pharm Sci* 80: 942–945.

ElSohly M A, Feng S, Murphy T P *et al.* (2001). Identification and quantification of 11-Nor-Δ^9-tetrahydrocannabinol-9-carboxylic acid, a major metabolite of Δ^9-tetrahydrocannabivarin. *J Anal Toxicol* 25: 476–480.

Garrett E R, Hunt C A (1974). Physiochemical properties, solubility and protein binding of Δ^9-tetrahydrocannabinol. *J Pharmac Sci* 63: 1056–1064.

Giroud C, Menetrey A, Augsburger M, Buclin T, Sanchez-Mazas P, Mangin P (2001). Δ^9-THC, 11-OH-Δ^9-THC and Δ^9-THCCOOH plasma or serum to whole blood concentrations distribution ratios in blood samples taken from living and dead people. *Forensic Sci Int* 123: 159–164.

Gosh S K, Poddar M K (1992). Effect of Δ^9-tetrahydrocannabidiol and theophylline on hepatic microsomal drug metabolizing enzymes. *Biochem Pharmacol* 44: 2021–2027.

Halldin M M, Andersson L K R, Widman M, Hollister L E (1982a). Further urinary metabolites of Δ^1-tetrahydrocannabidiol in man. *Arzneim Forsch/Drug Res* 32: 1135–1138.

Halldin M M, Carlsson S, Kanter S L, Widman M, Agurell S (1982b). Urinary metabolites of Δ^1-tetrahydrocannabidiol in man. *Arzneim Forsch/Drug Res* 32: 764–768.

Halldin M M, Widman M, Bahr C V, Lindgren J E, Martin B R (1982c). Identification of *in vitro* metabolites of Δ^1-tetrahydrocannabidiol formed by human livers. *Drug Metab Dispos* 10: 297–301.

Harvey D J (1985). Mass spectrometry of the cannabinoids and their metabolites. *Mass Spectrom Rev* 6: 135–229.

Harvey D J (1992). Cannabinoids. In: Desteno D M, ed. *Mass Spectrometry: Clinical and Biomedical Applications*, Vol 1. New York: Plenum Press: 207–257.

Harvey D J, Brown N K (1990). In vitro metabolism of cannabidiol in seven common laboratory mammals. *Res Commun Substance Abuse* 11: 27–37.

Harvey D J, Paton W D M (1984). Metabolism of the cannabinoids. *Rev Biochem Toxicol* 6: 221–264.

Harvey D J, Martin B R, Paton W D M (1978). Comparative *in vivo* metabolism of delta-1-tetrahydrocannabinol (delta-1-THC), cannabidiol (CBD) and cannabinol (CBN) in several species. In: Frigerio A, ed. *Recent Developments in Mass Spectrometry in Biochemistry and Medicine*, Vol 1. New York: Plenum Press: 161–184.

Harvey D J, Martin B R, Paton W D M (1980). Identification of *in vivo*, liver metabolites of delta-1-tetrahydrocannabinol, cannabidiol and cannabinol produced by the guinea-pig. *J Pharm Pharmacol* 32: 267–271.

Hively R L, Mosher W A, Hoffmann F W (1966). Isolation of *trans* Δ^6-tetrahydrocannabinol from marijuana. *J Am Chem Soc* 88: 1832–1833.

Hollister L E (1973). Cannabidiol and cannabinol in man. *Experientia* 29: 825–826.

Hollister L E (1988). Cannabis – 1988. *Acta Psychiatr Scand Suppl 345* 78: 108–118.

Hollister L E, Gillespie H K (1973). Δ^8- and Δ^9-Tetrahydrocannabinol. Comparison in man by oral and intravenous administration. *Clin Pharmacol Ther* 14: 353–357.

Hollister L E, Gillespie H K, Ohlsson A, Lindgren J E, Wahlen A, Agurell S (1981). Do plasma concentrations of Δ^9-tetrahydrocannabinol reflect the degree of intoxication. *J Clin Pharmacol* 21: 171S–177S.

Huestis M A, Henningfield J E, Cone E J (1992a). Blood cannabinoids. II. Models for the prediction of time of marijuana exposure from plasma concentrations of Δ^9-tetrahydrocannabinol (THC) and 11-nor-9-carboxy-Δ^9-tetrahydrocannabinol (THCCOOH). *J Anal Toxicol* 16: 283–290.

Huestis M A, Henningfield J E, Cone E J (1992b). Blood cannabinoids. I. Absorption of THC and formation of 11-OH-THC and THCCOOH during and after smoking marijuana. *J Anal Toxicol* 16: 276–282.

Huestis M A, Sampson A H, Holickly B J, Henningfield J E, Cone E J (1992c). Characterization of the absorption phase of marijuana smoking. *Clin Pharm Ther* 52: 31–41.

Hunt C A, Jones R T (1980). Tolerance and disposition of tetrahydrocannabinol in man. *J Pharmacol Exp Ther* 215: 35–44.

Hunt C A, Jones R T, Herning R I, Bachman J (1981). Evidence that cannabidiol does not significantly alter the pharmacokinetics of tetrahydrocannabinol in man. *J Pharmacokinet Biopharm* 9: 245–260.

Jaeger W, Benet L Z, Bornheim L Z (1996). Inhibition of cyclosporine and tetrahydrocannabidiol metabolism by cannabidiol in mouse and human microsomes. *Xenobiotica* 26: 275–284.

Johansson E, Halldin M M (1989). Urinary excretion half-life of Δ^1-tetrahydrocannabinol-7-oic acid in heavy marijuana users after smoking. *J Anal Toxicol* 13: 218–223.

Johansson E, Ohlsson A, Lindgren J E, Agurell S, Gillespie H, Hollister L E (1987). Single-dose kinetics of deuterium-labelled cannabinol in man after intravenous administration and smoking. *Biomed Environ Mass Spectrom* 14: 495–499.

Johansson E, Agurell S, Hollister L E, Halldin (1988). Prolonged apparent half-life of Δ^1-tetrahydrocannabinol in plasma of chronic marijuana users. *J Pharm Pharmacol* 40: 374–375.

Johansson E, Halldin M M, Agurell S, Hollister L E, Gillispie H K (1989). Terminal elimination plasma half-life of Δ^1-tetrahydrocannabinol (Δ^1-THC) in heavy users of marijuana. *Eur J Clin Pharmacol* 37: 273–277.

Johansson E, Gillespie H K, Halldin M M (1990). Human urinary excretion profile after smoking and oral administration of [^{14}C]Δ^1-tetrahydrocannabinol. *J Anal Toxicol* 14: 176–180.

Karniol I G, Shirakawa I, Kasinski N, Pfeferman A, Carlini E A (1974). Cannabidiol interferes with the effects of Δ^9-tetrahydrocannabidiol in man. *Eur J Pharmacol* 28: 172–177.

Keimowitz A R, Martin B R, Razdan R K, Crocker P J, Mascarella W, Thomas B F (2000). QSAR analysis of Δ^8-THC analogues: relationhip of side-chain conformation to cannabinoid receptor affinity and pharmacological potency. *J Med Chem* 43: 59–70.

Kelly P, Jones R T (1992). Metabolism of tetrahydrocannabinol in frequent and infrequent marijuana users. *J Anal Toxicol* 16: 228–235.

Kliewer S A, Wilson T M (2002). Regulation of xenobiotic and bile acid metabolism by the nuclear pregnane X receptor. *J Lipid Res* 43: 359–364.

Kumar R N, Chambers W A, Pertwee R G (2001). Pharmacological actions and therapeutic uses of cannabis and cannabinoids. *Anaesthesia* 56: 1059–1068.

Law B, Mason P A, Moffat A C, Gleadle R I, King L J (1984). Forensic aspects of the metabolism and excretion of cannabinoids following oral ingestion of cannabis resin. *J Pharm Pharmacol* 36: 289–284.

Lemberger L, Weiss J L, Watanabe A M, Galanter I M, Wyatt R J, Cardon P V (1972). Temporal correlation of the psychologic effects and blood levels after various routes of administration. *N Engl J Med* 286: 685–688.

Lindgren J E, Ohlsson A, Agurell S, Hollister L, Gillespie H (1982). Clinical effects and plasma levels of 9-tetrahydrocannabinol (9-THC) in heavy and light users. *Psychopharmacology* 74: 208–212.

McArdle K, Mackie P, Pertwee R, Guy G, Whittle B, Hawksworth G (2001). Selective inhibition of Δ^9-tetrahydrocannabinol metabolite formation by cannabidiol in vitro. *Toxicology* 168: 133–134.

McArdle K, Mackie P, Pertwee R, Guy G, Whittle B, Hawksworth G (2003). Cannabidiol (CBD) differentially inhibits Δ^9-tetrahydrocannabinol (THC) metabolism by human P450s and induces CYP3A23 and CYP2B1/2 *in vivo* in rat. *Toxicology* **192**: 90–91.

McBurney L J, Bobbie B A, Sepp L A (1986). GC/MS and EMIT analysis of Δ^9-tetrahydrocannabinol metabolites in plasma and urine of human subjects. *J Anal Toxicol* 10: 56–64.

McLeod H (1999). Pharmacokinetics for the prescriber. In: Petrie J C, ed. *Medicine, Clinical Pharmacology*, Vol 27. Abingdon: The Medicine Publishing Company Ltd: 10–14.

Martin B R, Agurell S, Nordvqvist M, Lindgren J E (1976). Dioxygenated metabolites of cannabidiol formed by rat liver. *J Pharm Pharmacol* 28: 603–608.

Martin B R, Jefferson R G, Winckler R *et al.* (2002). Assessment of structural commonality between tetrahydrocannabinol and anandamide. *Eur J Pharmacol* 435: 35–42.

Mathews J M, Etheridge A S, Black S L, De Costa K S (2000). Cannabidiol inhibits multiple cytochrome P450 isozymes *in vivo* in rat and *in vitro* in human microsomes: unexpected inhibition of CYP2D isoforms. In: Hinson J A, ed. *Drug Metabolism Reviews*, Vol 32. New York: Marcel Dekker: 79.

Matsunaga T, Kishi N, Tanaka H, Watanabe K, Yoshimura H, Yamamoto I (1998). Major cytochrome P450 enzyme responsible for oxidation of secondary alcohols to the corresponding ketones in mouse hepatic microsomes: oxidation of

7-hydroxy-Δ^8-tetrahydrocannabidiol to 7-oxo-Δ^8-tetrahydrocannabinol. *Drug Metab Dispos* 26: 1045–1047.

Matsunaga T, Kishi N, Higuchi S, Watanabe K, Ohshima T, Yamamoto I (2000). CYP3A4 is the major isoform responsible for oxidation of 7-hydroxy-Δ^8-tetrahydrocannabinol to 7-oxo-Δ^8-tetrahydrocannabinol in human liver microsomes. *Drug Metab Dispos* 28: 1291–1296.

Matsunaga T, Tanaka H, Higuchi S *et al.* (2001). Oxidation mechanism of 7-hydroxy-Δ^8-tetrahydrocannabidiol and 8-hydroxy-Δ^9-tetrahydrocannabidiol to the corresponding ketones by CYP3A11. *Drug Metab Dispos* 29: 1485–1491.

Mattes R D, Shaw L M, Edling-Owens J, Engleman K, ElSohly A (1993). Bypassing the first-pass effect for the therapeutic use of cannabinoids. *Pharmacol Biochem Behav* 44: 745–747.

Mechoulam R, Devane W A, Glaser R (1999). Cannabinoid geometry and biological activity. In: Nahas G G, Sutin K M, Harvey D J, Agurell S, eds. *Marihuana and Medicine*. New Jersey: Humana Press: 65–90.

Mitra G, Poddar M K, Ghosh J J (1976). In vivo and in vitro effects of delta-9-THC on rat liver microsomal drug metabolising enzymes. *Toxicol Appl Pharmacol* 35: 523–530.

Muangmoonchai R, Smirlis D, Wong S C, Edwards M, Phillips I R, Shepherd E A (2000). Xenobiotic induction of cytochrome P450 2B1(CYP2B1) is mediated by the orphan nuclear receptor constitutive androstane receptor (CAR) and requires steroid co-activator 1 (SRC-1) and the transcription factor Sp1. *Biochem J* 355: 71–78.

Narimatsu S, Matsubara K, Shimonishi T, Watanabe K, Yamamoto I, Yoshimura H (1988). Enzymatic oxidation of 7-hydroxylated Δ^8-tetrahydrocannabinol to 7-oxo-Δ^8-tetrahydrocannabinol by liver microsomes of the guinea pig. *Drug Metab Dispos* 16: 156–161.

Narimatsu S, Watanabe K, Matsunga T *et al.* (1990a). Cytochrome P-450 isozymes in metabolic activation of Δ^9-tetrahydrocannabidiol by rat liver microsomes. *Drug Metab Dispos* 18: 943–948.

Narimatsu S, Akutsu Y, Matsunga T, Watanabe K, Yamamoto I, Yoshimura H (1990b). Purification of a cytochrome P-450 isozyme belonging to a subfamily of P450IIB from liver microsomes of guinea pigs. *Biochem Biophys Res Commun* 172: 607–613.

Narimatsu S, Watanabe K, Yamamoto I, Yoshimura H (1991). Sex difference in the oxidative metabolism of Δ^9-tetrahydrocannabidiol in the rat. *Biochem Pharmacol* 41: 1187–1194.

Ohlsson A, Lindgren J E, Wahlen A, Agurell A, Hollister L E, Gillespie B A (1980). Plasma delta-9-tetrahydrocannabinol concentrations and clinical effects after oral and intravenous administration and smoking. *Clin Pharmacol Ther* 28: 409–416.

Ohlsson A, Lindgren J E, Wahlen A, Agurell S, Hollister L E, Gillespie H K (1982). Single dose kinetics of deuterium-labelled Δ^1-tetrahydrocannabinol in heavy and light cannabis users. *Biomed Mass Spectrom* 9: 6–10.

Ohlsson A, Lindgren J E, Anderson S, Agurell S, Gillespie H, Hollister L E (1984). Single dose kinetics of cannabidiol in man. In: Agurell S, Dewey W L, Willette R, eds. *The Cannabinoids: Chemical, Pharmacological and Therapeutic Aspects*. New York: Academic Press: 219–225.

Ohlsson A, Lindgren J E, Anderson S, Agurell S (1986). Single dose kinetics of deuterium-labelled cannabidiol in man after smoking and intravenous administration. *Biomed Environ Mass Spectrom* 13: 77–83.

Perez-Reyes M, Di Guiseppi S, Owens S M (1981). The clinical pharmacology and dynamics of marihuana cigarette smoking. *J Clin Pharmacol* 21: 201S–207S.

Perez-Reyes M, Di Guiseppi S , Davies K H, Schindler V H, Cook C E (1982). Comparison of effects of marihuana cigarettes of three different potencies *Clin Pharmacol Ther* 31: 617–624.

Pertwee R G (1999a). Prescribing cannabinoids for multiple sclerosis: current issues. *CNS Drugs* 11: 327–334.

Pertwee R G (1999b). Pharmacology of cannabinoid receptor ligands. *Curr Med Chem* 6: 635–664.

Pertwee R G (2001). Cannabinoid receptors and pain. *Progr Neuropharmacol* 63: 569–611.

Reeve V C, Robertson W B, Grant J *et al.* (1983). Hemolyzed blood and serum levels of Δ^9-THC: Effects on the performance of roadside sobriety tests. *J Forensic Sci* 28: 963–971.

Reiter A, Hake J, Meissner C, Rohwer J, Friedrich H J, Oehmichen M (2001). Time of drug elimination in chronic drug abusers. Case study of 52 patients in a 'low-step' detoxification ward. *Forensic Sci Int* 119: 248–253.

Roth M D, Marques-Magallanes J A, Yuan M, Sun W, Tashkin D P, Hankinson O (2001). Induction and regulation of the carcinogen-metabolizing enzyme CYP1A1 by marijuana smoke and Δ^9-tetrahydrocannabinol. *Am J Respir Cell Mol Biol* 24: 339–344.

Samara E, Bialer M, Mechoulam R (1988). Pharmacokinetics of cannabidiol in dogs. *Drug Metab Dispos* 16: 469–472.

Shimada T, Yamazaki H, Mimura M, Inui Y, Guengerich M (1994). Interindividual variations in human liver cytochrome P-450 enzymes involved in the oxidation of drugs, carcinogens and toxic chemicals: studies with liver microsomes of 30 Japanese and 30 Caucasians. *J Pharmacol Exp Ther* 270: 414–423.

Spatzeneggar M, Jaeger W (1995). Clinical importance of hepatic cytochrome P450 in drug metabolism. *Drug Metab Rev* 27: 397–417.

Turner C E, ElSohly M A, Boeren E G (1980). Constituents of *Cannabis sativa* L., XVII: A review of the natural constituents. *J Nat Prod* 43: 169–234.

Wahlqvist M, Nilsson I M, Sandberg F, Agurell S (1970). Binding of Δ^1-tetrahydrocannabinol to human plasma proteins. *Biochem Pharmacol* 19: 2579–2584.

Wall M E, Perez-Reyes M (1981). The metabolism of Δ^9-tetrahydrocannabidiol and related cannabinoids in man. *J Clin Pharmacol* 21: 178S–189S.

Wall M E, Brine D R, Perez-Reyes M (1976). Metabolism of cannabinoids in man. In: Braude M C, Szara S, eds. *Pharmacology of Marihuana*. New York: Raven Press: 93–113.

Wall M E, Sadler B M, Brine D, Taylor H, Perez-Reyes M (1983). Metabolism, disposition and kinetics of delta-9-tetrahydrocannabinol in men and women. *Clin Pharmacol Ther* 34: 352–363.

Watanabe K, Narimatsu S, Yamamoto I, Yoshimura H (1987). Self-catalysed inactivation of cytochrome P450 during microsomal metabolism of cannabidiol. *Biochem Pharmacol* 36: 3371–3377.

Watanabe K, Matsunaga T, Narimatsu S *et al.* (1991). Catalytic activity of cytochrome P450 isozymes purified from rat liver in converting 11-oxo-delta 8-tetrahydrocannabinol to delta 8-tetrahydrocannabinol-11-oic-acid. *Biochem Pharmacol* 42: 1255–1259.

Watanabe K, Narimatsu S, Matsunaga T, Yamamoto I, Yoshimura H (1993). A cytochrome P450 isozyme having aldehyde oxygenase activity plays a major role in metabolizing cannabinoids by mouse hepatic microsomes. *Biochem Pharmacol* 46: 405–411.

Watanabe K, Matsunga T, Yamamoto, I, Funae Y, Yoshimura H (1995). Involvement of CYP2C in the metabolism of cannabinoids by human hepatic microsomes from an old woman. *Biol Pharm Bull* 18: 1138–1141.

Widman M, Nilsson M, Nilsson JL, Agurell S, Borg H, Granstrand B (1973). Plasma protein binding of 7-hydroxy-Δ^1-tetrahydrocannabinol: an active Δ^1-tetrahydrocannabinol metabolite. *J Pharm Pharmacol* 25: 453–457.

Widman M, Agurell S, Ehrnebo M, Jones G (1974). Binding of (+)- and (−)-Δ^1-tetrahydrocannabinols and (−)-7-hydroxy-Δ^1-tetrahydrocannabinol to blood cells and plasma proteins in man. *J Pharm Pharmacol* 26: 914–916.

Williams P L, Moffat A C (1980). Identification in human urine of Δ^9-tetrahydrocannabinol-11-oic acid glucuronide: a tetrahydrocannabinol metabolite. *J Pharm Pharmacol* 32: 445–448.

Yamamoto I, Narimatsu S, Watanabe K, Shimonishi T, Yoshimura H, Nagano T (1983). Human liver microsomal oxidation of Δ^8-tetrahydrocannabidiol. *Chem Pharm Bull* 31: 1784–1787.

Yamamoto I, Narimatsu S, Shimonishi T, Watanabe K, Yoshimura H (1984). Differences in epoxides formation and their further metabolism between delta 9- and delta 8-tetrahydrocannabinols by human liver microsomes. *J Pharmacobiodyn* 7: 254–262.

Yamamoto I, Gohda, H, Narimatsu S, Yoshimura H (1988). Identification of canna-bielsoin, a new metabolite of cannabidiol formed by guinea-pig hepatic microsomal enzymes, and its pharmacological activity in mice. *J Pharma-cobiodyn* 11: 833–838.

Yisak W, Agurell S, Lindgren J E, Widman M (1978). In vivo metabolites of cannabinol identified as fatty acid conjugates. *J Pharm Pharmacol* 30: 462–463.

9

Clinical studies of cannabis-based medicines

Philip J Robson and Geoffrey W Guy

The clinical literature on cannabis and its extracts reviewed below is limited by two important factors: the political, ethical and methodological difficulties inherent in conducting human research on an illegal, 'pariah' drug and the lack of quality test articles for clinical trials. Plant materials have tended to be of dubious quality, content and stability, and synthetic cannabinoid analogues often failed to represent the pharmacological attributes of the natural substance. A further complication has been the lack of objectivity that many 'experts' have brought to the cannabis debate. Poorly controlled research produces ambiguous results that may be interpreted by the reader according to pre-existing prejudices. It has been remarked (Hall *et al.*, 1994) that anecdotes about cannabis seem to be more readily accepted when they point to adverse rather than positive effects.

In recent years the attitude to medicinal cannabis has changed radically in the UK and some other countries, notably Canada. In Britain this mood was given focus in 1998 when, following a comprehensive review of the available data, a House of Lords Select Committee concluded that an urgent expansion of research into the therapeutic potential of cannabis and its derivatives was justified (House of Lords Select Committee on Science and Technology, 1998). A similar conclusion has been reached by a number of other independent organisations in the UK including the British Medical Association, Pain Society, Pharmaceutical Society, Department of Health, and Home Office. Calls for action have been voiced in mainstream medical journals (Robson, 1998, 2001). Politicians in many countries, aware of changing public attitudes, now see the recreational and therapeutic uses of cannabis as entirely separate issues, and regulatory authorities are generally eager to receive and assess the evidence of clinical utility. Much support has been forthcoming from patients' groups such as the MS Society, Alliance for Cannabis Therapeutics, and INSPIRE (representing patients with spinal cord injury).

Until recently, there has been a marked lack of enthusiasm from major pharmaceutical companies to rise to this challenge. The decision by the UK Government to grant GW Pharmaceuticals the licences necessary to initiate cultivation and devise extraction procedures equal to the task of producing standardised plant extracts of proven content and stability was both timely and judicious, coinciding as it did with a renewed interest generally in plant-based medicines. It is also relevant that many researchers and patients have concluded that the whole plant is more effective as a medicine than delta-9-tetrahydrocannabinol (THC) alone, especially in the form of synthetic analogues. Some of this apparent superiority may simply be related to speed of onset from smoked material or patients' enjoyment of intoxication, but there is now much evidence for the therapeutic potential of cannabinoids other than THC, as well as non-cannabinoid plant constituents such as terpenes and flavonoids. Synergistic interactions between various plant components also seem to play a part (McPartland and Russo, 2001). It is also true that major advances over the past 15 years or so in understanding the structure and function of the endocannabinoid system (Chapter 5) have opened up many exciting possibilities for safe and effective synthetic medicines.

In the remainder of this chapter we will first summarise the existing clinical literature including unpublished information from the extensive GW Pharmaceuticals patient database, then go on to discuss practical issues relating to formulation of cannabis-based medicinal extracts (CBME) and clinical trial design, and finish by outlining current research programmes along with some preliminary outcome data.

Review of existing clinical evidence for therapeutic potential

Antiemetic properties

Many cytotoxic drugs used in the treatment of malignant disease are powerful emetics, and the distress caused by drug-induced nausea and vomiting is the major limiting factor in determining patients' acceptance of cancer chemotherapy (Carmichael, 1992). Controlled trials in previous decades established that natural and synthetic forms of THC were invariably superior to placebo (Chang *et al.*, 1979; Orr and McKernan, 1981; Jones *et al.*, 1982). Controlled comparisons of THC with the antiemetics available in the 1970s and 1980s suggested that it is either equivalent in effect (Ungerleider *et al.*, 1982) or superior (Einhorn,

1981; Orr and McKernan, 1981; Penta *et al.*, 1981; Niiranen and Mattson, 1985; Dalzell *et al.*, 1986; Levitt, 1986; Niederle *et al.*, 1986; Pomeroy *et al.*, 1986; Chan *et al.*, 1987; Formukong *et al.*, 1989; Plasse *et al.*, 1991). Commonest unwanted effects included somnolence, dry mouth, ataxia, dizziness, dysphoria and postural hypotension. Oral THC and nabilone often produced more unwanted effects than comparison drugs, yet THC was nevertheless preferred by patients (Einhorn, 1981; Ungerleider *et al.*, 1982; Niiranen and Mattson, 1985; Dalzell *et al.*, 1986). Levonantradol produced a higher frequency of dysphoric effects than nabilone or THC (Levitt, 1986) and has since disappeared without trace. An optimal balance of efficacy and unwanted effects is best achieved with relatively modest doses of THC (i.e. 7 mg/m^2 or less) (Levitt, 1986; Plasse *et al.*, 1991).

Children seemed to respond well to nabilone (Dalzell *et al.*, 1986; Chan *et al.*, 1987) and to be tolerant of adverse effects, but confirmation is required. A small pilot study (Abrahamov *et al.*, 1995) indicated a positive response to Δ^8-THC in eight children receiving highly emetic antineoplastic therapy for various blood cancers. Vomiting was noted in 60% of children receiving metoclopramide, but when Δ^8-THC was given orally 2 hours before chemotherapy and repeated 6-hourly for 24 hours, no vomiting occurred on any of the 480 occasions this strategy was applied. Two children reported unwanted effects: both were 'slightly irritable' and one (age 4) showed 'slight euphoria'.

There are many unanswered questions about the potential role of cannabinoids as antiemetics in modern therapeutics (Hall *et al.*, 1994): For which types of emesis are they most effective? What is the appropriate dose and route of administration? What drug combinations are likely to enhance their effects? Is tolerance likely to occur? Most crucially, there are no comparisons to date of cannabinoids with the newer specific 5-HT$_3$ antagonists (granisetron, ondansetron, tropisetron). However, the combination of an antiemetic effect alongside other attributes (e.g. analgesia, muscle relaxation, sedation) may provide a compelling case for exploration of a potential role for cannabis extracts in conditions such as AIDS, cancer or perioperative pain.

Multiple sclerosis (MS) and other neurological conditions

> Drug therapy of muscle spasticity is generally only moderately effective and is limited by adverse effects. (Panegyres, 1992)

Spasticity is a central feature of MS, spinal cord injury (SCI) and cerebral palsy. Neuropathic pain is a common symptom and in MS dozens of very painful muscle spasms can occur each day. Tremor, ataxia and lower urinary tract problems also contribute to the high incidence of anxiety and depression in these conditions.

THC and other cannabinoids have been shown (Baker *et al.*, 2000) to ameliorate both tremor and spasticity in a well-validated animal model of MS (experimental allergic encephalomyelitis). Antagonism of the CB_1 receptor greatly worsened these signs, indicating a role for endogenous cannabinoids in the control of tremor and spasticity.

There are many anecdotal reports (e.g. Hodges, 1992; Grinspoon and Bakalar, 1993) that cannabis can relieve some of the most distressing symptoms of MS and SCI, including spasticity, muscle pain, tremor, spasms on walking, paraesthesiae, leg weakness, trunk numbness, facial pain, impaired balance, nystagmus, anxiety and depression (Consroe *et al.*, 1996). Malec *et al.* (1982) reported that 21 out of 24 SCI patients with spasticity who had tried cannabis found that it alleviated their symptoms.

Open or single-blind observations in a small number of patients have given some support to these reports (Dunn and Davis, 1974; Petro, 1980; Clifford, 1983; Consroe *et al.*, 1986; Meinck *et al.*, 1989; Breneissen *et al.*, 1996). A recent survey of MS patients in the UK and US found that between 30 and 97% experienced relief in symptoms with cannabis, depending on the particular symptoms (Consroe *et al.*, 1997). In descending order of improvement, these were: spasticity, chronic pain, acute paroxysmal phenomena, tremor, emotional dysfunction, anorexia/weight loss, fatigue states, double vision, sexual dysfunction, bowel and bladder dysfunctions, vision dimness, dysfunctions of walking and balance, and memory loss.

Two small placebo-controlled studies (Petro and Ellenberger, 1981; Ungerleider *et al.*, 1987) both demonstrated that THC in doses between 5 and 10 mg orally was significantly superior to placebo in relieving spasticity with minimal adverse effects, and nabilone (1 mg on alternate days for one month) was better than placebo in a study of a single case (Martyn *et al.*, 1995). Improvement in nocturia, muscle spasm and general well-being was also noted in this patient. However, cannabidiol (CBD) was 'neither symptomatically beneficial nor toxic' in 10 patients with Huntington's disease at a dose of 10 mg/kg per day (Consroe *et al.*, 1991). A single dose of smoked THC impaired both posture and balance in comparison with placebo in 10 MS patients and 10 normal subjects (Greenberg *et al.*, 1994), a not-unexpected occurrence with any skeletal muscle relaxant.

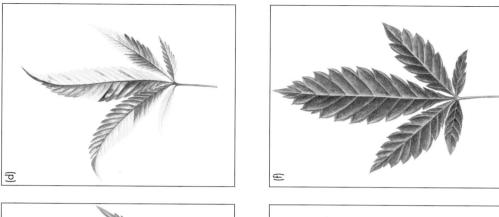
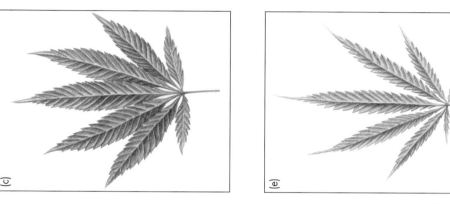
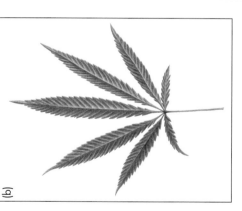
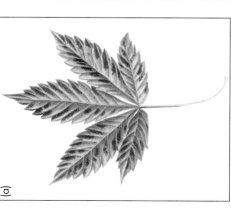

Plate 1 A comparison of the leaf morphologies of a selection of cannabis varieties. **(a)** *Cannabis sativa* subspecies *indica* var. 'Afghan'. **(b)** *Cannabis sativa* subspecies *ruderalis*. **(c)** *Cannabis sativa* hybrid cross of *indica* and *sativa* subspecies, variety G1 – a GW high-THC variety. **(d)** *Cannabis sativa* hybrid cross of *indica* and *sativa* subspecies, variety Gloria – a variegated GW variety. **(e)** *Cannabis sativa* subspecies *sativa* G5 M16 – a clone line of a GW high-CBD variety. **(f)** *Cannabis sativa* subspecies *indica* var. M77 – a GW high-CBC variety. (Illustrations by Valerie Bolas.)

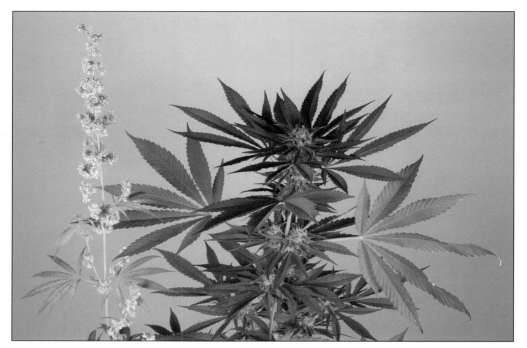

Plate 2 A glasshouse grown male (staminate) cannabis plant (left) and (pistillate) female (right), both in full flower. (Photo courtesy of Peter Smith.)

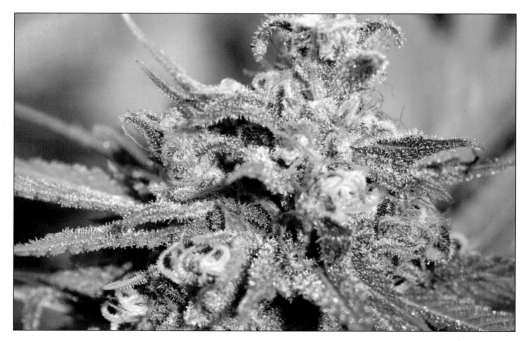

Plate 3 Close-up view of a mature female cannabis inflorescence. The plant sparkles with its covering of glandular trichomes. (Photo courtesy of Peter Smith.)

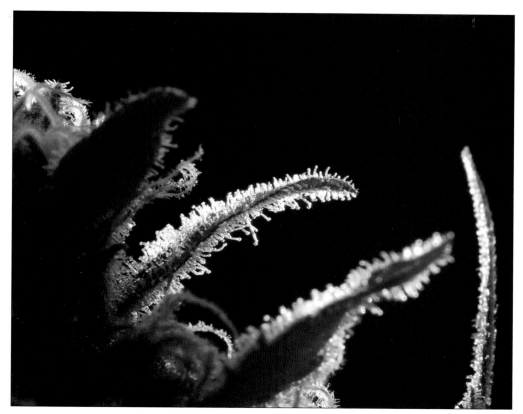

Plate 4 The tip of a female inflorescence of high-THC medicinal cannabis illuminated from behind. The bracts that surround the individual flowers are covered in a dense pubescence of glandular trichomes. These trichomes each have a resin head at the tip. (Photo courtesy of Peter Smith.)

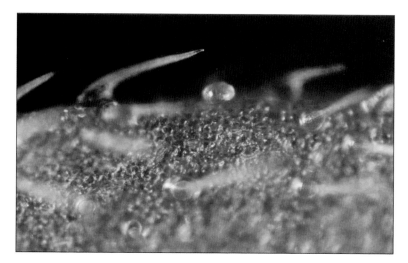

Plate 5 A cannabis seedling leaf. Through the microscope, a capitate sessile trichome can be seen on the surface at the edge of the leaf. This is surrounded by non-glandular trichomes – simple leaf hairs. (Photo courtesy of David Potter.)

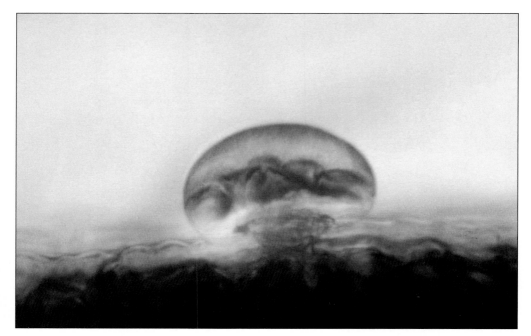

Plate 6 Close-up view of the same capitate sessile trichome. Approximately 50 μm in diameter, the glandular head contains a mixture of cannabinoids and terpenes. These are produced in the secretory cells. These are clearly visible at the base of the glandular head. (Photo courtesy of David Potter.)

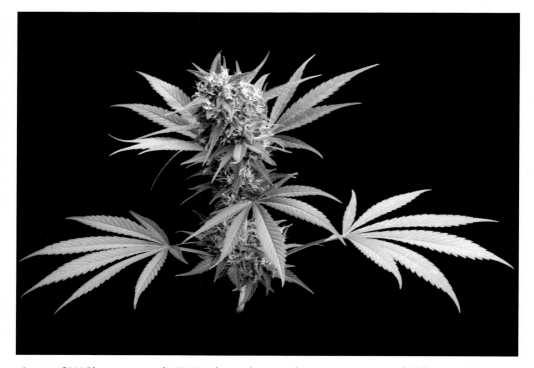

Plate 7 GW Pharmaceutical's THC-rich purple cannabis variety G116 in full flower. (Photo courtesy of Peter Smith.)

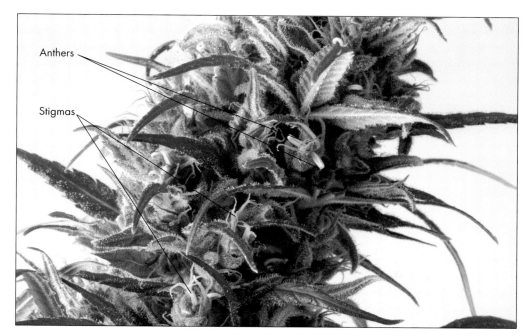

Anthers

Stigmas

Plate 8 A female cannabis inflorescence with immature anthers. If pollen from these anthers reaches the stigmas, self-pollination can be effected. (Photo courtesy of Peter Smith.)

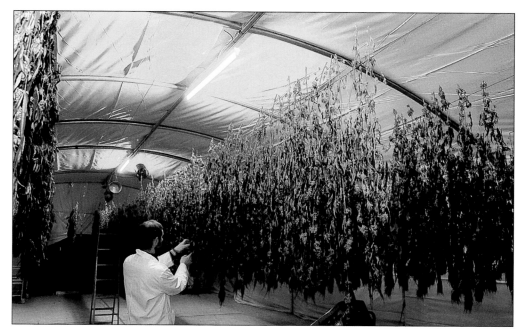

Plate 9 Harvested plants hang to dry in a dehumidified room for 7 days. (Photo courtesy of Peter Smith.)

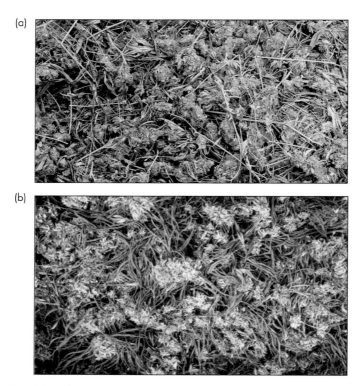

Plate 10 (a) Dried THC botanical raw material – variety G1. **(b)** Dried CBD botanical raw material – variety G5. (Photos courtesy of Peter Smith.)

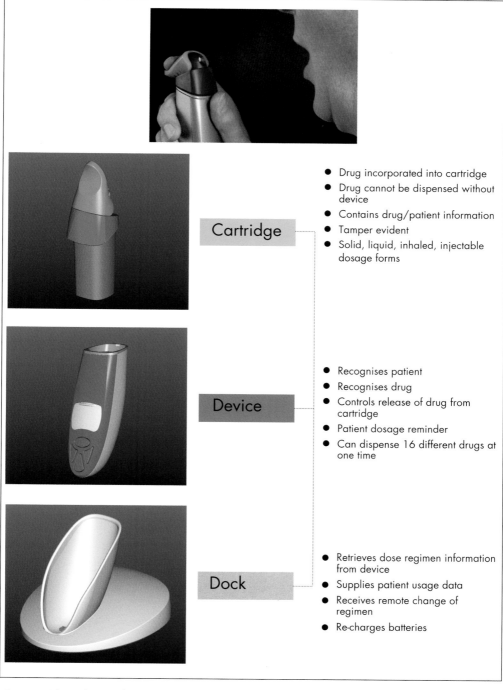

Cartridge
- Drug incorporated into cartridge
- Drug cannot be dispensed without device
- Contains drug/patient information
- Tamper evident
- Solid, liquid, inhaled, injectable dosage forms

Device
- Recognises patient
- Recognises drug
- Controls release of drug from cartridge
- Patient dosage reminder
- Can dispense 16 different drugs at one time

Dock
- Retrieves dose regimen information from device
- Supplies patient usage data
- Receives remote change of regimen
- Re-charges batteries

Plate 11 The Advanced Dispensing System.

Chronic pain (see also Chapter 10)

Once again, there is no shortage of anecdotal reports of the analgesic activity of cannabis in a range of painful conditions including bone and joint pain, migraine, cancer pain, menstrual cramps and labour pain (e.g. Grinspoon and Bakalar, 1993). Cannabinoids have been shown to have analgesic properties in thermal, mechanical and chemical-induced models of pain in animals (Segal, 1986; Formukong *et al.*, 1989), with non-opiate mechanisms appearing to predominate. Allodynia and hyperalgesia were reduced in rodent models of chronic pain. A dose-dependent antinociceptive effect of cannabis was demonstrated in healthy volunteers (Greenwald and Stitzer, 2000).

Five small placebo-controlled trials in severe pain (cancer-related, postoperative or neurogenic) (Noyes *et al.*, 1975a,b; Jain *et al.*, 1981; Maurer *et al.*, 1990; Holdcroft *et al.*, 1997) showed that oral THC produces a dose-related analgesic effect superior to that of placebo and comparable in potency to codeine, though possibly of longer duration. Higher doses (>15 mg) were associated with frequent adverse effects such as sedation, 'mental clouding' and slurred speech. A recent meta-analysis (Campbell *et al.*, 2001) cast doubt on the future role of cannabinoids in the management of pain, but the validity of this conclusion has been challenged (Grotenhermen, 2001; Iversen, 2001).

Emerging evidence implies that cannabis may benefit neuropathic pain. The 1997 National Institute of Health workshop on medical cannabis concluded: 'Neuropathic pain represents a treatment problem for which currently available analgesics are, at best, marginally effective. Since delta-9-THC is not acting by the same mechanism as either opioids or NSAIDs, it may be useful in this inadequately treated type of pain.'

Growing and colleagues (1998) also concluded that cannabis had potential as a treatment for neuropathic pain. They noted: 'A few animal studies support the idea that cannabinoids may have analgesic action in neuropathic pain. Given that this is the type of pain for which current treatments are least satisfactory, this would appear to be an area of greatest potential for cannabis, perhaps as an adjuvant to a regime of standard analgesics.'

An example of this condition is phantom limb pain, which afflicts roughly 30% of all amputees and is typically served poorly by standard analgesics. The UK House of Lords Science and Technology Committee (1998) concluded that 'pain which originates from damaged nerves might respond to cannabinoids. ... An example of such pain is phantom limb pain following amputation. ... [There is] anecdotal evidence that cannabis can relieve this pain [and] ... trials of cannabis should be undertaken in such patients.'

New research also demonstrates that the endocannabinoid anandamide helps modulate pain. Scientists at the University of Naples demonstrated (Calignano et al., 1998) in rats that anandamide is released when cells are damaged. Rats treated with a cannabinoid receptor antagonist demonstrated a prolonged and enhanced reaction to pain. Moreover, anandamide in conjunction with the endogenous compound PEA (palmitylethanolamide) has been observed to reduce pain 100-fold (Calignano et al., 1998).

Effects upon appetite and weight

The appetite-stimulating effect of cannabis often reported by recreational users ('the munchies') has been confirmed using both smoked marijuana and oral THC in controlled studies in both fasting and non-fasting human volunteers (Hollister, 1971; Foltin et al., 1986). The research literature relevant to the effects of exogenous and endogenous cannabinoids on appetite and weight in animals and humans has been comprehensively reviewed by Kirkham and Williams (2001).

Open studies in cancer patients (Plasse et al., 1991; Nelson et al., 1994) suggested that THC has a positive effect on appetite and weight. In a double-blind study in 54 patients with various cancers Regelson et al. (1976) found that oral THC (0.1–0.4 mg/kg daily) produced a significant gain or preservation of weight in comparison with placebo. THC also improved depression and 'tranquillity' scores, but somnolence, dizziness and disassociation were troublesome in a quarter of the patients.

Many patients with acquired immune deficiency syndrome (AIDS) have reported anecdotally a wide range of symptom relief with illicit cannabis. These include reduction in nausea, improved appetite, reduced anxiety, relief of aches and pains, improved sleep, and inhibition of oral candidiasis (Plasse et al., 1991; Grinspoon and Bakalar, 1993). Progressive weight loss is a major problem in this condition and there are many explanations for this, including intestinal malabsorption, infestation of the mouth or oesophagus by opportunistic pathogens, side-effects of antiretrovirals and other medication, metabolic disturbances and clinical depression. In a controlled trial in 88 AIDS patients, oral THC (5 mg daily) was significantly superior to placebo in improving appetite and reducing nausea (Beal et al., 1995). THC seemed to improve mood better than placebo ($p = 0.06$), and there was a tendency toward weight gain. THC produced significantly more adverse effects than placebo, the most frequent being euphoria, dizziness, 'thinking abnormalities' and sedation, but 75% of these fell into the mild or moderate categories.

Of relevance to this indication, Kaslow *et al.* (1989) monitored the progress of nearly 5000 HIV-positive men for 18 months and found no evidence that use of psychoactive substances (including cannabis) had any discernible effect upon T-helper lymphocyte counts or progression to AIDS.

The study team who conducted the 1999 US Institute of Medicine Review concluded that 'For patients such as those with AIDS or who are undergoing chemotherapy, and who suffer simultaneously from severe pain, nausea, and appetite loss, cannabinoid drugs might offer broad-spectrum relief not found in any other single medication.' They also concluded that cannabis's 'short-term immuno-suppressive effects are not well established but, if they exist, are not likely great enough to preclude a legitimate medical use.'

Another condition frequently associated with decreased appetite and malnutrition is senile dementia of Alzheimer type. Eleven patients with Alzheimer's disease were treated for 12 weeks on an alternating schedule of dronabinol (THC) and placebo (six weeks of each treatment). The dronabinol treatment resulted in substantial weight gains and decline in disturbed behaviour (Volicer *et al.*, 1997). No serious side-effects were observed. One patient had a seizure and was removed from the study, but the investigators were unsure whether this was attributable to the dronabinol.

Inflammatory disorders

Antipyretic and anti-inflammatory activity of cannabinoids have been reported in a variety of animal models (Formukong *et al.*, 1989) and again there are numerous anecdotal reports of benefit from illicit cannabis in a range of inflammatory conditions (GW Pharmaceuticals survey – information on file, and see below).

The first scientific evidence of potential benefit in this domain was reported recently by Malfait *et al.* (2000). In a well-validated animal model of rheumatoid arthritis (RA) (murine collagen-induced arthritis, classical acute and chronic relapsing varieties) CBD was shown to protect against clinical progression and to protect joints against severe damage. Mechanism of action was found to have both anti-inflammatory and immunomodulatory components.

Seizure disorders

Epilepsy is one of the most prevalent neurological disorders, affecting around 1% of the world's population, and the historical role for cannabis in treatment is well described (O'Shaugnessy, 1843; Reynolds, 1890). Modern anticonvulsant drugs fail to provide satisfactory control in up to 30% of epileptic patients.

The effects of cannabinoids in animal models are complex (Karler and Turkanis, 1981; Consroe and Snider, 1986). CBD has powerful anticonvulsant effects apparently unlimited by tolerance, but shows distinct species differences. THC is proconvulsant in some models (especially in huge doses) but anticonvulsant in others. The mode of action remains uncertain.

There are numerous anecdotal reports of beneficial effects of cannabis in human epileptics, and two single case reports. Keeler and Reifler (1967) described a man with grand mal epilepsy who was convulsion-free for six months off medication but then suffered three fits after smoking cannabis on seven occasions over a three-week period, though the fits were unrelated to periods of intoxication. Consroe and colleagues (1975) in contrast reported a young man who converted poor seizure control into complete alleviation by adding 2–5 cannabis cigarettes nightly to his conventional medication.

Only one controlled trial (Cunha *et al.*, 1980) has been conducted. CBD (200–300 mg daily for up to 4.5 months added to standard therapy) was compared with placebo in a double-blind, parallel group design in 15 poorly controlled patients with 'secondary generalised epilepsy'. Half the CBD patients remained 'almost free' of fits throughout the experiment and all but one of the others showed 'partial improvement'. All but one of the placebo patients remained unchanged. A quarter of the patients reported somnolence whilst receiving CBD but this was the only reported adverse effect.

Asthma

Small controlled studies in asthmatic volunteers conducted in the 1970s (Tashkin *et al.*, 1976, 1977; Williams *et al.*, 1976) showed that oral, smoked and aerosolised THC had significant bronchodilator activity comparable to that of salbutamol, though slower in onset. This was at the cost of dose-related tachycardia and intoxication at higher doses. Unfortunately, the aerosol then available had an irritant effect, resulting in cough and discomfort. There is a theoretical possibility of a synergistic combination with beta$_2$-adrenoceptor agonists since cannabinoids do not appear to act via the sympathetic nervous system (Graham, 1986). Nabilone does not seem to have a useful bronchodilator action (Archer *et al.*, 1986).

Anxiety, insomnia and other psychiatric conditions

Two small controlled studies (Fabre and McLendon, 1981; Ilaria *et al.*, 1981) involving a total of 31 psychiatric outpatients showed that nabilone (1–3 mg daily) was significantly superior to placebo at relieving anxiety over 7 or 14 days of treatment. Dizziness, dry mouth and drowsiness were reported by some patients, but both sets of authors concluded that nabilone appeared to be an effective anxiolytic and that further investigation was justified. Zuardi and colleagues have conducted a series of studies on CBD after finding that it appeared to antagonise the anxiogenic effects of THC along with some other marijuana-like effects in healthy volunteers (Zuardi *et al.*, 1982). CBD produced a selective anxiolytic effect in the elevated plus-maze model in rats (Guimaraes *et al.*, 1990) and in a subsequent experiment in healthy volunteers (Zuardi *et al.*, 1993) it was found that CBD (300 mg orally) exhibited anxiolytic effects in comparison with placebo in a simulated public speaking task.

CBD was also found to have a profile resembling that of an atypical antipsychotic agent in a rodent model predictive of antipsychotic activity (Zuardi *et al.*, 1991). In a report of a single case, CBD (in doses up to 1500 mg/day) was found to improve psychotic symptoms without toxic effects in a psychotic patient whose response to haloperidol was negated by intolerable adverse effects (Zuardi *et al.*, 1995).

Isolated controlled studies suggested that CBD (160 mg) may be an effective hypnotic (Carlini and Cunha, 1981), and that THC (0.1 mg/kg) may have antidepressant properties in cancer patients (Regelson *et al.*, 1976).

Glaucoma

Glaucoma is the commonest cause of blindness in the Western world. Raised intraocular pressure (IOP) is usually due to an obstruction to the outflow of aqueous humour at the front of the eye, and the many different variations of defect can be divided into open- and closed-angle varieties. By far the commonest is primary open-angle (chronic simple) glaucoma.

It has been long established that topical or systemic THC reduces IOP in various animal models (Adler and Geller, 1986) and in human volunteers (Hepler *et al.*, 1976; Perez-Reyes *et al.*, 1976; Jones *et al.*, 1981), though the mechanism of action has yet to be clarified. Reductions to 30% below baseline are typical but conjunctival engorgement and tear reduction were often noted. THC, Δ^8-THC, and 11-hydroxy-THC were more effective than cannabinol, and CBD appeared to be without effect. In the study by Jones and colleagues (1981) tolerance to the IOP reduction seemed to develop after dosing for several days.

In the 1970s anecdotal reports of the relief of symptoms by smoked marijuana appeared and individuals successfully argued in the US for legal access to the drug (Grinspoon and Bakalar, 1993). Hepler and colleagues (1976) carried out a pilot study of smoked marijuana and oral THC (15 mg) in 11 glaucoma patients. Seven of these showed a reduction in IOP averaging 30% while four did not respond.

Two small controlled studies of smoked and topical THC confirmed a significant reduction in IOP in comparison with placebo. Smoked THC (2%) was compared with placebo in a double-blind parallel group study in 18 patients with glaucoma of varying aetiology (Merritt *et al.*, 1980). IOP was significantly reduced in comparison with placebo, maximally from an average of 30 mmHg to 21 mmHg between 1.5 and 2.5 hours after dosing. Unfortunately, these effects were accompanied by reductions in blood pressure, increases in heart rate and 'alterations in mental status', which limited the clinical usefulness of the active medication. Merritt and colleagues went on to investigate the effect of THC eyedrops in a double-blind comparison with placebo in eight patients (Merritt *et al.*, 1981). Dose-related reductions in IOP were recorded using 0.05% and 1% drops with minimal adverse effects. Interestingly, parallel reductions were noted in the untreated eye, leading the authors to speculate on a systemic mode of action.

It is now apparent that IOP is not the only pathological mechanism in glaucoma. Impaired autoregulation in arteries supplying the optic nerve head may interfere with perfusion and cause neural damage (Prunte *et al.*, 1998). The discovery that CB_1 receptors are present in microvasculature (Sugiura *et al.*, 1998) and the ability of endogenous cannabinoids to produce vasodilation (Sugiura *et al.*, 1998) suggests the possibility that exogenous cannabinoids may alleviate this deficit. Antioxidant and NMDA receptor neuroprotective properties of cannabinoids (Hampson *et al.*, 1998) raise the hope that they might improve survival of ischaemic retinal ganglion cells.

Migraine

A century ago, William Osler gave his opinion that cannabis was 'probably the most satisfactory remedy' for migraine. Some patients and physicians are once again showing interest in examining the potential of cannabis to treat symptoms of migraine. Russo (1998) concluded that 'cannabis … presents the hypothetical potential for quick, effective, parenteral treatment of acute migraine.' He judged cannabis a 'far safer alternative' than many prescription antimigraine drugs, and reported that a large percentage of migraine sufferers fail to respond to or cannot tolerate standard therapies.

Serotonin activity may be an important target for new migraine medicines, and Volfe *et al.* (1985) reported that THC (but not CBD) may inhibit the release of serotonin from normal platelets when incubated with plasma from migraine patients.

A possible link between cannabinoids and migraine is suggested by the abundance of cannabinoid receptors in the periaqueductal grey (PAG) region of the brain. The PAG is part of the neural system that suppresses pain and is thought to be involved in the generation of migraine headaches (Goadsby and Gundlach, 1991). The link between cannabinoids and migraine might be elucidated by examining the effects of cannabinoids on PAG (Lichtman *et al.*, 1996). Recent results indicating that both cannabinoid receptor subtypes are involved in controlling peripheral pain (Calignano *et al.*, 1998) suggest that the link is possible. Further research is warranted.

Brain injury/stroke

Emerging research indicates that certain cannabinoids may exhibit neuroprotective properties. Researchers at the National Institute for Mental Health (NIMH) reported that THC and CBD are potent antioxidants in animals (Hampson *et al.*, 1998). CBD was selected because it is non-psychoactive, fast acting and apparently non-toxic. They found that it protected rat brain cells that had been exposed to toxic levels of glutamate better than standard antioxidants such as vitamins C and E. There is speculation that this finding may have relevance to humans exposed to high levels of glutamate following brain injury.

Dexanabinol (HU-211), a synthetic drug similar to CBD, is apparently active in animal models of cerebral ischaemia (Lavie *et al.*, 2001) and autoimmune encephalitis (Achiron *et al.*, 2000). A press announcement (7 October 1998) by the Pharmos Pharmaceutical Company in Israel announced that it reduced mortality and eased intracranial pressure in 67 patients suffering from severe head injuries. The company expects to begin large-scale human trials on the drug in Europe and America in 2004.

Antitumour effects

Cannabinoids have been reported to inhibit tumour growth *in vivo* and *in vitro* in a range of models and to increase animal survival (Harris *et al.*, 1976). A small body of research indicates that cannabinoids may help protect against the development of certain types of tumours. One study (Harris *et al.*, 1976) examined the effects of THC, Δ^8-THC and cannabinol on cancer cells in mice lungs. The authors reported that cannabinoids reduced the size of the tumours by 25–82%, depending on dose and duration of treatment, with a corresponding increase in survival time. An unpublished study within the US National Toxicology Program found that mice and rats given high doses of THC over long periods of time appeared to have greater protection against malignancies than untreated controls. Researchers concluded that in both mice and rats, 'the incidence of benign and malignant neoplasms ... were decreased in a dose dependent manner' (James, 1997).

De Petrocellis *et al.* (1998) reported that anandamide 'potently and selectively inhibits the proliferation of human breast cancer cells in vitro' by interfering with their DNA production cycle. Non-mammary tumour cells were not affected by anandamide.

Miscellaneous possibilities

There is considerable evidence from animal models (Hine *et al.*, 1975; Bhargava, 1976; Lal *et al.*, 1981; Chesher and Jackson, 1985) that THC and its analogues inhibit many of the signs and symptoms of opioid withdrawal. Anecdotal reports from withdrawing addicts suggest this may also occur in humans.

A handful of documented case studies suggest that cannabis produces beneficial effects on Tourette's syndrome (Sandyk and Awerbuch, 1988; Hemming *et al.*, 1993; Muller-Vahl *et al.*, 1997). Muller-Vahl *et al.* (1999) reported that in an open trial a 25-year-old patient treated with 10 mg of THC experienced marked improvement of both vocal and motor tics. Improvement began 30 minutes after dosing, total tic severity was down from 41 before treatment to 7 at 2 hours, and benefit lasted for about 7 hours. No adverse effects were reported.

Mechoulam (1986) has drawn attention to the lack of modern research directed at possible antihelmintic and oxytocic applications.

GW Pharmaceuticals patient database

The founding of GW Pharmaceuticals in 1998 caused considerable media interest, and many people who hoped to participate as subjects in the medicinal research programme contacted the company requesting information. Three thousand, five hundred and sixteen individuals who contacted GW Pharmaceuticals between 1998 and 2001 were asked to complete an extensive questionnaire detailing their current or previous experience of illicit cannabis as a medicine, and 2458 (70%) complied. Of these, 1517 (62%) were female, and 1671 (68%) had never tried cannabis but hoped to gain access to a legal supply.

Of the 787 individuals who were either current (470) or previous (317) users, the majority suffered from MS or other neurological conditions, with the next largest category being various forms of arthritis. Many patients recorded multiple diagnoses. This distribution reflects the pattern of publicity and the interest of well-organised patient groups such as the MS Society, so the sample is highly selected and should not be taken as representative of the general pattern of medicinal cannabis use in the UK.

The average age of current users was 46 years with a range of 20–82, and just over half of these reported daily intake. Modal consumption was one or two cannabis cigarettes ('spliffs') daily, though a quarter of the subjects were smoking three or more spliffs each day.

Of previous users, 68% cited practical issues of supply as their reason for discontinuation, made up of 38% being unable to maintain a reliable source of supply and a further 30% finding the cost of black market material unacceptable (average price approximately £100 for an ounce of variable quality material). Only a small minority of ex-users reported that they had abandoned cannabis because of lack of efficacy (6%) or unwanted effects (13%).

Looking at the cannabis-experienced group as a whole, cannabis was considered to be more effective than other available treatment by 69% of subjects, and of these 42% considered the difference to be marked. Only 3% of subjects had found cannabis to be inferior to standard treatments. This finding is unsurprising in a sample selected, presumably, on the basis of dissatisfaction with standard treatment, but it does suggest that cannabis may provide benefit in otherwise refractory cases. Reports from this sample also confirm that perceived benefits from cannabis go further than specific symptom relief – 93% said it made them feel better overall, and this effect was marked in 68% of the sample. It remains possible, of course, that this relates to the intoxicating effects of smoked cannabis, but this is at odds with clinical experience with MS patients in the Oxford trials – most have no desire at all for intoxication, regarding it as an unwanted effect that would interfere with their ability to proceed normally with their working and family lives.

Unwanted effects associated with cannabis are shown in Table 9.1. These were not spontaneously reported but were derived from a checklist of predictable effects (i.e. forced choice). It is interesting to note that some adverse effects commonly associated with cannabis (e.g. dry mouth, drowsiness, anxiety, impaired coordination, dizziness/vertigo) appear to have a greater prevalence with standard treatments. Only 3% of subjects thought that adverse effects were worse after cannabis than standard treatments, with the majority (59%) rating standard treatments worse.

Although this database is highly selected and cannot be assumed to be representative of the experiences of medicinal cannabis users in general, it is the largest such group currently assembled and gives further support to the hypothesis that cannabis may have therapeutic efficacy for refractory symptoms with an acceptable adverse effect profile.

Delivery systems for cannabis medicinal extracts

Although the lungs are an excellent route for the absorption of cannabinoids, smoking is out of the question as a method of delivering a medicine for several reasons. Most patients are non-smokers of tobacco and would have considerable practical difficulties in achieving satisfactory smoke inhalation, and the act of smoking is socially unacceptable these days in most public places. More importantly, pyrolysis releases a host of toxic materials in both gaseous and particulate phases. Indeed differences in smoking methods result in the delivery of as much as four times the volume of tar from a marijuana cigarette than would be generated by a tobacco cigarette of equivalent weight. Aerosols and vaporisers offer promise as alternative methods of lung delivery and, although these present major pharmaceutical challenges, a number are under development. They share with the smoked route the potential disadvantage of peak and trough effects as a result of a spiky pharmacokinetic profile.

An obvious alternative is to take the drug by mouth, and there are two cannabinoids currently licensed in oral formulations (dronabinol and nabilone). Unfortunately, the very low water solubility of key

Table 9.1 Numbers of patients reporting unwanted effects with medicinal cannabis in comparison to other therapy

	Number of patients reporting effect				
	With medicinal cannabis		With other therapy		
Effect	*Current* (n – 470)	*Previous* (n – 317)	*Current* (n – 470)	*Previous* (n – 317)	*Never* (n – 1671)
Red eyes	87	24	29	9	38
A feeling of well-being	321	159	42	26	120
A floating sensation	92	61	45	17	76
Dry mouth/dehydration	139	40	241	145	601
Increased appetite	238	77	26	22	102
Laughter, giggling fits	132	59	3	9	17
A desire to speak more freely	145	58	12	8	39
An altered sense of time	86	40	38	10	48
Increase in keenness of senses	111	32	5	3	21
Muscle relaxation	401	202	122	76	314
Drowsiness	137	68	202	115	512
A stimulating feeling	165	63	19	6	39
A depressed feeling	10	4	156	60	243
A quicker pulse/palpitations	24	14	68	27	108
Anxiety	18	6	112	48	186
Panic	10	8	54	26	95
Flashing lights/ hallucinations	11	8	17	14	59
Difficulty in coordination	23	20	81	43	175
Dizziness or vertigo	16	20	97	38	197
Total	2166	963	1369	702	2990

The questionnaire provided a list of effects including most of the main accepted undesirable effects associated with use of cannabis. Patients indicated whether they had experienced these effects with cannabis and/or with other therapy. Please note that a minority of the 'never' group did not address this question at all.

cannabis constituents aggravates still further the normal variability of absorption from the gastrointestinal tract, resulting in poor predictability of both the timing and intensity of peak effects. This makes life very difficult for patients who may wish to titrate the dose against the intensity of their symptoms, as is the norm for most individuals who smoke cannabis medicinally. This requirement is all the more compelling given the wide variation in individual sensitivity to both the therapeutic and unwanted effects of cannabis derivatives. An additional drawback is the production of larger quantities of reputedly unhelpful metabolites such as 11-OH-THC as a result of the hepatic first pass phenomenon (see Chapter 8). The oral route is obviously useless in patients with nausea and vomiting. Skin patches and intranasal formulations have not been a success to date, and suppositories, whilst viable pharmaceutically, are unlikely to be welcomed by most patients.

These difficulties have stimulated interest in both liquid and solid oromucosal preparations. GW Pharmaceuticals have piloted the use of sublingual drops and propellant-powered aerosols in studies in healthy volunteers, but the best results in terms of pharmacokinetic profile and subject preference have been obtained using a pump action spray (PAS). Figure 9.1 illustrates the range of pharmacokinetic profiles that are attainable by alterations in the excipients, and which could potentially be tailored for speed of onset and duration of action to fit individual therapeutic requirements. For example, patients with chronic pain might require a preparation with a fairly flat but predictable profile to maintain steady state over the full 24 hours without peaks and troughs (Figure 9.1, PAS A), with a vaporiser or inhaled aerosol to tackle occasional break-through pain. On the other hand, for postoperative pain a more rapid onset and offset might be preferable (Figure 9.1, PAS B). When larger doses are required (for example, with CBD-rich preparations) solid dose forms such as pastilles or sublingual tablets may provide the answer.

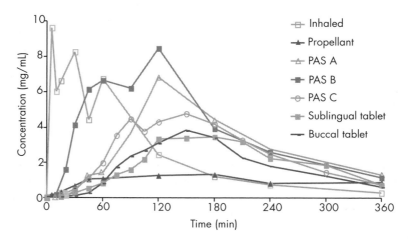

Figure 9.1 Pharmacokinetic profiles for a range of THC preparations. Mean THC data normalised to 10 mg. Venous blood samples were taken via an indwelling catheter from dorsum of hand or antecubital fossa. PAS, pump action spray.

One of the challenges inherent in restoring a pariah drug such as cannabis to medical respectability in certain countries (e.g. the USA) lies in convincing doctors and regulators that the preparation will not be abused by the patient or diverted on to the black market. A potential solution to this problem, also pioneered by GW Pharmaceuticals, is the Advanced Dispensing System (see Plate 11).

Practical issues in initiating a clinical research programme

Despite the fact that cannabis has a medicinal track record extending back thousands of years, the modern clinical researcher is faced with many unknowns. Which extracts are appropriate for which symptoms in which disease states? Which formulations are best suited to which type of patient? What doses should be chosen and what is the optimal pattern of delivery? What is the most appropriate clinical trial methodology and how is the problem of individual variability in response to be tackled? And to what extent do the perceived risks of recreational use impinge on the medicinal arena? These questions will be dealt with in turn based on the authors' experience of having initiated from scratch a clinical trial programme to explore the potential of standardised plant extracts (see Chapters 2 and 3).

Choice of extract for initial study

There is a great deal of solid scientific data pointing to the therapeutic potential of THC, but unfortunately this is also the principal psychoactive component of the plant. So are there any other substances among the hundreds produced by the plant that may either damp down some of the unwanted effects of THC or add a therapeutic element of their own? The starting point for answering this question is to accept that the thousands of patients who have claimed that naturally occurring cannabis relieves their symptoms cannot all be wrong. There is good scientific evidence that many other substances produced by the plant have therapeutic properties in their own right and that synergistic interactions are likely (McPartland and Russo, 2001). The other cannabinoid which is usually present to a significant degree in black market cannabis is cannabidiol (CBD), in a concentration often comparable with that of THC itself.

CBD has a number of potentially therapeutic effects in its own right (see Chapters 5 and 7) including anti-inflammatory, anti-convulsant, muscle relaxant, analgesic, antipsychotic, antiemetic and anxiolytic properties. By inhibiting cytochrome P450 3A11 in the liver it may also reduce hydroxylation of THC to its 11-hydroxy metabolite, a substance that is reputed to possess four times the intoxication potency of THC itself (Browne and Weissman, 1981). There is some evidence that it may inhibit the anxiogenic effects of THC in humans (Zuardi *et al.*, 1982) and that small alterations in the ratio of CBD to THC significantly alter its modulatory effect on such THC-related phenomena as distortion of time estimation, subjective intoxication and tachycardia (Karniol and Carlini, 1973). Preliminary clinical data also suggest that combining CBD with THC alters susceptibility of certain symptoms and has an impact upon the prevalence of adverse effects (Robson *et al.*, 2002), but much more work is required to delineate these subtle differences with any confidence.

Design of initial clinical studies

The practical information that exists to guide modern medicinal use is extremely limited. Specifically, what is an appropriate starting and maintenance dose, and what is the most suitable dosing regime? These questions pose particular difficulty since marked individual variation in response to both recreational and medicinal cannabis is well recognised.

Studies in healthy volunteers can give some limited guidance, and GW Pharmaceuticals carried out a number of these in preparation for its clinical programme. Of particular interest were observations of dose/effect relationships for well-known markers of cannabis activity, including tachycardia, postural hypotension and subjective intoxication. More specific effects on cognitive function were assessed through measures of memory, attention, motor coordination and reaction time. These studies provided some broad guidelines as to suitable doses but could only take what patients would regard as toxic effects for their end-points. Once again, large individual variation in response was noted.

Double-blind, randomised, placebo-controlled clinical trials (RCTs) will always form the final mechanism through which the relative merits of any new medicine can be assessed with confidence, but there are some essential prerequisites: target conditions must be accurately defined, appropriate doses and formulations of test articles must be identified, and the validity and reliability of outcome measures assured. In approaching these difficulties, uncontrolled pilot studies are vulnerable to several types of subject and observer bias, the confounding effect of natural fluctuations of the disorder, and the impact of the placebo effect. An alternative strategy that has a long tradition in psychological research is to carry out a series of randomised, placebo-controlled, crossover studies in single subjects ('n of 1' trials).

In this design, each patient acts as his or her own control in testing the trial medicines against placebo. As with RCTs, strict inclusion and exclusion criteria can be applied, uniform treatment procedures and validated outcome measures adopted, and appropriate statistical testing selected. In this way, not only can beneficial and adverse effects in individual patients be placed in the context of the response to placebo, but also common characteristics may emerge which can be generalised to the target population. Johannessen (1991) provides an example of how this approach proved useful in the evaluation of cimetidine. Guyatt and colleagues at McMaster University have described their considerable experience in the application of the 'n of 1' design (e.g. Guyatt *et al.*, 1990a,b). A number of statistical approaches to data generated by 'n of 1' studies have been applied successfully (Edgington, 1984). Where one or more test articles appear to produce an apparently significant effect, re-challenge under similar controlled conditions within the same subject is a statistically powerful manoeuvre.

The Institute of Medicine study team supported (1999) the 'n of 1' approach for cannabinoid clinical research, making the following comment:

> The challenge of integrating the ideal of standardized and rigorous processes for treatment evaluation with everyday clinical practice has encouraged interest in single-patient trials. Methods for such trials have been established and tested in a variety of clinical settings, usually under everyday conditions. They are particularly valuable when physicians or patients are uncertain about the efficacy of treatment for symptomatic diseases. Controls can be incorporated even in this kind of trial. Such trials can be double blinded and can involve cross-over designs in which the patient is treated with alternating treatments, such as placebo-drug-placebo or one drug followed by another drug. As with any other clinical trial, a single-patient trial should be designed to permit objective comparison between treatments.

Preliminary evaluations of cannabis extracts lend themselves to this strategy for the following reasons: target conditions such as MS are heterogeneous in their symptom profile; the necessary prerequisites for RCTs listed above have yet to be identified, and 'n of 1' studies can be expected to generate this information; target symptoms within the defined clinical conditions are temporarily reversible, so repeated treatment periods are feasible; cannabis extracts are expected to have a prompt onset of action, so treatment periods can be of manageable length; placebos matched to test articles are available. New information from individual patients can rapidly inform appropriate modifications to trial design.

Patients, dosing and outcome measures

If cannabis-based medicinal extracts are to regain a place in conventional therapeutics they will have to overcome the pariah status that has resulted from frustrated attempts to prohibit the recreational use of cannabis for many decades. In this context it is not enough for CBMEs merely to be as good as standard treatments – they must offer some tangible advantage to justify their very existence.

For this reason, and also because the existing evidence for clinical utility reviewed above is primarily anecdotal, the starting point is to look for medical conditions for which the standard treatments are either not fully effective or dangerously toxic. MS and other neurological conditions where muscle spasticity and neuropathic pain are key features are good examples of such disorders. Early GW Pharmaceuticals trials have selected patients with these conditions who have tried every accessible conventional treatment and still find themselves burdened with refractory, life-impairing symptoms. Rather than withdraw existing treatments on entry into trials, efforts were made to stabilise intake and the CBME (or placebo) then added in on top.

The first patients to enter the research were recruited by local clinicians or drawn from the GW Pharmaceuticals database described above. They were screened to ensure eligibility and to rule out undiagnosed conditions that may affect outcome measures, such as urinary tract infections or high blood pressure. For inclusion in the early studies, MS and other neurological patients had to be experiencing at least one of the following symptoms to a clinically significant degree despite receiving appropriate standard treatments: neuropathic pain, spasticity, muscle spasms, lower urinary tract disturbance (e.g. urgency, incontinence, frequency, nocturia), or tremor. Patients were not enrolled if they had a past history of serious drug or alcohol misuse, any medical condition that CBME might possibly aggravate, such as schizophrenia, uncontrolled cardiovascular disorders or epilepsy, or impairment of their liver or kidney function to the point that metabolism or excretion of CBME might be impaired. Research was conducted under the auspices of licences from the UK Home Office and Department of Health, and was approved by local or regional Research Ethics Committees. It was carried out according to the standards agreed under the internationally agreed Guidelines for Good Clinical Practice, and all patients gave written informed consent to participate.

In devising the dosing schedules for the trials, it was necessary to take into account the likelihood of wide individual variation in sensitivity to CBMEs, and the need for patients to differentiate for themselves the separate thresholds for symptom relief and intoxication with THC-containing medicines. A system was therefore developed by which the initial exposure to CBME would take place in clinic with continuous medical and nursing supervision, and following this the patient would discover his or her own optimal dosing regime by a process of gradual self-titration against symptom relief or emergence of unwanted effects. Specially trained research nurses monitored the patients' progress by telephone during the home dosing period and arranged extra assessments if necessary. During the initial clinic dosing early patients underwent continuous monitoring of cardiovascular function, and plasma samples were taken to investigate the relationship between blood levels of CBME and objective effects. After baseline measures and an open run-in period on THC:CBD 1:1 CBME patients entered a randomised, double-blind, crossover comparison of THC:CBD 1:1 CBME, THC-rich CBME, CBD-rich CBME, and placebo. Some early results are summarised below.

Choice of outcome measures for clinical trials in conditions such as MS poses particular difficulties because most rely entirely on the subjective reports of the patients, while those with more objectivity (such as the Ashworth Scale for spasticity) tend to be markedly unreliable. To counter this, early patients were subjected to a wide range of standardised measures of symptoms and disability (e.g. Barthel ADL Index, Rivermead Mobility Index, Ashworth Scale, General Health Questionnaire, nine-hole peg test, Short Orientation-Memory-Concentration test); numerical rating scales of symptom severity administered in clinic at the end of each treatment period by a research nurse who had no previous contact with that patient; and visual analogue scales (VAS) measuring symptoms and general well-being (alertness, relaxation, optimism, energy, sleep, intoxication) completed by patients in a daily diary throughout the entire period of study.

Once patients had completed each acute study it was considered essential for ethical reasons to allow them the option of continuing to receive CBME long term within a research context if there was good evidence that significant clinical benefit had been obtained. At the same time as satisfying a humanitarian requirement, such chronic studies provide vital information on the safety and tolerability of these medicines over months or even years of dosing. In practice, it was found that a large majority of the patients who completed acute studies chose to progress to long-term maintenance (see below).

Safety issues for cannabis-based medicines

Effects on cognition

It is well known that cannabis and THC produce a range of acute effects in recreational users and experimental subjects. These have been reviewed by Solowij (1998) and can be summarised as follows: intoxication, with euphoria, sensory enhancement, increased social conviviality, and a sense of relaxation and contentment; perceptual effects including distorted time and space estimation and alteration in sensory modalities; impairment in both sustained and divided attention; impairment in reaction time, motor control and dexterity; impairment in various aspects of memory and higher cognitive function including associative and abstractive processes, planning and organisational strategies. As is the case with many other prescription and over-the-counter drugs, patients receiving cannabis-based medicines should therefore be warned to avoid driving and other potentially hazardous tasks at any time they feel impaired. For a full account of the potential effects of cannabis and its derivatives on driving, see Chapter 12.

An important question is whether any of these acute cognitive deficits are capable of persisting after cannabis has been discontinued and fully eliminated from the body. Despite a large and rapidly expanding scientific literature it is unfortunately still impossible to answer this question with confidence, and this is largely due to methodological shortcomings in much of this research. Gonzalez *et al.* (2002) proposed seven 'minimal criteria' by which to assess the scientific credibility of studies exploring non-acute cognitive effects of cannabis: inclusion of subjects with a history of 'primarily' cannabis use; inclusion of an appropriate control group; use of valid neuropsychological outcome measures; cannabis group demonstrably drug-free on day of testing; study reports length of abstinence from cannabis before test day; study addresses possibility of other recreational drug use in cannabis group; study addresses other potentially confounding factors such as coexisting psychiatric or neurological problems. Only 13 out of 40 eligible studies met these basic criteria. Control group matching is crucial, since it is known that age, gender, ethnicity and years spent in education affect neuropsychological performance. Heavy cannabis users may be recruited from patients requesting psychiatric help in connection with their cannabis use, producing important selection bias. Additionally, studies often incorporate multiple outcome measures without controlling for this in the statistical analysis, and if there is one statistically significant finding among 20 non-significant results it tends to be the former which is highlighted. Unfortunately, as the authors point out, negative results are quickly disseminated in both the scientific and lay media without any allowance being made for these serious shortcomings.

Another problem lies in distinguishing reversible residual effects (due to slow metabolism of cannabis components or withdrawal phenomena) from irreversible effects. Pope *et al.* (2002) carried out neuropsychological testing in 77 current heavy users and 87 controls. The former showed significant memory deficits at 0, 1 and 7 days of abstinence but by day 28 were virtually indistinguishable from the control subjects. No significant association was found between duration of cannabis use and cognitive performance after 28 days of abstinence. This is a diametrically opposite result to that obtained by Solowij *et al.* (2002), who found that deficits on several neuropsychological measures were correlated with lifetime duration of cannabis exposure. In seeking to explain such discrepancies, Pope *et al.* (2002) point out that even well-controlled studies depend on the assumption that, after adjustment for more obvious confounding factors, short-, longer term and non-users of cannabis are comparable on *all* factors other than exposure to cannabis. Additionally, the acute effects of cannabis in heavy users may impact on outcome measures through a negative effect on school attendance and social integration.

Grant *et al.* (2003) carried out a meta-analysis of studies that have attempted to address non-acute cognitive effects, which failed to demonstrate a substantial, systematic or detrimental effect of cannabis use on neuropsychological performance. They concluded: 'The small magnitude of effect sizes from observations of chronic users of cannabis suggests that cannabis compounds, if found to have therapeutic value, should have a good margin of safety from a neurocognitive standpoint under the more limited conditions of exposure that would likely obtain in a medical setting.'

Dependency potential

Another important question is whether cannabis and its derivatives have a capacity to induce dependence, either physical or psychological. Properties of THC that may have a bearing on this have been investigated in numerous animal models but the degree to which these predict human behaviour outside the laboratory is questionable. Perhaps of more relevance in the case of a drug with such wide current human use is to examine what actually happens in the real world.

The evidence for cannabis dependence has been reviewed by Johns (2001). The generally accepted components of a dependence syndrome are a declining response on chronic dosing (tolerance), a clear-cut withdrawal syndrome when the drug is stopped, difficulty in keeping consumption under control, and a preoccupation with the drug which interferes with the normal activities of living.

Tolerance to the subjective effects of marijuana has been noted (Georgotas and Zeidenberg, 1979), and there is some evidence (Wisbeck *et al.*, 1996) that a minority (16%) of regular recreational smokers experienced at least one of the following symptoms related to their cannabis use: irritability, insomnia, tremor, sweating, GI disturbance or appetite change. Thomas (1993) reported that around a third of cannabis users experienced some difficulty in controlling their use of the drug. Unfortunately, all of this research is dogged by serious methodological problems including highly selected samples, non-validated measures, poor response rates in community surveys, and a host of confounding variables. However, it seems reasonable to accept that psychological dependence will occur in a small minority of regular cannabis smokers. The existence of a clear-cut physical dependence syndrome is much less convincing on the basis of the published literature. If it exists at all it is probably mild and fleeting and is likely to consist of a few days of sleep disturbance and somatic symptoms of anxiety in heavy daily users who abstain abruptly.

In an interview study (Robson and Bruce, 1997) the dependence potential of various street drugs was assessed in 201 problem and 380 'social' drug users using the well-validated Severity of Dependence Scale (SDS). Scores (maximum = 15) in the problem group were 12.9 for heroin, 9.6 for other opioids, 6.1 for amphetamine and 5.5 for crack cocaine. Cannabis SDS score was 2.6 and comparable with those of LSD (3.1) and ecstasy (1.3), two drugs which are generally not associated with physical or psychological dependence. In the parallel sample of social users, the cannabis SDS was similar at 3.4.

If the concept of cannabis dependence is a slippery one in recreational users it is even more difficult to tie down in patients taking CBME long term to relieve symptoms. If such a patient is abruptly denied a medicine which has relieved previously intractable symptoms it would hardly be surprising if he or she yearned for that drug and became preoccupied with re-establishing supply. Experience in the therapeutic setting with much more powerfully addictive drugs than cannabis is encouraging: for example, opioid dependency is a very unusual outcome when patients are treated with these agents for the relief of pain and other symptoms (Porter and Jick, 1980).

Cannabis and psychosis

It is generally accepted that large doses of cannabis (or, possibly, smaller doses in susceptible individuals) may rarely produce a short-term psychotic illness in people with no pre-existing history of psychiatric illness (Thomas, 1993). This may consist of confusion, delusional ideas and hallucinations, and typically remits completely and rapidly on abstinence from the drug.

Of greater potential importance is the suggestion originating in a paper by Andreasson *et al.* (1987) that recreational cannabis use may represent an independent risk factor for the development of schizophrenia in later life. This has subsequently been the subject of increased research interest and, unfortunately, sensationalised reports in the lay media. The existence and significance of this association remains controversial and the methodology and interpretation of many of the scientific papers upon which it is based have been criticised by independent observers in the *British Medical Journal* and elsewhere. Issues raised include presence of clinical or subclinical psychiatric illness in subjects prior to cannabis consumption; lack of a clear temporal link between cannabis use and subsequent psychiatric illness; poor reliability of the diagnosis of schizophrenia; confusion between acute toxic states and functional mental illness; confusion of association with causation; confounding effects of other recreational drugs and environmental risk factors for mental illness; unreliability of self-report of an illegal activity; lack of a correlation in epidemiological studies between prevalence of cannabis consumption and schizophrenia. The consensus view, represented by Degenhardt and Hall (2002), seems to be that cannabis use is probably capable of precipitating psychotic disorders in vulnerable individuals and of exacerbating symptoms in those with existing mental illness, but that the existing evidence does not support the claim that cannabis can cause schizophrenia in previously healthy subjects.

A recent review paper (Arseneault *et al.*, 2004) whose authorship includes Professor Robin Murray, an acknowledged expert in the field, examined the causal association between recreational cannabis and psychosis. The review identified five studies that included a well-defined sample drawn from population-based registers or cohorts and used prospective measures of cannabis use and adult psychosis. The authors estimated on the basis of these studies that cannabis smoking by young adolescents confers an overall twofold increase in the relative risk for later schizophrenia. However, they point out that 'cannabis use appears to be neither a sufficient nor a necessary cause for psychosis. It is a component cause, part of a complex constellation of factors leading to psychosis.' They further conclude: 'Although the majority of young people are able to use cannabis in adolescence without harm, a vulnerable minority experiences harmful outcomes. The epidemiological evidence suggests that cannabis use among psychologically vulnerable adolescents should be strongly discouraged by parents, teachers and health practitioners alike.'

In a personal communication with one of the authors of this chapter (PJR) in which the significance of these findings for medicinal cannabis research were discussed, Professor Murray offered the following opinion:

> My position on the question of medicinal cannabis derived products [as opposed to recreational use] is that the two are relatively separate fields. Most of the evidence concerning recreational cannabis use and psychosis suggests that one needs to take large quantities over a prolonged period to run any increased risk. However, it is very difficult to quantify what the required amounts are. Furthermore, it is clear that those who have some personality or familial predisposition are more vulnerable than the average person. We are in the middle of genotyping one of our samples to see whether those who carry one of the fashionable schizophrenia susceptibility genes are more vulnerable to cannabis-related psychosis.
>
> The issue of why adolescents seem to be more vulnerable than those starting later in life is quite unclear; it could be that they are biologically sensitive because of some developmental stage of brain development or it could be that starting very young is associated with continued higher levels of use.
>
> I think it will be some years before we have evidence to answer the type of question that you ask. I would think you should simply adopt an empirical approach and monitor the occurrence of any psychiatric side-effect in your trials.

Recently completed human research

A consecutive series of double-blind, randomised, placebo-controlled single patient crossover trials has recently been reported from Oxford (Wade *et al.*, 2003). Twenty-four patients with MS (18), spinal cord injury (4), brachial plexus injury (1) or neurofibromatosis (1) received whole plant extracts of THC CBME, CBD CBME, THC:CBD 1:1 CBME, or placebo self-administered by oromucosal spray at doses determined by titration against symptom relief or unwanted effects within the range 2.5–120 mg per 24 hours. Patients recorded symptom, well-being and intoxication scores on a daily basis using visual analogue scales, completed standard measures of disability, mood and cognition on regular clinic visits, and recorded adverse events. Results are shown in Tables 9.2 and 9.3. At the nursing assessments, all three CBMEs improved spasticity in comparison with placebo and both THC CBME

Table 9.2 Results from a study of the effects of cannabis on neurogenic symptoms in patients with MS: data from two-weekly assessments (20 patients)

Symptom	Baseline	CBD CBME	THC CBME	CBD:THC	Placebo
Spasticity[a]	6.2 (2.9)	**3.8 (2.0)**	**3.8 (2.0)**	**4.1 (1.8)**	5.4 (2.3)
Spasm[b]	5.5 (2.4)	4.6 (2.2)	**3.4 (1.8)**	**3.6 (1.6)**	4.9 (2.5)
Fatigue[a]	5.2 (2.1)	4.6 (2.4)	4.2 (2.2)	5.2 (2.5)	5.0 (2.4)
Pain[a]	5.6 (3.3)	3.8 (2.9)	3.5 (2.8)	3.9 (2.9)	4.4 (3.2)
Incontinence[a]	2.9 (3.3)	1.4 (1.4)	1.2 (1.8)	1.8 (2.8)	1.4 (2.1)
Urgency[a]	4.1 (3.6)	3.2 (3.0)	3.0 (2.7)	3.5 (3.4)	3.3 (3.1)

Numerical rating scales: Mean (SD) score at each assessment point.
[a]Scores 10 (bad) – 0 (good).
[b]Frequency/24 h.
Bold indicates values with statistically significant difference from placebo at $p < 0.05$.
Adapted from Wade et al. (2003).

Table 9.3 Results from a study of the effects of cannabis on neurogenic symptoms in patients with MS: data from daily diary visual analogue scales (20 patients)

Symptom (n)	Baseline	CBD CBME	THC CBME	CBD:THC	Placebo
Spasticity (8)	29.0 (16.1)	47.8 (18.5)	57.3 (22.2)	43.8 (15.6)	42.3 (18.1)
Spasm (16)	40.9 (18.5)	54.6 (19.1)	58.4 (22.3)	55.8 (24.4)	47.3 (22.6)
Pain (12)	30.1 (17.8)	**54.8 (22.6)**	54.6 (27.4)	51.3 (27.0)	44.5 (22.7)
Bladder (10)	44.2 (22.1)	60.5 (28.4)	56.4 (30.0)	55.7 (30.3)	54.9 (28.8)
Tremor (8)	36.4 (16.4)	38.3 (22.9)	42.8 (23.7)	40.3 (27.0)	40.6 (21.1)
Alertness (20)	47.5 (20.1)	56.9 (22.6)	60.4 (21.4)	58.3 (23.2)	56.5 (19.3)
Appetite (20)	46.8 (23.6)	43.4 (25.4)	**45.6 (26.3)**	44.4 (26.0)	39.0 (25.9)
Happiness (20)	52.7 (23.5)	58.6 (22.2)	60.5 (20.1)	61.0 (21.0)	55.3 (16.6)
Relaxation (20)	52.2 (22.2)	59.9 (23.6)	60.1 (22.5)	60.1 (22.6)	54.8 (19.7)
Optimism (20)	54.3 (24.5)	58.7 (21.8)	59.6 (20.1)	58.6 (21.9)	54.0 (16.7)
Energy (20)	40.9 (20.3)	50.1 (19.3)	52.3 (19.1)	50.9 (18.5)	50.5 (16.9)
Well-being (20)	48.2 (21.3)	55.2 (19.9)	58.0 (17.2)	56.8 (19.5)	52.9 (15.1)
Sleep (20)	47.3 (19.7)	57.9 (25.1)	61.7 (25.4)	**65.3 (22.6)**	59.0 (24.4)
Refreshed (20)	38.5 (17.9)	51.6 (23.5)	52.7 (25.7)	55.2 (24.7)	51.0 (23.8)

Mean (SD) score over last 7 days of each two-week period.
Scores range from 0 (worst possible) to 100 (best possible).
Bold indicates values with statistically significant difference from placebo at $p < 0.05$.
CBME, cannabis-based medicinal extract.
Adapted from Wade et al. (2003).

and THC:CBD CBME improved muscle spasm. Diary records show that THC CBME significantly improved VAS scores of pain, muscle spasm and spasticity; THC:CBD CBME significantly improved spasm and sleep; and CBD CBME significantly improved pain. Four patients withdrew due to unwanted effects, which are summarised in Table 9.4. The authors concluded that CBME can improve neurogenic symptoms unresponsive to standard treatments, and that unwanted effects were predictable and generally well tolerated.

This has been followed up with a parallel group, double-blind, randomised placebo-controlled study in 160 patients with MS experiencing significant problems from at least one target symptom: spasticity, muscle spasms, bladder problems, neuropathic pain or tremor (Wade DT, personal communication). Whole plant extract containing THC and CBD in

Table 9.4 Results from a study of the effects of cannabis on neurogenic symptoms in patients with MS: adverse events possibly, probably or definitely related to trial medication

	CBD CBME (n = 21)	THC CBME (n = 20)	CBD:THC (n = 20)	Placebo (n = 21)
Headache	1	3	1	2
Nausea	1	1	1	3
Diarrhoea	1	2	1	1
Fall	1	1	1	1
Sleepiness	0	1	2	1
Vomiting	0	1	1	2
Anxiety	0	0	0	2
Cough	0	1	1	0
Depressed mood	1	1	0	0
'Drug toxicity'	0	1	1	0
Fatigue	0	0	1	1
Impaired balance	0	1	1	0
Influenza symptoms	0	0	1	1
Sore mouth	1	1	0	0
Thirst	1	0	1	0
Disturbed attention	0	1	0	0
Dizziness	0	0	0	1
Hypoaesthesia	1	0	0	0
Hypotension	0	0	0	1
Patients with one or more adverse events	7 (33%)	11 (55%)	6 (30%)	10 (48%)

CBME, cannabis-based medicinal extract.
Adapted from Wade *et al.* (2003).

equal proportions in an oromucosal spray delivering 2.5 mg of each cannabinoid in a single activation were compared with a matched placebo spray. After initial dosing in clinic, patients were given instructions on how to titrate the dose upwards at home to a maximum of 48 sprays/24 hours, aiming for optimal balance of symptom relief and unwanted effects. Treatment period was six weeks, and preliminary analysis indicates a significant improvement in a subjective measure of spasticity.

Berman and colleagues (2003) examined the effect of THC CBME and THC:CBD CBME on the severe and intractable neuropathic pain which frequently results from traumatic brachial plexus avulsion. Characteristically, an extremely distressing and disruptive crushing and burning pain, often accompanied by shooting pain, is felt in the distal part of the damaged limb. Opioids, anticonvulsants and tricyclic antidepressants are partially effective at best. Forty-eight patients were studied in a randomised, double-blind, placebo-controlled crossover design with two-week treatment periods. Patients continued on all previous stable medicines including analgesics. At the beginning of each treatment period patients self-titrated to obtain an optimal balance between pain relief and unwanted effects. Primary outcome measure was BS-11 scores of pain at the end of week 2 of each treatment period. Results are shown in Table 9.5.

Both CBMEs significantly decreased pain and improved sleep. Although the effect size is only modest, it was felt by the investigator to be clinically significant. The authors pointed out that at an average daily intake of only eight sprays patients may not have maximally titrated their CBME dose within the allotted two weeks. They concluded that,

Table 9.5 Efficacy of two cannabis-based medicinal extracts for relief of central neuropathic pain from brachial plexus avulsion

	Baseline	Placebo	THC	THC:CBD
Pain BS-11	6.7	6.7	6.1 ($p < 0.005$)	6.1 ($p < 0.002$)
VAS	60.9	52.9	43.6 ($p < 0.04$)	45.1 ($p < 0.09$)
McGill total intensity	17.3	15.5	13.4 ($p < 0.04$)	13.8 ($p < 0.14$)
Sleep quality BS-11	4.8	5.2	6.0 ($p < 0.001$)	5.9 ($p < 0.01$)
GHQ-12	13.4	13.5	12.3 ($p < 0.18$)	10.9 ($p < 0.02$)
Sprays/24 h	n/a	9.2	7.3	6.9

p-values are shown compared to week 2 of the placebo period.
BS-11, Box Scale 11; GHQ-12, General Health Questionnaire 12; VAS, visual analogue scale.
From Berman *et al.* (2003).

given the refractory nature of brachial avulsion pain, CBME appears to represent 'a significant advance in treatment'.

Rog and Young (2003) have investigated the impact of THC:CBD CBME on central neuropathic pain in MS, a problem that afflicts up to 52% of patients with this condition. They compared CBME with placebo in a five-week randomised, double-blind, parallel group study in 66 patients, of whom 64 (96.9%) completed the trial. Mean number of sprays daily after completed titration was 9.6 for the active medicine and 19.1 for placebo.

Clinically and statistically significant reductions of pain in favour of CBME in comparison with placebo were noted for both BS-11 measures (-1.25; 95% CI -2.11, -0.39; $p = 0.005$) and the Neuropathic Pain Scale (-6.82; 95% CI -13.28, -0.37; $p = 0.039$). Sleep disturbance was also significantly improved by CBME in comparison with placebo (-1.39; 95% CI -2.27, -0.5; $p = 0.003$). On a seven-point Patient's Global Impression of Change Scale, those treated with CBME were 3.9 times more likely (95% CI 1.51, 10.06; $p = 0.005$) to feel 'much improved' or 'very much improved' than those receiving placebo. Thirty patients (88.2%) on CBME and 22 (68.8%) on placebo had at least one adverse event, none of which were serious. A range of standard tests for mood and cognitive function revealed no significant differences between CBME and placebo, with the sole exception of the long-term storage component of the Selective Reminding Test which showed a significant difference in favour of placebo ($p = 0.009$).

A consistent theme in all studies on CBME so far conducted is an improvement in the quality (and, when measured, quantity) of sleep. This could primarily be the result of relief of nocturnal symptoms or a primary hypnotic effect, and a sleep laboratory study in healthy subjects (Nicholson et al., 2004) has thrown some light on this question. The effects of THC CBME (15 mg) and THC:CBD CBME (5 mg:5 mg and 15 mg:15 mg) on nocturnal sleep, early morning performance, memory and sleepiness were studied in eight healthy subjects (four males, four females) in a randomised, double-blind, placebo-controlled crossover trial. The electroencephalogram, electro-oculograms and electromyogram were recorded during the sleep period, and performance, sleep latency and subjective assessments of sleepiness and mood were assessed the following morning. There was no evidence that 15 mg THC (a standard clinical dose) significantly altered the normal sleep process (as would be the case with hypnotics such as the benzodiazepines), but the next day there were residual effects on memory (immediate and delayed word recall), sleep latency was decreased, and subjects reported increased anxiety and sleepiness. CBD appeared to have dose-dependent alerting properties since it increased wakefulness during sleep and counteracted the residual sedative effect and memory impairment associated with THC the morning after dosing. These results suggest that improvements in sleep seen in clinical studies are more likely to be due to symptom relief than a primary hypnotic effect.

An important study exploring the effects of oral synthetic THC (Marinol) and a cannabis extract (Cannador) on spasticity and other symptoms related to multiple sclerosis has been funded by the Medical Research Council and the results have been recently published (Zajicek *et al.*, 2003). This was a randomised, placebo-controlled trial involving 33 UK centres and 630 patients, and the primary outcome measure was change in overall spasticity score as represented by the Ashworth Scale (a measure of biological impairment, as opposed to disability or handicap), which is dependent on an estimation by a clinician.

The results of the study were mixed. There was no change in the Ashworth score following 15 weeks of treatment with either THC or Cannador, but there were significant improvements for both active treatments in subjective measures of spasticity, muscle spasms, pain and sleep, and also in an objective measure of mobility. The authors noted an unexpected reduction in hospital admissions for relapse in the two active treatment groups. The known interaction of cannabinoids with the immune system, and the fact that MS is regarded as an autoimmune condition, led them to comment that this finding was worthy of further investigation. Minor unwanted effects were frequently reported in all three treatment groups, with a higher prevalence for the active treatments. The small number of serious adverse events were evenly spread across the three groups.

The limitations of the Ashworth Scale in measuring such a complex phenomenon as spasticity are well known (Hinderer and Gupta, 1996) and are acknowledged by the authors. They also note that the evidence in support of the currently available standard drug treatments for spasticity (and many other MS-related symptoms) is weak. An accompanying editorial (Metz and Page, 2003) recommended that 'future studies … should not rely totally on the Ashworth scale' and noted that poor bioavailability of oral cannabinoids may also have influenced the outcome. Precise titration of dose to allow for wide variations in individual response was not possible with a twice-daily dosing regime.

In a press release on 7 November 2003, the Chief Executive of the Multiple Sclerosis Trust made the following comment on the results of this study:

> It is frustrating that the results of the study are somewhat equivocal. We are pleased that the CAMS study confirms the strong anecdotal evidence of the benefit of cannabis for some people with MS. It is particularly encouraging that patients receiving cannabis perceived an improvement in both spasticity and pain, when compared with those on placebo, and that no significant side effects were reported. However, it is clear that the primary assessment tool used to measure spasticity, the Ashworth Scale, has failed to capture the full impact of this aspect of MS. Spasticity is a complex collection of symptoms encompassing pain and stiffness, some of which can only accurately be assessed using subjective measures. However, overall, we believe that this study, combined with others which demonstrate symptomatic improvement, provides convincing evidence that cannabis may be clinically useful in treating some of the symptoms of MS.

Future directions for clinical research

At the time of writing, the utility of CBME THC:CBD in combating neuropathic pain and other neurogenic symptoms such as spasticity and bladder dysfunction in MS and spinal cord injury is being further explored in several randomised, placebo-controlled trials which are scheduled for completion in 2004. The effectiveness of two CBMEs in the treatment of cancer pain is being investigated in a large, multicentre, placebo-controlled study, and an MRC-funded group under the direction of Dr Anita Holdcroft is conducting a trial of THC in post-operative pain.

Although many effective remedies already exist for most post-operative pain, the immediate postoperative period still poses therapeutic challenges. Patient-controlled analgesia using i.v. morphine administered in response to the patient's own electronic signals is highly effective but the main dose-limiting adverse effect is opiate-induced nausea and vomiting. This is not only unpleasant and painful for the patient but may also disrupt wound repair. Not only does THC offer powerful antiemetic activity, but it also produces analgesia by a different pharmacological mechanism to morphine which may result in a synergistic effect. For this reason, pilot studies in perioperative pain following hysterectomy and total hip replacement have recently commenced and initial results are very encouraging. In animal studies

(Cichewicz and Welch, 2002), adding THC to morphine has the fascinating result of virtually eliminating two of the major drawbacks associated with opiates, namely tolerance and physical dependence. If this remarkable finding could be replicated in humans it would have very important implications for the everyday treatment of chronic pain.

The exciting discovery of anti-TNF activity and immune modulation by CBD *in vitro* and *in vivo* in a murine model of rheumatoid arthritis (RA) (Malfait *et al.*, 2000) provides support to the anecdotal accounts from patients that cannabis eases the symptoms of many inflammatory conditions. At the time of writing, pilot studies in RA and Crohn's disease are underway.

The possibility that cannabis extracts may not only reduce intraocular pressure in glaucoma but may also ameliorate other pathological effects such as those resulting from impairment or damage to retinal microvasculature (see above) has been the inspiration for a pilot study in glaucoma.

Patients with intractable diseases that impair respiratory function often experience the unpleasant symptom of 'air hunger'. Anecdotal reports suggest that cannabis may alleviate this without depressing respiration and thereby aggravating the primary condition, as would be the case with existing remedies such as opiates. The likely reason for this is the virtual absence of CB_1 receptors in the pontomedullary part of the brainstem, the location of the respiratory oscillator. A pilot study in patients with chronic obstructive airways disease will explore the potential of CBME in relieving air hunger while carefully monitoring respiratory function.

Early studies from Oxford reported above (Wade *et al.*, 2003) indicated that CBD CBME may have a powerful analgesic effect in its own right. As a non-psychoactive cannabinoid, CBD lends itself to fixed dosing regimes rather than self-titration, and it is currently under investigation in a placebo-controlled crossover study of three doses in the treatment of neuropathic pain associated with MS.

CBD also shows promise in the treatment of functional psychoses such as schizophrenia and bipolar disorder, and as a neuroprotective agent when the brain suffers an insult such as trauma or hypoxia. These possibilities will be explored in human studies during 2004.

A robust observation among recreational cannabis users is a powerful appetite-stimulating effect ('the munchies'), and this has been demonstrated repeatedly in both healthy volunteers and patients with appetite impairment and weight loss (see above). A team of scientists from

Reading University are conducting a three-year project to investigate the physiological and behavioural components of this effect in more detail.

Finally, there is the speculative but intriguing possibility that cannabis extracts may have an impact not only on the symptoms of the diseases discussed above but, in some cases, on the disease process itself. This may be the result of the neuroprotective and anti-inflammatory activity that has been demonstrated in numerous animal models for THC, CBD and other cannabis constituents (see Chapters 6 and 7). The research needed to test this important and exciting hypothesis in humans poses daunting methodological challenges, but will inevitably become an increasing preoccupation during the next few years.

References

Abrahamov A, Abrahamov A, Mechoulam R (1995). An efficient new cannabinoid anti-emetic in pediatric oncology. *Life Sci* 56: 2097–2102.

Achiron A, Miron S, Lavie V *et al.* (2000). Dexanabinol (HU-211) effect on experimental autoimmune encephalomyopathy: implications for the treatment of acute relapses of multiple sclerosis. *J Neuroimmunol* 102: 26–31.

Adler M W, Geller E B (1986). Ocular effects of cannabinoids. In: Mechoulam R, ed. *Cannabinoids as Therapeutic Agents*. Boca Raton, FL: CRC Press: 51–70.

Andreasson S, Allebeck P, Engstrom A, Rydberg U (1987). Cannabis and schizophrenia: a longitudinal study of Swedish conscripts. *Lancet* 2: 1483–1486.

Archer R A, Stark P, Lemberger L (1986). Nabilone. In: Mechoulam R, ed. *Cannabinoids as Therapeutic Agents*. Boca Raton, FL: CRC Press: 85–103.

Arseneault L, Cannon M, Witton J, Murray R (2004). The causal association between cannabis and psychosis: an examination of the evidence. *Br J Psychiatry*, 184: 110–117.

Baker D, Pryce G, Croxford *et al.* (2000). Cannabinoids control spasticity and tremor in a multiple sclerosis model. *Nature* 404: 84–87.

Beal J E, Olson R, Lefkowitz L *et al.* (1995). Dronabinol as a treatment for anorexia associated with weight loss in patients with AIDS. *J Pain Symptom Management* 10: 89–97.

Berman J, Lee J, Cannon A *et al.* (2003). Efficacy of two cannabis based medicinal extracts for relief of central neuropathic pain from brachial plexus avulsion: results of a randomised controlled trial. Paper presented at the Pain Society Annual Scientific Meeting, Glasgow, 1–4 April 2003.

Bhargava H (1976). Inhibition of naloxone-induced withdrawal in morphine dependent mice by THC. *Eur J Pharmacol* 36: 259–262.

Breneissen R, Egli A, Elsohly M A *et al.* (1996). The effect of orally and rectally administered delta-9-THC on spasticity: a pilot study with two patients. *Int J Clin Pharmacol Ther* 34: 446–452.

Browne R G, Weissman A (1981). Discriminatory stimulus properties of delta-9-THC: mechanistic studies. *J Clin Pharmacol* 21: 227S–234S.

Calignano A, La Rana G, Loubet-Lescoulie P *et al.* (1998). Control of pain by endogenous cannabinoids. *Nature* 394: 277–281.

Campbell F A, Tramer M R, Carroll D, Reynolds D J M, Moore R A, McQuay H J (2001). Are cannabinoids an effective and safe option in the management of pain? A qualitative systematic review. *BMJ* 323: 13–16.

Carlini E A, Cunha J M (1981). Hypnotic and anti-epileptic effects of cannabidiol. *J Clin Pharmacol* 21: 417–427.

Carmichael J (1992). The principles of cancer chemotherapy. In: Grahame-Smith D G, Aronson J K, eds. *Oxford Textbook of Clinical Pharmacology*, 2nd edn. Oxford: Oxford University Press: 505–516.

Chan H S L, Correia J A, Macleod S M (1987). Nabilone versus prochlorperazine for control of cancer chemotherapy-induced emesis in children: a double-blind, crossover trial. *Pediatrics* 79: 946–952.

Chang A E, Shiling D J, Stillman R C *et al.* (1979). Delta-9-THC as an antiemetic in cancer patients receiving high-dose methotrexate. *Ann Intern Med* 91: 819–830.

Chesher G B, Jackson D M (1985). The quasi-morphine withdrawal syndrome: effect of cannabinol, cannabidiol, and THC. *Pharmacol Biochem Behav* 23: 13–15.

Cichewicz D L, Welch S P (2002). The effects of oral administration of delta-9-THC on morphine tolerance and physical dependence. *Abstracts of the ICRS 12th Annual Symposium on the Cannabinoids.*

Clifford D B (1983). THC for tremor in multiple sclerosis. *Ann Neurol* 13: 669–671.

Consroe P, Snider S R (1986). Therapeutic potential of cannabinoids in neurological disorders. In: Mechoulam R, ed. *Cannabinoids as Therapeutic Agents.* Boca Raton, FL: CRC Press: 21–49.

Consroe P F, Wood G C, Buchsbaum H (1975). Anticonvulsant nature of marihuana smoking. *JAMA* 234: 306–307.

Consroe P, Sandyk R, Snider S R (1986). Open label evaluation of cannabidiol in dystonic movement disorders. *Int J Neurosci* 30: 277–282C.

Consroe P, Laguna J, Allender J *et al.* (1991). Controlled clinical trial of cannabidiol in Huntington's disease. *Pharmacol Biochem Behav* 40: 701–708.

Consroe P, Musty R, Rein J *et al.* (1996). The perceived effects of smoked cannabis on patients with multiple sclerosis. *Eur Neurol* 38: 44–48.

Consroe P, Musty R, Rein J, Tillery W, Pertwee R G (1997). The perceived effects of smoked cannabis on patients with multiple sclerosis. *Eur Neurol* 38: 44–48.

Cunha J M, Carlini E A, Pereira A E *et al.* (1980). Chronic administration of cannabidiol to healthy volunteers and epileptic patients. *Pharmacology* 21: 175–185.

Dalzell A M, Bartlett A M, Lilleyman J S (1986). Nabilone: an alternative antiemetic for cancer chemotherapy. *Arch Dis Child* 6(1): 502–505.

Degenhardt L, Hall W (2002). Cannabis and psychosis. *Curr Psychiat Rep* 4: 191–196.

De Petrocellis L, Melck D, Palmisano A *et al.* (1998). The endogenous cannabinoid anandamide inhibits human breast cancer cell proliferation. *Proc Natl Acad Sci USA* 95: 8375–8380.

Dunn M, Davis R (1974). The perceived effects of marijuana on spinal cord injured males. *Paraplegia* 12: 175.

Edgington E S (1984). Statistics and single case analysis. *Progr Behav Modif* 16: 83–119.

Einhorn L H (1981). Nabilone: an effective antiemetic in patients receiving cancer chemotherapy. *J Clin Pharmacol* 21: 64S–69S.

Fabre L F, McLendon D (1981). The efficacy and safety of nabilone (a synthetic cannabinoid) in the treatment of anxiety. *J Clin Pharmacol* 21: 377S–382S.

Foltin R W, Brady J V, Fischman M W (1986). Behavioural analysis of marijuana effects on food intake in humans. *Pharmacol Biochem Behav* 25: 577–582.

Formukong E A, Evans A T, Evans F J (1989). The medicinal use of cannabis and its constituents. *Phytother Res* 3: 219–231.

Georgotas A, Zeidenberg P (1979). Observations on the effects of heavy marijuana smoking on group interaction and individual behaviour. *Compr Psychiatry* 20: 427–432.

Goadsby P J, Gundlach A L (1991). Localization of [^{3}H]-dihydroergotamine binding sites in the cat central nervous system: Relevance to migraine. *Ann Neurol* 29: 91–94.

Gonzalez R, Carey C, Grant I (2002). Nonacute (residual) effects of cannabis use: a qualitative analysis and systematic review. *J Clin Pharmacol* 42: 48–57S.

Graham J D P (1986). The bronchodilator action of cannabinoids. In: Mechoulam R, ed. *Cannabinoids as Therapeutic Agents*. Boca Raton, FL: CRC Press: 147–158.

Grant I, Gonzalez R, Carey C L, Natarajan L, Wolfson T (2003). Non-acute (residual) neurocognitive effects of cannabis use: a meta-analytic study. *J Int Neuropsychol Soc* 9: 679–689.

Greenberg H S, Werness S A, Pugh J E et al. (1994). Short-term effects of smoking marijuana on balance in patients with multiple sclerosis and normal volunteers. *Clin Pharmacol Ther* 55: 324–328.

Greenwald M K, Stitzer M L (2000). Antinociceptive, subjective and behavioural effects of smoked marijuana in humans. *Drug Alcohol Depend* 59: 261–275.

Grinspoon L, Bakalar J B (1993). *Marihuana, the Forbidden Medicine*. New Haven, CT: Yale University Press.

Grotenhermen F (2001). Cannabinoid receptor agonists will soon find their place in modern medicine (letter). *BMJ* 323: 1250.

Growing L, Ali R L, Christie P, White J M (1998). Therapeutic use of cannabis: clarifying the debate. *Drug Alcohol Rev* 17: 445–452.

Guimaraes F S, Chiaretti T M, Graeff F G, Zuardi A W (1990). Antianxiety effet of cannabidiol in the elevated plus-maze. *Psychopharmacology* 100: 558–559.

Guyatt G H, Heyting A, Jaeschke R (1990a). N of 1 randomised trials for investigating new drugs. *Controlled Clin Trials* 11: 88–100.

Guyatt G H, Keller J L et al. (1990b). The n of 1 randomised controlled trial: clinical usefulness. *Ann Intern Med* 112: 293–299.

Hall W et al. (1994). *The Health and Psychological Consequences of Cannabis Use*. National Drug Strategy Monograph Series No. 25. Canberra: Australian Government Publishing Service.

Hampson A, Grimaldi M, Aselrod J *et al.* (1998). Cannabidiol and delta-9-tetrahydrocannabinol are neuroprotective antioxidants. *Proc Natl Acad Sci USA* 95: 8268–8273.

Harris L S, Muinson A E, Carchman R A (1976). Anti-tumoral properties of cannabinoids. In: Braude Mc, Szara S, eds. *The Pharmacology of Marihuana*, Vol 2. New York: Raven Press: 773–776.

Hemming M, Yellowlees P M (1993). Effective treatment of Tourette's syndrome with marijuana. *J Clin Pharmacol* 7: 389–391.

Hepler R S, Frank I M, Petrus R (1976). Ocular effects of marihuana smoking. In: Braude MC, Szara S, eds. *The Pharmacology of Marihuana*, Vol 2. New York: Raven Press: 815–824.

Hinderer S R, Gupta S (1996). Functional outcome measures to assess interventions for spasticity. *Arch Phys Med Rehabil* 77: 1083–1089.

Hine B, Friedman E, Torrelio M *et al.* (1975). Morphine-dependent rats: blockade of precipitated abstinence by THC. *Science* 187: 443–445.

Hodges C (1992). Very alternative medicine. *Spectator* 1 August: 18.

Holdcroft A, Smith M, Jacklin A (1997). Pain relief with oral cannabinoids in familial Mediterranean fever. *Anaesthesia* 52: 483–486.

Hollister L E (1971). Hunger and appetite after single doses of marihuana, alcohol, and dextroamphetamine. *Clin Pharmacol Ther* 12: 44–49.

House of Lords Select Committee on Science and Technology (1998). *Cannabis: The Scientific and Medical Evidence*. The House of Lords Session 1997–8, 9th report. London: Stationery Office.

Ilaria R L, Thornby J I, Fann W E (1981). Nabilone, a cannabinoid derivative, in the treatment of anxiety neurosis. *Curr Ther Res* 29: 943–949.

Institute of Medicine (1999). The medical value of marijuana and related substances. In: Joy J E, Watson S J, Benson J A, eds. *Marijuana and Medicine: Assessing the Science Base*. Washington DC: National Academy Press: chapter 4.

Iversen L (2001). Few well controlled trials of cannabis exist for systematic review. *BMJ* 323: 1250.

Jain A K, Ryan J R, McMahon F G *et al.* (1981). Evaluation of intramuscular levonantrodol and placebo in acute postoperative pain. *J Clin Pharmacol* 21: 320S–326S.

James J (1997). Unpublished federal study found THC-treated rats lived longer, had less cancer. *AIDS Treatment News* 263.

Johannessen T (1991). Controlled trials in single subjects. *BMJ* 303: 173–178.

Johns A (2001). Psychiatric effects of cannabis. *Br J Psychiatry* 178: 116–122.

Jones R T, Benowitz N L, Herning R I (1981). Clinical relevance of cannabis tolerance and dependence. *J Clin Pharmacol* 21: 143S–152S.

Jones S E, Durant J R, Greco F A *et al.* (1982). A multi-institutional phase III study of nabilone vs placebo in chemotherapy-induced nausea and vomiting. *Cancer Treatment Rev* 9: 45–48S.

Karler R, Turkanis SA (1981). The cannabionoids as potential antiepileptics. *J Clin Pharmacol* 21: 437S–448S.

Karniol I G, Carlini E A (1973). Pharmacological interaction between cannabidiol and delta-9-THC. *Psychopharmacologica* 33: 53–70.

Kaslow R A, Blackwelder W C, Ostrow D G *et al.* (1989). No evidence for a role of alcohol or other psychoactive drugs in accelerating immunodeficiency in HIV-1-positive individuals. *JAMA* 261: 3424–3429.

Keeler M H, Reifler C B (1967). Grand mal convulsions subsequent to marihuana smoking. *Dis Nerv Syst* 18: 474–475.

Kirkham T C, Williams C M (2001). Endogenous cannabinoids and appetite. *Nutr Res Rev* 14: 65–86.

Lal H, Bennett D A, Shearman G T *et al.* (1981). Effectiveness of nantradol in blocking narcotic withdrawal signs through non-narcotic mechanisms. *J Clin Pharmacol* 21: 361S–366S.

Lavie G, Teichner A, Shohami E *et al.* (2001). Long term cerebroprotective effects of dexanabinol in a model of focal cerebral ischaemia. *Brain Res* 901: 195–201.

Levitt M (1986). Cannabinoids as antiemetics in cancer chemotherapy. In: Mechoulam R, ed. *Cannabinoids as Therapeutic Agents.* Boca Raton, FL: CRC Press.

Lichtman A H, Cook S A, Martin B R (1996). Investigation of brain sites mediating cannabinoid-induced antinociception in rats: Evidence supporting periaqueductal gray involvement. *J Pharmacol Exp Ther* 276: 585–593.

McPartland J, Russo E (2001). Cannabis and cannabis extracts: greater than the sum of their parts? *J Cannabis Ther* 1: 103–132.

Malec J, Harvey R F, Cayner J J (1982). Cannabis effect on spasticity in spinal cord injury. *Arch Phys Med Rehabil* 63: 116–118.

Malfait A M, Gallily R, Sumariwalla P F *et al.* (2000). The non-psychoactive cannabis-constituent cannabidiol is an oral anti-arthritic therapeutic in murine collagen-induced arthritis. *Proc Natl Acad Sci USA* 97: 9561–9566.

Martyn C N, Illis L S, Thom J (1995). Nabilone in the treatment of multiple sclerosis. *Lancet* 345: 579.

Maurer M, Henn V, Dittrich A *et al.* (1990). Delta-9-THC shows antispastic and analgesic effects in a single case double blind trial. *Eur Arch Psychiatry Clin Neurosci* 240: 1–4.

Mechoulam R (1986). The pharmacohistory of cannabis sativa. In: Mechoulam R, ed. *Cannabinoids as Therapeutic Agents.* Boca Raton, FL: CRC Press: 1–19.

Meinck H M, Schonle P W, Conrad B (1989). Effect of cannabinoids on spasticity and ataxia in multiple scleroris. *J Neurol* 236: 120–122.

Merritt J C, Crawford W J, Alexander P C *et al.* (1980). Effect of marihuana on intraocular and blood pressure in glaucoma. *Ophthalmology* 87: 222–228.

Merritt J C, Olsen J L, Armstrong J R *et al.* (1981). Topical delta-9-THC in hypertensive glaucomas. *J Pharmac Pharmacol* 33: 40–41.

Metz L, Page S (2003). Oral cannabinoids for spasticity in multiple sclerosis: will attitude continue to limit use? (Editorial) *Lancet* 362: 1513.

Muller-Vahl K, Kolbe H, Dengler R (1997). Gilles de la Tourette-Syndrom: Einflub von Nikotin, Alkohol und marihuana auf die linkische Symptomatikt. *Nervenarz* 68: 985–989.

Muller-Vahl K, Schneider U, Kolbe H *et al.* (1999). Treatment of Tourette's syndrome with delta-9-tetrahydrocannabinol. *Am J Psychiatry* 156: 495.

Nelson K, Walsh D, Deeter P *et al.* (1994). A phase-II study of delta-9-THC for appetite-stimulation in cancer-associated anorexia. *J Palliative Care* 10: 14–18.

Nicholson A N, Robson P J, Stone B M, Turner C (2004). Effect of delta-9-tetrahydrocannabinol and cannabidiol on nocturnal sleep and early morning behaviour in young adults. *J Clin Psychopharmacol*, in press.

Niederle N, Schutte J, Schmidt C G (1986). Crossover comparison of the antiemetic efficacy of nabilone and alizapride in patients with nonseminomatous testicular cancer receiving cisplatin therapy. *Klin Wochenschr* 64: 362–365.

Niiranen A, Mattson K (1985). A cross-over comparison of nabilone and prochlorperazine for emesis induced by cancer chemotherapy. *Am J Clin Oncol* 8: 336–340.

Noyes R Jr, Brunk S F, Baram D A (1975a). Analgesic effects of delta-9-THC. *J Clin Pharmacol* 15: 139–143.

Noyes R Jr, Brunk S F, Avery D A (1975b). The analgesic properties of delta-9-THC and codeine. *Clin Pharmacol Ther* 18: 84–89.

Orr L E, McKernan J F (1981). Antiemetic effect of delta-9-THC in chemotherapy-associated nausea and emesis as compared to placebo and compazine. *J Clin Pharmacol* 21: 76S–80S.

O'Shaugnessy W B (1843). On the *Cannabis indica* or Indian hemp. *Pharmacol J* 2: 594.

Panegyres P K (1992). The drug therapy of neurological disorders. In: Grahame-Smith D G, Aronson J K, eds. *Oxford Textbook of Clinical Pharmacology*, 2nd edn. Oxford: Oxford University Press: 441–442.

Penta J S, Poster D S, Bruno S, Macdonald J S (1981). Clinical trials with anti-emetic agents in cancer patients receiving chemotherapy. *J Clin Pharmacol* 21: 11S–22S.

Perez-Reyes M, Wagner D, Wall M E, Davis K H (1976). Intravenous administration of cannabinoids and intraocular pressure. In: Braude M C, Szara S, eds. *The Pharmacology of Marihuana*. New York: Raven Press: 829–832.

Petro D J (1980). Marihuana as a therapeutic agent for muscle spasm or spasticity. *Psychosomatics* 21: 81–85C.

Petro D J, Ellenberger C (1981). Treatment of human spasticity with delta-9-THC. *J Clin Pharmacol* 21: 413S–416S.

Plasse T F, Gorter R W, Krasnow S H *et al.* (1991). Recent clinical experience with dronabinol. *Pharmacol Biochem Behav* 40: 695–700.

Pomeroy M, Fennelly J J, Towers M (1986). Prospective randomised double-blind trial of nabilone versus domperidone in the treatment of cytotoxic-induced emesis. *Cancer Chemother Pharmacol* 17: 285–288.

Pope H G, Gruber A J, Hudson J I, Huestis M A, Yurgelun-Todd D (2002). Cognitive measures in long-term cannabis users. *J Clin Pharmacol* 42: 41–47S.

Porter J, Jick H (1980). Addiction rare in patients treated with narcotics (letter). *N Engl J Med* 302: 123.

Prunte C, Orgul S, Flammer J (1998). Abnormalities of microcirculation in glaucoma: facts and hints. *Curr Opin Ophthalmol* 9: 50–55.

Regelson W, Butler J R, Schulz J *et al.* (1976). Delta-9-THC as an effective antide-pressant and appetite-stimulating agent in advanced cancer patients. In: Braude M C, Szara S, eds. *The Pharmacology of Marihuana*. New York: Raven Press: 763–776.

Reynolds J R (1890). Therapeutic uses and toxic effects of cannabis indica. *Lancet* 1: 637–638.

Robson P (1998). Cannabis as medicine: time for the phoenix to arise? *BMJ* 316: 1034–1035.

Robson P (2001). Therapeutic aspects of cannabis and cannabinoids. *Br J Psychiatry* 178: 107–115.

Robson P, Bruce M (1997). A comparison of 'visible' and 'invisible' users of amphet-amine, cocaine and heroin: two distinct populations? *Addiction* 92: 1729–1736.

Robson P, Wade D T, Makela P M, House H (2002). Cannabis medicinal extracts, including cannabidiol, alleviated neurogenic symptoms in patients with mul-tiple sclerosis and spinal cord injury. *Abstract 56: International Cannabinoid Research Society, 12th Annual Symposium on the Cannabinoids*.

Rog D, Young C (2003). Presentation to the European Committee for Treatment and Research in Multiple Sclerosis, Milan, 20 September 2003.

Russo E (1998). Cannabis for migraine: the once and future prescription? An his-torical and scientific review. *Pain* 76: 3–8.

Sandyk R, Awerbuch G (1988). Marijuana and Tourette's syndrome. *J Clin Psychopharmacol* 8: 444–445.

Segal M (1986). Cannabinoids and analgesia. In: Mechoulam R, ed. *Cannabinoids as Therapeutic Agents*. Boca Raton, FA: CRC Press.

Solowij N (1998). Acute effects of cannabis on cognitive functioning. In: *Cannabis and Cognitive Functioning*. Cambridge: Cambridge University Press: 29–38.

Solowij N, Stephens R S, Roffman R A *et al.* (2002). Cognitive functioning of long-term heavy cannabis users seeking treatment. *JAMA* 287: 1123–1131.

Sugiura T, Kodaka T, Nakane S (1998). Detection of an endogenous cannabimimet-ic molecule, 2-arachidonoylglycerol, and cannabinoid CB1 receptor mRNA in human vascular cells: Is 2-arachidonoylglycerol a possible vasomodulator? *Biochem Biophys Res Commun* 243: 838–843.

Tashkin D P, Shapiro B J, Frank I M (1976). Acute effects of marihuana on airway dynamics in spontaneous and experimentally produced bronchial asthma. In: Braude M C, Szara S, eds. *The Pharmacology of Marihuana*. New York: Raven Press.

Tashkin D P, Reiss S, Shapiro B J *et al.* (1977). Bronchial effects of aerosolised delta-9-THC in healthy and asthmatic subjects. *Am Rev Respir Dis* 115: 57–65.

Thomas H (1993). Psychiatric symptoms in cannabis users. *Br J Psychiatry* 163: 141–149.

Ungerleider J T, Andyrsiak T, Fairbanks L *et al.* (1982). Cannabis and cancer chemotherapy: a comparison of oral delta-9-THC and prochlorperazine. *Cancer* 50: 636–645.

Ungerleider J T, Andyrsiak T, Fairbanks L *et al.* (1987). Delta-9-THC in the treat-ment of spasticity associated with multiple sclerosis. *Adv Alcohol Subst Abuse* 7: 39–50.

Volfe Z, Dvilansky A, Nathan I (1985). Cannabinoids block release of serotonin from platelets induced by plasma from migraine patients. *Int J Clin Pharmacol Res* 5: 243–246.

Volicer L, Stelly M, Morris J, McLaughlin J, Volicer B J (1997). Effects of dronabinol on anorexia and disturbed behavior in patients with Alzheimer's disease. *Int J Geriatr Psychiatry* 12: 913–919.

Wade D T, Robson P J, House H, Makela P M, Aram J (2003). A preliminary controlled study to determine whether whole-plant cannabis extracts can improve intractable neurogenic symptoms. *Clin Rehabil* 17: 21–29.

Williams S J, Hartley J P, Graham J D (1976). Bronchodilator effect of delta-9-THC administered by aerosol to asthmatic patients. *Thorax* 31: 720–723.

Wisbeck G A, Schuckit M A, Kalmijn J A (1996). An evaluation of the history of a marijuana withdrawal syndrome in a large population. *Addiction* 91: 1469–1478.

Zajicek J, Fox P, Sanders H *et al.* (2003). Cannabinoids for treatment of spasticity and other symptoms related to multiple sclerosis (CAMS study): multicentre randomised placebo-controlled trial. *Lancet* 362: 1517–1526.

Zuardi A W, Shirakawa I, Finkelfarb E, Karniol I G (1982). Action of cannabidiol on the anxiety and other effects produced by delta-9-THC in normal subjects. *Psychopharmacology* 76: 245–250.

Zuardi A W, Rogdrigues J A, Cunha J M (1991). Effects of cannabidiol in animal models predictive of antipsychotic activity. *Psychopharmacology* 104: 260–264.

Zuardi A W, Cosme R A, Graeff F G, Guimaraes F S (1993). Effects of ipsapirone and cannabidiol on human experimental anxiety. *J Psychopharmacol* 7: 82–88.

Zuardi A W, Morais S L, Guimaraes F S, Mechoulam R (1995). Antipsychotic effect of cannabidiol. *J Clin Psychiatry* 56: 485–486.

10

Cannabis in the treatment of chronic pain

William Notcutt

Chronic pain affects approximately 1 person in 12. For those who are over the age of 65 the incidence rises beyond 1 in 4. All the current analgesics have their problems. Non-steroidal anti-inflammatory drugs (NSAIDs) cause over 2000 deaths per year in the UK. Opioids are commonly not only ineffective for neurogenic pain but also cause side-effects such as drowsiness, nausea, vomiting, constipation or pruritus (or a combination). Antidepressants and anticonvulsants are widely used but often give rise to drowsiness, dry mouth and other symptoms. Ketamine is dysphoric or even hallucinogenic at analgesic doses. There are other, non-pharmacological methods for managing pain that are widely used. Sadly, having tried all the therapeutic options, many patients are left to continue their lives with inadequate or minimal control of their pain.

There is a need for new pharmacological approaches to pain management. Over the last 20 years most of the improvements and developments have been in drug delivery (patient controlled analgesia, slow release formulations, epidural infusions, transdermal patches, etc.). The remainder of the improvements have been in the development of new variations of old drugs. The recognition that cannabis may provide a wholly new approach to pain control has stimulated the drive to develop this as a medicine.

This chapter will explore the use of cannabis for pain, covering the following topics:

- Historical perspective
- Understanding pain
- Outline of the assessment and management of chronic pain
- Experience with sublingual cannabis-based medicines.

History

Over the centuries cannabis remained an important constituent of a wide range of medicines used to relieve pain, provide anaesthesia and 'cure' a variety of other diseases. In 1763 the *New English Dictionary* stated that cannabis root applied to the skin eases inflammation.

The first strong evidence for the analgesic properties of cannabis emerged in the latter part of the nineteenth century. In India, Dr O'Shaughnessy had observed its use and wrote of its analgesic and anticonvulsant properties. He popularised it on his return to Europe. Hundreds of papers followed from him and others, citing its use for neuralgic pain of arm, sciatica, inflammation of knee, facial neuralgia, rheumatic pain, toothache, facial pain, neuritis, migraine, dysmenorrhoea, muscle spasticity, etc. This list has close parallels with current thinking on the potential therapeutic uses.

The use of opiates and aspirin grew at the end of the nineteenth century and generally provided reliable analgesia. Consequently, the use of cannabis for pain declined. It was difficult to obtain a reliable response because of the variability of the cannabinoid content of the plants, and because of problems with preparation, storage and delivery to the patient. Consequently cannabis became little more than a mild sedative and/or tranquilliser, which was then supplanted by the benzodiazepines. Finally, in the UK in 1971, its use as a medicine was proscribed and it was categorised as a Schedule 1 drug. Little clinical research was undertaken in the twentieth century.

Since the 1960s there has been an explosion of knowledge about pain. The basic science has been studied in depth and the mechanisms for the production of acute and chronic pain are slowly being unravelled. Added to this is an understanding of the mode of action of opiates and other analgesics. Simultaneously there has been the growth of pain management as a specialty.

In parallel there has been a growth in the scientific knowledge base of cannabinoids. Sadly, clinical research has been almost non-existent, primarily because of legal and political restrictions, but also because of the absence of standardised pharmaceutical preparations.

In the last 20 years in the UK it has been patients with multiple sclerosis (MS) that have led the call for cannabis to be available as a medicine. Individually, many patients had found that cannabis had helped pain, spasticity, muscular spasms, bladder pain and dysfunction. Others, however, have experienced acute adverse effects, probably because of the unpredictability of the dose they have taken. As time has passed more patients have declared their use of cannabis for a variety of chronic pain problems and for other medical conditions. In the USA it has been the AIDS lobby that has been heavily active in promoting cannabis as a medicine. It is not widely recognised that AIDS can produce a variety of pain syndromes and other distressing symptoms that might be relieved by cannabis (see Table 10.1).

In the UK there has been some interest in the clinical use of nabilone, a synthetic cannabinoid that has been available for some 25 years. Its effect is similar to that of Δ^9-tetrahydrocannabinol (THC), particularly in its side effects. It is licensed for the treatment of intractable vomiting induced by chemotherapy but its use was limited because of dysphoria and the lack of a parenteral preparation. Although it fell into almost total disuse with the advent of the 5-HT_3 antagonist antiemetics, renewed interest in nabilone for pain relief has developed out of the growing body of anecdotal reports on the benefits of cannabis for pain.

Pain clinicians are faced with a large number of patients who have failed to respond to conventional therapy. These are some of the most challenging patients that any specialty of medicine has to cope with. These clinicians are well used to using a variety of cental nervous system (CNS) drugs in varieties of combinations and they are usually not averse to trying novel therapy in desperate circumstances. Indeed our current methods for treating neuropathic pain evolved because of such approaches.

In a recent study by the author and colleagues, nabilone was administered to more than 60 patients, most of whom had intractable pain from MS. However, we also used it for patients who had other intractable neurogenic pain and severe spinal pain. Results for the first 43 patients have been published (Notcutt *et al.*, 1997).

Our experience was no more than an indication for future study. Approximately a third of patients gained benefit and continued using the drug for varying periods. One patient with trigeminal anaesthesia dolorosa had her pain permanently eliminated. Improvement in sleep was an unexpected but frequently stated benefit. However, a further third found that side-effects outweighed any benefits. The symptoms of drowsiness and dysphoria were the major problems and a dry mouth was also often noted.

The oral route for cannabinoids does not produce predictable absorption and there is also a significant first pass effect. Nabilone as 1 mg capsules was too much for many patients. Therefore we restricted it to night-time use only on initial use. All but one of those patients who had previously used cannabis for their pain preferred it to nabilone. They found that their cannabis use was more controllable and the side-effects less pronounced.

We did not develop our work with nabilone, as dose management was a problem that we could not overcome for many patients. The close similarity of nabilone to Δ^9-THC in effect concerned us, even though some patients could tolerate the drug. The impending arrival of cannabis-based medicinal extracts (CBME) was the logical way forward.

The publication of the 1997 BMA report on *The Therapeutic Uses of Cannabis* (British Medical Association, 1997), closely followed by the House of Lords Select Committee on Science and Technology (1998) and then the Institute of Medicine report (1999) from the USA, gave the establishment's seal of approval and encouragement for clinical research in this area.

Two further steps were required. First there was a need for extracts of cannabis to be prepared to acceptable levels of preparation, purity, quality and standardisation for them to be identified as medicines. Secondly, the extracts needed to be delivered into the patient by a recognised route. Initially the inhalational route was proposed but this presented too many technical problems. By changing to the sublingual route using a spray formulation, the first pass effect was minimised, reliable absorption could take place and the onset of effect was sufficiently rapid for accurate titration to be achieved.

Apart from intravenous injection, inhalation of cannabis remains the quickest route of absorption and therefore is probably the easiest to titrate by. However, the inhalation of the smoke (and associated carcinogens) from the burning of dried plant material is unacceptable, harmful and totally unnecessary in modern medical practice. Serious studies on the medicinal properties of cannabis cannot be undertaken on cannabis cigarettes (joints, etc.). However, this route is likely to remain a popular and convenient route where medicinal extracts are not available.

The history of the medicinal use of cannabis might have been very different had not a decision been taken in 1971 in the UK to remove it from medicinal use.

Understanding pain

The understanding of pain has grown rapidly over the last 35 years. Of critical importance were the Gate Control Theory and the discovery of the endogenous opioid system of receptors and ligands. Subsequently some of the complex neurochemistry, particularly at peripheral and spinal level, has been unravelled. At the same time the understanding of the psychology of pain has developed. It is not practical to give here a detailed review and therefore this chapter will focus on the aspects of the basic science that are particularly relevant to cannabinoids in their use for chronic pain. While some of the sites of cannabinoid action have been discovered, we are still far from a comprehensive understanding of the role of this system in the pain process.

Cannabinoid physiology and pain

Working from the periphery inwards, the first site of involvement of the cannabinoid system on the pain pathway lies outside the nervous system. The mast cell, which releases bradykinin as part of the inflammatory response, has CB_2 receptors as part of its control mechanism (Figure 10.1). As anandamide shares arachidonic acid as a precursor to the prostaglandins it is not surprising that cannabinoids may prove to have an important role in inflammatory pain.

Pain neural pathways

When inflammation occurs, the nociceptors (pain receptors) not only transmit pain but are also hypersensitised, thereby amplifying the

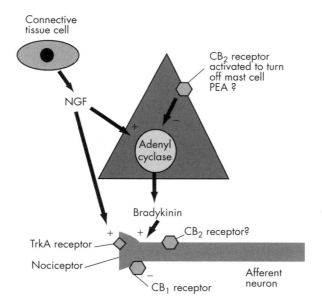

Figure 10.1 Cannabinoids and the mast cell. The mast cell is activated by nerve growth factor (NGF) released from connective tissue cells that have been involved in tissue damage and/or inflammation. Bradykinin is released, which excites peripheral nociceptive (pain) neurons. At the same time the CB_2 receptor is switched on to damp down the activity of the cell. The endocannabinoid PEA (palmitoylethanolamide) is probably involved here. On the peripheral nociceptor there are CB_1 receptors and possibly CB_2.

peripheral stimulation. This phenomenon has two forms – primary and secondary hyperalgesia. This effect has been looked at in detail in bladder inflammation and endocannabinoids have been found to have a controlling function (Jaggar *et al.*, 1998). This is further supported by the presence of CB_1 and possibly CB_2 receptors on primary afferent nociceptors, possibly exerting an antihyperalgesic effect.

The nociceptors transmit to the dorsal horn of the spinal cord, where processing of the incoming signals takes place. Descending pathways from the brain may inhibit or amplify the signals and this is a way in which depression, anxiety, fear, distraction, etc. influence the pain perceived. At the same time a range of other peripheral sensory inputs, both somatic and visceral, may affect pain processing. Hence, for example, skin stimulation (massage, acupuncture, transcutaneous nerve stimulation, etc.) and hormonal changes in the menstrual cycle can alter pain.

The rostro-ventro-medial (RVM) nucleus in the brainstem is an important source of descending modulation of nociceptive input to the spinal cord (Figure 10.2) (Meng *et al.*, 1998). It has also been shown to be a site of endocannabinoid action. It projects directly to the dorsal horn of the spinal cord, and is the final common pathway for many of the pain-modulating brain regions that feed into it. The modulation of the nociceptive pathways is tonically active. CB_1 receptors are located

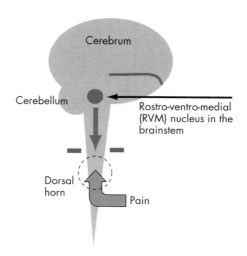

Figure 10.2 The rostro-ventro-medial nucleus is a site of endocannabinoid action. It projects to the dorsal horn of the spinal cord exerting an inhibitory effect on incoming pain signals.

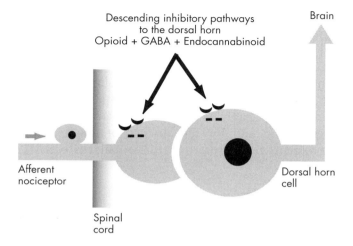

Descending inhibitory pathways
to the dorsal horn
Opioid + GABA + Endocannabinoid

Brain

Afferent
nociceptor

Dorsal horn
cell

Spinal
cord

Figure 10.3 Inhibitory pathways exist to control the flow of pain signals into the central nervous system. They descend from the brainstem and endocannabinoids are one of several neurotransmitters involved.

both pre- and postsynaptically on primary afferents and spinal neurons (Figure 10.3). Cannabinoid inhibition of dorsal root ganglion neurons has been demonstrated (Johanek *et al.*, 2001; Millns *et al.*, 2001).

Endocannabinoid tone

It has been suggested that a reduction in endocannabinoid levels may produce a reduction in tonic inhibition of the nociceptive input, thereby contributing to the development of hyperalgesia and chronic pain. In addition, the expression of the c-fos gene in the dorsal horn in inflammation has been shown to be suppressed by cannabinoids. However, it has also been shown that the analgesic effect is probably not mediated directly through opioid receptors (Hamann and Di Vadi, 1999). Thus endocannabinoid activity seems to be emerging as an integral part of pain signal processing.

There may well be other sites deeper in the CNS at which cannabinoids affect the processing of pain. For example, there is good evidence that cannabinoids are effective in the management of migraine (Russo, 1998). This may be through an effect on nociceptive pathways in the brain, or through interactions with serotonergic pathways. The antiemetic action is likely to be an interaction with either the chemoreceptor trigger zone or with the vomiting centre in the brainstem. The effect of cannabinoids on the cerebellum causes a change in muscle tone, thereby influencing the pain experienced from spasticity and muscle spasms.

One of the major problems with analgesics such as morphine is the effect on respiration mediated through opiate receptors in the vital centres of the brainstem. The respiratory rate slows as opiate levels rise and as pain is controlled. CB_1 receptors are sparse in this area of the brainstem and this probably accounts for the lack of effect of cannabinoids on respiration and for the absence of any reports of deaths directly due to acute respiratory or cardiovascular effects.

Aetiology of chronic pain

Pain is categorised into two major types:

- Nociceptive pain – pain from diseased/injured non-neural tissue (e.g. chronic spinal pain, degenerative arthritis, irritable bowel syndrome, chronic cystitis, etc.)
- Neuropathic pain – pain due to damage of neural tissue (e.g. phantom limb pain, peripheral neuropathy, prolapsed disc, paraplegia, MS, thalamic or central post-stroke pain, etc.).

Two additional categories may be used:

- Psychogenic pain, where the pain apparently has no organic basis. Although almost all pain has some organic origin, psychological factors can become the dominant problem. This term is over-used by non-pain clinicians, often in a pejorative manner, for the patient who does not fit 'normal' stereotypes.
- Idiopathic pain, where the cause of the pain is uncertain. (e.g. chronic pelvic pain, chronic perineal pain, atypical facial pain, etc.).

Additionally many pain problems may have a mixed aetiology. Many patients with nociceptive pain develop neurophysiological changes over time that are similar to those seen with neuropathic pain.

While it is possible to explore and understand the neurophysiology, pain remains a very individual phenomenon. Multiple pathophysiological mechanisms underlie both nociceptive pain and neuropathic pain.

- Different mechanisms may coexist in a single patient and might change over time (Hansson *et al.*, 2001).
- Different mechanisms for pain genesis probably exist within a single clinical diagnostic group.
- Different patients with similar or identical diagnoses may need very different treatment strategies (Loeser, 2000).

Table 10.1 The complexity of pain in multiple sclerosis

Aetiology of pain	Central neural damage (neuropathic pain)
	Somatic muscle spasm, spasticity
	Visceral muscle spasm (e.g. bladder)
	Mechanical (spinal)
	Mechanical (immobility)
	Unrelated to MS
Aggravated by	Psychosocial factors: depression, immobility, employment loss, burden on family, etc.
	Variable progression of disease
	Other potential neurological disturbances of vision, coordination, strength, sensation, speech and swallowing, bladder control, sexuality, cognitive function, etc.

Many patients have more than a single pain problem and it can be difficult to be precise over the aetiology of each. The patient with a prolapsed intervertebral disc may have mechanical back pain as a result of the degenerate disc, and neuropathic pain as a result of nerve root compression. Patients with MS can have a multitude of pain problems with a variety of aetiological, temporal and descriptive characteristics, making analysis for a clinical trial very difficult (Table 10.1). AIDS presents similar problems (Table 10.2).

Table 10.2 Pain syndromes in ambulatory AIDS

151 Patients – 1–7 pains (ave 2.7) total – 405
  Headache – 46% of patients, 17% of pains
  Joint pain – 31% of patients, 12% of pains
  Polyneuropathy – 28% of patients, 10% of pains
  Muscle pains – 27% of patients, 12% of pains
Causes
  Direct effect of AIDS conditions   30%
  Pre-existing unrelated conditions   24%
  Therapy for AIDS   4%
  Undetermined   37%
Pathophysiology
  Somatic 45%
  Visceral 15%
  Neuropathic 19%
  Idiopathic 4%
  Headache 17%

From Hewitt *et al.* (1997).

Psychosocial factors

Pain, depression and adaptive behaviour

Depression is a common, almost normal, occurrence in patients with intractable pain and diseases such as MS (Feinstein, 1997). Anxieties about diagnosis, disability, the future, etc. are additional complicating factors. Any improvement in pain may influence mood and vice versa.

There are also social and behavioural aspects to pain. Employment (loss or gain), marital disharmony, bereavement, financial problems are all examples of factors that can have an important influence on pain. The longer a group of patients is studied, the more likely it is that such events will occur. If they occur during a double-blind, placebo-controlled crossover trial then they can profoundly influence the outcomes.

Patients who have had pain for a long time are likely to have developed various adaptive behaviours that enable them to cope with life. Primary, secondary and tertiary gain may be involved. The behavioural patterns of an individual and their surrounding family environment may be so distorted that change back to 'normality' can be little short of impossible.

Pain assessment and management

Measuring and assessing pain

Pain is a combination of physical, psychological and social factors. There is no direct objective measure of physical pain, unlike pulse rate, blood sugar, etc. The commonest subjective measure is the visual analogue scale (VAS), whereby the intensity of a pain is assessed by the patient on a 100-mm line defined as 'no pain' at one end and the 'worst pain imaginable' at the other. Pain control, sleep, activities, side-effects, etc. can also be similarly assessed objectively. The presence of more than one pain adds to complexity of interpretation.

Pain relief and quality of life

If a patient gets substantial benefit from an analgesic then they may increase their activity. This might generate more pain, returning them to the same level as they were before. Thus the pain measure records no change but they show an overall improvement in quality of life. Similarly, if sleep improves, then the ability to cope with pain improves. These changes in the quality of life alter the patient's perception of their pain, making comparisons of intensity of pain very complex.

While measurement of a physical symptom is difficult, the dimension of mood has to be acknowledged and there is a wide range of established and validated questionnaire tools for this. Quality of life questionnaires provide a broad evaluation of change in a patient's life. Perhaps this is the most important outcome for any patient.

Managing chronic pain

In the past, pain management revolved around the administration of an analgesic agent by injection or by a pill to eliminate the pain, whether acute or chronic. Over the last 20 years the approach to the patient has broadened and the goals are more realistically defined (Table 10.3). A range of therapeutic methods ranging from the pharmacological and physical through to the psychological and behavioural may be used, usually in a variety of appropriate combinations (Table 10.4). The main aim of the management of chronic pain is to restore function and rehabilitate the patient. Reducing the pain is a normal objective but a more important goal is to restore the patient's control over their problem and situation.

Measurement of end-points

The use of a single drug as the lone therapeutic technique for the management of chronic pain usually has little impact. Similarly, merely measuring the intensity of the pain has limited scope in the evaluation of a therapy for chronic pain. This makes the study of a new therapy within a multifaceted therapeutic background complex. It is not surprising that there are far fewer conventional randomised, double-blind, placebo-controlled clinical trials in chronic pain than in other therapeutic areas such as cardiovascular medicine, where end-points can be expressed in objective numerical terms. Furthermore, picking the most difficult patients to study at the outset of studying a new drug adds to the difficulty.

Table 10.3 Example of a set of goals for the management of chronic pain

Controlling the pain so that:
you can sleep
you can rest more comfortably
you can move more easily and be more active
you can participate in family life
you can return to normal life

Table 10.4 Review of the main options used in the treatment of chronic pain

Therapeutic approaches to chronic pain
Information
 Understanding the cause of the pain and the diagnosis
Pharmacotherapy
 Analgesics, NSAIDs, opioids
 Ketamine, capsaicin
 Tricyclic antidepressants
 Membrane stabilisers – anticonvulsants
 Steroids
Stimulation
 TNS, acupuncture, spinal cord stimulation
Physical
 Physiotherapy, osteopathy, etc.
 Rehabilitation
Psychological
 Counselling, Cognitive Behavioural Therapy, hypnosis, etc.
Social intervention
 Occupational therapy, aids for living
 Retraining, re-employment

NSAIDs, non-steroidal anti-inflammatory drugs; TNS, transcutaneous nerve stimulation.

Starting to study cannabis medicines for pain

While some simple studies on the acute effects of THC on pain were carried out in the mid-1970s by Noyes and others, no substantial studies on chronic pain had been undertaken until the current generation started in 2000. Since May 2000 my colleagues and I have studied a group of 34 patients with chronic pain and other neurological problems (Notcutt *et al.*, 2004). We have observed patients both during acute administration and over prolonged periods of regular use (up to 40 months). We now have more than 80 patient-years of experience. Others have also embarked on studies of CBME for pain and other neurological problems. This final section is based on the experience gained from our own current research programme.

Designing the study

When designing our first studies on CBME we had to take into account the following factors:

- The problem of heterogeneity of pain (see above 'Aetiology of chronic pain')

- The biophysical, psychological and social dimensions of chronic pain
- The variability of the previous and current therapy
- The variable sites of action of cannabinoids
- The variable psychoactive effect
- The likely variable dose/benefit and adverse effect profile: (a) between healthy volunteers and patients, (b) between patients themselves (as with morphine and most other psychoactive drugs)
- The problem of the novelty of the agents and the route of administration.

Consequently we embarked on single-patient studies using an 'n of 1' methodology whereby each patient acts as their own control (Guyatt *et al.*, 1990). This provides an essentially observational study (Black, 1996) with some quantitative rigour. Others have used this approach for single cases of cannabinoid use (Martyn *et al.*, 1995; Holdcroft *et al.*, 1997; Hamann and Di Vadi, 1999).

Cannabinoids studied

We investigated three extracts: high THC, high CBD (cannabidiol) and a 1:1 mixture of THC and CBD. The extracts were derived from cloned plants bred for high THC or CBD yield. Each extract contained a target cannabinoid (THC or CBD), which was present to the extent of more than 95% of the total cannabinoid content. The remaining 5% consisted of 1–3% of the alternative principal cannabinoid (CBD or THC) respectively. The residue consists of 'other cannabinoids'. These have not been fully characterised, but include cannabinol (CBN), cannabichromene (CBC), cannabigerol (CBG) and the carboxylic acid precursors of these cannabinoids.

The rationale for using CBD came from the knowledge that many patients using illicit cannabis medicinally prefer strains with a substantial proportion of this cannabinoid. Whether this reflects greater effectiveness or a lower side-effect profile (Zuardi *et al.*, 1982) is not established. Therefore we suspected that a 1:1 mixture of THC and CBD might be optimal but that we would need to compare it to high THC- and high CBD-containing extracts alone.

Patient selection

Currently the CBME is being studied in patients 'at the end of the road', the fate of many new drugs during their initial evaluation. Unfortunately, it is difficult to make substantial impact on the pain of such patients. Greater benefits might be seen if the CBME were to be used earlier in the development of a pain syndrome or when the pain is less intense. From our knowledge of the physiology it may be appropriate to use CBME in the acute setting to prevent or control hyperalgesia and the descent into chronic pain.

When faced with desperate patients there is a great temptation to 'try anything'. Until we have much greater experience, common sense needs to be used in the selection of patients and caution must be taken for those who are frail, elderly, severely incapacitated, on a variety of medications, etc.

We have focused primarily on patients with neuropathic pain but there is no basis to exclude patients with nociceptive pain. I have seen many patients in my pain relief clinics with nociceptive pain who are deriving benefit from their use of illicit cannabis. Improvement in sleep and muscle relaxation are common results. Unfortunately most patients do not fit into tidy, narrow diagnostic groups based on pain aetiology (see above).

Contraindications

Cannabis and cannabinoids seem to have a very low physical toxicity. As yet there is limited knowledge on the contraindications to the use of cannabinoids as almost all information is derived from anecdotes and from studies on recreational users. As experience grows these may change. Our current contraindications are as listed below.

Absolute contraindications

- There is evidence that cannabis might precipitate a psychotic illness, particularly in those who are at risk of developing such a disorder in the future. Therefore until there is sufficient evidence, a history of psychosis should remain an absolute contraindication (Hall, 1999).
- There is evidence that there may be an interaction with levodopa and similar anti-parkinsonism drugs. Therefore use of this group of drugs is currently considered to be an absolute contraindication.
- Drugs using cytochrome P450 3A4 enzyme as their exclusive mode of metabolism (theoretically fentanyl could be a problem), until further experience is gained.

Relative contraindications

- The effects on the cardiovascular system are varied and cannot be reliably predicted. While this may be of minor importance to a healthy person there may be a risk in the presence of significant hypertension or ischaemic heart disease.
- Many patients are on a range of drugs that may affect both the CNS and the cardiovascular system. As yet we have little knowledge about the interaction of most drugs or herbal medicines with cannabinoids. The metabolism of anticoagulants such as warfarin may be affected.
- Assessing the effects of CBME on patients presenting with a complex range of symptomatology (physical, psychological and social) can present almost impossible problems. Frail and elderly patients may prove extremely sensitive to the side-effects.
- Patients who are intolerant of a wide range of psychoactive drugs. Currently it is impossible to separate the therapeutic from the psychoactive effects. Therefore extreme caution and slow titration is essential for this group.
- We already have concerns on the use of morphine and other psychoactive drugs in patients with actual or suspected substance misuse. Control of the use of such drugs is usually very difficult. Some too will have a history of recreational use of cannabis and may see the prescribing of CBME as a route to a regular source of high-grade material. The physician has the responsibility here in ensuring that the prescribed medicine will be used for its specified purpose. The presence in a patient's household of an individual who is a substance misuser/recreational user should also be taken into account. The presentation of the medication in a package which is tamper evident and not easy to divert for illicit use is therefore crucial.

Preparing the patient

As with all other treatments, the patient needs to be counselled beforehand. There are probably extra factors that need to be taken into account with CBME, particularly as there is so much myth and ignorance about the effects of cannabis.

Patients who have never used cannabis before may be anxious about using the drug for the first time. The experience of a mild 'high' or dysphoria may cause anxiety and even some panic. Therefore, on the first occasion when they increase the dose, we advise patients to ensure that there is someone with them. If they develop side-effects then they should lie down as these will pass off within 1–2 hours. The development of appropriate titration schedules should minimise this.

Many patients may come with a previous positive experience of using cannabis illicitly for their illness. Such patients cannot only identify the benefits, but can also manage the side-effects. However, their experience with CBME may not be exactly the same due to different composition, strength and delivery route of the illicit cannabis. We have used the same titration regime for all. However, when a supervised titration has been undertaken, the regular user can start at a higher level.

As with morphine, patients need to understand the issue of addiction. We advise that they will not become addicted if they use cannabis medicine appropriately. However, they are informed that they might experience mild withdrawal symptoms if they discontinue suddenly, having used the medication for a prolonged period (anxiety, depression, sleep and appetite disturbances, irritability, tremors, perspiration, nausea, muscle twitching, restlessness, weight loss, gastrointestinal upsets). These symptoms are described by recreational users and may be different when cannabis is used medicinally (Felder and Glass, 1998). Future clinical studies may define these more accurately.

Currently we advise our patients to be discreet over who they tell about their use of CBME. This avoids prurient interest, but more importantly, it reduces the risk of burglary. There is a potential for such patients to become a target if it becomes widely known that they have a supply of high-quality cannabis-based medicine in the home.

Titration

As early as 1890 a titration was proposed but this related to oral, poorly standardised preparations:

> The tincture of the Pharmacopoeia contains one grain in about twenty minims, and this is convenient for use with children; but for the adult, where a gradually increasing dose is required, a tincture with a strength of one grain in ten drops is more useful. The dose should be given in minimum quantity, repeated in not less than four or six hours, and gradually increased by one drop every third or fourth day, until either relief is obtained, or the drug is proved, in such case, to be useless. With these precautions I have never met with any toxic effects, and have rarely failed to find, after a comparatively short time, either the value or the uselessness of the drug. J Russell Reynolds (1890)

When we started our study of CBME for chronic pain we faced five main challenges in designing a titration schedule:

- The CBME had not been used clinically
- The sublingual route was novel
- Experience with other analgesics suggested that the dose range might be very wide
- The onset of complications might similarly be very variable
- The intensity of the side-effects might be variable and potentially distressing.

We drew on the experience gained from Phase I studies of sublingual CBME, from my own experience with the synthetic cannabinoid nabilone and from the experience of patients smoking cannabis illicitly for medicinal purposes.

The initial dosing schedule was one spray every 15 minutes under direct supervision. We anticipated that absorption would achieve a peak clinical effect at about 15–20 minutes. The spray was repeated until either a satisfactory effect was achieved or side-effects appeared or a total of eight sprays were reached.

One spray of CBME contains either 2.5 mg THC or 2.5 mg CBD or 2.5 mg THC + 2.5 mg CBD (1:1 mixture) (+ other trace cannabinoids, etc. as described above).

Our initial group of patients all had current or previous experience of using cannabis medicinally. We perceived that this would give us an initial 'feel' for the CBME with a group of patients who knew the benefits and would tolerate the side-effects. Our initial regime proved too rapid for some and as a result we extended the interval between doses to 30 minutes.

While our initial goal had been to titrate to benefit, we soon altered our goal. We realised that cannabinoids do not necessarily function in the same way as morphine in providing rapid analgesia. Therefore we recognised that such a titration was primarily to ensure tolerability and secondarily to show a clinical benefit.

Having undertaken a slow titration over a period of 2 hours we instructed the patients to use 50–75% of that total dose as their starting dose when they returned home. (For example, if they managed three sprays over 1 hour, their starting dose would be two sprays, taken together, 4–6 hourly as required.) A schedule for further dose escalation emerged:

- Increases in the number of sprays/dose are advised at 2-day intervals.
- If the daytime doses are ineffective then these should be increased by one spray per dose.

- If sleep is still a problem increase the night-time dose by one spray every 2 days.
- If side-effects (drowsiness, dysphoria, high feeling, etc.) start to appear after an individual dose then the dose should be stepped down to the previous level.
- Most of our patients have responded within a total of 16 sprays/day.

If patients were not titrated under supervision, then an acceptable starting point would be one spray, 4 hourly for 2 days. The dose escalation schedule above could then be instituted.

The sublingual route proved to be an effective way of administrating the drug. The onset of effect and side-effect was rapid enough at about 20–30 minutes (the onset of epidural analgesia used after surgery is 15–20 minutes; oral morphine takes about 30 minutes). For most patients titration was accurate enough. For those who proved very sensitive to the effects of CBME, a 1.25 mg dosage increment needs to be developed to allow finer control of dosing.

Results of 'n of 1' studies

Our studies have been designed to find some initial pathways into clinical research on CBME. The 'n of 1' methodology proved to be a satisfactory way of studying patients in depth. It allowed flexibility to look at individual problems while retaining some of the rigour of the double-blind, placebo-controlled crossover. At the end of each patient study the results of a variety of parameters were assessed and a clinical judgement made on the results.

While most of the patients fell into diagnostic groups there was no real similarity between individuals. The study can be criticised for bias for these were all patients who were desperate to find something to help them with their symptoms and all were self-selecting, as they had volunteered for the study. Therefore we took care not to quantify benefits or side-effects or to extrapolate beyond the limits of our study design.

Improvement in pain was the major objective and some patients showed clear evidence of the benefit of CBME. As an example, patient no. 8 complained of severe spasm-like pains in her urethra and in her pelvic floor that were distinct from one another. These were caused by a cystectomy and other pelvic surgery resulting from complications of the MS that she had had for over 20 years. Figure 10.4 shows her response to THC, CBD, a 1:1 mixture of THC:CBD and placebo. The VAS scores in the evening were recorded in a diary over 12 weeks. The first two weeks

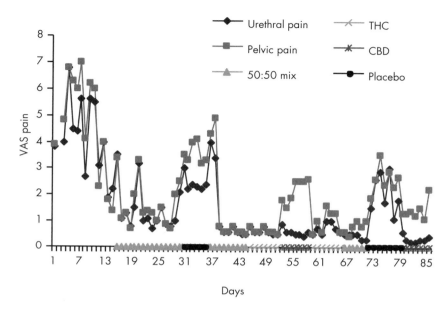

Figure 10.4 Response shown by patient no. 8 to THC, CBD, a 1:1 mixture of THC:CBD and placebo. The visual analogue scores (VAS) of her two pains measured in the evening are plotted for each day. The first 14 days are a baseline on no CBME. For the next 14 days the patient used the 1:1 mixture of THC:CBD in an open label fashion. Having demonstrated benefit, she then used the cannabis-based medicinal extract (CBME) in a double-blind, placebo-controlled, crossover fashion. The type of CBME used is indicated along the x-axis.

were the baseline period. The next two weeks were a run-in open label introduction to CBME using 1:1 THC:CBD. Having demonstrated benefit, she underwent eight one-week periods using different CBMEs, double blind. The changes in pain are demonstrated. The 1:1 mixture seems to be more effective for pain control than THC alone and was associated with a substantial improvement in her sex life.

Not every patient showed such a change in pain levels. Patient no. 7 suffered with chronic leg and back pain. She had had two laminotomies for disc prolapse and then nerve root scarring. Her pain scores showed no change over the course of the study (Figure 10.5). When we looked at her sleep, it became clear that this improved substantially with the use of the 1:1 mixture (Figure 10.6). While the hours of sleep did not change, the quality did and this was of great benefit to her. Later, when she continued to use the CBME in a long-term safety extension study she gradually reduced her morphine intake from 120 mg/day to 10 mg/day.

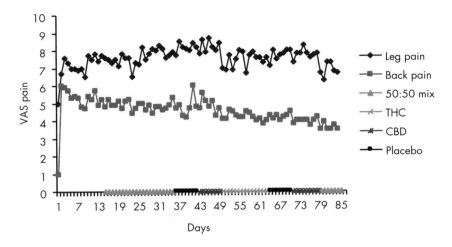

Figure 10.5 Response shown by patient no. 7 to THC, CBD, a 1:1 mixture of THC:CBD and placebo. The visual analogue scores (VAS) of her two pains measured in the evening are plotted for each day. The first 14 days are a baseline on no CBME. For the next 14 days the patient used the 1:1 mixture of THC:CBD in an open label fashion. Having demonstrated benefit, she then used the cannabis-based medicinal extract (CBME) in a double-blind, placebo-controlled, crossover fashion. The type of CBME used is indicated along the x-axis.

Pain clinicians recognise that sleep improvement can make a substantial improvement in a patient's ability to manage their pain. The importance of this benefit of CBME on sleep was underestimated at the start of the study. Some believe that one of the main benefits of tricyclic antidepressants in the management of pain is through an improvement in sleep.

Other benefits have been seen. Improvement in bladder control in patients with MS is valuable, particularly if nocturia and frequency are relieved. Some patients have had improvement in mobility and exercise tolerance, enabling increases in activity. These were rarely dramatic changes, recognising the underlying diagnoses and the intractability of the symptoms of these patients. Reduction in depression and improvement in quality of life were also demonstrated (as measured by standard assessment tools) but the cause for this is probably multifactorial.

The ability to distance themselves from the pain has also been beneficial for some. While not seeing any significant change in intensity, the distance allows the patient to cope better and gives back some control.

Changes in neural function have been seen. For example, a remission of severe allodynia in relation to a complex regional pain syndrome

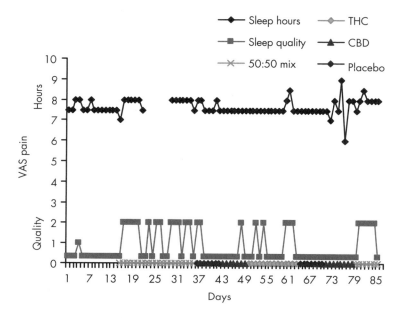

Figure 10.6 Quantity and the quality of sleep for patient no. 7 following treatment with THC, CBD, a 1:1 mixture of THC:CBD and placebo. The sleep quality is scored: 2 = Good, 1 = Fair, 0 = Poor. The quantity of sleep is measured in hours.

was seen. While these changes were noted they were not studied in detail. Return of neural function has been observed by others with the use of gabapentin for pain.

Overall, THC and the 1:1 mixture of THC:CBD seemed the most effective as analgesics. We could demonstrate little benefit from CBD in our group of patients but this extract may be useful in other circumstances such as inflammatory arthropathy (Malfait *et al.*, 2000).

While some patients do get marked acute analgesic effects at onset of the CBME, most patients experience slower and more long-lasting effects, closer to those that are seen when a tricyclic antidepressant such as amitriptylline is used for pain management.

The commonest goal of chronic pain management is to move the patient to a state where they are in greater control of their problem, physically, psychologically and socially (Table 10.4). The improvement of many patients was in quality of life issues (mood, sleep, activity, relaxation, bladder function, distancing, etc.). Perhaps this reflects the ubiquitous nature of the endocannabinoid system. Merely looking at pain as an outcome measure is too narrow a focus.

Acute side-effects

The first description of the use of sublingual cannabis was by C R Marshall in 1897 in *The Lancet* (cited by Iverson, 2000). It is not possible to know the exact dose that he took but it was probably large. He gives an excellent description of the side effects.

> On the afternoon of Feb. 19th last ... I took 0.1–0.15 gramme of the pure substance from the end of a glass rod. It was about 2.30 pm. The substance very gradually dissolved in my mouth; it possessed a peculiar pungent, aromatic, and slightly bitter taste, and seemed after some time to produce a slight anaesthesia of the mucous membranes covering the tongue and fauces. I forgot all about it and went on with my work. Soon after ... about 3.15 – I suddenly felt a peculiar dryness in the mouth, apparently due to an increased viscidity of the saliva. This was quickly followed by paraesthesia and weakness in the legs, and this in turn by diminution in mental power and a tendency to wander aimlessly about the room. I now became unable to fix my attention on anything and I had the most irresistible desire to laugh. ... but the lucid intervals gradually grew shorter and I soon fell under the full influence of the drug. I was now in a condition of acute intoxication, my speech was slurring, and my gait ataxic. I was free from all sense of care and worry and consequently felt extremely happy. ... The most peculiar effect was a complete loss of time relation: time seemed to have no existence: I appeared to be living in a present without a future or a past.

Marshall's colleagues became increasingly worried about him and eventually sent for medical help, but by the time the doctor arrived at around 5:00 p.m. Marshall had begun to recover and by 6:00 p.m. he was on his way home after a cup of coffee and suffered no ill-effects afterwards. He repeated the experiment three weeks later, using 50 mg and achieved similar but milder effects.

When considering side-effects, context is important in two respects. First, there is the absence of recorded deaths directly caused by the drug itself. However, there have undoubtedly been deaths from accidents where cannabis has played a part. Second, 1 in 1200 patients on long-term NSAIDs will die from gastrointestinal complications (equates to approximately 2000 deaths/year in the UK) (Tramer *et al.*, 2000).

The 'high'

Most people expect that patients who use cannabis as a medicine will be spending half of their lives 'high' or 'stoned'. Patients who use cannabis illicitly for the relief of pain commonly state that they want to avoid this effect and they control their intake to their analgesic or sleep needs. It is of no benefit for a patient to go from state of being prostrate with pain to being cataleptic with cannabis.

The terms 'high' or 'stoned' belong to the hippy era and should be avoided in the context of medicinal cannabis. Euphoria, dysphoria, etc. are more appropriate descriptors of these effects.

Furthermore, there are many health professionals who perceive that a mild psychoactive effect from the drug is somehow wrong. This only seems to be of concern to those who do not treat patients in pain or distress. In the past, the use of diamorphine was said to confer a mildly euphoric state for the dying patient and this was seen to be beneficial. In the *British National Formulary* 41 (BNF, 2001) on morphine it is written: 'In addition to relief of pain, morphine also confers a state of euphoria and mental detachment.' Many other psychoactive drugs are used for mood-altering effects. Elevating the mood of a patient whose life is miserable because of chronic, untreatable pain would seem to be a worthwhile goal.

There is also a desire by some to find a form of cannabis that is stripped of psychoactive effects, but this goes against the experience with morphine. Any drug that has multiple sites of action within the CNS is unlikely to be obtained in a form that does not affect consciousness, mood or cognition in some way. No one has achieved this with opiates after a century of research.

During acute dosing under direct observation we have observed dysphoric and 'euphoric' effects. These were seen on a few occasions in our earlier patients. With modification of the dosing schedules, these have been minimised. The patients were briefed on the early signs (light-headedness, dizziness, mild anxiety) and halted their use of the spray when they started to observe any such effects. This is a particular problem for those naïve to cannabinoids and where there is a certain amount of expectation. After a few doses there seems to be a growth in confidence and perhaps a tolerance for these effects. However, some patients remained tolerant only of low doses of the CBME. Most clinicians who prescribe psychoactive drugs commonly see similar effects. Overall the current regime is probably adequate for most patients as it covers a wide range of dosing requirements.

Occasionally patients may experience some panic as they experience the onset of these side-effects. However they should not be severe if the patient has been instructed properly in titration and in the possibility of the effect. First use of the drug should be undertaken with someone else present, especially if the patient is frail. The patient should lie down if they feel at all unwell or strange. They need to know that the effects normally pass off within 2 hours. If necessary, the use of a benzodiazepine such as midazolam could be considered in extreme circumstances.

When we have observed postural hypotension, this has always been associated with a dose escalation that was too rapid. It responds to simple routine measures and is short lived. Therefore if patients feel very light-headed, faint or dizzy they should be instructed to lie down and to expect the resolution of the symptoms within 1–2 hours. Postural hypotension is a common side-effect of a range of hypotensive and other drugs.

A dry mouth has been noted by several patients when using CBME. Unfortunately many patients continue to use other medications which have this potential. Other oral side-effects are a stinging from the spray due to the excipients. One of our patients developed acute reddening, papules and tiny ulcers under her tongue after uneventfully using the spray for many weeks. Others have observed this (P Robson, personal communication). Development of the formulations may resolve this and the unpleasant taste that many patients currently complain of.

Long-term use

Patients with chronic pain commonly take medication over a prolonged period (months, years). It is therefore necessary to observe patients using cannabinoids over the long term to discover what the problems are. At the present time patients can only use CBME if they are part of a clinical trial, because of the regulations on studying new drugs and because of the need for Home Office licences. We set up an extension study to monitor the progress of the patients who had shown benefit in the 'n of 1' study. It would have been unethical to have conducted the initial study and then not provided the opportunity for the patients to continue to obtain benefit.

When patients start to use CBME over a long period of time they do not stop being patients with pain problems. They will continue to need supervision of their drug use at some level (secondary or primary care). We encourage them to customise their use of CBME until they reach an optimal level. This may reflect their daily activities, including sleep time.

There are many factors that can effect the benefit that they may have initially obtained from the CBME.

Disease progression

Some patients, particularly those with MS, can have progression of their disease, exacerbating current pains and disabilities and introducing new problems. Assessment of the benefits of CBME has to continue against this background and changes in therapy may be necessary. We have observed this in three of 14 patients with MS. Another patient with a degenerative neurological problem steadily deteriorated until she died. Conversely, one patient improved to a point of not requiring further CBME.

Other issues can arise. One patient had an accident in falling out of his wheelchair and exacerbated his back pain. Another patient with a complex regional pain syndrome planned an amputation of her leg, more for cosmetic reasons than for pain.

Emotional changes

Chronic pain and ill-health remain depressing problems. For some patients improvements can be dramatic and life transforming. For others, the benefits of the CBME may be limited. Against a background of severe unremitting pain, depression and anxiety are not far away and can be precipitated by a wide range of factors.

Social upheavals

Two of our first 34 patients had a spouse die during the study. Another patient decided to initiate divorce proceedings against his wife, who we later discovered had a severe obsessive-compulsive disorder. Redundancy, severe house damage, problems with children, illness in close relatives, the birth of a daughter and other substantial upheavals have all occurred to patients during the study. Whilst this might seem to be exceptional, a review of an equivalent number of personal acquaintances revealed similar levels of social crisis.

So far we have not observed any adverse long-term effects that can be attributed to the use of CBME. Those patients who demonstrated good-quality benefit from the initial study have continued to show good benefit over the long term. However, numbers are small and the duration of our experience is less than 2 years/patient. There are few epidemiological studies on long-term use, and those that we have relate to illicit, recreational use (Sidney *et al.*, 1997; Lyketsos *et al.*, 1999). However, there is no strong evidence of harm from cannabinoids themselves.

Influence of cannabis on driving

For many patients with chronic pain, driving is an essential need to enable them to maintain as high a level of independence as possible. From the start we have attempted to address this issue using the best knowledge available.

In recent years there has been increasing concern about the influence of prescribed psychoactive medication on driving. Studies on cannabis have shown two principal effects (Sexton *et al.*, 2000). First, drivers may have difficulty in 'tracking', the ability to follow a line accurately around the corner. Second, reaction times to a sudden event are increased. However, drivers who have used cannabis are aware of the effects of the drug and will take steps to compensate (unlike the situation with alcohol). Thus the deleterious effects on driving are offset by slower speed. Sadly, we have almost no knowledge of the effect of severe pain as a distraction to driving.

Users of CBME need to know that this may impair their ability to drive a car safely and may make them unfit to drive. It is an offence to drive whilst unfit because of a physical disability or whilst intoxicated by alcohol or any other drug, prescribed or otherwise. Based on the experience gained from acute dosing we advise patients that they may be unfit to drive for at least 2 hours after taking the study medication, but also that it may be longer. Therefore they have to determine their own level of fitness to drive.

Final comments

Although our experience has been limited, CBMEs have proved no more difficult to use than conventional psychoactive medication used for pain. If they are used in less extreme circumstances they may well show different effects to those that we have seen so far.

As time goes by I anticipate that cannabis derivatives will find a place as alternatives or supplements to the established conventional pain management therapies (Table 10.5).

Further extracts and routes of administration are likely to emerge and find uses. However, it will take many years to truly evaluate their place. Moving beyond pain there may be other clinical uses as research uncovers the function and importance of the endocannabinoid system.

Table 10.5 Potential for cannabis-based medicinal extracts: pain and associated uses

Phantom limb, CRPS, spinal cord injury and other neuropathic pain states
Chronic nociceptive pain
Arthritis
Fibromyalgia
Migraine
Adjuvant to opioid analgesia in palliative care – anxiolytic, antiemetic, analgesic
Muscle spasticity – somatic and visceral

Acute pain – including spinal pain
Prevention of 'wind-up'

Sedation in intensive care
Premedication
Appetite stimulant – AIDS, malignancy

CRPS, complex regional pain syndrome.

Morphine was purified in 1806, and the syringe as a delivery system was first used in 1853. Research into morphine continues to this day. I suspect that clinical research into cannabinoids is going to continue for many years to come.

Acknowledgements

I would like to acknowledge the contributions of my colleagues Mario Price, Samantha Newport, Roy Miller, Sue Simmons, Cathy Sansom and Cheryl Phillips to the clinical information presented above.

As we have worked in Great Yarmouth, we have also collaborated with colleagues undertaking their own research programmes on CBME in Oxford and at the National Hospital for Nervous Diseases in London. Some of their experiences have contributed to our own studies.

References

Black N (1996). Why we need observational studies to evaluate the effectiveness of health care. *BMJ* 312: 1215–1218.
BNF (2001). *British National Formulary*, 41. London: British Medical Association and Royal Pharmaceutical Society: 210.
British Medical Association (1997). *Therapeutic Uses of Cannabis*. Amsterdam: Harwood Academic.
Feinstein A (1997). MS, depression and suicide. Clinicians should pay more attention to psychopathology. Editorial. *BMJ* 315: 691–692.

Felder C C, Glass M (1998). Cannabinoid receptors and their endogenous agonists. *Annu Rev Pharmacol Toxicol* 38: 179–200.

Guyatt G H, Heyting A, Jaeschke R *et al.* (1990). N of 1 randomized trials for investigating new drugs. *Controlled Clin Trials* 11: 88–100.

Hall W (1999). Cannabis use and psychosis. *Drug Alcohol Rev* 17: 433–444.

Hamann W, Di Vadi P P (1999). Analgesia with nabilone not via opioid receptors. *Lancet* 353: 560.

Hansson P, Lacerenza M, Marchettini P (2001). Aspects of clinical and experimental neuropathic pain: The clinical perspective. In: Hansson P *et al.*, eds. *Neuropathic Pain: Pathophysiology and Treatment*. Seattle: IASP Press: chapter 1.

Hewitt D J, McDonald M, Portenoy R K, Rosenfeld B, Passik S, Breitbart W (1997). Pain syndromes and etiologies in ambulatory AIDS patients. *Pain* 70: 117–123.

Holdcroft A, Smith M, Jacklin A *et al.* (1997). Pain relief with oral cannabinoids in familial mediterranean fever. *Anaesthesia* 52: 483–488.

House of Lords Select Committee on Science and Technology (1998) *Cannabis: The Scientific and Medical Evidence*. The House of Lords Session 1997–8, 9th report. London: Stationery Office.http://www.publications.parliament.uk/pa/ld199798/ldselect/ldsctech/151/15101.htm

Institute of Medicine (1999). *Marijuana and Medicine: Assessing the Science Base*. Washington, DC: Institute of Medicine. http://www.nap.edu/html/marimed/.htm

Iverson L (2000). *The Science of Marijuana*. New York: Oxford University Press: 31.

Jaggar S I, Sellaturay S, Rice A S (1998). The endogenous cannabinoid anandamide, but not the CB2 ligand palmitoylethanolamide, prevents the viscero-visceral hyper-reflexia associated with inflammation of the rat urinary bladder. *Neurosci Lett* 253: 123–126.

Johanek L, Heitmiller D, Turner M, Nader N, Hodges J, Simone D (2001). Cannabinoids attenuate capsaicin-evoked hyperalgesia through spinal and peripheral mechanisms. *Pain* 93: 303–315.

Loeser J D (2000). The future: Will pain be abolished or just pain specialists? In: *Pain: Clinical Updates*, Vol VIII. Seattle, WA: International Association for the Study of Pain: 6.

Lyketsos C G, Garrett E, Liang K Y, Anthony J C (1999). Cannabis use and cognitive decline in persons under 65 years of age. *Am J Epidemiol* 149: 794–800.

Malfait AM, Gallily R, Sumariwalla PF *et al.* (2000). The non-psychoactive cannabis constituent cannabidiol is an oral anti-arthritic therapeutic in murine collagen-induced arthritis. *Proc Natl Acad Sci USA* 97: 9561–9566.

Martyn C N, Illis L S, Thom J (1995). Nabilone in the treatment of multiple sclerosis. *Lancet* 345: 579.

Meng I D, Manning B H, Martin W J, Fields H L (1998). An analgesia circuit by cannabinoids. *Nature* 395: 381–383.

Millns P J, Chapman V. Kendall D A (2001). Cannabinoid inhibition of the capsaicin-induced calcium response in rat dorsal root ganglion neurones. *Br J Pharmacol* 132: 969–971.

Notcutt W G, Price M, Chapman G (1997). Clinical experience with nabilone for chronic pain. *Pharmac Sci* 11: 551–555.

Notcutt W, Price M, Miller M *et al.* (2004). Cannabis based medicinal extracts for chronic pain: Results from 34 'N of 1' ttudies. *Anaesthesia*, in press.

Russell Reynolds J (1890). Therapeutical uses and toxic effects of *Cannabis indica*. *Lancet* I(March 22): 637–638.

Russo E (1998). Cannabis for migraine treatment: the once and future prescription? An historical and scientific view. *Pain* 7: 3–8.

Sexton B F, Tunbridge R J, Brook-Carter N (2000). The influence of cannabis on driving. *Transport Res Lab Rep* 477.

Sidney S, Beck J E, Tekawa I S *et al.* (1997). Marijuana use and mortality. *Am J Public Health* 87: 585–590.

Tramer M R, Moore R A, Reynolds D J, McQuay H J (2000). Quantitative estimation of rare adverse events which follow a biological progression: a new model applied to chronic NSAID use. *Pain* 85: 169–182.

Zuardi A W, Finkelfarb E, Bueno O F (1982). Action of cannabidiol on the anxiety and other effects produced by THC in normal subjects. *Psychopharmacology* 76: 245–250.

11

The forensic control of cannabis

Alex Allan

Herbal cannabis *Cannabis sativa* L. (Indian hemp, marijuana) and cannabis resin (hash, hashish) are presently controlled by United Kingdom laws as Class B in Schedule 2 of the Misuse of Drugs Act (1971), and as a Schedule 1 substance in the 1970 Drug Abuse Prevention and Control Act in the USA (Phillips, 1998). However, tetrahydrocannabinol (THC) and preparations containing it are controlled as Class A. Many other countries have similar laws, being signatories to the various UN conventions on drug control.

In March 2002 the Advisory Council on the Misuse of Drugs (ACMD), chaired by Professor Sir Michael Rawlins, studying the position of cannabis in society in the UK for the Home Office of the UK Government, has proposed among other recommendations that all cannabis preparations be downgraded to Class C in recognition of the more relaxed attitude developing in society and that it is not as harmful as other Class B drugs, for example amphetamine or barbiturates (UK Government, 2002). However, the Council stresses that it does possess harmful properties and that this warrants the continuation of controls. Some police forces in the UK have already treated the possession of cannabis for personal use as a non-arrestable offence under Section 24 of the Police and Criminal Evidence Act 1984 (PACE), as it would be if it were Class C, and merely issued cautions. In parts of London only a verbal warning is given, perhaps acknowledging the increasingly widespread use, especially in the younger sector of the population, i.e. 22% of 16–29 year olds being users. Atha and Blanchard (1997) report a self-reported user survey on the extent to which users had fallen foul of the law and found that 88.5% of these offences involved cannabis. These relaxations in the UK official view of cannabis have lagged behind the attitude of the authorities to cannabis in the Netherlands in particular, which have permitted so-called cannabis cafés to function since the mid-1980s but still prosecute for supply or importation.

The United Nations International Narcotics Control Board (INCB) provides the view that countries that have signed the 1961 Single

Convention on Narcotic Drugs and later UN Conventions are still obliged to regulate the possession and use of cannabis and indeed other illicit substances in a framework of control and legislation (INCB, 2001). Cannabis was included in Schedule I of the 1961 Single Convention and also Schedule IV, the latter requiring stringent control measures because drugs in this schedule were considered to be particularly open to abuse and to produce ill effects, which should not be offset by therapeutic advantages. The INCB reminds countries that are planning to relax their laws for political reasons or medical uses more than it thinks prudent, that the World Health Organization should be informed and involved in the health and medical evaluation in accordance with Article 3 of the 1961 Convention. This will enable any developments to be carried out within the framework of international law.

The introduction of cannabis-based medicines may make the job of the forensic scientist more challenging than it is now, requiring them to distinguish between licit and illicit use. However various accommodations have already been made to permit the growth of hemp for industrial uses. For example in the UK, the Misuse of Drugs Regulations (1985) permits the lawful cultivation of cannabis under licence subject to various conditions. The type of cannabis grown is restricted to particular hemp cultivars that have a THC content of less than 0.3%, and this may be checked by the authorities to ensure compliance (Phillips, 1998). Sometimes stolen hemp plants are passed off as 'street' cannabis to unsuspecting users who are then liable to prosecution for possession, no matter how little THC the cannabis contains!

Phillips (1998) referred to the legal aspects of the control of cannabis in the methodology for the interdiction, identification and confirmation of the various forms of *Cannabis sativa*. The present chapter attempts to bring up to date some of the newer scientific aspects of cannabis analysis in terms of identification of the material and to show how the analytical capabilities for the measurement of cannabinoids and metabolites in body fluids have developed and improved over the last 20–30 years. These developments have enabled legislators in some countries to incorporate proscribed limits for the active principle, THC, into their Road Traffic Legislation.

The developments in analytical techniques and the growing understanding of the action of THC and other cannabinoids in the body have also permitted forensic analysts to attempt to distinguish between the various cannabis-based products and to assess to what extent their use may influence behaviour.

Analytical aspects of cannabis control

Present situation in the UK

The analytical forensic techniques currently used in the UK to confirm whether a suspect seizure is *C. sativa* or not reflect a pragmatic cost-effective approach due to the pressure on police budgets. There is emphasis on hard drugs and the competitive nature of the market for the supply of these services in England and Wales. The initial test employed is usually the Duquenois colour test (also known as the Negms test, with the Levine modification, which relies on the formation of a purple colour following reaction of the suspect material with hydrochloric acid and vanillin, and the transfer of this colour from the aqueous layer to an added chloroform layer. This is reasonably specific but may be subject to occasional false positives from coffee, so further testing is necessary for an unambiguous assignment.

The confirmation may be carried out by microscopic examination in which the scientist examines the plant material for the presence of hairs, particularly the cystolithic and glandular hairs characteristic of *C. sativa*. This is useful for identification but does not enable the scientist to distinguish between cannabis seizures of differing potency. When this is required, gas chromatography–mass spectrometry (GC/MS) may be employed to assess the percentage of THC present.

GC/MS is probably the most widespread and useful technique employed today in forensic control of drugs. This two-stage piece of equipment is employed often in bench-top size and is predominantly computer-controlled. A separation stage, gas chromatography, permits the differential separation of the analytes in the vapour phase; these are carried at elevated temperature by a carrier gas such as helium over a thin film of absorptive gum on the inner surface of a capillary column several metres long. Confirmation is achieved when the GC column eluant is passed into a mass spectrometer, which operates under high vacuum, and in which the analyte is ionised by a beam of electrons, producing fragmentation patterns that are characteristic of that molecule.

Thin-layer chromatography (TLC) is still employed for traces of material or hash oil: an ethanolic extract is run on a silica gel-coated plate sprayed with diethylamine and eluted by a mixture of solvents, toluene (75 parts), *n*-hexane (30 parts) and diethylamine (3 parts). The eluted spots of three of the major components of cannabis, viz. THC, cannabidiol (CBD) and cannabinol (CBN), are visualised by spraying with an azo dye Fast Blue BB, producing the colours red, orange and violet respectively, and are compared with reference material. The more polar precursor cannabinoid acids remain on the baseline in this system. For an identification to be confirmed, the relative distance the spots of each compound have eluted should be the same for the unknown material and the reference.

Two-dimensional (2D) TLC has also been used but is only useful for profiling a single specimen, due to the sequential solvent running steps, since only one sample can be run easily on the same plate (Phillips, 1998).

GC/MS may also be employed for identification, especially when only trace amounts are available, and also to quantify the THC content of illicitly produced cannabis. This technique may also be used to distinguish between legally grown hemp and the higher THC content illicit herbal cannabis material.

Trends in potency of cannabis

This section is included to illustrate the trends of higher potency cannabis seized over the last 20 years, and perhaps reflects an increasing awareness of cannabis and other drugs by the general population, no doubt assisted by widespread illicit supplies and the freely available information about drugs on the internet and in the media.

A survey of the cannabis resin and cannabis content of 2204 unsmoked reefers was carried out in the Republic of Ireland over the period from 1980 to 1996 and was compared with similar surveys in the UK (Buchanan and O'Connell, 1998). The object of the exercise was to assist the courts in the Republic to determine whether a quantity of cannabis or cannabis resin was for personal use or potentially for dealing. They found the average weight of resin in the 2025 cigarettes containing this material to be 102 mg with quite a wide, but approximately bell-shaped, distribution (from 0–19 mg to 760–779 mg) (Figure 11.1).

The survey also showed that the average weight of resin in these cigarettes per year varied little over the period. The average weight of herbal cannabis found in the analysis of the 179 remaining cigarettes was 260 mg but this varied considerably per year over the period considered.

A statistical analysis of potency trends (Δ^9-THC and other cannabinoid content) in confiscated marijuana in the USA over a period of 18 years from 1980 to 1997 has been reported (ElSohly et al., 2000). The authors used GC to measure the THC concentration primarily but also recorded the percentages of CBD, cannabichromene (CBC) and CBN in marijuana, sinsemilla, ditchweed, hashish and hash oil. They found that the mean THC level increased from 1 to 2% in 1980–1981,

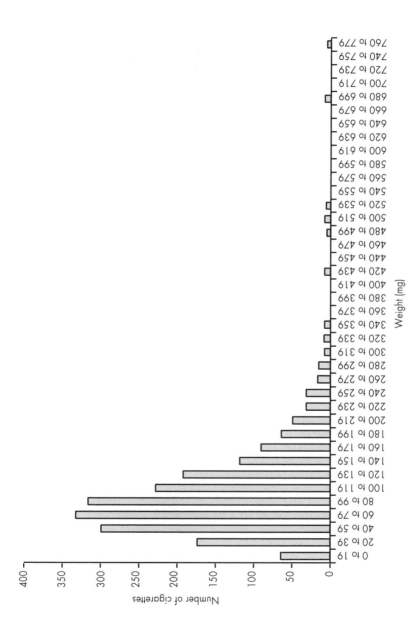

Figure 11.1 The weight distribution (mg) of cannabis resin in 2025 unsmoked hand-rolled cigarettes surveyed in the Republic of Ireland (1980–1996). With permission of the Forensic Science Society.

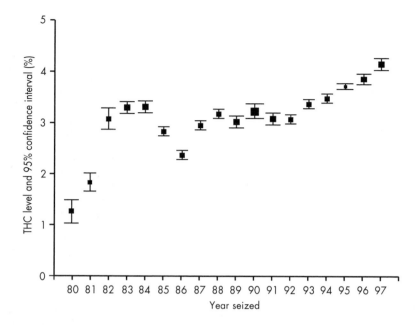

Figure 11.2 The mean THC level and 95% confidence interval for marijuana samples seized in the USA from 1980 to 1997 by year of seizure. With permission of ASTM International.

and to 4% by 1997, although not uniformly. For sinsemilla (the flowering tops of female plants without seeds, the mean THC concentration increased from just over 6% in 1980 to just under 12% by 1997, but with some wide variations, especially in the latter years of the period. This makes it difficult to draw safe conclusions (see Figures 11.2 and 11.3).

With the large numbers of samples analysed, the authors confirm with a high degree of confidence the trend that other studies had suggested – that there seems to be a general increasing potency of cannabis. This has probably arisen due to the development and selection of increasingly potent strains facilitated by the optimum growth conditions produced by hydroponic cultivation. This trend clearly has implications for health and other authorities.

Analytical techniques

Some interesting new techniques and developments of existing ones to analyse cannabis are described in the following examples to illustrate the changing nature of the science used in cannabis control.

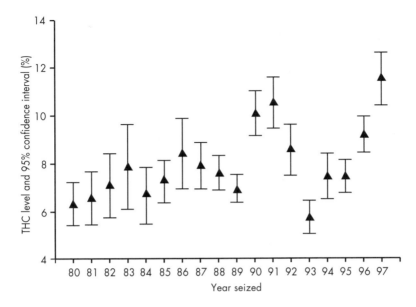

Figure 11.3 The mean THC level and 95% confidence interval for sinsemilla seized in the USA from 1980 to 1997 by year of seizure.

US sentencing guidelines determine the degree of punishment for possession of cannabis (marijuana) with the intent to manufacture, basing the severity of sentence on the number of *C. sativa* plants (including cuttings) where 50 or more plants are involved (Taylor *et al.*, 1994). Having 100–999 plants carries a 5-year sentence for possession, which increases to 10 years for more than 1000 plants. Each plant, no matter the stage of development, is considered to be equivalent to 1 kg of marijuana, therefore viable cuttings are included in the count. Stem cuttings of the female plant are used for propagation because female flowering tops produce the highest concentration of THC, making more potent cannabis; hence the viability of stem cuttings, with or without adventitious roots, is determined. The authors found that stem cuttings with a single root 1–2 mm in length can be classified as plants, but assuming the intention of the Congressional lawmakers was to include viable cuttings, then cuttings at the earlier, callous stage should also be included in the count for sentencing.

In order to improve on time-consuming two-stage analyses such as microscopy and GC/MS for the forensic analysis of cannabis products, a rapid method involving supercritical fluid chromatography with atmospheric pressure chemical ionisation mass spectrometry has been proposed (Bäckström *et al.*, 1997). Liquid carbon dioxide, modified with methanol increasing from 2% to 7% in 15 minutes, was used as the mobile phase through a 25-cm, 4.6-mm internal diameter column with cyanopropyl-silica packing. This enabled four of the major cannabinoids, Δ^8-THC, Δ^9-THC, CBD and CBN, to be separated in less than 8 minutes, following a 30-minute extraction step in ethanol and centrifugation for 5 minutes. THC could be rapidly confirmed and quantified by the procedure, which produced better separation and less waste eluant than high-performance liquid chromatography (HPLC) and was more convenient and faster than GC/MS, although this method had slightly poorer separation.

Restriction profiling

A method for the identification of C. *sativa* using restriction profiling of the internal transcribed spacer II (ITS2), a spacer flanking the 5.8S tandem repeat gene of the nuclear ribosomal DNA, has been proposed to enable identification to take place when only badly aged or poor condition plant material is available (Siniscalco Gigliano, 1998; Siniscalco Gigliano and Di Finizio, 1998). Using polymerase chain reaction (PCR) amplification of the DNA for 30 cycles, this method is sensitive enough to allow 50 mg of plant material to be confirmed as C. *sativa* with a high degree of confidence, or it can also be used as a screening method to eliminate non-C. *sativa* species. Furthermore, the procedure permits the comparison to be performed without a sequencer. Various restriction endonucleases, seven in all, were selected to generate characteristic fragments from the ITS2 region (218 base pairs) and its contiguous neighbouring lengths to include a total original DNA base pair length of approximately 600. The purified fragments were then compared by electrophoresis on a 2% agarose gel with the similarly digested control C. *sativa*.

Capillary chromatographic separation

Capillary electrochromatography (CEC) of cannabinoids has been proposed to enable the analyst to realise the advantages of HPLC and capillary zone electrophoresis (CZE) (Lurie *et al.*, 1998). Baseline separation of seven cannabinoids was demonstrated, though with rather poor area reproducibility unless the areas were calculated relative to cannabinol. The benefits of CEC include the ability to rapidly analyse a wide range of polar and thermally labile compounds together with less polar compounds, unlike conventional HPLC, CZE or indeed gas chromatography (GC)-based methodologies, all of which can only handle a proportion of these various molecules easily. The object of CEC analysis was to enable the cannabinoids of various cannabis products to be compared conveniently for intelligence purposes. Lurie *et al.* (1998) refer to strategic intelligence – the determination of country of origin – and tactical intelligence – the determination of whether two or more seizures originate from the same source to link them for example to a dealer or a distributor. The advantage of CZE is that it has good separation efficiency, and HPLC has the advantages of being able to handle both highly polar compounds and thermally labile compounds with considerable loading of analyte using well-understood chromatography. Using reversed-phase CEC allows the analyst to take advantage of the electrosmotic flow characteristics of the mobile phase in CZE, in which there are no frictional column wall effects to slow the analyte down, unlike the laminar flow of normal pressure-driven HPLC columns which produces peak broadening of the analyte, and so obtains a 5–10 times improvement in separation efficiency.

Useful increases in linearity and sensitivity could be obtained by using a 32-second injection time at 5 kV fixed voltage with a high-sensitivity ultraviolet (UV) detector cell. They also noted that separation efficiencies of the order of 200 000 plates per metre could be achieved on a 40-cm packed bed length (CEC Hypersil™ C_{18}, 3 μm column), enabling the comparisons of complex mixtures such as these to be achieved much more readily, even under isocratic conditions, than with a gradient HPLC run of the same duration.

Immunoassays

The use of a monoclonal antibody immunoassay has been proposed to distinguish cannabis from other plant species without recourse to GC or HPLC methodology or when the plants have been significantly degraded by ageing or heating, thus extending the use of immunoassay tests traditionally used for body fluids, to extracts of the cannabinoids from plants (Tanaka and Yukihiro, 1999).

Immunoassays permit the analysis of low concentrations of a substance in a complex matrix, recognising only the shape of the molecule (or very closely related shapes) against which the antibody used has been raised. This sensitive competitive enzyme-linked immunosorbent assay (ELISA) was developed from a monoclonal antibody (MAb) with a broad specificity to the phenolic cannabinoids to cater for the

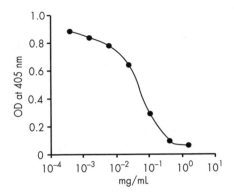

Figure 11.4 The standard curve of *Cannabis sativa* extracts (THCA strain) showing the immunoassay optical density response versus the concentration of the extracts in mg/mL. With permission of Elsevier Science.

complexity resulting from two main phenotypes of *C. sativa*; that with Δ^1-tetrahydrocannabinolic acid (Δ^1-THCA) as the major cannabinoid component and the cannabidiolic acid (CBDA) phenotype. Figure 11.4 illustrates the response in the immunoassay of the optical density versus the logarithm of the concentration of the THCA strain extracts. Note the higher sensitivity of the assay at the lower concentrations. Further complexity in cannabinoid content is caused by the other major cannabinoids such as THC, CBN and CBD, as well as the wide range of more minor cannabinoids including the homologues. Ageing due to oxidative changes and the effect of light increases the range of compounds present in the plant material, thus making a broad-specificity analysis necessary. Nevertheless the ELISA test was found to be less reactive with most other plant species tested (apart from *Xylosma japonicum*), including the closely related *Moraceae* species, even when compared with degraded cannabis samples as shown in Table 11.1.

Geographical origin of seized samples

In terms of determining possible country of origin, recent preliminary work using near-infrared reflectance in diffuse reflectance mode enabled the analyst to distinguish between the flowering tops of samples of *C. sativa* from Turkey, Thailand, India and South Africa (Kudo *et al.*, 2000). Although the technique is rapid and non-destructive, frequent surveys would be needed to keep the database current.

Table 11.1 Reactivities of the cannabis monoclonal antibody MAb-4A4 against *Cannabis* plants and Moraceae plants

Plant name	Inhibition (%)
Cannabis sativa (THCA strain)	100
Cannabis sativa (CBDA strain)	111
Heated *Cannabis sativa* (CBDA strain)	61
Weathered *Cannabis sativa* (CBDA strain)	50
Morus bombycis	4
Morus forma spontanea	26
Broussonetia kaempferi	24
Humulus japonicus	32
Humulus lupulus	6
Ficus erecta	18
Ficus wightiana	24
Ficus elastica	22
Ficus retusa	22

These discrimination procedures are based on the organic composition of the plant, especially their cannabinoid components and the overall appearance of physical features; however a different approach – the examination of trace metal ratios, has been suggested as a forensic tool to indicate geographical origin (Landi, 1997). The rationale behind this lies in the various strains of cannabis adapted naturally and cultivated to suit greatly differing soil and climatic conditions throughout the world, producing plants of wide morphological and biochemical characteristics.

Four commercial cultivars of fibre/hemp-producing *C. sativa* were grown in six populations in four fields in northern Italy, chosen so that they had only slightly different soil and climatic conditions. Analysis by atomic absorption spectroscopy (AAS) of the leaves and flowering tops of the female plants was undertaken to compare trace metal content of these parts, in order to examine the ranges of metals expected in the populations and to see if multi-element discriminant analysis could distinguish the six populations. The authors found significant differences, particularly in the Ca, Mg, Cu, Mn, Fe, Zn and Mo concentrations between both the leaves and the flowering tops, for all six populations. They also found that if variable mixes of these parts of the plant were used to simulate different marijuana production, the elemental composition of this would change according to the proportion of each part. However, they also found that multivariate statistical analysis would discriminate between even the mixed flowering top and leaf products due to the differences in their elemental composition, which was in the following order: Ca > Mo > K = Fe > Zn > Mn > Cu = Na > Mg. It was concluded that further work would be justified to see whether or not these conclusions were generally applicable.

Last but not least, in forensic proceedings it may often be useful to examine not only the cannabis in large seizures of resin but also to compare the wrappings in order to link separate seizures and secure a prosecution for dealing or importation of the cannabis. This typically is done by comparison of the striations on the polythene and other extruded wrapping material found on these items using polarised light, by physical fitting of the pieces or by comparison of any welds or seams.

Determination of cannabinoids in body fluids for forensic purposes

This section presents a selection from the large volume of literature published on the determination of the possible influence or impairment of behaviour by cannabinoids in body fluids for forensic purposes and attempts to give an overview of the range of studies from the 1970s through to the present day. This period has culminated in the wide availability of immunoassay techniques and automated GC/MS in particular, thus enabling analyses of body fluids to be carried out relatively economically and rapidly to try to quantify and elucidate the actions of cannabis on individuals. Conclusions may then be drawn as to possible effects on behaviour and driving ability for courts and investigation purposes. These two techniques remain the most widely used for the screening of body fluids for the presence of cannabinoids and the latter provides the necessary unequivocal standard of proof required for forensic purposes in many countries.

Newer developments of hyphenated mass spectrometry techniques such as GC/MS/MS, LC/MS and LC/MS/MS play an increasing part in the analyses of cannabinoids when, for example, intact metabolite conjugates are analysed or when better sensitivity and selectivity are required. Methods to speed up analysis and increase throughput of laboratories will also be seen from the examples described below. Furthermore, scientific developments are described from the early days of establishing and validating methodology on complex, difficult-to-use equipment or with convoluted procedures through to modern computer-driven methodology that has become more accessible, reliable, sensitive, selective and versatile.

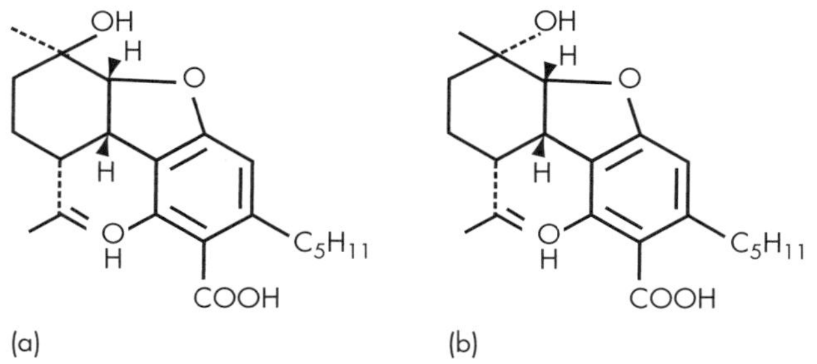

Figure 11.5 The structure of cannabielsoic acid isomers.

Analytical methodology

Mass spectrometry has played a crucial role in the analysis of cannabis, although initially due to the cost, complexity of instrumentation and lack of availability, use was not widespread. A typical example of the earlier work involving MS was the elucidation of the structure of pyrolytic products of cannabidiol (Heerma *et al.*, 1974). The object of the exercise was to determine if the psychotomimetic activity of cannabis resin was due to substances other than THC, since the effects seemed to be produced even in the near absence of this active principle (another consideration was the possible overestimation of THC in seizures of cannabis). Several compounds were found in addition to unchanged CBD, which remained in about 90% yield. These were isolated by preparative gas chromatography and the structures were determined by mass spectrometry and compared with reference mass spectra of known cannabinoids. One of the major pyrolysis products when oxygen was present was found to be cannabielsoin arising from the decarboxylation of cannabielsoic acid. A small amount of THC was isolated, presumably contributing to the psychotomimetic activity of the resin when smoked in a reefer. The structure of cannabielsoic acid is shown in Figure 11.5.

Development of hyphenated techniques

The late 1970s saw hyphenated techniques, in particular reversed-phase HPLC-radioimmunoassay (HPLC/RIA) being introduced in the UK in a forensic context. This followed work on earlier immunoassay work developed at the University of Surrey (Law *et al.*, 1979). The Home Office Central Research Establishment, the research facility of the Government-operated Forensic Science Service in England and Wales, implemented this technique following validation by GC/MS for the analysis of THC and its metabolites in body fluids. The method, which consisted of injecting blood or urine samples (protein precipitated in the case of blood) and collecting fractions of the HPLC eluant, followed by analysis by RIA, was designed to allow a rapid, relatively cheap, forensically valid methodology to be implemented at a time when GC/MS analysis was much more expensive, not very sensitive and time consuming, i.e. before the days of readily accessible data systems, autosamplers (for automated injection and batching on the GC) and robust capillary GC columns.

The application of this technique to some forensic casework in the UK was reviewed and illustrated by the analysis of body fluids in two deaths and discussion of whether or not prior possession of cannabis had occurred when carboxy-THC was found in the urine, for example (Law, 1981).

A commercial TLC methodology has been used in conjunction with two different sensitivity enzyme immunoassays (EIA) to provide a forensically acceptable screen and confirmation procedure for urinary cannabinoids (Sutheimer et al., 1985). The procedure for the confirmation of carboxy-THC and therefore cannabis use was simple and cheap. The combination of TLC with the lower sensitivity EIA (cut-off at 100 ng/mL cross-reactivity of urinary cannabinoids) afforded an almost 100% chance of confirmation and even with the higher sensitivity immunoassay (20 ng/mL cut-off), more than 95% of the positives were confirmed by TLC.

The introduction of a low-cost ion-trap mass spectrometer enabled development of the analysis of carboxy-THC in urine following solid-phase extraction (McMurdy et al., 1986). However, it subsequently transpired that various instrumental difficulties ensured that the benchtop quadrupole mass spectrometers being developed at about the same time were more popular in forensic analyses.

The mass spectrometry of the cannabinoids and their metabolites has been reviewed thoroughly, demonstrating the pivotal role MS has played in elucidating their structures (Harvey, 1987). The author also predicts the use of MS/MS, with its extreme selectivity, by fragmentation of individual ions, to investigate the problem of cannabinoid accumulation in adipose tissue of chronic users and possible deleterious effects on health.

In contrast to the widespread use of immunoassay screening followed by GC/MS for unambiguous confirmation of carboxy-THC in urine, a cheap method based on high-performance TLC following optimised solid-phase extraction has been proposed (Brandt and Kovar, 1997). The method relies on the use of UV spectroscopy and Fourier-transform infrared spectroscopy (UV/FTIR) coupling, avoiding the need for potentially hazardous visualisation sprays such as the Fast Blue B salts. Detection limits are in the 20 ng/mL range, but only measurable between narrow limits (14.4–43.2 ng/mL).

Solid-phase microextraction (SPME) of cannabinoids in water and saliva using commercially available poly(dimethylsiloxane) SPME fibres has been investigated in order to determine whether or not this direct, solvent-free extraction method may be applied to biological matrices (Hall *et al.*, 1998). The authors found that the extraction from saliva could be significantly improved by pretreatment with glacial acetic acid to precipitate the proteins, which were then discarded following centrifugation. The method compared directly with liquid/liquid extraction in terms of relative standard deviation and was much faster. It also lends itself to automation.

Continuing the theme of automated extraction procedures, a robotic solid-phase extraction and GC/MS analysis of THC in blood has been described to cope rapidly with the greatly increasing workload in a toxicology laboratory in Utah analysing the blood of drivers resulting from a new 'any-amount' law (Stonebraker *et al.*, 1998). A detection limit of 1 ng/mL for THC was obtained by the use of trifluoroacetic acid derivatives and negative chemical ionisation in the mass spectrometer. When combined with modification of the eluting solvents for THC and carboxy-THC, considerable time and other savings in terms of glassware were achieved compared with the previously used manual extraction method.

An automated solid-phase extraction of THC and carboxy-THC from whole blood that used GC with conventional electron impact (EI) mass spectrometry has also been described (D'Asaro, 2000). Extensive method validation was reported and the limits of quantification were 1 ng/mL for THC and 2 ng/mL for carboxy-THC for this procedure, which was developed to analyse the blood of suspected impaired drivers in Arizona.

The enhanced selectivity of THC and metabolite detection in serum by means of an MS/MS method with an ion trap has been reported, circumventing some of the disadvantages of the instrument in the normal 'scan' mode (Weller *et al.*, 2000). Furthermore the introduction of relatively low-cost MS/MS using ion traps rather than more expensive multisector instruments such as triple quadrupoles has enabled wider applicability of the technique. THC was identified down to

0.25 ng/mL, hydroxy-THC 0.5 ng/mL and carboxy-THC down to less than 2.5 ng/mL with quantification down to 2, 5 and 8 ng/mL respectively. However within-run and day-to-day precision was still not as good as quadrupole instruments, ranging from 4.2 to 10.4%, causing these somewhat high quantification limits. Nevertheless the lack of interference in the monitored daughter ions from the parent or precursor ions allowed these very good detection limits to be achieved and ensured confirmation of the substances.

The rapid simultaneous determination of both carboxy-THC and its glucuronide in urine using MS/MS on a triple quadrupole with liquid chromatography has been reported (Weinmann *et al.*, 2000). Because the glucuronide is not amenable to GC, it is usually hydrolysed to the free carboxy-THC before analysis by GC/MS. This is not necessary with liquid chromatography and the monitoring of both the conjugate and free acid may allow the refinement of a 'cannabis impairment factor' mooted for the serum of drivers. The authors planned to evaluate the ratios of the free acid to the conjugate in urine and eventually serum to see if it was possible to determine whether or not chronic or single use of cannabis had occurred, based on the different elimination rates of these two metabolites.

Finally as an example of improved detection in difficult matrices, the monitoring of carboxy-THC in hair has been reported by the application of high-volume GC injection combined with negative ion mass spectrometry to achieve the necessary sensitivity (Moore *et al.*, 2001). A disadvantage of chemical ionisation MS such as negative ionisation is the preponderance of ion current on the molecular ion and lack of characteristic confirmatory ions required for a forensic identification, however this was addressed by the use of the trifluoroacetyl-hexafluoroisopropyl derivative and two ionisation reagent gases, methane and ammonia. Fragmentation produced two ions for methane and three for ammonia. The use of 25-µL injection volumes further helped the achievement of detection limits of 0.3 pg/mg of hair, of which 20 mg was required for the analysis. Carboxy-THC was found in the hair of daily users and a weekly user but not in the hair of a monthly user or those living with daily users (all self-reported).

Interpretation of cannabis use in a forensic context

We have seen that in the late 1970s and early 1980s somewhat non-specific methods such as immunoassays were used, and to get more information, convoluted hyphenated techniques were developed to analyse the various cannabis components and metabolites in body fluids. Developments in GC/MS and falling costs enabled more sensitive, reliable and cost-effective methods for the quantification and identification of cannabis analytes in body fluids (and other items) to be implemented widely and led to an increased exploration in the effects and implications of cannabis (and other illicit drugs) on behaviour. This facilitates an assessment of whether or not the sample donor was under the influence of cannabis at the time of an incident. This assessment may be applied to either the accused party or the victim of a crime, or both, depending on sampling delay.

To illustrate these trends, several papers and articles are summarised below as examples of the types of analyses and interpretations developed to attempt to answer these questions.

The clinical effects, including the perceived 'high', and preliminary monitoring of the kinetics of plasma Δ^9-THC after administration by various routes (smoking, intravenously and oral consumption) were studied in 11 male subjects aged between 18 and 35 years using GC/MS for the analysis (Ohlsson *et al.*, 1980). They observed that reddened conjunctivae were a reliable indication of cannabis use although not necessarily related to perceived 'high', this effect being observed when the plasma concentration of THC exceeded 5 ng/mL. Pulse rate was considered to be a somewhat less reliable sign of use: the highest increase (median +40 beats per minute, range +25 to +100) occurred with intravenous THC at the highest median levels of 100 ng/mL; smoking produced a median increase of 34 bpm (range 0 to +80) at a median THC level of 45 ng/mL and the lowest increase 26 bpm (range +4 to +68) was recorded with oral THC at a median THC level of 4.5 ng/mL. The correlation between the perceived 'high' and the logarithm of the plasma THC levels was not particularly strong; this was thought to be due to the lipophilicity of the drug causing rapid removal from the blood while brain levels were still rising, thus producing a delayed effect. Differences in plasma THC levels produced by the various routes of administration were also considered and attempts made to explain the differences.

Forensic aspects of the metabolism and excretion of cannabis were considered following oral ingestion of cannabis resin by combined HPLC/RIA (Law, 1983; Law *et al.*, 1984a). The authors found that the glucuronide conjugate of carboxy-THC (O ester) was the major metabolite detected in the urine and the free acid was not detected to any significant extent. They suggested that the total cannabinoid content of the blood or urine was not useful in interpretation but that the parent drug/metabolite ratios and the metabolite/metabolite ratios may be of more use for indicating recent cannabis use. In particular they suggested that a total metabolite/THC ratio of less than 20 indicated recent oral cannabis consumption.

Passive smoking of cannabis was also considered by these authors to address the legal defence that positive cannabinoid findings in blood and urine of defendants were due to inadvertent inhalation from side-stream smoke (Law *et al.*, 1984b). Four subjects remained in an unventilated small room (approximately 28 m³ in volume) while six volunteers smoked one reefer cigarette each at their normal rate and then left. The four subjects remained in the room for a total of 3 hours and urine samples of these and the six smokers were analysed. The urine samples of the non-smokers showed significant cannabinoid content (up to 6.8 ng/mL) for up to 6 hours after exposure, but the blood, which was taken up to 3 hours after exposure started, exhibited no cannabinoid cross-reactivity. These data were compared with those from other studies and the conclusion drawn that it would be unlikely to find cannabinoids in the blood of passive inhalers. However in extreme conditions, detectable urinary cannabinoids can be produced and such findings must therefore be interpreted with caution. The high lipophilicity of THC presumably leads to the rapid removal from the bloodstream so that it remained undetectable with the techniques used.

The presence and analysis of cannabinoids in urine arising out of 'passive smoking' has been reviewed in terms of pharmacokinetics and metabolism (Moffat, 1986). Because of the lipophilicity of THC, it has a high volume of distribution (10 L/kg) and a long half-life of 20–36 hours. These characteristics also apply to the metabolites; carboxy-THC has a half-life of 22 hours and its glucuronide has a half-life of 21 hours. These properties lead to the metabolites being detectable for a considerable time, up to several weeks in urine in some cases. Analysis of the urine revealed that the glucuronide was the major urinary metabolite and that the free, unbound carboxy acid is present as a minor metabolite unless storage conditions are poor. Moffat also cautions that the urine should be hydrolysed before analysis to liberate the unbound acid. The criteria for the detection of cannabis metabolites in urine due to passive inhalation are discussed; a sensitive screening test is required and RIA fits this bill (2 ng/mL cut-off) rather than EIA, which is a tenth as sensitive; the conditions for detectable levels of metabolite are somewhat extreme; prolonged exposure to high concentrations of reefer smoke in a small, confined space such as a car or small, ill-ventilated room being required.

Further studies of repeat passive inhalation of sidestream smoke from various numbers of reefers were conducted on volunteers who sat in a small, unventilated room (Cone *et al.*, 1987). In particular the volunteers who were exposed to extreme conditions, i.e. cannabis smoke from 16 marijuana cigarettes for 1 hour for 6 consecutive days, showed some evidence of accumulation of cannabinoids in their bodies, unsurprisingly perhaps in the light of the long half-lives of the cannabinoids. There was also some evidence of the experience of 'highs' by these volunteers. The authors did note that these extreme conditions were unlikely to be tolerated in real life because of smoke irritation of the eyes. The volunteers who were exposed to the smoke from only four cigarettes per day produced positive findings only occasionally and the urine samples were more frequently negative. They concluded that the amount of absorption depended on the concentration of THC in the room. The authors used EIA, RIA and GC/MS for the analyses.

The excretion patterns of cannabis metabolites have been analysed in 86 male and female chronic users after last use (Ellis *et al.*, 1985). The authors used two commercial EIA tests to perform semi-quantitative and qualitative cannabinoid screening on urine samples taken from Navy service personnel with a minimum of three positive cannabinoid findings after admission to the Naval Drug Rehabilitation Center. Of the subjects admitted to the facility, 97.7% were male and they ranged in age from 18 to 34 years (mean 22.8 years old) and had a 8.9-year mean history of cannabis use (range 2–21 years). The study followed each individual until he or she had 10 consecutive negative results (less than the lowest calibrator of 20 ng/mL cross-reactivity in the semi-quantitative test) on their daily urine screens. The 86 individuals presented with positive results for a mean time of 17 days before their first negative result, with a high range up to 46 days. The mean time for 10 consecutive negative results (<20 ng/mL cut-off) was 27 days and ranged up to 77 days. The researchers concluded that a single urine test was of no practical value in predicting last use or extent of cannabis use, although they did note that broadly speaking the length of time the urine samples remained positive correlated with self-reported light, moderate or heavy use but with considerable overlap. A biphasic elimination pattern was also noted, the latter being slower than the initial rate.

The use of GC/MS and EIA enabled the THC and metabolic profile of THC in plasma and urine to be established, enabling time since use of cannabis resin to be estimated (McBurney *et al.*, 1986). THC levels above 2–3 ng/mL in the plasma indicated smoking within 6 hours. For the urine, levels of the 8β,11-dihydroxy-THC metabolite above 15–20 ng/mL indicated smoking within the previous 4–6 hours.

A prolonged apparent half-life of THC in the plasma of chronic marijuana users (daily use of more than one reefer) has been noted following work with deuterium-labelled THC using GC/MS in the selected ion mode to maximise sensitivity (Johansson *et al.*, 1988). A mean plasma half-life of 4.1 days ± 1.1 days was obtained by analysing the plasma concentrations of THC for 13 days in three volunteers who each smoked deuterium-labelled THC in four cigarettes (two per day for 2 days). The results agreed with animal models and are consistent with the lipophilic THC being absorbed into fat tissues. The authors also surmised that, although the plasma THC levels were not high enough to give any psychoactive effects, they could nevertheless contribute to side-effects produced by long-term use.

The pharmacokinetics and metabolism of THC were reviewed with the emphasis on humans (Agurell *et al.*, 1986). Particular attention was paid to those metabolites which displayed psychotomimetic properties similar to THC. (*Note*: The authors use the biogenetically based monoterpene numbering system, in which Δ^1-THC is equivalent to Δ^9-THC in the dibenzopyran system which is predominantly used and adopted by *Chemical Abstracts* – the use of the two different systems causes confusion, particularly when dealing with the metabolites, but the dibenzopyran system cannot be used for cannabinol (Figure 11.6).)

Of particular interest to forensic investigations is the section reviewing the relationship between plasma levels of the drug and its metabolites and effects such as the 'high'. The authors conclude that there is a temporal dissociation between the plasma concentration of THC and the psychological and physiological effects. The origin of this time lag was not clear and several causes were discussed. Slow penetration across the blood–brain barrier, then slow distribution in the brain and slow start up in biochemical reactions once at the appropriate receptors all figured prominently as possible causes. 11-Hydroxy-THC (7-hydroxy-THC in the monoterpene system) is the primary metabolite of THC and was thought to have about the same psychoactivity as the parent compound in humans, but proved only important in terms of overall effects when cannabis was ingested orally, due to the higher concentrations produced relative to THC via this route. Carboxy-THC, the major urinary metabolite in humans, was inactive.

Contrary to the conclusions regarding the time lag of the THC effects behind plasma concentrations, work carried out by the Addiction

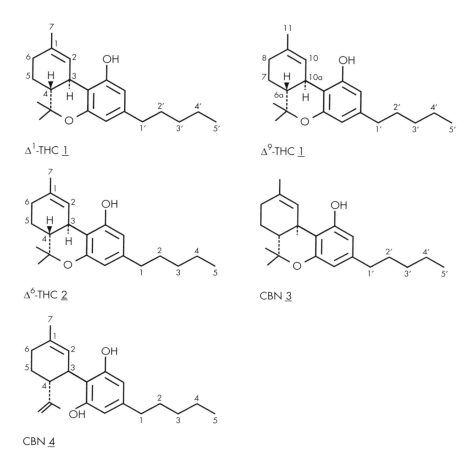

Figure 11.6 The monoterpene (Δ^1-THC) and dibenzopyran (Δ^9-THC) numbering systems for THC and some other cannabinoids.

Research Center, National Institute on Drug Abuse in Baltimore, Maryland, demonstrated that the time lag was artefactual (Huestis *et al.*, 1992a). They claimed that rapid collection of blood and careful monitoring of behavioural and physiological effects showed that any delay was, at worst, only minutes and the effects appeared rather to be concurrent with the appearance of THC in the blood. The blood levels of THC peaked at 9 minutes.

Further work was carried out by the Addiction Research Center to monitor the metabolite levels during experiments on once weekly cannabis use with this rapid collection protocol to get a complete pharmacokinetic profile of THC and its metabolites in plasma (Huestis *et al.*, 1992b). It was shown that the effects of THC again peaked quickly before smoking had ceased, then fell quickly and that the hydroxy-THC levels were much lower than THC levels, peaking after smoking had ceased. The carboxy-THC level rose slowly and plateaued for an extended period. The time to peak was nearly 2 hours. The authors also extended these studies and proposed the use of two models to predict the time of cannabis exposure from plasma concentrations of THC and carboxy-THC (Huestis *et al.*, 1992c). The equation relating the time, *T*, with the THC plasma concentration used for model 1, obtained by linear regression analysis of the data was:

$$\text{Log } T = -0.698 \log[\text{THC}] + 0.687$$

For model 2, the equation incorporated the carboxy-THC concentration thus:

$$\text{Log } T = (0.576 \times \log[\text{THCCOOH}]/[\text{THC}]) - 0.176$$

Equations were also calculated for the 95% confidence limits of these calculations of time of use. These models enabled the exposure time to be predicted with 90 and 89% accuracy respectively, to assist the forensic scientist to interpret the plasma levels.

Other authors examined 5 years' worth of GC/MS data for blood THC levels and compared this with blood or urine carboxy-THC concentrations in order to try to determine if any relationship existed to assist in impairment interpretations (Moody *et al.*, 1992). They concluded, however, that as with previous observations, an accurate estimate of the THC concentration (and possible impairment) from the metabolite concentration was virtually impossible because of inter-individual differences, due not least to genetic polymorphism of the isoenzyme of the cytochrome P450 responsible for the metabolism of THC.

Whole blood and plasma or serum levels of THC, 11-hydroxy-THC and carboxy-THC have been studied to determine whether or not someone was under the influence of cannabis at the time of a crime (Giroud *et al.*, 2001). This work refined that of Heustis and others and it was applied to whole blood, the usual sample available in forensic cases, especially when the samples are taken post-mortem, using a plasma/whole blood ratio of 1.6:1. It was found that the evidential value of post-mortem values in prediction of influence is less reliable due to changes in drug concentrations after death.

Predicting the time of use of cannabis based on urinary THC concentrations in particular, measured by GC/MS, has been investigated (Manno *et al.*, 2001). The authors propose that a concentration of 'free' THC in the urine of greater than 1.5 ng/mL, following hydrolysis of the THC-glucuronide, indicates use of cannabis during the 8 hours prior to sampling and is much more useful in this respect than carboxy-THC measurements alone.

'Marinol', which contains synthetic Δ^9-THC as an active ingredient, was introduced in to the US as a medicine for the control of nausea and vomiting in patients undergoing chemotherapy, and as an appetite stimulant in AIDS patients. It was thought necessary to develop an analytical procedure to distinguish between use of illicit and licit THC and a GC/MS method was proposed based on Δ^9-tetrahydrocannabivarin (Δ^9-THCV – the C3 side-chain homologue of THC), a substance present in natural cannabis (ElSohly *et al.*, 1999). The presence of THCV and its metabolites, thought to be produced in an analogous manner to THC which has a C5 side-chain, should then identify illicit cannabis use. This paper produced some controversy in the literature because of a claimed lack of evidence for the assertions (Sedgwick, 2000). However, further work on THCV, including a clinical study, demonstrated that the proposition by ElSohly *et al.* was verified (ElSohly *et al.*, 2001a,b). Hence carboxy-THCV was only present in the urine of illicit cannabis users and not in the urine of patients prescribed synthetic THC.

Because of the introduction of medicines derived from cannabis plants in the UK, it could be difficult to distinguish between legal and illegal products in body fluids and doubtless similar methodologies are going to be needed to determine the two sources when necessary.

Finally, to put into context the lack of acute toxic aspects of cannabis, this aspect is illustrated by the very few reports in the literature of fatalities due to its use, in comparison with alcohol or other drugs of abuse such as heroin. A case of fatal ingestion of 'bhang', an Indian preparation of *C. sativa*, has been reported recently (Gupta *et al.*, 2001). However, the individual involved, a 25-year-old male who drank a glass of 'bhang' as part of a religious festival, may have had predisposing factors. He had rheumatic heart disease affecting some of his heart valves and had some time previously undergone open-heart surgery on one of the damaged valves. At the post-mortem examination it appeared that he had only consumed a normal dose of 'bhang', a bolus of crushed hemp amounting to about 2 g in water, and his heart was approximately twice the expected size with the left atrium particularly enlarged.

Cannabis and driving

The use of illicit drugs by drivers is generating particular interest at the moment in the UK because of the debate in the media about the effects on ability to drive safely. As cannabis is the most commonly used illicit drug, it is important to know whether, and to what extent, cannabis use may be causing problems in terms of road safety. If problems are identified, then the legislature will be required to address the issues involved and forensic analytical capabilities will necessarily play a role in any enforcement that is required of new or indeed existing laws. This issue, and others pertinent to cannabis and driving, are discussed in Chapter 12.

Quality control of analytical procedures

Two examples are touched upon to illustrate some of the analytical issues associated with THC and cannabis analysis. A particular problem is the relative instability of Δ^9-THC. It is light sensitive and very hydrophobic, therefore care must be taken to see that it is not lost during storage and analysis. One study examined the stability of Δ^9-THC in glass and in plastic containers (Christophersen, 1986). It was found that samples of spiked blood in plastic containers lost between 60% and 100% of the THC content during storage. When comparing identical blood samples stored in plastic and glass containers, the final THC concentration in plastic containers varied between 0 and 87% of that in the glass containers. The authors therefore recommend that any vessels used for storage of such blood samples be investigated for THC loss.

A contribution to the improvement of accuracy in the quantitation of Δ^9-THC in illicit drug substances by GC with flame-ionisation detectors (GC-FID) has been proposed (Poortman-van der Meer and Huizer, 1999). To take account of Δ^9-THC that is potentially unstable and variations in the strength of purchased standard solutions from that stated, together with introduced analytical errors, the authors proposed a procedure using the comparative signal response based on the effective carbon number response factors for CBD and CBN to predict the response expected for THC and verify its concentration. This allowed them to use the more stable CBD and/or CBN to measure the THC content of cannabis seizures.

Conclusions

With improving analytical technology and increasing understanding of the effects of cannabis on behaviour, authorities will rely more and more on forensic analysts and their scientific armoury to measure THC, its metabolites and perhaps other cannabinoids to satisfy the particular forensic requirements of their legislation. Clearly this picture will be more complicated if a country permits the use of medicinal cannabis while still restricting the non-medicinal use.

References

Agurell S, Halldin M, Lindgren J-E *et al.* (1986). Pharmacokinetics and metabolism of Δ^1-tetrahydrocannabinol and other cannabinoids with emphasis on man. *Pharmacol Rev* 38: 21–43.

Atha M J, Blanchard S (1997). Regular users. Self-reported drug consumption patterns and attitudes towards drugs among 1333 regular cannabis users. Independent Drug Monitoring Unit, Wigan, UK.

Bäckström B, Cole M D, Carrott M J *et al.* (1997). A preliminary study of the analysis of *Cannabis* by supercritical fluid chromatography with atmospheric pressure chemical ionisation mass spectroscopic detection. *Sci Justice* 37: 91–97.

Brandt C, Kovar K-A (1997). Determination of 11-nor-Δ^9-tetrahydrocannabinol-9-carboxylic acid in urine by use of HPTLC-UV/FTIR on-line coupling. *J Planar Chromatogr* 10: 348–352.

Buchanan B E, O'Connell D (1998). Survey on cannabis resin and cannabis in unsmoked hand rolled cigarettes seized in the Republic of Ireland. *Sci Justice* 38: 221–224.

Christophersen A S (1986). Tetrahydrocannabinol stability in whole blood: plastic versus glass containers. *J Anal Toxicol* 10: 129–131.

Cone E J, Johnson R E, Darwin W D *et al.* (1987). Passive inhalation of marijuana smoke: Urinalysis and room air levels of delta-9-tetrahydrocannabinol. *J Anal Toxicol* 11: 89–96.

D'Asaro J A (2000). An automated and simultaneous solid-phase extraction of Δ^9-tetrahydrocannabinol and 11-nor-9-carboxy-Δ^9-tetrahydrocannabinol from whole blood using the Zymark RapidTrace™ with confirmation and quantitation by GC/EI-MS. *J Anal Toxicol* 24: 289–295.

Ellis G M, Mann M A, Judson B A *et al.* (1985). Excretion patterns of cannabinoid metabolites after last use in a group of chronic users. *Clin Pharmacol Ther* 38: 572–578.

ElSohly M A, Feng S, Murphy T P *et al.* (1999). Δ^9-Tetrahydrocannabivarin (Δ^9-THCV) as a marker for the ingestion of cannabis versus Marinol®. *J Anal Toxicol* 23: 222–224.

ElSohly M A, Ross S A, Mehmedic Z *et al.* (2000). Potency trends of Δ^9-THC and other cannabinoids in confiscated marijuana from 1980–1997. *J Forens Sci* 45: 24–30.

ElSohly M A, Feng S, Murphy T P *et al.* (2001a). Identification and quantitation of 11-nor-Δ^9-tetrahydrocannabivarin-9-carboxylic acid, a major metabolite of Δ^9-tetrahydrocannabivarin. *J Anal Toxicol* 25: 476–480.

ElSohly M A, deWit H, Wachtel S R *et al.* (2001b). Δ^9-Tetrahydrocannabivarin as a marker for the ingestion of marijuana versus Marinol®: Results of a clinical study. *J Anal Toxicol* 25: 565–571.

Giroud C, Ménétrey A, Augsburger M *et al.* (2001). Δ^9-THC, 11-OH-Δ^9-THC and Δ^9–THCCOOH plasma or serum to whole blood concentrations distribution ratios in blood samples taken from living and dead people. *Forens Sci Int* 123: 159–164.

Gupta B D, Jani C B, Shah P H (2001). Fatal 'bhang' poisoning. *Med Sci Law* 41: 349–352.

Hall B J, Satterfield-Doerr M, Parikh A R, Brodbelt J S (1998). Determination of cannabinoids in water and human saliva by solid-phase microextraction and quadrupole ion trap gas chromatography/mass spectrometry. *Anal Chem* 70: 1788–1796.

Harvey D J (1987). Mass spectrometry of the cannabinoids and their metabolites. *Mass Spectrom Rev* 6: 135–229.

Heerma W, Terlouw J K, Laven A *et al.* (1974). Structure elucidation of pyrolytic products of cannabidiol by mass spectrometry. In: Frigerio A, Castagnoli N, eds. *Mass Spectrometry in Biochemistry and Medicine*. New York: Raven Press: 219–227.

Huestis M A, Sampson A H, Holicky B J *et al.* (1992a). Characterization of the absorption phase of marijuana smoking. *Clin Pharmacol Ther* 52: 31–41.

Huestis M A, Henningfield J E, Cone E J. (1992b). Blood cannabinoids. I. Absorption of THC and formation of 11-OH-THC and THCCOOH during and after smoking marijuana. *J Anal Toxicol* 16: 275–282.

Huestis M A, Henningfield J E, Cone E J (1992c). Blood cannabinoids. II. Models for the prediction of time of marijuana exposure from plasma concentrations of Δ^9-tetrahydrocannabinol (THC) and 11-nor-9-carboxy-Δ^9-tetrahydrocannabinol (THCCOOH). *J Anal Toxicol* 16: 283–290.

INCB (2001). *Report*. Vienna: International Narcotics Control Board: Sections 208–230.

Johansson E, Agurell S, Hollister L E, Halldin M (1988). Prolonged apparent half-life of Δ^1-tetrahydrocannabinol in plasma of chronic marijuana users. *J Pharm Pharmacol* 40: 374–375.

Kudo M, Moffat A C, Watt R A (2000). The use of near-infrared reflectance spectroscopy for the identification of the geographical origins of *Cannabis sativa*. *J Pharm Pharmacol* 52(Suppl): 295.

Landi S (1997). Mineral nutrition of *Cannabis sativa* L. *J Plant Nutr* 20: 311–326.

Law B (1981). Cases of cannabis abuse detected by analysis of body fluids. *J Forens Sci Soc* 21: 31–39.

Law B (1983). Radioimmunoassay methods for the forensic analysis of cannabinoids in biological fluids. PhD thesis, University of Surrey, UK.

Law B, Williams P L, Moffat A C (1979). The detection and quantification of cannabinoids in blood and urine by RIA, HPLC/RIA and GC/MS. *Vet Hum Toxicol* 21(Suppl): 144–147.

Law B, Mason P A, Moffat A C *et al.* (1984a). Forensic aspects of the metabolism and excretion of cannabinoids following oral ingestion of cannabis resin. *J Pharm Pharmacol* 36: 289–294.

Law B, Mason P A, Moffat A C *et al.* (1984b). Passive inhalation of cannabis smoke. *J Pharm Pharmacol* 36: 578–581.

Lurie I S, Meyers R P, Conver T S (1998). Capillary electrochromatography of cannabinoids. *Anal Chem* 70: 3255–3260.

McBurney L J, Bobbie B A, Sepp L A (1986). GC/MS and EMIT analyses for Δ^9-tetrahydrocannabinol metabolites in plasma and urine of human subjects. *J Anal Toxicol* 10: 56–64.

McMurdy H H, Lewellen L J, Callahan L S, Childs P S (1986). Evaluation of the ion trap detector for the detection of 11-nor-Δ^9-THC-9-carboxylic acid in urine after extraction by bonded-phase adsorption. *J Anal Toxicol* 10: 175–177.

Manno J E, Manno B R, Kemp P M *et al.* (2001). Temporal indication of marijuana use can be estimated from plasma and urine concentrations of Δ^9-tetrahydrocannabinol, 11-hydroxy-Δ^9-tetrahydrocannabinol, and 11-nor-Δ^9-tetrahydrocannabinol-9-carboxylic acid. *J Anal Toxicol* 25: 538–549.

Moffat A C (1986). Monitoring urine for inhaled cannabinoids. *Arch Toxicol* Suppl 9: 103–110.

Moody D E, Monti K M, Crouch D J (1992). Analysis of forensic specimens for cannabinoids. II. Relationship between blood Δ^9-tetrahydrocannabinol and blood and urine 11-nor-Δ^9-tetrahydrocannabinol-9-carboxylic acid concentrations. *J Anal Toxicol* 16: 297–301.

Moore C, Guzaldo F, Donahue T (2001). The determination of 11-nor-Δ^9-tetrahydrocannabinol-9-carboxylic acid in hair using negative ion gas chromatography-mass spectrometry and high-volume injection. *J Anal Toxicol* 25: 555–558.

Ohlsson A, Lindgren J-E, Wahlen A *et al.* (1980). Plasma delta-9-tetrahydrocannabinol concentrations and clinical effects after oral and intravenous administration and smoking. *Clin Pharmacol Ther* 28: 409–416.

Phillips G F (1998). Analytical and legislative aspects of cannabis. In: Brown D T, ed. *Cannabis: The Genus Cannabis*. Amsterdam: Harwood Academic Publishers: 71–113.

Poortman-van der Meer A J, Huizer H (1999). A contribution to the improvement of accuracy in the quantitation of THC. *Forens Sci Int* 101: 1–8.

Sedgwick B (2000). Δ^9-Tetrahydrocannabivarin (THCV) as a marker of cannabis use: Is the methodology forensically acceptable? *J Anal Toxicol* 24: 73–75.

Siniscalco Gigliano G (1998). Identification of *Cannabis sativa* L. (Cannabaceae) using restriction profiles of the Internal Transcribed Spacer II (ITS2). *Sci Justice* 38: 225–230.

Siniscalco Gigliano G, Di Finizio A (1998). The *Cannabis sativa* L. fingerprint as a tool in forensic investigations. *Bull Narcot* XLIX & L: 129–137.

Stonebraker W E, Lamoreaux T C, Bebault M *et al.* (1998). Robotic solid-phase extraction and GC-MS analysis of THC in blood. *Am Clin Lab* 17(6): 18–19.

Sutheimer C A, Yarborough R, Hepler B R, Sunshine I (1985). Detection and confirmation of urinary cannabinoids. *J Anal Toxicol* 9: 156–160.

Tanaka H, Yukihiro S (1999). Monoclonal antibody against tetrahydrocannabinolic acid distinguishes *Cannabis sativa* samples from different plant species. *Forens Sci Int* 106: 135–146.

Taylor R, Lydon J, Andersen J D (1994). Anatomy and viability of *Cannabis sativa* stem cuttings with and without adventitious roots. *J Forens Sci* 39: 769–777.

UK Government (2002). Home Office. http://www.drugs.gov.uk/newsandevents/pressreleases/cannabis_acmd/view (accessed 26 March 2002).

Weinmann W, Vogt S, Goerke R *et al.* (2000). Simultaneous determination of THC-COOH and THC-COOH-glucuronide in urine samples by LC/MS/MS. *Forens Sci Int* 113: 381–387.

Weller J-P, Wolf M, Szidat S (2000). Enhanced selectivity in the determination of Δ^9-tetrahydrocannabinol and two major metabolites in serum using ion-trap GC-MS-MS. *J Anal Toxicol* 24: 359–364.

12

A review of cannabis and driving skills

David Hadorn

This chapter reviews some of the attempts to define the complex effects of cannabis on driving behaviour. The effects of cannabis are put into context with recreational and prescription drugs.

Because cannabis and alcohol both affect cognitive function, it is often assumed that cannabis negatively affects driving skills, like alcohol. However, a surprisingly strong and consistent body of evidence has shown that this is not the case. Analyses of responsibility for traffic collisions have repeatedly determined that drivers with only cannabis in their systems (i.e. no alcohol) were if anything *less* culpable than drug-free drivers, whereas alcohol was confirmed as a major causal factor in producing traffic collisions. In prospective studies using driving simulators or road tests, cannabis was shown to produce mild levels of impairment in subjects' ability to keep cars in the centre of the lane and to maintain a constant following distance. However, cannabis subjects were aware of this impairment and compensated by driving more cautiously, e.g. by maintaining slower speeds and longer following distances. These studies also found that alcohol consistently produced significantly more impairment than cannabis, including more aggressive driving (e.g. faster speeds, riskier overtaking). Unlike cannabis subjects, however, alcohol subjects had no insight into their impairment and thus made no attempt to compensate.

Forensic control of cannabis and driving

Proponents of cannabis use would say that the evidence for impairment of driving ability following cannabis use is not clear and that it is difficult to establish a causal link between cannabis use and vehicular fatalities in the epidemiological studies carried out so far. In many instances of crashes resulting in fatalities there is poly-drug use and combinations of drugs with alcohol to further complicate the picture, making it difficult to attribute crashes to use of a particular substance (although the link has been established for alcohol). However, the important question still remains as to whether or not a driver under the influence of the psychomotor, cognitive and other effects of cannabis is safe to drive in a busy urban environment while having to deal with and process the rapidly changing information from traffic situations and road conditions, and control the vehicle satisfactorily. There is considerable evidence that cannabis does impair ability to perform the multiple functions required to drive a car safely. Although the deleterious effects of cannabis are manifestly not as severe as those of alcohol, they are more complex due to its sedative and stimulant properties; nevertheless several countries have proscribed the use of cannabis by drivers and have introduced legislation to that effect. The impetus behind these measures seems to be several fold – the increasing use of cannabis, especially by younger and therefore more inexperienced drivers; the increasing volume of traffic, dependence on personal vehicles for transport and concomitant increase in accidents; studies highlighting the effects of cannabis on brain function and increased public awareness of the hazards associated with driving and substance abuse; and not least the costs to society and individuals of road traffic casualties.

Laboratory studies of cognition and motor performance

From the technical aspect, the trend has been towards better and cheaper analytical facilities, especially over the last 10–15 years, because of the improvement in the capabilities of drug testing laboratories to deal reliably with the low concentrations of the active substances in body fluids. In particular this is a consequence of the diminishing cost of mass spectrometers due to the developments of personal computer-based data stations and the spread of large-scale administrative drug testing schemes such as employee screening, forcing the costs down to produce robust and reliable methodology (Harvey, 1987).

Some of the numerous papers on this matter are summarised below to give an idea of the issues involved and the author refers the reader to the primary literature for more detailed information.

The effect of increasing doses of tetrahydrocannabinol (THC) in smoked marijuana on peripheral vision has been studied in relation to its effect on driving skills (Moskowitz *et al.*, 1972). Progressive peripheral and central vision performance decrements were demonstrated according to the dose, which was 0, 50, 100 and 200 µg of THC per kg of bodyweight. The deterioration of peripheral light-detecting ability was in contrast to previous studies where no deficit in function was found. The authors believe that the earlier studies did not demand as much of their subjects in terms of complexity or attentiveness and that their study is more representative of the demanding tasks and skills required in driving, flying or operating complex machinery.

A double-blind Swiss study examined the effects of 350, 400 or 450 µg of THC per kg of body weight on car driving skills, comparing the effects of a placebo and the orally administered drug on 54 volunteers, both male and female professionals such as doctors and psychologists, with an average age of 34 years (Kielholz *et al.*, 1973). As well as the usual physical indicators of cannabis use, such as infused conjunctivae, increased pain sensitivity, raised pulse rate, raised diastolic blood pressure and increased heart rate, self-assessed effects of the THC group included changes in motor functions, coordination, impairment of abilities to concentrate and adjust to the environmental situation, and dysphoric/euphoric experiences. These changes in the user's physiological and psychological condition may affect driving ability, especially when there is simultaneous stress such as the requirement to take rapid decisions and actions. The authors noted that adaptability was reduced, reaction time was prolonged and an increase in the frequency of wrong or inadequate responses was observed. They also observed that the smooth automatic responses required to drive a car safely were disturbed. The extent of the impairment was a function of the initial attitude, mood and personality structure of the subject.

Significant after-effects were noted for 8–10 hours after consumption of cannabis and some effects such as impairment of concentration, headache, faintness and tremor were present in some subjects for up to 24 hours after intake.

The Canadian Commission of Inquiry into the Non-Medical Use of Drugs (LeDain Commission) studied and reported the effects of cannabis and alcohol on car driving and psychomotor tracking (Hansteen *et al.*, 1976). The Commission concluded that cannabis can adversely affect psychomotor performance such as pursuit tracking, hand and body steadiness, braking stop time and start time, and other factors important to driving ability in a dose-related manner such as short-term memory, vigilance, signal detection and tasks requiring divided attention, but were unable to determine whether or not cannabis did contribute to crashes. They cautioned that until further data were obtained, driving under the influence of cannabis, like alcohol, should be avoided.

The study of ethanol, marijuana and other drug use in single-vehicle accidents in North Carolina was reported for 600 driver fatalities (Mason and McBay, 1984). This study found that, like other epidemiological studies, the biggest decrement in driving performance can be attributed to use of alcohol but a similar link had not been found for other drugs. They found that using a specific radioimmunoassay (RIA) method, with an arbitrary cut-off set at 3 ng/mL, THC was detected in 7.8% of drivers and that these were usually young white males with a higher incidence of multiple drug use than the other drivers. The mean blood THC concentration was found to be 8.7 ng/mL (standard deviation 8.25) with a range of 3.1–37 ng/mL. The authors also looked at carboxy-THC levels and compared them with the blood THC concentration to see if they could estimate when cannabis had been used in relation to the crash. The cannabis drivers had ethanol findings and mean blood ethanol concentrations similar to those determined for all the drivers in the study. The authors thought that as many as 28 drivers (4.7%), or as few as 9 (1.5%), could have experienced some cannabis-induced effects or the combined effects of cannabis and alcohol but probably only one driver would have been significantly impaired by cannabis use alone. However, negative reporting when the blood THC concentration in victims was less than 3 ng/mL could have resulted in the exclusion of some drivers still experiencing the effects of cannabis, although the authors concluded that this number would have been small, and such low THC concentrations would not be associated with significant adverse effects.

Another Canadian survey examined the incidence of ethanol and cannabis occurrence in 1394 fatally injured road users comprising 1169 drivers and 225 pedestrians in Ontario from 1982 to 1984 (Cimbura et al., 1990). The authors employed an initial RIA screen to indicate the presence of cannabinoids then confirmed and quantified any THC by gas chromatography–mass spectroscopy (GC/MS). This study followed on from an earlier, smaller, one in Ontario from April 1978 to March 1979 that showed that cannabis was the second most frequently detected psychoactive substance, the first being alcohol. The later study also showed that cannabis was the second most common substance, after alcohol, occurring in the blood and urine of these road traffic accident victims. Although the rate of cannabinoid occurrence was similar in both studies, at 12% for the former and 12.7% for the latter, the incidence of THC detection increased from 3.7% to 10.9% over this period. It is not clear why this was so and it was attributed to possible differences in the studies and methodologies. It was also noted that out of the 127 THC positive drivers, 124 were males.

Ethanol alone was found in 47.9% of the driver fatalities, THC alone in 1.7% and the two together in 9.2% showing that like other studies, the two in combination may produce an enhancement of the deleterious effects of either alone. Interestingly it was also noted that motorcyclists and moped riders had a much higher rate of THC occurrence, at 22.4%, than other motorists, for example car drivers at 8.9%. Van and lorry drivers presented with the lowest incidence of THC at 5.8%, presumably because more of these motorists were driving as part of their occupations than the others.

The authors stress that the presence of THC or indeed any other psychoactive substance in the blood of the deceased drivers does not demonstrate a causal link. However they comment that the presence of THC may very well show recent cannabis use and therefore the driver may be experiencing the pharmacological actions of cannabis, which should be taken into consideration when attributing cause.

A study in the state of Rheinland-Pfalz in Germany surveyed the incidence of cannabis use amongst impaired road users in 1987 (Becker *et al.*, 1992). They looked at 8654 road users aged 18–35, average age 26, who had been tested for blood alcohol because of impairment of ability to drive and randomly selected 500 males and 150 females for further analysis by immunoassay for cannabis. They found a positive rate (greater than 20 ng/mL carboxy-THC equivalent cross-reactivity) of 7.7% (95% confidence limits 5.5–10.4%) for the males and 2.7% (95% confidence limits 0.7–6.8%) for the females, and recommended that blood tests for illicit and medicinal drugs be carried out on impaired road users who presented with little or no alcohol in their bloodstreams.

In the UK and some other European countries such as the Netherlands, prosecution of certain road traffic laws requires evidence of impairment of driving ability. This applies to substances other than alcohol, which is subject to proscribed limits (e.g. 80 mg% in the UK for blood and 50 mg% in the Netherlands). In Britain, for a prosecution under Section 4 of the Road Traffic Act (1988) to stand a chance of success in the courts, it is necessary to demonstrate that the driver was impaired. This may be accomplished by witness statements, either from civilians or more usually police officers, testifying that the driving behaviour was abnormal; by field impairment tests carried out by a suitably trained police officer or by the Police Surgeon (Forensic Medical Examiner) or both; and for the forensic toxicologist to identify and measure a substance that may interfere with or impair the ability to drive safely. For a Dutch prosecution to succeed under Article 8 of the legislation (Wegenverkeerswet, 1994) a further element is necessary; it needs to be demonstrated that the driver ought to have known that the drug would have affected driving ability. If the defendant denies the charges, then there this is plenty of scope for argument in court as to whether or not driving ability is impaired sufficiently, if at all, to warrant a guilty verdict because of the often subjective nature of the impairment assessment, notwithstanding the standardised nature of field impairment testing being introduced in the UK.

To avoid these difficulties the Belgian and German Parliaments have introduced laws that make it illegal to drive a vehicle if certain substances including cannabis are present in the body. These are substances known to cause driving impairment and their presence is demonstrated by analysis of the blood and/or urine of the driver. A Dutch study reviewed the forensic significance of the results obtained from the toxicological analysis of impaired drivers in European states. In the Netherlands, which has similar laws in this respect to the UK, the situation was compared with Belgium and Germany. The numbers of drivers who would have fallen foul of the law if proscribed drug limit legislation were introduced into the Netherlands was determined (Smink *et al.*, 2001). In addition to several other illicit substances, the Belgian law specifies a limit for cannabinoids of 50 ng/mL in urine following the initial immunoassay-based screening test and in plasma the confirmatory test has a limit of 2 ng/mL for THC. The German laws (Section 24a des Strassenverkeersgesetzes, May 1998, an administrative road traffic regulation and Section 316 StGB, a criminal law) effectively use the analytical detection limit for THC of 0.1 ng/mL as the driving limit for this substance; action can be undertaken at 0.11 ng/mL of THC in blood.

It was also noted that over the period of this Dutch survey (January 1995 to December 1998), the rate of cannabis-positive drivers increased from 8% of the total analysed in 1995 to 29% in 1998, while the annual numbers and percentages of drugs-positive drivers stayed broadly the same. The authors were unable to offer a full explanation for this phenomenon but suggested it may be due to an increase in poly-drug use. They also found that out of 1665 blood and urine samples analysed for drugs during this period, nearly 11% were positive for cannabis in combination with at least one other drug. Interestingly they also found that poly-drug use accounted for 42% of the cases and cocaine was the most commonly occurring drug in combination, unlike the experiences of other countries where cannabis was the most prevalent.

When the authors applied the Belgian Law, which forbids the use of amphetamines including 'ecstasy'-related compounds, cannabinoids, cocaine or opiates, to their results they found that 24% of Dutch drivers (24/102) could have been prosecuted automatically by exceeding the limit for cannabis. Their opinion was that this would therefore avoid the need for discussion in court. It should be noted that the UK laws do have the advantage of being able to cater for the incidents of impairment by drug or substances not proscribed in a particular law. For example the author has dealt with cases of volatile substance impairment (toluene and butane) and γ-hydroxybutyrate (GHB) abuse, substances on which no prosecution could be carried out under present Belgian laws.

In the US, Utah state legislature passed a similar 'any-amount' law in 1994 allowing the driver to be charged with driving under the influence if any controlled drug or metabolite was detected (Stonebraker *et al.*, 1998). The implications for the forensic toxicologist are briefly described above.

Some recently performed work in the UK on the influence of different doses of cannabis on the ability to drive car simulators has been reported and is to be published in the literature (Sexton *et al.*, 2001). The authors attempted with this study to combine different aspects of previous studies; the experimental aspects of performance decrements or changes with the sociological aspects – what factors influence the decision to drive. It was concluded that cannabis has a measurable effect on psychomotor performance, particularly affecting tracking ability such as controlling the vehicle accurately around bends for example (i.e. similar to the effects generally observed in earlier studies). They noted that drivers at traffic lights under the influence of the highest cannabis dose reacted 0.5 s faster than placebo-ingesting drivers. They suggested that this might be due to disturbance of these driver's internal clocks causing them to heighten their attention ready for the change of lights. Alternatively, in a similar manner to alcohol at low doses, the stimulant effects may be encouraging the drivers to take more risks, thus they advised that further investigation would be necessary. They were of the opinion that the ability to carry out divided tasks was not as severely affected as with alcohol, and drivers recognised that they were impaired and compensated by driving more cautiously.

Three basic approaches can be used to arrive at estimates of the impact of cannabis on driving performance: (1) studies of the effects of cannabis on sensory, motor and coordination skills that are considered relevant to driving, (2) retrospective analyses that document the presence or absence of cannabis in the blood of victims of traffic collisions, and (3) prospective studies in which known amounts of cannabis are consumed by volunteers, followed by an assessment of their driving skills, either in a driving simulator or under actual driving conditions. We will consider each approach in turn.

A substantial literature exists concerning the effects of cannabis on cognitive performance and motor skills in laboratory settings (Chesher and Starmer, 1983; Solowij, 1998; UK Department for Transport, 2000). This literature has revealed varying degrees of impairment on skills of perception and motor response. These have been mostly mild, but of sufficient degree in many studies to warrant concern that cannabis might negatively affect driving skills.

However, studies of actual driving skills have consistently revealed lesser degrees of impairment than would have been predicted based on these laboratory studies. This initially unexpected finding is discussed by the UK Department for Transport (DFT) in its report *Cannabis and Driving*:

> It is notable that the studies based on laboratory tests tend to indicate more effects of cannabis consumption than those using simulation and road observation methods. The higher incidence of effects under laboratory test conditions relative to the 'natural' conditions of simulation and road studies has been attributed to (i) reduced error variance from greater control of test conditions; (ii) higher task demand under novel test conditions; (iii) irrelevance or non-equivalence of laboratory test to component of driving; (iv) greater latitude for compensatory effort under 'natural' conditions; and (v) self-selection under 'natural' conditions not to be exposed to risk (e.g., not drive). (UK Department for Transport, 2000)

Similarly, Robbe and O'Hanlon concluded that 'performance decrements obtained under artificial and non-life threatening conditions in the laboratory do not automatically predict similar decrements in driving situations that are closer to real-world driving.' (Robbe and O'Hanlon, 1993).

In view of the questionable relevance of laboratory-based findings to actual driving skills, most contemporary analyses of cannabis and driving focus on studies obtained under more realistic and relevant conditions. We will follow this practice.

Retrospective analyses of traffic collisions

Many studies have examined blood obtained from victims of traffic accidents in an attempt to derive evidence for or against an impairing effect of cannabis on driving skills, however this approach is highly problematic for several reasons. The most fundamental problem is that blood tests for cannabis do not provide a valid indication of the level of cannabis-induced impairment (if any), nor even an indication of recent use. When cannabis is smoked, blood levels of THC rise immediately and then drop rapidly, often before a smoking session is completed. Blood levels fall to 5–10% of their initial level within 1 hour of use, whereas the cognitive effects of cannabis often persist for several hours. Moreover, due to their lipophilic nature, cannabinoids are deposited in fatty tissues, from which they are slowly released, resulting in detectable levels of cannabinoids for days or weeks after last ingestion.

Some studies (see below) have attempted to estimate the time of last use by reference to the relative blood levels of free THC versus its major metabolite (when smoked), THC acid. More recent use is supposed to be associated with increased relative levels of free THC versus THC acid. Another approach to estimating time since last use relies on quantitative measures of THC, with higher levels taken to mean more recent use. Unfortunately, neither approach has been validated prospectively, nor does any particular reason exist to believe that time since last use is linearly correlated with impairment. In any case, most studies do not report or differentiate between THC and its metabolites, nor is the time elapsed between the index traffic collision and blood drawing always reported. Even if all such factors could be controlled, there is no known link between cannabinoid blood levels and impairment. One difficulty in elucidating such a link is the observation that people who use cannabis heavily for prolonged periods can develop tolerance to the somatic and psychological effects of THC, irrespective of concentration (Hunt and Jones, 1980; Mason and McBay, 1984; Peck *et al.*, 1986).

Accordingly, the most definite conclusion that can be reached from such studies is that some proportion of people involved in traffic collisions (within a specified sampling frame) have used cannabis within the past several days to weeks. Without much more information than is currently available, it is impossible to interpret any given observed proportion of cannabis-positive tests as incriminating or exonerating cannabis as a causal factor in traffic collisions.

Several additional considerations further hamper the ability of retrospective blood-test studies to provide causal information about the effect of cannabis on driving. Chief among these is that approximately two-thirds of drivers who had THC in their bloodstream also tested positive for alcohol, leaving very few drivers who tested positive only for cannabis. Another confounding factor is demographic: cannabis users tend to be young males, who as a group are known to have a proclivity for risk-taking behaviours, including dangerous driving (Williams *et al.*, 1985; Ferguson and Horwood, 2001).

A final obstacle to the interpretation of retrospective studies of blood test results is the universal absence of an appropriate control group. Ideally, control blood samples would be obtained from 'random' drivers passing by the same locations at approximately the same times as the drivers involved in the collisions. However, for obvious logistical and ethical reasons this is never done. These considerations led the UK Department for Transport to conclude that studies relying on blood tests for cannabis cannot meaningfully assess the effects of cannabis on risk of collision 'given the absence of valid baseline data for cannabis detected in the non-involved population'.

In an attempt to circumvent the absence of a proper control group, several retrospective studies have attempted to assign responsibility for collisions, comparing and contrasting blood test findings among those individuals deemed culpable from those deemed not culpable. In effect, drivers deemed non-culpable are considered a control group of sorts insofar as the results of their drug tests are considered representative of all drivers within the timeframe and geographical location of the study. However, culpability judgements are inevitably imperfect, and many individuals deemed non-culpable are nonetheless likely to bear a substantial burden of responsibility for failing to avoid the collisions. After all, the vast majority of potential collisions are avoidable (and avoided) through appropriate defensive driving techniques. Nevertheless, attempts to assign culpability are essential if retrospective studies are to have any relevance at all to the question at hand. Accordingly, we do not consider retrospective studies that did not assign culpability.

Several culpability studies have been performed, all of which have concluded, to varying degrees, that cannabis-using drivers are no more responsible for producing traffic crashes than drug-free drivers, and indeed usually less so. In marked contrast, all studies found that alcohol-using drivers were significantly more culpable than drug-free drivers.

Two major government-funded studies are typical. A study by Terhune *et al.* (1992), sponsored by the US DOT/NHTSA, examined blood samples taken from 1882 drivers killed in car, truck and motorcycle accidents in seven states during 1990–1991. Only 17 of these drivers had cannabinoids in their bloodstream without concomitant alcohol, precluding a statistically significant conclusion. Nevertheless, the investigators concluded that 'the THC-only drivers had a responsibility rate below that of the drug-free drivers ... there was no indication that cannabis by itself was a cause of fatal crashes' (Terhune *et al.*, 1992). In this study, alcohol was found in 51.5% of the drivers deemed responsible for fatal accidents. Two-thirds of cannabis- and other-drug-using drivers also tested positive for alcohol and the responsibility rate for the alcohol-plus-THC combination was 95%.

An Australian review of 2500 injured drivers conducted by Hunter *et al.* in May 1998 found that 22.6% of the sample tested positive for at least one drug, including alcohol, while 10.3% were positive for at least one drug excluding alcohol. Cannabinoids were found in 7.1% of the sample as the sole drug and in a further 3.7% in combination with one or more other drugs. The authors concluded, 'Overall, there was no significant increase in culpability for cannabinoids alone. There was some suggestion of a biphasic effect for cannabinoids, with a slight protective effect at lower concentrations, accompanied by an increase in the proportion culpable at higher concentrations.'

Chesher and Longo recently tabulated the essential design features and findings of these and other culpability studies (Tables 12.1 and 12.2) (Chesher and Longo, 2002). These investigators concluded: 'The prominent features to be noted here include the significant and dominant role of alcohol in crashes. One also notes the nonsignificant role of cannabis.' The authors caution that methodological differences across studies (e.g. in how culpability was assessed and how blood samples were obtained and interpreted) limit the extent to which these can be compared. Nevertheless, the uniformity of the studies' findings is certainly indicative of a lack of major negative impact on driving.

With regard to the concomitant effect of alcohol and cannabis, Chesher and Longo conclude: 'In all cases the culpability rate of drivers was not significantly different between those in the alcohol alone group and those with alcohol plus cannabis. This suggests that the increased crash risk reported for alcohol plus cannabis was due to the alcohol effect which clouded any evidence for an interaction between these drugs.'

In a previous analysis of these same culpability studies, Bates and Blakeley (1999) arrived at a similar conclusion: 'There is no evidence that consumption of cannabis alone increases the risk of culpability for traffic crash fatalities or injuries for which hospitalisation occurs, and may reduce those risks ... it is not possible to exclude the possibility that the use of cannabis (with or without alcohol) leads to an increased risk of road traffic crashes causing less serious injuries and vehicle damage.'

Table 12.1 Summary of culpability studies on motor vehicle accidents involving cannabis: effect of time delay on results

Study	Cannabinoids detected (alone or in combination with alcohol)	Time delay between crash and blood sample collection
Non-fatally injured drivers		
Terhune et al., 1992	39 drivers tested positive for cannabinoids, 39 with THC, 17 of whom were in the cannabis-only group. RIA screen with GC/MS confirmation	Crash occurred less than 4 h before arrival at hospital. Distribution of time delay 20.3% <1 h; 41.9% 1–2 h, 31.2% >2 h, 6.2% unknown. Authors found no differences in the THC distribution of the earlier and later samples. Concluded that at the time of blood sample collection the THC concentrations of most drivers were decreasing at a low rate
Hunter et al., 1998	255 drivers tested positive for cannabinoids. 85 with THC; 50 of these were in the cannabis-only group. RIA screen with GC/MS confirmation	Distribution of time delay: 15.1% <1 h, 39.4% 1–2 h, 20.3% 2–3 h, 9.8% 3–4 h, 5.6% 4–5 h, 8.9% >5 h
Fatally injured drivers		
Warren et al., 1981	47 drivers tested positive for cannabinoids. 14 with THC, 2 of whom were in the cannabis-only group. RIA screen only	Drivers were dead on arrival at hospital, or died shortly thereafter. No information on time delay
Williams et al., 1985	151 drivers tested positive for cannabinoids: 151 with THC, 19 of whom were in the cannabis-only group. RIA screen with GC/MS confirmation	Drivers died on impact or within 2 h of the crash. No information on time delay
Donelson et al., 1985	38 drivers tested positive for cannabinoids. 38 with THC, 4 of whom were in the cannabis-only group	Drivers died within 1 h of the crash. No information on time delay

(*continued*)

Table 12.1 *Continued*

Study	Cannabinoids detected (alone or in combination with alcohol)	Time delay between crash and blood sample collection
Terhune *et al.*, 1992	56 drivers tested positive for cannabinoids. 56 with THC, 19 of whom were in the cannabis-only group. RIA screen with GC/MS confirmation	The majority of drivers (94%) died within 2 h of the crash and 6% died within 4 h. Authors concluded that survival time had little impact on drug prevalence rates. Distribution of time delay for drivers who died within 2 h of the crash: 41.2% <8 h, 13% 8–12 h, 26.8% 12–24 h, 20% over 24 h. Authors suggested time delay may have affected drug prevalence rates (and drug concentrations) but did not attempt to calculate concentrations at time of crash
Drummer and Chu, 1999	106 drivers tested positive for cannabinoids. 2 with THC, both of whom were in the cannabis-only group. RIA screen with GC/MS confirmation	No information on selection criteria for drivers, or on time delay

Note: Screening methods alone are not reliable. Further definitive testing is essential for identification and quantification of drug(s).
RIA, radioimmunoassay; GC/MS, gas chromatography – mass spectroscopy.
From Chesher and Longo (2002).

Table 12.2 Summary of culpability studies on motor vehicle accidents involving alcohol, cannabis and no drugs (as controls)

Culpability study	Total n	Drug-free drivers		Alcohol only		Cannabis alone		Alcohol and cannabis	
		n	% culpable	n	% culpable	n	% culpable	n	% culpable
Fatally injured drivers									
Warren et al., 1981	401	124	58	172	See notes	14	See notes	33	See notes
Williams et al., 1985	440	78	71	130	82 (S)	19	63 (NS)	132	95 (S)
Donelson et al., 1985	1169	148	64	188	86 (S)	4	75[a]	29	76[a]
Terhune et al., 1992	1882	799	69.8	745	<0.10 BAC = 75.8 (NS) >0.10 BAC = 93.9 (S)	19	57.9 (NS)	97	94.6 (S)
Drummer and Chu, 1999	1045	479	79.8	262	<0.10 BAC = 74 (NS) >0.10 BAC = 98.5 (S)	43	60 (NS)	63	93.1 (S)
Non-fatally injured drivers									
Terhune et al., 1992	497	273	34.3	74	<0.10 BAC = 59.9 (NS) >0.10 BAC = 79.8 (S)	17	52.9 (NS)	22	45.5 (NS)
Hunter et al., 1998	2500	1766	53.5	214	48.7	178	50.6 (NS)	74	93 (S)

Note: Statistical significance determined using chi-square with the exception of Drummer who used Fisher's exact test. S = statistically significant compared with drug-free drivers ($p < 0.05$), NS = not statistically significant compared with drug-free drivers.
BAC, blood alcohol concentration (%).
All of these studies examined other drugs in addition to alcohol and cannabis. This will explain any arithmetical differences that might appear.
The culpability rate for all cannabis-positive drivers (no breakdown between those with and those without alcohol) was 90%. This was 1.7 times greater than the culpability rate for drug-free drivers. However 49% of cannabis-positive drivers also tested positive for alcohol. No information provided on statistical significance for any of the between-group comparisons. No analysis for cannabis alone.
The number of drivers who tested positive for cannabis alone was too small for any meaningful comparison with the drug-free drivers. No information provided on statistical significance for alcohol alone, cannabis alone, or for alcohol + cannabis.
Note that culpable drivers included those who were fully culpable and those who were culpable/contributory. Authors used five categories of culpability.
[a]When including drivers who were culpable/contributory for both drug-free and cannabis-alone groups, the culpability rate was significantly higher in the cannabis group than that of drug-free drivers (73.4% versus 42.5%, $p < 0.05$).
From Chesher and Longo (2002).

One culpability study not included in the above analyses was performed by the State of Washington, which found that only about 6% of drivers killed in automobile crashes between September 1992 and August 1993 tested positive for cannabis and not also alcohol (Logan, 1994). The report concluded that alcohol was by far the 'dominant problem' in drug-related accidents. Individuals who used cannabis alone were found to be, if anything, less culpable than non-drug-users. The report concluded:

> There was no indication that marijuana by itself was a cause of fatal accidents … In the absence of alcohol, no drug or drug group evidenced a driver responsibility rate significantly different from the drug free control group. When drugs were combined with alcohol, no drug or drug group exhibited a responsibility rate significantly different from alcohol itself. The THC-only drivers had a responsibility rate below that of the drug free drivers, as was found previously by Williams and colleagues (1985). While the difference was not statistically significant, there was no indication that cannabis by itself was a cause of fatal crashes.

The UK Department for Transport recently reviewed all extant culpability analyses of cannabis and driving (UK Department for Transport, 2000), and concluded that:

> Current methodologies can only determine the presence of cannabinoids, not evidence of impairment. Thus, not only is it problematic to estimate the percentage of accident involvements *associated* with cannabis use alone, there is no evidence that impairment resulting from cannabis use *causes* accidents. Attempts to alleviate these problems by calculating risk of culpability for an accident (rather than the risk of having an accident) suggest that cannabis may actually *reduce* responsibility for accidents. It is evident that further epidemiological research is needed. [emphasis in original].

Thus, although one cannot reliably link the presence of cannabinoids in the blood to increased risk of collision, the findings of culpability-assessed retrospective studies consistently indicate a lower than expected rate of cannabinoids in the blood of collision-involved drivers. This rather unexpected finding has been confirmed in several prospective studies of actual driving skills in road simulators or under actual driving conditions, a subject to which we shall now turn.

Prospective driving studies

A series of studies conducted since the late 1960s has tested subjects' ability to drive under simulated or actual on-road conditions, measuring parameters such as speed, ability to stay in centre of lane, headway (distance maintained from car ahead), and overtaking behaviour.

The only study performed under actual driving conditions in traffic was sponsored by the US Department of Transportation, National Highway Traffic Safety Administration and performed by Robbe and O'Hanlon in 1993 in the Netherlands (Robbe and O'Hanlon, 1993). In a preliminary study, investigators determined that marijuana users prefer doses of up to 300 μg/kg to achieve their desired psychoactive effect, and that this dosage 'slightly impairs the ability to maintain a constant headway while following another car' under actual driving conditions. The road tracking impairment researchers found that this dosage 'was within a range of effects produced by many commonly used medicinal drugs and less than that associated with a blood alcohol concentration of 0.08% in previous studies employing the same test.' These investigators concluded:

> Marijuana, when taken alone, produces a moderate degree of driving impairment which is related to the consumed THC dose. The impairment manifests itself mainly in the ability to maintain a steady lateral position on the road, but its magnitude is not exceptional in comparison with changes produced by many medicinal drugs and alcohol. Drivers under the influence of marijuana retain insight in their performance and will compensate, where they can, for example, by slowing down or increasing effort. As a consequence, THC's adverse effects on driving performance appear relatively small. ... Of the many psychotropic drugs, licit and illicit, that are available and used by people who subsequently drive, marijuana may well be among the least harmful.

The UK Department for Transport recently reviewed seven simulator studies and 10 road trials (including the study by Robbe and O'Hanlon described above) that examined the effects of cannabis and, usually, alcohol on driving skills (UK Department for Transport, 2000). This review built on (and concurred with) an earlier analysis of these same studies by Smiley (1999). Tables prepared for the DFT report are reproduced here (Tables 12.3 and 12.4); these list the methods and major findings of these studies.

Table 12.3 Tabulated summary of simulator studies of cannabis and driving

Study	Design[a]	Dose[b]	Time[c] (h)	Task[d]	Measures[e]	Effect[f]
Crancer et al., 1969	n = 36 WS Cannabis Placebo Alcohol	314 µg/kg 0 0.10 BAC	0.5 2.5 4.0	**Environment:** Filmed driving (23 min), operating speedometer, non-interactive **Task:** Operate vehicle controls as appropriate to scene, adjust speedometer to keep within range set to scene speed limit	Speed outside range Inappropriate use of controls (errors) relative to scene: accelerator, brake signal, total errors	**Cannabis:** Only increased errors for speedometer out-of-range after 0.5 hours since consumption **Alcohol:** Increased out-of-range errors **Cannabis:** No control errors **Alcohol:** Increased all errors over entire period
Dott, 1972	n = 12 WS Cannabis Cannabis Placebo	157 µg/kg 314 µg/kg 0	0.5	**Environment:** View of model cars on a moving belt **Task:** Attempt passing manoeuvres with oncoming traffic (in some cases passing opportunities were signalled as an 'emergency', if a rapid response was required in that situation)	Number of emergency passes abandoned. (Decision) time from event to start of pass attempt: emergency cases, non-emergency cases	**Cannabis:** Both cannabis doses increased number of abandoned emergency pass attempts. Decision time increased, but only for non-emergency cases

(continued)

Table 12.3 Continued

Study	Design[a]	Dose[b]	Time[c] (h)	Task[d]	Measures[e]	Effect[f]
Ellingstad et al., 1973	n = 256 BS Cannabis Cannabis Placebo (non-users) Placebo (users) Alcohol Alcohol	161 μg/kg 318 μg/kg – – 0.5% BAC 0.10% BAC	0.5	**Environment:** Filmed presentation of over-taking (with minimum safety margin), followed by film clip of overtaking stages, non-interactive **Task:** Indicate point last moment that would overtake from clips	Accepted time for over-taking depicted in film clip	**Cannabis:** Both cannabis doses increased distance (time) accepted to over-take, with fewer 'unsafe' cases accepted, relative to other treatment conditions
Moskowitz et al., 1976	n = 23 WS Cannabis Cannabis Cannabis Placebo	50 μg/kg 100 μg/kg 200 μg/kg 0	0.25	**Environment:** Car cab with filmed presentation (45–70 min), semi-interactive (brake and accelerator affected presentation speed) **Task:** Vehicle control to follow road contour. Subsidiary visual choice reaction time task	**Vehicle control:** Mean speed, SD speed, SD lane position **Subsidiary task:** Responses, reaction time	**Cannabis:** No effect of cannabis dose on any control measures **Cannabis:** Increased reaction time for subsidiary task (and initial increase in incorrect responses)
Moskowitz et al., 1976	n = 10 WS Cannabis Placebo Alcohol	200 μg/kg 0 0.075% BAC	0.25	As above	**Visual search pattern:** Frequency and duration of eye glances	**Cannabis:** No effect of cannabis dose **Alcohol:** Alcohol increased duration and frequency of glances *(continued)*

Table 12.3 Continued

Study	Design[a]	Dose[b]	Time[c] (h)	Task[d]	Measures[e]	Effect[f]
Smiley et al., 1981	$n = 45$ BS Alcohol Alcohol Placebo WS (at each level of BS) Cannabis Cannabis Placebo	0.05% BAC 0.08% BAC 0 100 µg/kg 200 µg/kg 0	0.25	**Environment:** Fully interactive driving simulator with car cab and simplified road scene (45 min), inclusion of curves and wind gusts (pursuit and compensatory tracking) **Task:** Vehicle control to navigate route. Subsidiary (random) visual choice reaction time task. Performance rewarded and errors (crashes) penalised	**Vehicle control:** SD speed, SD lane position, SD headway, correct turns, crashes **Subsidiary task:** Reaction time	**Cannabis:** Cannabis increased speed and lane position variability during curves and wind gusts, and increased variability of headway and lane position when car following (particularly at high dose). Cannabis also resulted in fewer correct turns. The high dose produced more crashes under emergency conditions **Alcohol:** Few effects other than increase in lane position variability **Cannabis:** Increased reaction time for high dose only **Alcohol:** No effect

(continued)

Table 12.3 *Continued*

Study	Design[a]	Dose[b]	Time[c] (h)	Task[d]	Measures[e]	Effect[f]
Stein et al., 1983	n = 12 BS Alcohol Placebo WS (at each level of BS) Cannabis Cannabis Placebo	0.10% BAC 0 100 μg/kg 200 μg/kg 0	0.5	**Environment:** Similar to Smiley et al. (1981) **Task:** Similar to Smiley et al. (1981) except that (i) no performance incentive; (ii) inclusion of speeding check; (iii) subsidiary task was not random, involving responses made to signs embedded in scene	**Vehicle control:** **Subsidiary task:**	**Cannabis:** Few effects other than decrease in mean speed and change in steering control style **Alcohol:** More crashes and speeding cases, as well as increased lane position and speed variability **Cannabis:** No effects **Alcohol:** More sign recognition errors and increased response times

[a]Indicates overall sample size and design: within subject (WS) or between subject (BS). Control conditions involved placebo treatment of cannabis without THC or drink without alcohol.
[b]Calculated as mg of THC per kg bodyweight and percentage blood alcohol content (% BAC).
[c]Time elapsed between end of consumption and start of task.
[d]Description of simulation environment, level of interaction with input to the simulation, and the assigned primary and subsidiary tasks.
[e]Dependent measures for primary and subsidiary tasks.
[f]Main effects of treatment on dependent measures.
Adapted from Smiley (1986, 1999); UK Department for Transport Report (2000).

Table 12.4 Tabulated summary of road trials of cannabis and driving

Study	Design[a]	Dose[b]	Time[c] (h)	Task[d]	Measures[e]	Effect[f]
Klonoff, 1974 Study 1	$n = 64$ BS Cannabis Cannabis Placebo (Task was completed in blocks of trials. Block 2 & 3 were used to predict expected score for block 4 using multiple regression. Treatment was made between block 3 & 4. Observed performance in block 4 was compared to expected value. Deviation from CI of expected indicated impairment.)	70 µg/kg 120 µg/kg 0 µg/kg	—	**Environment:** Closed circuit **Tasks:** (a) Drive car through slalom courses and avoid contact with demarcating cones (b) Braking response to simulated emergency event (c) Determine if gap wide enough to accept car	Number of cones hit Braking distance Correct gap judgement	**Cannabis:** More cones were hit with cannabis, and most often with high dose **Cannabis:** No effect of cannabis **Cannabis:** Only high dose impaired gap judgement

(continued)

Table 12.4 Continued

Study	Design[a]	Dose[b]	Time[c] (h)	Task[d]	Measures[e]	Effect[f]
Klonoff, 1974 Study 2	n = 38 WS Cannabis Placebo BS dose	See BS 0 µg/kg 70 or 120 µg/kg	–	**Environment:** City street driving (27 km) **Task:** Drive in a mock attempt to pass driving test in presence of examiner	Normalised driving exam score	**Cannabis:** Only the high dose resulted in impairment, primarily in terms of judgement and concentration
Hansteen et al., 1976	n = 16 WS Cannabis Cannabis Placebo Alcohol	21 µg/kg 0 BAC 88 µg/kg 0 BAC 0 µg/kg 0 BAC 0.07% BAC 0 µg/kg	<25 h 3.0 h	**Environment:** Closed circuit (0.7 km) **Task:** Drive car as quickly as possible through slalom course and avoid contact with demarcating poles and cones	**Vehicle control:** Number of cones hit Observed awkward or superfluous movements	**Cannabis:** Only the high dose resulted in more hit cones. Only slight effect at 3 h **Alcohol:** More cones hit. Only slight effect at 3 h **Cannabis:** No effect **Alcohol:** Increased impairment

(continued)

Table 12.4 Continued

Study	Design[a]	Dose[b]	Time[c] (h)	Task[d]	Measures[e]	Effect[f]
					Mean speed (lap time)	**Cannabis:** Only the high dose resulted in a small reduction in mean speed (increased lap time). Only slight effect at 3 h **Alcohol:** No effect
Casswell, 1979	$n = 13$ WS		~40 min	**Environment:** Closed circuit (0.7 km) **Task:** Drive car as quickly as possible through slalom course and avoid contact with demarcating poles and cones **Subsidiary task:** Auditory signal detection	**Primary task:** Mean speed	**Cannabis:** Without alcohol, lower mean speed **Alcohol:** Increased speed alone and in (low dose) combination with cannabis
	Session 1a	0.10% BAC 0 µg/kg				
	Session 1b	0% BAC 89 µg/kg				
	Session 2a	0% BAC 0 µg/kg			Lateral position variability	**Cannabis:** No effect without alcohol **Alcohol:** Increased lateral position variability alone and in combination with cannabis
	Session 2b	0% BAC 89 µg/kg				
	Session 3a	0.05% BAC 44 µg/kg				
	Session 3b	0.05% BAC 44 µg/kg				

(continued)

Table 12.4 Continued

Study	Design[a]	Dose[b]	Time[c] (h)	Task[d]	Measures[e]	Effect[f]
Caswell, 1979					Steering wheel reversals	**Cannabis:** No effect without alcohol **Alcohol:** Decreased reversals variability alone and in combination with cannabis
					Subsidiary task: Reaction time	**Cannabis:** Slowed reaction time alone and in combination with high alcohol dose **Alcohol:** No effect of alcohol alone or in combination with low dose cannabis

(continued)

Table 12.4 *Continued*

Study	Design[a]	Dose[b]	Time[c] (h)	Task[d]	Measures[e]	Effect[f]
Attwood et al., 1981	n = 8 WS: Cannabis Alcohol Combined Double placebo	200 μg/kg 0% BAC 0 μg/kg 0.08% BAC 100 μg/kg 0.04% BAC 0 μg/kg 0% BAC	–	**Environment:** Closed runway (2 km) **Task:** Maintenance of speed, lateral position, and headway. Stopping vehicle (smoothly) at traffic signal. Decision to overtake with oncoming traffic	**Vehicle control:** e.g. speed, lateral position, headway, acceleration	No univariate effects (based on experiment-wise error rate): only multivariate discriminate analysis indicated that drugs (alcohol, cannabis) differed from control in terms of overall driving performance. Non-robust effects may be due to low n and absence of subsidiary task that would other-wise increase demand in a manner representing actual driving in traffic

(continued)

Table 12.4 Continued

Study	Design[a]	Dose[b]	Time[c] (h)	Task[d]	Measures[e]	Effect[f]
Peck et al., 1986	$n = 84$ BS: Cannabis Alcohol Combined Placebo	270 µg/kg 0% BAC 0 µg/kg 0.08% BAC 270 µg/kg 0.08% BAC 0 µg/kg 0% BAC	4 times at <25 h and hourly	**Environment:** Closed circuit **Task:** Vehicle control on route, gap acceptance, stopping at signal, forced lane changes, slalom section, field sobriety test, and standard laboratory tests of tracking and time estimation	**Vehicle control:** Driving examination. Sobriety test scores. Laboratory test scores	No univariate effects (based on experiment-wise error rate): only multivariate discriminate analysis indicated that drugs (alcohol, cannabis) differed from control. Effect of cannabis significant for all periods, but greatest in first. Alcohol effect greater than cannabis. Combined effect greater than either drug alone.
Smiley et al., 1986	$n = 16$ BS Alcohol Placebo WS (at each level of BS) Cannabis Cannabis Placebo and Alcohol (as a separate condition)	0.05% BAC 0% BAC 100 µg/kg 200 µg/kg 0 µg/kg 0.08% BAC	Over a 3-h period	**Environment:** Closed circuit under 'party like' conditions in evening **Primary task:** Respond to situations 'representative' of normal driving and alcohol/drug-involved accidents **Subsidiary task:** Visual target detection	**Vehicle control:** Mean headway, SD headway	**Cannabis:** Only the larger dose increased mean headway distance and variability **Alcohol:** No effect

(continued)

Table 12.4 Continued

Study	Design[a]	Dose[b]	Time[c] (h)	Task[d]	Measures[e]	Effect[f]
					Mean speed	**Cannabis:** No effect **Alcohol:** Increased speed
					Subsidiary task: Target detections	**Cannabis:** No effect **Alcohol:** Reduced detection at low dose, but increased at larger dose
Robbe and O'Hanlon, 1993 Study 2	$n = 23$ WS Cannabis Cannabis Cannabis Placebo	100 µg/kg 200 µg/kg 300 µg/kg 0 µg/kg	40 min 100 min	**Environment:** Closed highway (11 km) **Task:** Maintain speed target speed (90 kph) and lateral position along route	**Vehicle control:** SD Lateral position Mean speed	**Cannabis:** Lateral position variability increased for all doses **Cannabis:** Mean speed was near target value (with non-significant decrease in speed with higher doses). In two cases, the instructor had to intervene under the high-dose condition because subjects did not attend to obstacle in road

Table 12.4 Continued

Study	Design[a]	Dose[b]	Time[c] (b)	Task[d]	Measures[e]	Effect[f]
Robbe and O'Hanlon, 1993 Study 2					**Laboratory tests:** Compensatory tracking Hand steadiness	**Cannabis:** No effect for tracking
						Cannabis: Steadiness decreased for all doses
					Subject opinion: Performance	**Cannabis:** Performance quality was perceived to be worse for all doses
					Effort	**Cannabis:** Perceived effort increased and was highest for the largest dose
Robbe and O'Hanlon, 1993 Study 3	$n = 15$ WS Level 1 Level 2 Level 3	100 µg/kg 0 µg/kg 200 µg/kg 0 µg/kg 300 µg/kg 0 µg/kg	50 min 175 min	**Environment:** Open highway in traffic (16 km) **Task:** Two trials of car following on open highway in traffic to maintain 50 m distance with lead car changing speed (at an interval rate of 0.02 Hz). One trial of standard driving test as in Study 2	**Vehicle control:** Reaction time to lead vehicle speed change	**Cannabis:** Reaction time increased except for highest dose, and was correlated with mean distance ($r = 0.76$). With mean headway as a covariate, the effect for reaction time is non-significant

(continued)

Table 12.4 Continued

Study	Design[a]	Dose[b]	Time[c] (h)	Task[d]	Measures[e]	Effect[f]
					Headway distance	**Cannabis:** Mean headway near to target, with increased headway only for low dose
					SD Lateral position	**Cannabis:** Lateral position variability increased with the larger doses, but not the lowest
					Mean speed	**Cannabis:** Mean speed was near target speed, with significant speed reduction (1.1 kph) only for middle dose
					Laboratory tests: Compensatory tracking Hand steadiness	**Cannabis:** The highest dose impaired tracking **Cannabis:** All doses impaired hand steadiness
					Body sway	**Cannabis:** Body sway affected cannabis, but insensitive to dose

(continued)

Table 12.4 Continued

Study	Design[a]	Dose[b]	Time[c] (h)	Task[d]	Measures[e]	Effect[f]
Robbe and O'Hanlon, 1993 Study 3					**Subject opinion:** Performance	**Cannabis:** Perceived quality of performance was reduced for both higher doses (approached significance), but not the lowest
					Effort	**Cannabis:** No significant effect on perceived effort
Robbe and O'Hanlon, 1993 Study 4	$n = 30$ BS Cannabis, Alcohol	100 µg/kg 0 µg/kg 0.05% BAC 0% BAC	35 min 95 min	**Environment:** City driving in traffic (17.5 km) **Task:** Follow prescribed route, including specific manoeuvres such as repeated Y-turn	Driving proficiency (Molecular judgement by instructor based on 'online' assessment of driving performance. Molar judgement by instructor based on retrospective assessment of driving performance)	**Cannabis:** No effect for molecular or molar judgements **Alcohol:** No effect of molecular judgements, but impaired performance for molar judgements of vehicle handling and actions in traffic. Vehicle handling was significantly worse for alcohol compared to cannabis

(continued)

Table 12.4 *Continued*

Study	Design[a]	Dose[b]	Time[c] (h)	Task[d]	Measures[e]	Effect[f]
					Laboratory tests: Hand steadiness	**Cannabis:** Decreased hand steadiness **Alcohol:** Alcohol improved steadiness, but only shortly after drinking
					Time perception (indicate end of estimated 30 second period with eyes closed)	**Cannabis:** Time period was foreshortened, but only at the end of the session **Alcohol:** No effect on time estimation
					Subject opinion: Performance	**Cannabis:** Rated quality of performance was reduced **Alcohol:** No effect
					Effort	**Cannabis:** The amount of reported effort increased **Alcohol:** No effect

[a]Indicates overall sample size and design: within subject (WS) or between subject (BS). Control conditions involved placebo treatment of cannabis without THC or drink without alcohol.
[b]Calculated as mg of THC per kg bodyweight and percentage blood alcohol content (BAC).
[c]Time elapsed between end of consumption and start of task.
[d]Description of road environment and the assigned primary and subsidiary tasks.
[e]Dependent measures for primary and subsidiary tasks.
[f]Main effects of treatment on dependent measures.
Adapted from Smiley (1986, 1998); UK Department for Transport (2000).

The Department for Transport analysis reported that the simulator studies and road trials were consistent in their findings, which were:

1. Cannabis produces a consistent, mild to moderate impairment in tracking ability (keeping in centre of lane) and an increased variability in speed and headway. These were in the same range as observed in the Robbe and O'Hanlon (1993) study (less than that seen with blood alcohol concentrations of 0.08%).

2. Subjects taking cannabis take longer to decide whether to overtake and in the distance required before overtaking is attempted. This finding can be interpreted as producing either an unwanted delay in decision time or a salutary 'moment of reconsideration' before undertaking an inherently dangerous manoeuvre.

3. Cannabis induces more cautious driving habits, including slower speeds and larger headways and distances required before overtaking. This caution is generally interpreted as a sign that subjects under the influence of cannabis are aware of their impairment and take steps to compensate, whereas subjects with alcohol in their systems have little or no insight into their impairment and thus take no steps to compensate.

In her earlier review, Smiley concluded similarly:

> Marijuana impairs driving behaviour. However, this impairment is mitigated in that subjects under marijuana treatment appear to perceive that they are indeed impaired. Where they can compensate, they do, for example by not overtaking, by slowing down and by focusing their attention when they know a response will be required. ... Effects on driving behaviour are present up to an hour after smoking but do not continue for extended periods. ... With respect to comparisons between alcohol and marijuana effects, these substances tend to differ in their effects. In contrast to the compensatory behaviour exhibited by subjects under marijuana treatment, subjects who have received alcohol tend to drive in a more risky manner. Both substances impair performance; however, the more cautious behaviour of subjects who have received marijuana decreases the impact of the drug on performance, whereas the opposite holds true for alcohol. (Smiley, 1998)

Subsequent to these analyses, Britain's Transport Research Laboratory conducted a government-sponsored study of 18 experienced marijuana users who were examined using a driving simulator after ingesting various doses of marijuana (Sexton *et al.*, 2002). Again, researchers found a reduction in average speed by participants after high or low doses of marijuana, suggesting drivers were aware of their impairment. Steering ability was found to decrease with higher doses, and reaction times increased with dose level, but not significantly so. The investigators concluded:

> Overall, it is possible to conclude that cannabis has a measurable effect on psychomotor performance, particularly tracking ability. Its effect on higher cognitive functions, for example divided attention tasks associated with driving, appear not to be as critical. Drivers under the influence of cannabis seem aware that they are impaired, and attempt to compensate for this impairment by reducing the difficulty of the driving task, for example by driving more slowly. In terms of road safety, it cannot be concluded that driving under the influence of cannabis is not a hazard, as the effects on various aspects of driver performance are unpredictable. However, in comparison with alcohol, the severe effects of alcohol on the higher cognitive processes of driving are likely to make this more of a hazard, particularly at higher blood alcohol levels.

Of interest in this regard is a recent finding that chronic exposure to cannabis, in the absence of acute administration, may improve driving performance after alcohol use (Wright and Terry, 2002).

In its evaluation of cannabis, conducted in 1997, the UK's House of Lords reached a conclusion similar to those already cited:

> Impairment in driving skills does not appear to be severe, even immediately after taking cannabis, when subjects are tested in a driving simulator. This may be because people intoxicated by cannabis appear to compensate for their impairment by taking fewer risks and driving more slowly, whereas alcohol tends to encourage people to take greater risks and drive more aggressively. (House of Lords Select Committee on Science and Technology, 1998)

Similarly, in its review of the cannabis-and-driving literature, the European Monitoring Centre for Drugs and Drug Addiction concluded in 1999:

> Where experimental studies are concerned, although there is some conflicting evidence, cannabis does not seem to significantly impair very basic perceptual mechanisms. However cannabis does impair more subtle aspects of perceptual performance such as attention and short-term memory, although these are typically observed at higher doses. Most experimental studies have used fairly low doses of cannabis and this may not reflect the doses ingested by heavy marihuana users. (European Monitoring Centre for Drugs and Drug Addiction, 1999)

The insight cannabis users appear to have concerning the extent of any impairment they are experiencing may have an even more salutary effect insofar as these individuals may be more likely to decline to drive while impaired, than people who are under the influence of alcohol. Robbe and O'Hanlon (1993) found that a majority of smokers (about 65%) were not willing to drive a car for relatively unimportant reasons shortly after smoking (Robbe and O'Hanlon, 1993). However, most said they would drive for a very urgent reason. Willingness to drive was correlated to amount consumed and urgency, but not to actual impairment.

The combination of mild impairment and insight concerning this impairment is clearly preferable to the moderate or severe impairment, without insight, produced by alcohol. For most driving situations, accordingly, cannabis cannot be considered a hazard to traffic safety. However, whether cannabis might produce deleterious effects in the setting of more complicated or emergency type driving conditions is unknown. This point is discussed in the UK Department for Transport report:

> It is not clear whether the compensatory action of impaired drivers is sufficient to maintain an adequate safety margin. The consideration of a 'safety margin' must relate both to the behavioural and cognitive domains. Not only must the compensation provide effective per-formance to achieve task goals relevant to safety, it must also provide efficient performance to cope with the task demands. Thus, even in the absence of overt impairment of behaviour, the level of effort invested to compensate for the effect of cannabis must not deplete mental resources to the extent that (unexpected) task demands cannot be managed. To the extent that drivers compensate for the effect of cannabis, they appear able to manage routine and low demand tasks, but the remaining cognitive resources may not be sufficient to cope with peak and unexpected demands (Smiley, 1998). Further research is required to examine the mechanism and limitation of these compensa-tory effects under different levels of task predictability and demand levels.

The body of evidence reviewed above is remarkable in its consistency. It must be concluded that what evidence exists supports the view that the effects of cannabis on driving skills stand in sharp contrast to those pro-duced by alcohol. Clearly the two substances produce their cognitive effects in markedly different ways.

One factor not considered in any studies to date is the possibility that cannabis may improve vision, especially at night. Jamaican fishermen have reported improved night vision after smoking cannabis and experiments confirmed that cannabis increases blood flow to the retina (Brady, 2000). Also, to the extent cannabis can substitute for other psychoactive substances, such as tranquillisers, narcotics and antidepressants, decrements in driving skills could be reduced.

Medicinal cannabis and driving

The studies reviewed above were all conducted with healthy volunteers. It is unclear how the findings from these studies apply to patients who use cannabis or cannabis-based medicines for the relief of pain, spasticity and other symptoms. It is quite possible that relief of such symptoms could improve driving skills. A newly approved study to be conducted at the University of California's Center for Medicinal Cannabis Research will evaluate the effect on driving skills of three doses of cannabis or placebo on patients treated with smoked cannabis for spasticity associated with multiple sclerosis and for HIV-related peripheral neuropathy. The results of this study will represent the first data on the effects on driving skills of cannabis taken for medicinal purposes.

Similar considerations apply to the problem of fatigue and driving. In the US approximately 40 000 non-fatal injuries and 1550 fatalities result each year from crashes in which driver drowsiness/fatigue was cited by police. (It is widely recognised that these statistics underreport the extent of these types of crashes.) Relevant impairments identified in laboratory and in-vehicle studies due to drowsiness include slower reaction time, reduced vigilance, and deficits in information processing (www.nhtsa.dot.gov/people/perform/human/drowsy.html). Cannabis-based medicines that improve sleep for patients with, for example, chronic pain or multiple sclerosis, can be expected to result in safer driving from this perspective.

The absence of evidence implicating cannabis and cannabinoids in traffic collisions is reflected in the rather mild label warning accompanying the pharmaceutical drug Marinol, which is pure THC dissolved in sesame oil inside a capsule. This agent is approved in the United States to treat nausea associated with chemotherapy, and for appetite enhancement in patients with HIV infection. In 1999, The Drug Enforcement Agency reclassified Marinol from a Schedule II to a Schedule III medication, and to date 41 of 50 states have followed suit. Marinol's package states: 'Patients receiving treatment with Marinol should be specifically warned not to drive, operate machinery, or engage in any hazardous activity until it is established that they are able to tolerate the drug and to perform such tasks safely' (www.marinol.com). This is similar to warnings for benzodiazepines, morphine and other sedatives and analgesics, despite the measurable deleterious effects of these agents on risk-taking, drowsiness, accidents and culpability (www.nhtsa.dot.gov/people/perform/human/drowsy.html). This leaves open the question whether the patient or carer is the judge of the patient's ability to drive, or operate machinery safely. In the UK, the highway code states that:

Motor vehicles: drink and drugs

Driving, or being in charge, when under influence of drink or drugs.

4. – (1) A person who, when driving or attempting to drive a motor vehicle on a road or other public place, is unfit to drive through drink or drugs is guilty of an offence.
(2) Without prejudice to subsection (1) above, a person who, when in charge of a motor vehicle which is on a road or other public place, is unfit to drive through drink or drugs is guilty of an offence.
(3) For the purposes of subsection (2) above, a person shall be deemed not to have been in charge of a motor vehicle if he proves that at the material time the circumstances were such that there was no likelihood of his driving it so long as he remained unfit to drive through drink or drugs.
(4) The court may, in determining whether there was such a likelihood as is mentioned in subsection (3) above, disregard any injury to him and any damage to the vehicle.
(5) For the purposes of this section, a person shall be taken to be unfit to drive if his ability to drive properly is for the time being impaired.
(6) A constable may arrest a person without warrant if he has reasonable cause to suspect that that person is or has been committing an offence under this section.
(7) For the purpose of arresting a person under the power conferred by subsection (6) above, a constable may enter (if need be by force) any place where that person is or where the constable, with reasonable cause, suspects him to be.
(8) Subsection (7) above does not extend to Scotland, and nothing in that subsection affects any rule of law in Scotland concerning the right of a constable to enter any premises for any purpose.

The likely effects of medicinal cannabis on driving skills are best considered in relation to such produced by other commonly used pharmaceutical products for similar conditions. The use of standardised measures of driving skills, especially Standard Deviation of Lateral Position (SDLP), permits cross-comparisons of different drugs in this regard.

No dose [of cannabis] significantly affected this group's car following performance but all elevated SDLP in the Road Tracking Test. Relative to the placebo level, mean SDLP rose by 1.1, 1.8 and 2.9 cm in rough proportion to the THC dose. Though all significant, these changes were very modest in comparison to those produced by alcohol and a number of medicinal drugs in previous investigations. ... THC's effects were also far less than those of some commonly used medicinal drugs. For example, after a week of receiving diazepam 5 mg (Valium), thrice daily, and lorazepam 2 mg (Ativan), twice daily, different groups of clinically anxious patients drove with mean SDLPs that were respectively 7 and 10 cm higher than baseline (O'Hanlon *et al.*, 1995). Thus, we concluded that THC taken alone in doses preferred by its users does not seriously affect driving performance. (Robbe and O'Hanlon, 1993)

Thus, deviations in centre-line position were 3–10 times higher with benzodiazapine drugs than with cannabis (Verster *et al.*, 2002). Studies have also demonstrated significantly impaired driving skills associated with the use of antihistamines (O'Hanlon and Ramaekers, 1995; Weiler *et al.*, 2000), zopiclone (Vermeeren *et al.*, 2002) and prochlorperazine (Betts *et al.*, 1991). Subjects did not 'appreciate the impairment' produced by prochlorperazine, in contrast to the findings with cannabis, discussed above.

The use and effects of antidepressive drugs (including tricyclic antidepressants, TCAs) on psychomotor performance have been investigated and considered to a limited extent (Van Laar *et al.*, 1995; Soyka *et al.*, 1998). Empirical studies have shown that the use of these drugs can increase the risk of driving accidents in elderly patients and that different drug groups showed different effects. TCAs in particular were shown to worsen cognitive and psychomotor performance in some patients and, in comparison, serotonin-type antidepressive drugs produced less behavioural toxicity. It is generally understood that TCAs do impair cognitive ability when driving but further studies are necessary to fully explore their effects.

In terms of effects on driving performance, a particular concern to legislators, and therefore analysts, is the willingness of many motorists to drive under the influence not only of cannabis but frequently of several substances. Additional research is required on the effects of other drugs and substances that may be taken concomitantly with cannabis, for example, antidepressants. This trend contrasts with the increasing approbation of society in many Western countries to alcohol and tobacco. This concern has prompted the development of robust and sensitive legally defensible analyses for the determination of THC and its metabolites in body fluids in even lower concentrations.

In conclusion, driving ability does not appear to be substantially impaired by cannabis. Any impairment is well within the range of (or lower than) what is currently produced by pharmaceutical agents which are commonly used for similar conditions.

References

Attwood D A, Williams R D, Madhill H D (1981). Effects of moderate blood alcohol concentration on closed-course driving performance. *J Stud Alcohol* 41: 623–634.

Bates M, Blakeley A T (1999). Role of cannabis in motor vehicle crashes. *Epidemiol Rev* 21: 222–232.

Becker J, Junker T, Koepf W *et al.* (1992). Incidence of cannabis consumption among impaired road users in Rheinland-Pfalz. *Sucht* 38: 238–243.

Betts T, Harris D, Gadd E (1991). The effects of two anti-vertigo drugs (betahistine and prochlorperazine) on driving skills. *Br J Clin Pharmacol* 32: 455–458.

Brady P (2000). Ganja medicine in Jamaica. Jamaican researchers have developed legal marijuana medicines. *Cannabis Culture Magazine* CC23: January 16.

Casswell S (1979). Cannabis and alcohol effects on closed course driving behaviour. In: *Proceedings of the Seventh International Conference on Alcohol, Drugs and Traffic Safety, Melbourne*. Canberra: Australian Government Printer.

Chesher G B, Longo M (2002). Cannabis and alcohol in motor vehicle accidents. In: Gotenhermen F, Russo E, eds. *Cannabis and Cannabinoids: Pharmacology, Toxicology, and Therapeutic Potential*. Binghamton, NY: Haworth Press: 101–110.

Chesher G B, Starmer G A (1983). Cannabis and human performance skills. Drug and Alcohol Authority Research, Grant Report Series, Sydney.

Cimbura G, Lucas D M, Bennett R C, Donelson A C (1990). Incidence and toxicological aspects of cannabis and ethanol detected in 1394 fatally injured drivers and pedestrians in Ontario (1982–1984). *J Forens Sci* 35: 1035–1041.

Crancer A Jr, Dille J M, Delay J C *et al.* (1969). Comparison of the effects of marihuana and alcohol on simulated driving performance. *Science* 164: 851–854.

Donelson A C, Cimbura G, Bennett R C, Lucas D M (1985). The Ontario monitoring project: Cannabis and alcohol use among drivers and pedestrians fatally injured in motor vehicle accidents from March 1982 through July 1984. Traffic Injury Research Foundation of Canada, Ottawa.

Dott A (1972). Effect of marihuana on risk acceptance in a simulated passing task. DHEW publication HSM-72-10010. Department of Health, Education, and Welfare, Washington DC.

Drummer O, Chu, M (1999). Stability of THC. Melbourne Victorian Institute of Forensic Medicine, Department of Forensic Medicine Monash University.

Ellingstad V, McFarling L, Struckman D (1973). Alcohol, marijuana and risk-taking. DOT-HS-191-2-301. University of South Dakota, Vermillion.

European Monitoring Centre for Drugs and Drug Addiction (1999). *Literature Review on the Relation between Drug Use, Impaired Driving and Traffic Accidents*. (CT.97.EP.14). Lisbon: EMCDDA.

Fergusson D M, Horwood L J (2001). Cannabis use and traffic accidents in a birth cohort of young adults. *Accid Anal Prev* 33: 703–711.

Hansteen R W, Miller R D, Lonero L *et al.* (1976). Effects of cannabis and alcohol on automobile driving and psychomotor tracking. *Ann NY Acad Sci* 282: 240–256.

Harvey D J (1987). Mass spectrometry of the cannabinoids and their metabolites. *Mass Spectrom Rev* 6: 135–229.

House of Lords Select Committee on Science and Technology (1998). *Cannabis: The Scientific and Medical Evidence.* The House of Lords Session 1997–8, 9th report. London: Stationery Office. http://www.publications.parliament.uk/pa/ld199798/ldselect/ldsctech/151/15101.htm

Hunt C A, Jones R T (1980). Tolerance and disposition of tetrahydrocannabinol in man. *J Pharmacol Exp Ther* 215: 33–44.

Hunter C, Lokan R, Longo M, White J, White M (1998). *The Prevalence and Role of Alcohol, Cannabinoids, Benzodiazepines and Stimulants in Non-Fatal Crashes.* Adelaide: Forensic Science, Department for Administrative and Information Services, South Australia.

Kielholz P, Hobi V, Ladewig D *et al.* (1973). An experimental investigation about the effects of cannabis on car driving behaviour. *Pharmakopyschiatry* 6: 91–103.

Klonoff H (1974). Marijuana and driving in real-life situations. *Science* 186: 317–324.

Logan B K (1994). *Drug and Alcohol Use in Fatally Injured Drivers in Washington State.* Seattle, WA: Washington State Toxicology Laboratory, Department of Laboratory Medicine, University of Washington.

Mason A P, McBay A J (1984). Ethanol, marijuana, and other drug use in 600 drivers killed in single-vehicle crashes in North Carolina. *J Forensic Sci* 29: 987–1026.

Moskowitz H, Sharma S, McGlothlin W (1972). Effect of marihuana upon peripheral vision as a function of the information processing demands in central vision. *Percept Motor Skills* 35: 875–882.

Moskowitz H, Ziedman K, Sharma S (1976). Visual search behaviour while viewing driving scenes under the influence of alcohol and marijuana. *Hum Factors* 18: 417–431.

O'Hanlon J F, Ramaekers J G (1995). Antihistamine effects on actual driving performance in a standard test: a summary of Dutch experience, 1989–94. *Allergy* 50: 234–242.

O'Hanlon J F, Vermeeren A, Uiterwijk M M *et al.* (1995). Anxiolytics' effects on the actual driving performance of patients and healthy volunteers in a standardized test. An integration of three studies. *Neuropsychobiology* 31: 81–88.

Peck R C, Biasotti A, Boland P N *et al.* (1986). The effects of marijuana and alcohol on actual driving performance. *Alcohol Drugs Driving Abstr Rev* 2: 3–4.

Robbe H W L, O'Hanlon J F (1993). Marijuana and actual driving performance. DOT-HS 808 078. Department of Transportation: Washington DC: 66.

Sexton B F, Tunbridge R J, Brook-Carter N *et al.* (2001). The influence of cannabis on driving. TRL report TRL477. Summary at: http://www.roads.dtlr.gov.uk/roadsafety/research16 (accessed 4 March 2002).

Sexton B F, Tunbridge R J, Brook-Carter N *et al.* (2002). The influence of cannabis on driving. TRL Limited, Berkshire, UK. http://www.trl.co.uk/1024/reports.asp?url=477.htm (accessed January 2004).

Smiley A (1986). Marijuana: on-road and driving simulator studies. *Alcohol Drugs Driving* 2: 121–134.

Smiley A (1999). Marijuana: on-road and driving-simulator studies. In: Kalant H *et al.*, eds. *The Health Effects of Cannabis.* Toronto: Center for Addiction and Mental Health: 173–188.

Smiley A M, Moskowitz H, Ziedman K (1981). Driving simulator studies of marihuana alone and in combination with alcohol. In: *Proceedings of the 25th Conference of the American Association for Automotive Medicine*: 285–291.

Smink B E, Ruiter B, Lusthof K J, Zweipfenning P G M (2001). Driving under the influence of alcohol and/or drugs in the Netherlands 1995–1998 in view of the German and Belgian legislation. *Forens Sci Int* 120: 195–203.

Solowij N (1998). *Cannabis and Cognitive Functioning*. Cambridge: Cambridge University Press.

Soyka M, Dittert S, Gartenmeier A, Schafer M (1998). Driving fitness in therapy with antidepressive drugs. *Versicherungsmedizin* 50: 59–66.

Stein A C, Allen R W, Cook M L et al. (1983). A simulator study of the combined effects of alcohol and marijuana on driving behaviour – phase II. Department of Transportation, Washington DC.

Stonebraker W E, Lamoreaux T C, Bebault M et al. (1998). Robotic solid-phase extraction and GC-MS analysis of THC in blood. *Am Clin Lab* July: 18–19.

Terhune K W, Ippolito C A, Hendricks D L et al. (1992). The incidence and role of drugs in fatally injured drivers. DOT-HS 808 065. US Department of Transportation, Washington DC.

UK Department for Transport (2000). Cannabis and driving: a review of the literature and commentary. Department for Transport, London: chapter 5.

van Laar M W, van Willigenburg A P, Volkerts E R (1995). Acute and subchronic effects of nefazodone and imipramine on highway driving, cognitive functions, and daytime sleepiness in healthy adult and elderly subjects. *J Clin Psychopharmacol* 15: 30–40.

Vermeeren A, Riedel W J, van Boxtel M P et al. (2002). Differential residual effects of zaleplon and zopiclone on actual driving: a comparison with a low dose of alcohol. *Sleep* 25: 224–231.

Verster J C, Volkerts E R, Verbaten M N (2002). Effects of alprazolam on driving ability, memory functioning and psychomotor performance. A randomized, placebo-controlled study. *Neuropsychopharmacology* 27: 260–269.

Warren R, Simpson H, Hilchie J et al. (1981). Drugs detected in fatally injured drivers in the province of Ontario. In: *Proceedings of the 8th International Conference on Alcohol Drugs and Traffic Safety*. Stockholm: Almqvist and Wiksell International: 203–217.

Wegenverkeerswet (1994) Road Traffic Law, Stb. 1995, 475.

Weiler J M, Bloomfield J R, Woodworth G G et al. (2000). Effects of fexofenadine, diphenhydramine, and alcohol on driving performance. A randomized, placebo-controlled trial in the Iowa driving simulator. *Ann Intern Med* 132: 354–363.

Williams A, Peat M, Crouch D et al. (1985). Drugs in fatally injured young male drivers. *Public Health Rep* 100: 19–25.

Wright K A, Terry P (2002). Modulation of the effects of alcohol on driving-related psychomotor skills by chronic exposure to cannabis. *Psychopharmacology* 160: 987–1026.

13

International control of cannabis: changing attitudes

Alice Mead

At the beginning of the nineteenth century, warfare, colonisation and expanding trade exposed Europeans to the traditions and products of foreign lands. At that time, the Western world knew cannabis primarily as hemp, a critical source of fibre for textiles and naval products. However, for many centuries throughout Asia, India, Africa and the countries of the Arabian Peninsula, its use had been deeply embedded in the culture. Called by a variety of names, cannabis played an important role in religious ceremonies, cultural rituals and other social practices; provided therapeutic relief for a variety of ailments; and served as a source of nutrition. In short, it was viewed as a valuable herb with multiple functions.

Travellers brought back fascinating tales about the habits and customs of these far-off places. As a part of this cultural adventuring, physicians were introduced to the medicinal aspects of cannabis. Dr W B O'Shaughnessy, a surgeon under the employ of the British East India Company, was intrigued to learn that, in India, cannabis was used successfully for a variety of medical conditions. He investigated the effects of cannabis on animals and later, on patients. His writings described the therapeutic benefits of cannabis in the treatment of a variety of conditions, including cholera, tetanus and epilepsy.

In France, Dr Jacques-Joseph Moreau de Tours used cannabis (in the form of hashish) as a tool to explore the nature of mental illness. To pursue his investigation, Moreau enlisted the aid of a number of writers, poets and other artists, who formed the Club des Hachichins. Some of those members wrote sensationalistic accounts that captured the imagination of the reading public. English and American writers produced similarly popular writings.

The writings of O'Shaughnessy and Moreau de Tours ignited widespread interest within the medical profession, particularly in Europe and, to a more limited extent, in the United States. In 1860, the Ohio

Medical Society produced a report listing a large number of medical conditions that had been successfully treated by cannabis. Physicians prescribed cannabis freely, and it could be purchased from pharmacies and patent medicine salesmen. Cannabis appeared in national pharmacopoeias, joining other herbal medicines. Cannabis preparations – tinctures, fluid extracts and tablets – were generally administered orally, as were most herbal products.

Hence, as the twentieth century approached, the Western world did not view cannabis as a dangerous threat. Indeed, when questions as to its safety did arise the only extensive report to examine the issue – the Indian Hemp Commission Report – concluded in 1894 that in India the use of cannabis was a long-established social custom that, in moderation, did not pose serious dangers. The Commission's findings have been summarised as follows (Abel, 1980):

1. Moderate use of cannabis drugs had no appreciable physical effects on the body. As with all drugs, excessive use could weaken the body and render it more susceptible to diseases. Such circumstances were not peculiar to cannabis, however.
2. Moderate use of cannabis drugs had no adverse effect on the brain, except possibly for individuals predisposed to act abnormally. Excessive use, on the other hand, could lead to mental instability and ultimately to insanity in individuals predisposed by heredity to mental disorders.
3. Moderate use of cannabis drugs had no adverse influence on morality. Excessive use, however, could result in moral degradation. Although in certain rare cases cannabis intoxication could result in violence, such cases were few and far between.

The Report recommended that, rather than prohibition, cannabis use should continue to be controlled through taxation and regulation. Since cannabis taxation already provided a substantial source of revenue for the English Government, that recommendation was followed.

However, ethnic prejudices and other social and political influences rapidly overtook such benign approaches, and, as the twentieth century unfolded, cannabis became a 'demon weed', the target of antipathy and scorn.

A case study: the United States

Nowhere was that drama more vividly enacted than in the United States. Furthermore, the influence of its cannabis policies extended across the Western world. But for the US, international cannabis control might have evolved in quite a different manner. Ironically, the US can also be considered the birthplace of renewed interest in the therapeutic potential of cannabis. Hence, it may be instructive to begin an historical review and analysis by focusing on the path of cannabis control in the US.

Despite its initial popularity in the 1800s, the 'respectability' of cannabis did not last long. First, it fell out of favour as a medicine and as an agricultural commodity. Second, in its smoked form, it became associated in the public mind with dangerous 'narcotics' – as well as with dangerous lower class groups – and consequently with addiction, crime and insanity.

Loss of support within the medical profession

By the end of the nineteenth century, opiates and other manufactured pharmaceuticals had largely eclipsed the use of cannabis preparations. Being water soluble, opiates could be administered by means of the new hypodermic needle, thereby affording extremely rapid analgesic effect. By contrast, cannabis was primarily administered by oral means, although cannabis cigarettes were used to a limited extent for treatment of asthma. As a result, its onset of action was slow, and patient responses varied considerably. The active ingredient had not yet been identified, and dosages could not be standardised. The potency of commercial preparations differed significantly from pharmacy to pharmacy (Abel, 1980). Researchers had not been able to identify animal tests that could reflect on the drug's activity in humans. Cannabis preparations were also highly unstable. Finally, manufactured medicines containing only a single active principle were considered superior to complex herbal remedies. By the early part of the twentieth century, cannabis products were infrequently used, despite the fact that they offered some clear advantages over opiates (Adams, 1973; Mikuriya, 1973).

Decline in industrial/agricultural use

Interest in the industrial uses of hemp had also declined. The advent of the Civil War, the disappearance of slavery and the need for large-scale farming operations gradually made hemp cultivation economically infeasible. Because the harvesting and processing of hemp were so labour intensive, the cost of hiring labour made hemp prices uncompetitive with those of other plant fibres. Cotton and wool could be more easily spun for clothing. Jute fibre was a more economic substitute for twine and carpet warps. Germany developed a process of producing paper from trees. With the advent of steamships, sails made from hemp fibre were no longer needed. Hemp cultivation declined and virtually disappeared by the end of the 1920s (Lupien, 1995).

Increasing concern with drug addiction

As the nineteenth century waned, social reform movements sought to abolish the use of narcotics and alcohol. Particularly in the United States, the gathering momentum of these crusades swept cannabis into their ambit. While these movements had important differences, they shared common features. Prohibition was their chosen vehicle of control, and inflammatory rhetoric, rather than objective science, was their justification (Bonnie and Whitebread, 1970, 1974).

Initially, concern focused on opium, coca, morphine and their derivatives. The medical use of these substances had not been benign. The medical profession, not fully aware of morphine's addictive character, freely prescribed it to patients, many of whom became addicted. Furthermore, morphine and cocaine were present in significant quantities in many patent medicines, which were readily available from pharmacies, general stores, and travelling salesmen. As a result, 'accidental' addiction was common, particularly among the middle class. Inhabitants of rural areas, forced to self-medicate because they lacked access to physicians, were more likely than city dwellers to use patent medicines. Women were more affected than men. Some have estimated that between 2 and 5% of the adult population was addicted to morphine (Whitebread, 1995). Such addiction was viewed with compassion and alarm, rather than disgust.

Pressure built for the enactment of federal legislation. The Federal Government responded with the federal Pure Food and Drug Act of 1906 (PFDA). This law (1) required that certain drugs could only be sold on prescription; (2) established the Food and Drug Administration (FDA) and afforded it the authority to approve food and drugs; and (3) required labels to apprise consumers of the product's morphine or cocaine content. The PDFA effectively prevented the sale of patent medicines and thereby significantly reduced the numbers of instances of accidental addiction.

A new menace

However, the public reacted quite differently when drug use was associated with an underclass, particularly one comprised of immigrants. In the latter part of the nineteenth century, Chinese immigrants flowed into the US, bringing with them foreign habits, including the use of opium. Such practices fell afoul of the social reform movement, which could not tolerate habits that conflicted with their values and that might prevent the new ethnic minorities from assimilating into the dominant culture. Anti-Chinese sentiment also grew, resulting in laws designed, on the one hand, to 'vex and annoy the heathen Chinese', and, on the other, to protect middle America (particularly its youth) from further corruption (Bonnie and Whitebread, 1974).

By the late 1880s, 20 states had passed laws designed to eradicate the practice of opium smoking. Most were enacted in states into which Chinese immigrants had migrated (Bonnie and Whitebread, 1974). These early prohibitory measures embodied a common theme in narcotics prohibition:

> The likelihood of prohibitory drug legislation is increased when the drug is identified with ethnic minorities. Whether motivated by an ideological preference for cultural homogeneity or by outright prejudice, drug legislation may be aimed at the lifestyle of the users rather than at use of the drug. (Bonnie & Whitebread, 1974)

At the turn of the century, another threat appeared. Morphine and cocaine had replaced opium and were expanding into the 'underbelly' of major cities. The threat of 'morphinism' became associated in the public mind with prostitutes, pimps, gamblers and blacks and thereby with urban crime. By 1912, most states had enacted laws requiring a prescription for the distribution of opiates and cocaine (Bonnie and Whitebread, 1974).

The Federal Government also took action by passing the Harrison Narcotics Act of 1914. Such action also served the dual purpose of maintaining the reputation of the US within the international community. While the Act dealt only with opium and cocaine, its structure would serve as the foundation for the later Marijuana Tax Act of 1937. However, its provisions effectively prevented an individual from lawfully purchasing or possessing narcotics for non-medical use. Furthermore, in the hands of law enforcement and the courts, the Act was interpreted to prevent physicians from prescribing maintenance doses of narcotics to addicts. As a result, scores of addicts were forced underground to obtain drugs, resulting in steep black market prices and a consequent increase in crime. The connection between criminal behaviour and drug addiction was thus forged in the public mind. The states hastened to respond. Over the next 17 years, most enacted laws prohibiting the possession of opiates and cocaine for non-medical use. Many of these laws carried onerous criminal penalties (Bonnie and Whitebread, 1974).

Association of cannabis with ethnic and unpopular groups

The patterns described above set the stage for cannabis prohibition. After around 1914, Mexican immigrants began to enter the south-western and Rocky Mountain states. Like the Chinese, they brought with them their customs and practices, including in this case the recreational use of smoked cannabis. Hostility toward these new non-white arrivals was evidenced by newspaper articles and law enforcement reports, which increasingly deplored the dangerous and irrational behaviours that cannabis smoking allegedly provoked within this population. It was during this time that cannabis became known under a new name – 'marihuana' or 'marijuana', a disparaging, value-laden term that has coloured all subsequent debates about the subject.

The response was the same as it had been with the 'narcotics problem': prohibitory state and local legislation was enacted. There was little debate within, or public attention given to, such legislative proceedings. Marijuana, the 'killer weed', was presumed to be another dangerous, habit-forming narcotic that provoked criminal conduct by those who consumed it, largely members of ethnic minorities or other despised classes (Bonnie and Whitebread, 1970).

The substitution theory

On the East Coast of the US, an additional, and different, concern had emerged. The medical use of cannabis had already been regulated in many states as part of the effort to increase regulatory control over pharmaceutical manufacturers, pharmacies and physicians. However, after enactment of the federal laws restricting the availability of opiates, cocaine and alcohol, fear grew that addicts would resort to cannabis to satisfy their cravings. As early as 1914, New York City amended its Sanitary Code to add cannabis to the City's list of prohibited drugs. This fear of substitution demonstrated the widely held (although unsupported) belief that cannabis was, like opiates and cocaine, addictive and dangerous.

The threat expands

The smoking of cannabis for recreational purposes was initially confined to states receiving the first influx of Mexican immigration. However, new areas were gradually exposed to the practice, and new groups began to adopt its use. Caribbean sailors and West Indian immigrants introduced the use of smoked cannabis to ports along the US Gulf Coast. In those areas, cannabis use became associated with a number of stigmatised groups, such as blacks and 'unsavoury' whites (including gamblers, prostitutes, pimps and drug addicts) (Bonnie and Whitebread, 1974).

New Orleans became a particular focus of concern. Sensationalised newspaper stories circulated, and cannabis was cloaked with the mantle of 'dangerous narcotic' (Bonnie and Whitebread, 1974). Black jazz musicians and their admirers also embraced cannabis. As their music was transported from New Orleans into the eastern states, the use of cannabis accompanied it. The media, anxious to increase newspaper and journal sales, spread lurid stories of allegedly cannabis-related crime perpetrated by blacks in major cities.

Cannabis was further introduced into the industrial regions of the US as waves of Mexican labourers migrated north. There, they – and their customs – were met with even greater animus and discriminatory treatment. Mexicans were arrested in disproportionately high numbers for a variety of 'status' offences, such as disorderly conduct, giving more fuel to the fire of belief that cannabis caused lawless behaviour.

Newspaper and other reports began to warn that cannabis was being peddled to young people, including high school students and younger children, and that its use was causing widespread addiction among American youths. This spectre drew temperance and women's groups into the fray. By 1933, 33 states had put in place laws prohibiting the use of cannabis for non-medical purposes.

Despite the expanding vilification of cannabis, there was still no objective scientific evidence of its harmfulness. Indeed a governmental commission, convened to study the issue, concluded that cannabis posed little, if any, risk to public health and safety. In 1925, investigating the effects of cannabis on American soldiers stationed in Panama, the Panama Canal Zone Report flatly stated: 'There is no evidence that marihuana as grown here is a "habit forming" drug in the sense in which the term is applied to alcohol, opium, cocaine, etc., or that it has any appreciably deleterious influence on the individuals using it.' Despite this report, cannabis continued to come under increasingly harsh attack and control.

The Federal Government becomes involved

Cannabis demonisation escalated significantly in the 1930s. Harry J Anslinger, the first Commissioner of the newly formed Federal

Bureau of Narcotics (FBN), began a relentless campaign to convince the nation that cannabis was a 'menace' threatening to enslave the country's youth and destroy its moral fabric. Apparently, his determination did not derive solely from his belief that cannabis posed special harms. Rather, he hoped to convince the nation that the scourge of drug use in general required eradication, and that the tool of such eradication should be a fabric of uniform state narcotics laws. He sought to use the 'new menace' of cannabis as a lever to inflame state legislatures and the public (Bonnie and Whitebread, 1974).

Anslinger's goal was to eliminate cannabis use altogether, including its 'insignificant' medical use. Intensively lobbying state legislatures, and enlisting women's groups and the media, Anslinger disseminated reports 'demonstrating' that cannabis use resulted in addiction, insanity and crime. Since there was no effective countervailing force to contest these contentions, his campaign was successful. Newspaper editorials around the country bemoaned the perils of cannabis. Ironically, Anslinger's inflammatory 'Reefer Madness' rhetoric, used to secure passage of uniform acts within the states, aroused widespread alarm and increased demand for federal legislation. Initially reluctant to pursue such a course, Anslinger ultimately acceded to the call for federal action. Asserting again that cannabis was a dangerous menace, Anslinger convinced Congress that public hysteria and concern had reached significant levels, and that the use of cannabis had increased sharply since 1934, despite the advent of state legislation. Hence, he argued, federal action was needed to ensure adequate enforcement of the state uniform laws.

The New Deal Congress was happy to oblige. The American Medical Association opposed this effort. The AMA, represented by Dr William Woodward, contended that, while cannabis was 'seldom used' as a medicine, there was no evidence that its medical use had caused or would cause addiction. Therefore, he argued against inhibiting such medical use, since further research might prove it to be of substantial value. Dr Woodward maintained that, if control of medical use was necessary, it should be achieved through the less onerous provisions of the Harrison Narcotics Act. Nevertheless, the Marijuana Tax Act of 1937 was readily passed. It had the effect that Anslinger had long sought to achieve: the Act's bureaucratic burdens and draconian penalties effectively discouraged all further medical use of cannabis. In 1941, cannabis was removed from the US Pharmacopoeia.

The stepping stone thesis

During the 1940s, the visibility of the 'marijuana problem' receded from the public eye. State and federal enforcement occurred, but the war effort diverted attention from such issues. Indeed, the Federal Government allowed the cultivation of hemp to provide a source of rope for the war effort.

Scientific reports sporadically surfaced during this time, challenging the prevailing federal views about the dangers of cannabis. For example, the LaGuardia Committee Report in 1944 seriously challenged the theories that cannabis use resulted in insanity, addiction, juvenile delinquency and crime. However, this and other reports were either ignored or dismissed by the FBN, now joined by a bullied AMA.

As a result of this increasing scientific interest and opposition, however, the Federal Government was forced to modify the nature of its assertions. Like the phoenix rising from its ashes, as one unfounded theory was defeated, another would rise to take its place. The cannabis–crime link receded to some degree. Indeed, this theory came back to plague the law enforcement community, as defendants successfully raised 'cannabis insanity' as a defence to conviction in criminal cases. The FBN thereafter disavowed the idea that cannabis use commonly led to insanity. The physical addiction thesis, after being seriously challenged by a reputable scientist, was replaced by the spectre of 'psychological' addiction.

In the 1950s, perceived increases in opiate use – especially among young people – revived public alarm. The Federal Government responded with new legislation enhancing the penalties for both trafficking and possession for personal use of all 'narcotics' (including cannabis). State legislatures followed suit. This virtually automatic escalation in penalties, which now included mandatory minimum sentences, was to become a predictable American response to the rising drug use problem.

Cannabis was not the primary target of this legislation. However, the Federal Government had a new rationale for including cannabis within the prohibitory scheme. Cannabis was now claimed to be the 'stepping stone' or 'gateway' to opiate and cocaine addiction. The stepping stone theory caused cannabis to be swept once and for all into the battle against dangerous addictive drugs. Possession of the drug, even for one's own use, became a felony, accompanied by sentences of lengthy incarceration (Bonnie and Whitebread, 1974).

Social turmoil of the 1960s and a new symbolism

With the advent of the 1960s, a new era dawned. Wrenching political events, disruptive social turmoil and scientific evidence challenged the viability of many cannabis myths. The civil rights and, especially, the anti-war movements mobilised a large number of young people who were distrustful of conventional authority, who challenged conventional norms and values, and who sought to expand their horizons and consciousness. Government, law enforcement, organised religion and even the medical profession were often targets of scorn or suspicion.

Cannabis use increased significantly on college campuses and elsewhere across the country during this time. As a result, two crucial developments took place. First, it became evident that moderate use of cannabis did not, in fact, result in serious harm. Second, the new cannabis users were not members of an insular minority group that could easily be made the targets of prohibitory legislation. Indeed, middle-class parents, once fearful of the 'killer weed', now voiced concern that cannabis prohibition itself would destroy their children's lives and careers. By the early 1970s, the vast majority of states had reduced criminal penalties for cannabis possession, and 11 had decriminalised its use (Bonnie and Whitebread, 1974). Gone was the dynamic that had existed throughout most of the twentieth century with regard to cannabis. No longer were the cannabis-using groups disenfranchised and invisible in the political process. A new type of dialogue began, involving scientists, physicians, social policy experts, and other objective and knowledgeable professionals. A presidential commission – the National Commission on Marihuana and Drug Abuse (the Shafer Commission) – was formed to conduct a study of cannabis and to make recommendations for legislative and administrative action. The Shafer Commission released its report, *Marihuana: A Signal of Misunderstanding*, in March 1972. The report debunked previous claims of cannabis's harm. The Shafer Commission specifically concluded that, at least in moderate use, cannabis did not cause toxicity, psychosis, criminal behaviour, physical dependence, genetic damage or progression to other drugs, and recommended the decriminalisation of cannabis possession.

The same events were occurring elsewhere in the world. In 1968 the report of the Hallucinogens Subcommittee of the Advisory Committee on Drug Dependence (the Wootton Report) and in 1970 the report of the Canadian Government Commission of Inquiry into the

Non-medical Use of Drugs (the LeDain Commission Report) disputed existing beliefs about the harmfulness of cannabis. Many thought a new era of cannabis decontrol was about to emerge.

However, the anticipated sea change did not take place. In 1970, Congress enacted the Controlled Substances Act (CSA). On the one hand, the CSA reduced some of the criminal penalties applicable to cannabis offences. On the other hand, the CSA classified cannabis, along with heroin and LSD, as a drug that (1) had a high potential for abuse, (2) had no accepted medical use in the US, and (3) was not safe for use under medical supervision. Its placement under Schedule I of the CSA prevented its medical use and effectively stymied meaningful clinical research activity.

Threatened by the rapid changes that were taking place, conventional society fought back, and cannabis was again the scapegoat. The Nixon administration declared a 'War on Drugs', coupled it to a war on crime, and issued a battle cry that would be heard around the world (Baum, 1996). Cannabis use was now associated with 'dropping out', sexual permissiveness and a general breakdown of society and conventional morals. It was said to cause an 'amotivational syndrome' that caused young people to become alienated and unproductive. Indeed, President Nixon rejected the findings and recommendations of the Shafer Commission even before they were made public.

The rhetoric and fervour of this campaign escalated throughout the following decades. This siege was lifted to some extent during the presidency of Jimmy Carter, but was renewed with vigour when Ronald Reagan was elected. Parent groups, concerned about data showing increased cannabis use among high school students, mobilised to fuel the fire and give the 'gateway' theory renewed vigour. Science seemed equivocal. When confronted with a scientific report dispelling an old cannabis myth, opponents of reform pointed to a contrary report (Nahas, 1974; Stenchever *et al.*, 1974). The nascent trend toward cannabis decriminalisation came to an end.

Throughout the 1980s and 1990s, anti-drug measures (largely applied to cannabis) expanded into the social fabric. Mandatory drug testing spread within the employment and education sectors. A positive drug test could have such diverse consequences as denial of a college scholarship, loss or denial of a job or promotion, expulsion from school, or revocation of a driver's licence – even if driving was not involved in the offence. Slogans such as 'zero tolerance' and 'Just Say No' permeated the popular culture.

A polarisation of attitudes and the cannabis rescheduling case

As new, more mainstream voices emerged in the political process, the dynamics of cannabis control were forever transformed. However, since the CSA had stymied clinical research, science (despite the Shafer Commission Report) could not play a significant role. The debate then hardened into a dispute between polar opposites. The first, represented most forcefully by newly formed advocacy groups such as the National Organization for the Reform of Marijuana Laws (NORML) and Amorphia, sought full-scale legalisation. These groups supported the Shafer Commission's decriminalisation recommendation as an intermediate step toward their ultimate goal.

The opposing position contended that, in the absence of greater knowledge about the effects of cannabis, no action should be taken that might substantially increase the drug's use. By removing some of the penalties for cannabis use, they argued, even a partial decriminalisation might send the wrong signal to the public, and in particular, to young people. Concluding that decriminalisation was merely a stepping-stone to legalisation, they opposed any degree of reform.

Vitriol and conflict, then, became the hallmarks of this polarisation. When the Shafer Commission report failed to achieve significant legislative support, the advocates shifted their efforts from the legislative to the administrative and judicial realms. In the spring of 1972, NORML and several other organisations filed a rulemaking petition under the CSA requesting that the Bureau of Narcotics and Dangerous Drugs (BNDD), the successor of the FBN and the predecessor of the current Drug Enforcement Administration (DEA), remove cannabis from within the purview of the CSA, or, in the alternative, to place it in Schedule V, the least restrictive schedule. The BNDD resisted the petition, arguing that its obligations under the Single Convention prevented the US from decontrolling cannabis.

The wrangling continued through various administrative and judicial proceedings for approximately 22 years. Because the petition sought rescheduling or decontrol under the CSA, the evidence and arguments inevitably examined the medical usefulness of cannabis, as well as its potential for harm and abuse. The advocates were initially successful. An administrative judge ruled that (1) international law would permit cannabis and cannabis resin to be rescheduled to Schedule II of the CSA and (2) there was sufficient acceptance among physicians of its medical use to justify such an action. The DEA Acting Administrator rejected the proposition that the medical evidence justified rescheduling, and, in the ensuing litigation, formulated very stringent criteria to determine whether or not a substance can be moved from Schedule I to Schedule II. Ultimately, the Court of Appeals upheld the DEA's determination. In 1994 the rescheduling effort failed, and cannabis remained in Schedule I. A subsequent rescheduling petition was filed in 1995, one year after the final disposition of the first petition. In 2001, that petition was denied. An additional rescheduling petition, filed in October 2002, is currently pending.

The original rescheduling litigation has come to represent the beginning of the medicinal cannabis movement in the US. However, the initial litigants had sought to decontrol cannabis entirely, and their broader organisational mission was committed to such legalisation. The original litigants were later joined by a group – the Alliance for Cannabis Therapeutics – established in 1980 for the purpose of making cannabis available for medical uses, and medical issues did ultimately become the primary focus of the proceedings. Nevertheless, in the US many view the medicinal cannabis issue as coupled inextricably with the legalisation effort.

Patients speak out

The legalisation advocates were not alone. Patients and physicians were also beginning to raise their voices. As seriously ill individuals discovered the medicinal benefits of cannabis, they mobilised to challenge the CSA's restrictions on its availability. A number of these patients successfully raised the defence of 'medical necessity' in criminal prosecutions in state courts in the 1970s. One of these patients, Robert Randall, later brought suit against the Federal Government, seeking lawful, medically supervised access to cannabis. As a result of a settlement, the Government essentially agreed to provide Mr Randall (and subsequently other similarly situated patients) with 'research grade' cannabis. The cannabis was produced on a five-acre farm operated by the University of Mississippi under contract with the National Institute on Drug Abuse (NIDA). To support research efforts, the Federal Government established a cultivation project at the University of Mississippi to provide research-grade cannabis for various projects around the country. The cannabis, which was supplied by the National Institute on Drug Abuse (NIDA) through its Drug Supply Program, was produced primarily to supply research programmes investigating the harmfulness and abuse potential of cannabis. These 'federal' patients ostensibly took part in research trials conducted under 'compassionate use' or 'single patient' investigational new drug (IND) applications submitted by the treating physicians, although no data were actually gathered.

By 1983, 34 states had enacted legislation to make cannabis available to cancer and glaucoma patients, ostensibly through research programmes. Although only six of these states were actually able to obtain herbal cannabis to conduct the trials, the results indicated that both cannabis and THC had therapeutic efficacy for patients undergoing cancer chemotherapy (Musty and Rossi, 2001).

Patient support for medicinal cannabis expanded further as AIDS began to ravage the gay population. Many suffered from AIDS wasting and, later, the nausea and vomiting associated with the use of AZT. More and more patients sought access to NIDA cannabis through the Compassionate Use IND program. Indeed, ACT established an initiative entitled Marijuana/AIDS Research Service (MARS) to assist patients and their physicians in preparing the documentation required for a compassionate use IND. The Federal Government, alarmed at these increasing numbers, determined that the IND programme had placed the Government in an untenable position and was sending the 'wrong signal' about cannabis to the public. In 1992, the Secretary of Health and Human Services closed the programme to new applicants. Patients who were already receiving cannabis were allowed to continue to do so for their lives. Patients whose INDs had been approved, but who had not yet received cannabis, were provided with Marinol (Werner, 2001).

The role of Marinol

As patients pushed for access to cannabis, the Federal Government, embroiled in its War on Drugs, sought to divert them away from the herbal, smoked material to the non-smoked, synthetic cannabinoid THC (dronabinol). Beginning in the 1970s, the National Cancer Institute (NCI) had funded preclinical and clinical research into THC. Ultimately, NCI provided 75% of the funding for the research efforts leading to its development as a prescription product. In 1985, a formulated dronabinol product, Marinol, was approved for the treatment of nausea and vomiting associated with cancer chemotherapy. In 1992, the FDA approved it for a second indication, the treatment of anorexia associated with weight loss in AIDS patients. Marinol was initially placed in Schedule II of the CSA and, in 1999, Marinol was moved into Schedule III (Joy et al., 1999). Once Marinol was available by prescription, the Federal Government contended that the use of smoked cannabis was unnecessary.

The advocates go to the people

The cannabis advocates and medicinal cannabis supporters did not retreat. In 1991, San Francisco voters were presented with Proposition P, which called upon the State to restore cannabis to the list of available medicines. It passed by a 78% vote. As public support grew, the state legislature passed bills that would have made cannabis available to seriously ill patients. The governor vetoed those bills. Faced with defeat in the state legislature, the advocates went directly to the people. In 1996, the states of California and Arizona passed initiatives authorising seriously ill patients, with the recommendation or approval of their physicians, to use (or cultivate for their own use) medicinal cannabis. California also passed a cannabis research bill, which established the Center for Medicinal Cannabis Research (CMCR), based at the University of California San Diego. The Center has moved forward vigorously. State funding for the past 3 years has enabled the Center to provide grants to a number of clinical investigators who plan to investigate the therapeutic efficacy of cannabis for several medical conditions. The Center's work has been cited favourably by the International Narcotics Control Board (INCB, 2002).

The movement gathered momentum. Over the next few years, seven more states followed suit, either through the initiative process or through legislative enactment. Oregon, Washington, Alaska, Maine, Colorado, Nevada passed initiatives; Hawaii enacted legislation. The District of Columbia also passed an initiative, which was overturned by an act of Congress. Maryland recently enacted legislation that significantly reduced the penalties for seriously ill patients who use medicinal cannabis. Similar measures are being considered in a number of other states. Dispensaries (called cannabis buyers' clubs or compassion clubs) sprang up to provide patients with an alternative to the unregulated and sometimes unsafe products of the black market.

The Federal Government responded harshly. These state laws did not affect cannabis's illegal status under federal law. The federal Controlled Substances Act prohibits the cultivation or use of cannabis for any purpose. The state initiatives do not directly conflict with this prohibition, since the initiatives merely revoke existing state criminal law sanctions as they apply to qualifying patients, their caregivers and their physicians. However, neither do the initiatives affect the status of cannabis as a prohibited drug under federal law. Hence, patients who use cannabis, and those who aid and abet the patient, are still in jeopardy of prosecution under the CSA. Asserting that the public had been subjected to 'cruel hoax', high-ranking federal officials threatened that physicians, if they recommended cannabis to patients, could face criminal prosecution and/or loss of their licences to prescribe controlled substances.

A firestorm of protest occurred among patients, the public and the medical profession. Patients and physicians filed suit against the Federal Government, contending that the constitutional right of free speech protected the physician–patient dialogue against federal interference. A federal appellate court ruled that the First Amendment did indeed protect a physician's right to discuss cannabis with patients and recommend its use to them. However, the court stressed that if a physician intends for the patient to use the recommendation as a means for obtaining marijuana, the physician would be guilty of aiding and abetting the violation of federal law (Conant v. Walters 2002). Many physicians, uncomfortable with such ambiguous guidelines, refuse even to discuss the subject with patients. Without a physician's recommendation, a patient cannot be covered by the state cannabis initiatives and thus can still be subject to prosecution even under state law.

Faced with such protests, the 'drug czar', former General Barry McCaffrey, commissioned the prestigious Institute of Medicine to conduct a thorough review of the scientific evidence on medicinal cannabis. In the spring of 1999, the IOM issued its long-awaited report, *Marijuana and Medicine: Assessing the Science Base* (Joy et al., 1999). It concluded, among other things, that cannabinoids have potential therapeutic value for pain relief, control of nausea and vomiting, and appetite stimulation. Reviewing the existing scientific evidence, the report rejected the theory that cannabis use causes serious harms, including antisocial behaviour or psychosis; addiction and dependence; reproductive or cardiovascular damage; or amotivational syndrome. Indeed, the authors concluded that, except for the harms associated with smoking, the adverse effects of cannabinoid use 'are within the acceptable risks associated with approved medications' (Joy et al., 1999). However, stressing that cannabis smoke delivers harmful substances, the report recommended that research should seek to develop rapid-onset, reliable and safe delivery systems for cannabinoid medicines.

Nevertheless, conducting such research remained problematic. Despite an ostensible liberalisation of federal policy concerning the availability of NIDA cannabis, it continued to be extremely difficult for investigators to obtain access to research-grade cannabis and to secure the DEA licences necessary to conduct cannabis studies.

The Federal Government did not relent. Despite the IOM Report, the Department of Justice pursued litigation it had initiated in 1998 to close a number of cannabis dispensaries in California. Appealing an intermediate federal court's ruling that federal law did not prohibit the dispensaries from distributing cannabis to patients who could demonstrate 'medical necessity', the Government took the case to the US Supreme Court. Ultimately in the spring of 2001, the Court rejected the medical necessity argument (US v. OCBC 2001). The Supreme Court did not address the question of whether or not the CSA was unconstitutional as applied to patients (and dispensaries who supply them) who use medicinal cannabis when other medications have failed. A number of cases are currently pending in federal courts in California raising this and other federal constitutional issues.

In 2002, the Federal Government began vigorously to enforce the CSA, closing dispensaries in California, seizing patient records and filing criminal charges, particularly against individuals who cultivated cannabis for distribution to such dispensaries. But the federal drug prohibitionists recently suffered a significant set-back. A well-known medicinal cannabis advocate, who had been deputised by a California city to grow medicinal cannabis for dispensaries, was recently convicted in a criminal action in federal court. Despite the conviction, the federal judge sentenced him to only one day in jail (which he had already served) apparently signalling the judge's belief that the prosecution had been misguided and unjust.

As of this chapter's writing, there appears to be little appetite within the US Government for any type of cannabis reform. However, as popular support for medicinal cannabis grows, it may become increasingly difficult for the Government to enforce its full prohibitionist agenda.

International legislation

From the outset, the United States played a pivotal role world wide in efforts to control cannabis. As a result, international and US domestic control measures proceeded in parallel, often reinforcing one other. In addition, as in the US, similar factors – misinformation about the actual effects of cannabis and antipathy toward the types of individuals who used it – influenced international initiatives.

Often, trade considerations or other geopolitical factors caused countries to accede to US pressures. In many cases, these concerns led Western countries, which had no serious domestic drug problems, to accept obligations to enact punitive and prohibitory legislation within their borders.

Ironically, many Western nations undertook such obligations just before the time that early cannabis 'demonisation' began to unravel. Then, having agreed to enact draconian measures of control, countries found that they had seriously limited their ability to respond to changing social forces. Nevertheless, as the controversy escalated in the late 1960s, many nations began to question the US leadership in this area, and a few sought to chart their own course.

As in the US, the first wave of international control focused on the dangers of opium, morphine and cocaine, but cannabis was quickly swept along.

The 1912 Hague Convention

Opium was the initial focus of international concern. The US convened an international conference in 1909 in Shanghai to address the opium issue, and in particular to assist China in eradicating its opium problem. Opium was not at the time a significant domestic US problem. However, the US had alienated China by enacting the Chinese Exclusion Act that excluded Chinese labourers from the US. In retaliation, China imposed an embargo against US manufactured goods. The US hoped that the Shanghai conference would convince China of US goodwill and effect an improvement in US–Chinese trade relations. In addition, the US had recently acquired the Philippines, and with it a Government opium supply monopoly. Despite the suppression of the monopoly, smuggling continued (Sinha, 2001).

As a result, in 1909 the International Opium Commission met in Shanghai to discuss primarily the importation of opium into China. The attendees did not have the authority to adopt an international treaty. Thus, they could only agree to make recommendations to their governments concerning international control of opium. Subsequently, at the urging of the US, a plenipotentiary conference took place in The Hague, resulting in the 1912 International Opium Convention. The treaty required the parties gradually to suppress the domestic production and trade, and to prohibit as soon as possible the importation and exportation of raw and prepared opium. The agreement also called upon the parties to prevent illegal importation and smuggling of opium into China and to restrict the use and sale of opium in the parties' leased territories, settlements and concessions in China. A few nations, including the US, put the Convention into force among themselves in 1915; the

Convention did not come into force broadly until it was made a part of the Versailles Treaty in 1919 (Sinha, 2001). Some commentators believe that the US hoped to foist the burden of controlling the poppy and the coca leaf onto manufacturing countries, and, in addition, that the US representatives sought to obtain an international mandate to pressure the US Government to enact domestic drug control laws (Sinha, 2001), such as the Harrison Narcotics Act. The treaty provided that the use of opium should be restricted to medical and scientific purposes, thus establishing a principle that was to form the foundation of all subsequent international agreements.

The Convention did not formally address the question of cannabis or hashish. However, both Italy and the US had sought to bring the production of, and traffic in, cannabis under international control. The delegates did sign a protocol which stated that the 'hemp question' should be studied from a 'statistical and scientific point of view', to determine whether domestic legislation or international agreement was necessary to prevent abuse (Abel, 1980).

The 1925 Geneva Convention

During the First World War drug controls issues at the international level were quiescent. However, the US soon pressured the League of Nations to convene another plenipotentiary conference. For the first time, cannabis was formally considered. South Africa, Egypt and Turkey proposed that cannabis be included in the list of narcotics that would be covered by the Convention. The South African Government was concerned that the use of cannabis or 'dagga' would 'turn its black population into an unruly mob' (Abel, 1980). Egypt had long sought to eradicate the use of hashish by Sufis and members of the lower class (Abel, 1980). The Egyptian delegate contended that hashish could be addictive, that its 'acute' use could cause violence, and that 'chronic hashishism' ultimately resulted in insanity. Indeed, he maintained that hashish use had caused most of the cases of insanity in Egypt. He also argued that if other drugs were suppressed by means of the Convention, hashish use would soon replace them and become 'a terrible menace to the whole world'.

The US and Canada strongly supported the idea that cannabis would be covered by the Convention. Canadian lawmakers' attitudes on cannabis had been significantly affected, not only by the country's proximity to the US, but also by the sensationalistic and popular writings of 'Janey Cantuck', the pen name of a Canadian feminist and the first woman judge in the British Empire (Abel, 1980).

The matter was referred to a subcommittee, composed largely of representatives from Western countries in which cannabis use was virtually unknown. The subcommittee recommended the complete prohibition of the production and use of cannabis resin. Another subcommittee drafted provisions requiring the parties:

- to impose domestic controls over galenical preparations (extracts and tinctures) of Indian hemp;
- to impose import/export control over Indian hemp and resin;
- to prohibit export of resin to countries that had prohibited its use, or, if such importation is permitted, to require the importing country to issue a special import certificate stating that the import was approved for medical or scientific purposes and that it would not be re-exported; and
- to prevent the illicit international traffic in Indian hemp and particularly in the resin.

These provisions were ultimately adopted and included in the Convention (the Wootton Report). The 1925 treaty did not prohibit domestic cultivation, production or distribution of cannabis. Nevertheless, despite the fact that they had no serious domestic cannabis problems, some Western countries enacted domestic legislation to make cannabis illegal. This took place in Great Britain, for example, with the passage of the Dangerous Drugs Act of 1925. Canada added cannabis to its list of regulated substances under its Opium and Narcotics Drug Act of 1929. Thus began cannabis prohibition, from 'the top down', in the Western world.

The 1931 and 1936 Geneva Conventions

Cannabis received little international attention during most of the next 10 years. In 1933, however, stories from the US began to filter into international discussions. The Advisory Committee on Traffic in Opium noted that a 'smuggling trade' in cannabis cigarettes had sprung up between the US and Canada. The Committee suggested that, as international control restricted the availability of opium and coca derivatives, addicts would resort to cannabis; therefore, the Committee advised that cannabis should be closely monitored (the Wootton Report).

The Committee's concern led it to make a special assessment of cannabis. The US submitted a memorandum describing a 'widespread habitual use of marihuana' and 'the alarming influence of [cannabis] addiction' on criminal conduct; it noted that 34 out of 46 states had legislated to suppress cannabis. Several other nations also pressed for greater controls. The Committee established a Subcommittee on Indian Hemp, making the US representative chairman. The Subcommittee examined the literature and explored the matter for several years but issued no report, indicating that more information was needed regarding the relation between the use of cannabis and hashish and crime, insanity, addiction and transition to other drugs such as heroin.

The 1925 Convention had only limited effectiveness because drugs were shipped through non-signatory countries. Consequently, a further conference was convened in Geneva. Harry J Anslinger, representing the US, made his first entrance upon the international scene. One commentator, noting the influence of Mr Anslinger on international drug control, stated that he was 'utterly devoted to prohibition and the control of drug supplies at the source' and 'widely recognized as having had one of the more powerful impacts on ... international drug control into the early 1970s (Sinha, 2001). The 1931 conference resulted in the Convention for Limiting the Manufacture and Regulating the Distribution of Narcotic Drugs, which established a manufacturing limitation system. Parties were required to provide the Permanent Central Opium Board (PCOB) with estimates of their national drug requirements for medical and scientific purposes. The PCOB was to establish manufacturing limits for each country.

During the remainder of the 1930s, international negotiations continued, with a focus on reducing illicit drug trafficking and imposing severe criminal sanctions on traffickers. In 1936, another conference was convened in Geneva, resulting in the Convention for the Suppression of the Illicit Traffic in Dangerous Drugs. The US urged that the treaty include provisions requiring parties to criminalise all domestic activities – cultivation, production, manufacture and distribution – relating to the non-medical and non-scientific uses of opium, coca and cannabis. However, the focus of the Convention continued to be limited to trafficking, and the US did not sign the treaty (Sinha, 2001).

The period 1936–1961

As a result of World War II and throughout the Cold War period of the 1950s, no major international treaties emerged, although a number of more minor protocols were concluded. By the end of the 1940s, the disparity of treaty provisions was creating confusion. At the suggestion of the US, the United Nations Commission on Narcotic Drugs (CND) undertook an effort to consolidate all previous treaties into a single international agreement.

Cannabis was now receiving considerable attention. During the next few years, the CND would receive reports from the US and a number of non-Western countries indicating that cannabis was an increasing problem. A former WHO official contended that cannabis was a 'dangerous drug from every point of view', as well as being a stepping-stone to heroin addiction. By 1954, WHO began to advise the CND that cannabis and cannabis preparations no longer served any useful medical purpose and were essentially obsolete (the Wootton Report).

Armed with such information, the CND completed the consolidation process. In 1961, the CND had finally produced a draft that could be considered by a plenipotentiary conference. That draft reflected the belief that cannabis was a dangerous narcotic whose threat equalled that of the most dangerous opiates, not the least because it could serve as a stepping-stone to the use of such drugs.

The 1961 Single Convention

The 1961 Single Convention on Narcotic Drugs (Single Convention) was completed just before the 'new dialogue' on cannabis would begin. Around the world, nations adopted prohibitory domestic legislation to implement their obligations under the Convention instrument. However, across the Western world, as in the US, social turmoil challenged old cannabis myths on which the Single Convention was founded. Thus, in many countries a gap quickly opened between the requirements of law and the demands of a changing social order.

The Single Convention maintained and strengthened existing controls. For example, it maintained the requirements of licensing, reporting of national estimates of drug requirements and statistical returns, and establishing limits on production and manufacture, etc. The Single Convention also extended control systems to the plants cultivated to provide the raw materials for narcotic drugs. Its preamble highlighted the foundational principle of previous international agreements: that parties must limit exclusively to medical and scientific purposes the production, manufacture, export/import, distribution, trade, use and possession of drugs. Countries in which the use of cannabis was 'traditional' were allowed to permit such non-medical use for a maximum of 25 years. After that time, however, all non-medical use was to be discontinued.

The Convention classified substances within four schedules. The most stringent levels of control applied to Schedules I and IV, which contained, among other things, opium, coca, cannabis and their derivatives. Schedules II and III were subject to less restrictive controls. At the urging of the US, cannabis and cannabis resin were placed (along with heroin) in Schedule IV, because (1) its abuse was allegedly widespread and (2) the WHO had determined that its medical uses were obsolete. However, cannabis tinctures and extracts were listed only in Schedule I.

Schedule IV substances may, but are not necessarily required to be, completely prohibited. With regard to such substances, a party must adopt any 'special measures of control which in its opinion are necessary having regard to the particularly dangerous properties' of the drug in question. In addition, a party must prohibit the manufacture, export and import of, trade in, possession or use of, a Schedule IV drug, except for amounts that are necessary for medical and scientific research, including clinical trials with the drug that are conducted 'under or subject to the direct supervision and control' of the party. This requirement applies only if a party holds the opinion that 'the prevailing conditions in its country render [such prohibition] the most appropriate means of protecting the public health and welfare'.

The treaty allowed parties to prohibit completely the cultivation of opium, coca or cannabis, if it concluded that the prevailing conditions rendered such prohibition 'the most suitable measure ... for protecting the public health and welfare and preventing the diversion of drugs into illicit traffic.' Countries that permitted cultivation were required to establish a national monopoly that would take possession of and distribute the crops. However, there was an exception for stocks held by manufacturers of medicinal preparations, nor did the governmental monopoly requirement apply to such preparations.

In addition, the Single Convention required the parties to enact punitive domestic legislation. Subject to its constitutional limitations, each party was required to adopt measures to ensure that activities (including cultivation, production, manufacture, extraction, preparation, possession, offering, offering for sale, distribution, purchase, sale, transport, importation and exportation) contrary to the treaty would be 'punishable offences', and that 'serious offences' would be liable to 'adequate punishment particularly by imprisonment or other penalties of deprivation of liberty'.

The 1971 Convention on Psychotropic Substances

Following the Single Convention, drug abuse continued to increase. Much of the abuse involved synthetic psychotropic substances that were not covered by the 1961 treaty. Accordingly, the need for further international control resulted in the Convention on Psychotropic Substances of 1971 (1971 Convention). The Single Convention served as a general pattern for the 1971 Convention.

Like the Single Convention, the 1971 Convention classified substances into four schedules, although the organisation of those schedules was different. For example, Schedule IV is the most stringent schedule in the Single Convention, whereas Schedule I holds that position in the 1971 Convention.

Tetrahydrocannabinols were initially placed in Schedule I. Dronabinol (one specific isomer of delta-9-tetrahydrocannabinol), was moved to Schedule II in 1991. Dronabinol may in the near future be moved to Schedule IV. Recently, the 33rd meeting of the World Health Organization's Expert Committee on Drug Dependence made such a recommendation.

Article 22 of the treaty again required the parties to treat acts contrary to the treaty as punishable offences, and to ensure that serious offences would generally result in incarceration or other deprivation of liberty. However, Article 22, paragraph (b), allowed nations to provide treatment, education, aftercare, rehabilitation and social reintegration either as an alternative to conviction or punishment, or in addition to punishment, when dealing with an individual drug abuser.

The 1972 Protocol Amending the Single Convention

In further response to the increasing problems of drug trafficking and abuse, the 1972 Protocol Amending the Single Convention on Narcotic Drugs was concluded. This protocol expanded the power and role of the INCB in the control of drug trafficking and of both licit and illicit opium production. The protocol also added a provision for treatment or other non-punitive alternative, which paralleled that in the 1971 Convention.

The 1988 Trafficking Convention

Despite these treaties, the rise in drug trafficking and drug abuse continued unabated. In 1988, another treaty – the 1988 Convention Against Illicit Traffic in Narcotic Drugs and Psychotropic Substances – was consummated. The 1988 Convention focused primarily on measures to combat international drug trafficking, e.g. to facilitate confiscation of illicit proceeds and to restrict the freedom of movement of drug traffickers. It required the parties to establish a host of criminal offences and punishments to implement the prohibitions of previous treaties and to ensure that sanctions – such as imprisonment or other forms of deprivation of liberty, pecuniary sanction and confiscation – take into account the 'grave nature' of such offences.

Despite its emphasis on the evils of drugs trafficking, the 1988 Convention also took a more explicitly punitive approach to demand side issues, i.e. it viewed the individual drug user as part of the criminal enterprise. The treaty explicitly provided that, subject to its constitutional principles and the basic concepts of its legal system, the parties must establish as a criminal offence, the possession, purchase or cultivation of drugs for personal consumption contrary to previous treaties. Thus, as one commentator has noted, the treaty implied 'that drug users are also to be considered criminals' (Sinha, 2001).

However, other alternatives continued to be recognised. The Convention permitted the parties to provide non-punitive measures, such as treatment, education, aftercare, rehabilitation or social reintegration, either as an alternative to, or in addition to, conviction or punishment for offences relating to personal consumption. By contrast, for other offences such measures could be provided only in addition to punitive sanctions, although the parties may also apply less punitive measures for minor offences.

The Conventions and cannabis use

It is generally agreed that the both the 1961 and 1971 Conventions afford nations a reasonable degree of flexibility in choosing among various options for cannabis control. However, the extent of permissible reform is a matter of debate. The Conventions do not specify exactly what a party must do to implement their provisions. The official commentary to the Single Convention indicates that the provision requiring parties to criminalise certain offences (including possession) may be interpreted to exclude the possession of drugs for personal consumption (Office of the UN Secretary General, 1973). Furthermore, even if possession is criminalised, it could be subject to minor penalties, such as a fine.

Finally, both the 1961 and 1971 Conventions provide that the obligations to enact punitive measures are subject to the parties' 'constitutional limitations'. Therefore, if a national court were to rule that an individual had a constitutional right to use (and perhaps even to be given access to) medicinal cannabis, that nation would be relieved of any obligation under the Conventions to criminalise or otherwise punish such activity. This in fact has recently occurred in Canada.

The treaties also authorise non-punitive measures. Both Conventions explicitly recognise that drug abusers, whose possession or even distribution may be motivated by their underlying addiction, need not be dealt with harshly. Each treaty provides that, as to offences committed by individual drug abusers, the parties may provide treatment or other non-punitive measures as an alternative to conviction or punishment, 'no matter how serious that offence may be' (Office of UN Secretary General, 1973, 1976). However, the official 1961 Commentary also stresses that, even if parties choose not to impose penal sanctions for personal possession and consumption, they must enact administrative measures to prevent the possession of drugs (1) without legal authority and (2) for other than medical and scientific purposes. The commentary further opines that possession of drugs for distribution must be made punishable by imprisonment or other types of deprivation of liberty.

The 1988 Convention is more difficult to interpret. Article 3 of that document requires parties to apply criminal sanctions to offences involving the possession, purchase or cultivation of drugs for personal consumption contrary to the provisions of the 1961 and 1971 Conventions. However, despite this provision, reform may be possible. First, the 1988 Convention specifies that a country's obligation in this regard is 'subject to its constitutional principles and the basic concepts of its legal system'. Second, criminal sanctions need only be applied to personal consumption activities that contravene the previous conventions. Third, Article 3 does not require that such offences be considered serious, i.e. they could be classified as misdemeanours or administrative violations (Krajeski, 2000). Finally, paragraph 4d allows the parties to provide alternatives to criminal punishment for individuals (not limited to drug abusers) who commit such consumption-related offences.

The above suggests that a nation has considerable latitude in structuring its control system for cannabis. Nevertheless, the weight of opinion appears to hold that this latitude does not include outright legalisation, in part because this would contravene the principle that psychoactive drugs should be produced, traded, distributed, used, etc., exclusively for medical and scientific purposes (Krajeski, 2000). Not all agree. The Australian Institute of Criminology opined in a 1994 report that only a system of 'free availability', in which cannabis would be treated like caffeine, would be prohibited by international treaties.

What types of cannabis reform are possible?

Many commentators have explored the scope and potential flexibility of these Conventions with regard to cannabis reform. A number of options have been examined, and the concept of 'decriminalisation' has been widely debated. In order to clarify the issues, it may be helpful to outline a number of approaches, other than total prohibition, that have been considered or implemented and that may (or may not) be allowable under the treaties.

Prohibition with an administrative expediency principle

In this system, criminal prosecution of certain cannabis offences may not be afforded a high priority. If arrests occur the cases may be disposed of by non-incarceration, e.g. by fine or dismissal, or diversion. However, there is still the potential for jail sentences, and such penalties are sometimes imposed. Furthermore, this system can lend itself to discriminatory application, unless national guidelines are clear and consistently enforced.

Depenalisation

Under this system, the penalties for cannabis offences, particularly for simple possession for personal use, do not involve the possibility of incarceration. Rather, sanctions involve a fine, caution or other option. These sanctions may or may not result in a criminal record. This was the approach taken by the 11 states in the US in the 1970s that are commonly said to have 'decriminalised' cannabis possession. Such possession was illegal, but violation of the law was treated like a minor traffic offence and resulted only in the imposition of a fine. Similar systems are in place within some Australian states and territories. As drug policy analyst Eric Single has noted, the specifics of depenalisation will vary with a country's legal structure (Single, 1998). These variations might include:

- elimination of incarceration as a sentencing option
- transfer of cannabis offences to the category of a civil (rather than criminal) offence, incurring only a fine
- automatic diversion of offenders to treatment or community service, either before or after trial
- 'fine only' options by which offenders are afforded an opportunity to avoid prosecution by payment of a fine. This is the approach taken by South Australia through its Expiation Notice procedure.

Various reports have suggested slightly different models. McDonald *et al.* (1994) suggest the following: (1) total prohibition with no expediency principle; (2) total prohibition with an expediency principle; (3) total prohibition with an administrative decision to caution certain categories of offenders and/or divert them into treatment programmes; (4) total prohibition with non-criminal sanctions, e.g. replacing criminal convictions with civil fines or other penalties; (5) partial prohibition, where criminal sanctions remain for some cannabis-related offences, such as trafficking; and (6) regulation.

Decriminalisation

This term has been liberally used to describe a variety of systems that depart to some extent from the full prohibition model. For this reason, many contemporary drug policy analysts no longer use the term. The term might more accurately apply to a system in which a cannabis offence, particularly possession for personal use, does not incur any penalties, civil or criminal, nor does it contravene any law.

As Professor Single has stressed, it is important to distinguish between measures that reduce the penalties for cannabis offences and measures that remove the offences themselves. This is particularly true since the existence of a criminal record, resulting from the fact that the offender has committed an actual crime, is often more harmful to the individual than the severity of the sentence or other sanction (Single, 1998).

Legalisation or regulation

This term contemplates a system, like that of governing the availability of alcohol and tobacco products, in which cannabis cultivation, production, sale, possession and use are fully lawful, although regulated in a variety of ways. Under such a system, lawful sources of supply would exist. Such sources could either be regulated and licensed by the government, but otherwise operate within the free market system, or they could be managed as government monopolies. Some policy analysts argue that only this option will reduce or eliminate the black market in cannabis (Drug Policy Forum Trust, 1997).

Other variations are also possible. Furthermore, even if cannabis were legalised, governmental agencies and private organisations may still conduct educational campaigns and other programmes to discourage its use. Indeed, this option facilitates the development of credible and realistic educational programmes, which are therefore more likely to be effective among young people. In addition, treatment programmes can be more effective when the underlying activity is no longer subject to punishment, especially criminal punishment.

Additional policy options

The above options may either be embodied in law (*de jure*) or merely implemented in practice (*de facto*). For example, the Dutch cannabis policy can be said to be an example of *de facto* decriminalisation. It has also been cited as an example of total prohibition with an expediency principle. However, since its non-prosecution policy has been embodied in formal guidelines, it probably is better characterised as *de facto* decriminalisation of certain cannabis-related activities. Italy's 'partial prohibition' policy has been adopted *de facto*.

Furthermore, such reforms may be limited in scope, e.g. may apply only to selected offences, such as possession for personal use, or only to selected drugs, such as cannabis (Single, 2001). For example, a 'partial prohibition' system would allow adults to possess and (under some definitions) cultivate, a limited amount of cannabis for private personal use and non-profit distribution among friends. The need explicitly to consider the legal status of cultivation has been demonstrated by a recent report indicating that in the UK, domestically cultivated cannabis now makes up nearly half of UK cannabis consumption, having overtaken Moroccan resin (hashish) (Hough *et al.*, 2003). Much of this cultivation is undertaken for personal use by the cultivator and their friends and not for larger scale commercial distribution. It has been said that a partial prohibition system would (1) save law enforcement and criminal justice resources, (2) avoid bringing the law into disrepute as a result of being so flouted; (3) remove the stigma of criminal convictions of otherwise law-abiding people and reduce their contact with criminals; (4) avoid discriminatory enforcement of law; and (5) permit educational messages (about harms associated with use and ways to minimise such harms) to be communicated (Drug Policy Forum Trust, 1997). Several European nations have adopted such a policy. Another possibility would be to decriminalise or legalise cannabis only for (limited) medical use. This is the approach taken by the US states that allow the use of medicinal cannabis.

Finally, if a country wishes to take an action inconsistent with treaty obligations, it could also (1) seek to amend the treaty or (2) denounce its obligations under the treaty. Although specific options will vary by country, one thing seems clear. Increasingly, both disinterested policy analysts and governmental policymakers desire to ensure that drug control measures are, like medical treatment and research, 'evidence-based'.

Do international treaties allow cannabis-based medicines to be legally available?

The Single Convention would govern the conditions under which a complex preparation derived from the cannabis plant could be available for medical use. New synthetic cannabinoids or cannabimimetic preparations, on the other hand, would be governed by the 1971 Convention (Office of the UN Secretary General, 1973, 1976). Both Conventions stress that controlled substances must be made available for – and their use limited to – medical and scientific uses. However, the terms 'medical' and 'scientific' are not defined. There are thus two issues: (1) what amount and type of scientific evidence must exist in order for a party to make a cannabis medicine available; and (2) what international and/or domestic legal changes must take place in order to permit such availability? For example, in its 2001 Report, the International Narcotics Control Board questioned whether or not heroin maintenance programmes have an adequate evidentiary foundation. The INCB flatly stated that, in its opinion, programmes establishing drug injection rooms do not.

What evidence must a country have to make cannabis available as a medicine?

The regulatory systems of most Western countries, as a condition of granting marketing approval for a product, require convincing evidence of its quality, safety and efficacy. Generally, such evidence must be collected from properly controlled clinical trials conducted in accordance with international regulatory standards, and it is unlikely that crude, non-standardised herbal cannabis, particularly in smoked form, could satisfy such demanding criteria. Therefore, if a cannabis product were to be approved as a medicine in accordance with a party's general regulatory requirements, it could be made available by prescription without violating the party's obligations under the Single Convention and without requiring the concurrence of the World Health Organization and the INCB.

However, the situation would be less clear if a party were to create a special exception from these requirements only for cannabis. The Official Commentary to the 1961 Single Convention stresses that the term 'medical purposes' is ambiguous:

> [It] does not necessarily have exactly the same meaning at all times and under all circumstances. Its interpretation must depend on the stage of medical science at the particular time in question; and not only modern medicine, sometimes also referred to as 'western Medicine,' but also legitimate systems of indigenous medicine such as those which exist in China, India and Pakistan, may be taken into account in this connexion. (Office of the UN Secretary General, 1973)

This would suggest that the existing principles of a country's system of medicine, but not a product-specific deviation from that system, would satisfy the Single Convention. Despite such uncertainty, several nations have concluded that the provisions of the Single Convention are flexible enough to allow a signatory to grant compassionate access to medicinal cannabis.

Believing that the development of a pharmaceutical-quality cannabis preparation may be years away, some countries have considered the possibility of such interim measures. A recent report of a select committee of the House of Lords, for example, called for the rescheduling of herbal cannabis to Schedule 2 of the Misuse of Drugs Regulations to allow its prescription by physicians on a named patient basis (House of Lords Select Committee on Science and Technology, 1998). The Government promptly rejected this recommendation. In Australia, the Report of the Working Party on the Use of Cannabis for Medical Purposes concluded that the language of the Single Convention would allow a medical 'certification' system. In such a system, certain types of patients can be certified (authorised) to use (and generally also to cultivate) cannabis for medical purposes if their physician recommends or prescribes such use. In the alternative, individual physicians or classes of physicians could be certified to prescribe cannabis to patients meeting specified criteria. The US Institute of Medicine recommended the short-term (less than six months) use of smoked cannabis for patients with debilitating symptoms under certain conditions (Joy *et al.*, 1999). As early as 1999, following a judicial decree, Canada began to allow certain patients to use herbal cannabis under its 'Section 56 exemption' programme.

The International Narcotics Control Board has questioned this approach. It has suggested that, when a country departs from its general regulatory system to permit, for example, medical access to a controlled substance before its quality, safety and efficacy have been adequately established, questions may arise as to the consistency of that action with the requirements of the Single Convention (INCB, 2002).

What legal changes are necessary to permit the use of medicinal cannabis?

The Single Convention sets forth a procedure by which a substance can be moved to a different 'schedule'. It also sets forth a specific procedure that must be followed in order to modify the scope of control of a substance, i.e. to schedule a previously uncontrolled substance; to move a substance from a lesser to a stricter level of control, or vice versa; or to delete a substance from a schedule and free it from control (Article 3). The procedure can be initiated by a party or by WHO and is ultimately concluded by the Commission on Narcotic Drugs. If the Commission does make a scheduling decision, the parties are obligated to implement, through national law, the regime of control that attaches to the schedule in question. However, the Single Convention does not require a party to place a substance in a particular schedule under its domestic regulatory scheme. Rather, the party must impose the specific level of control called for under the treaty.

A fortiori, this procedure does not prohibit a party from unilaterally changing the domestic scheduling of a particular substance, even if WHO and CND have not rescheduled the substance under the Single Convention (and even if the Article 2 procedure has not been initiated), so long as the domestic scope of control continues to meet the minimum requirements of the treaty. Nowhere in the 1961 Commentary do the comments state or imply that international rescheduling is a condition precedent to national rescheduling. This is particularly true with regard to cannabis tinctures and extracts. Since they are listed only in Schedule I, along with morphine, hydrocodone and oxycodone, an approved pharmaceutical product could be made available by prescription under domestic law.

As with the Single Convention, the 1971 Convention only requires a party to subject a substance to the specific regime of control delineated by the relevant treaty schedule. Nothing in the text of the treaty, nor in the 1971 Commentary, states or even suggests that a party is prohibited from changing the domestic scheduling of a substance unless and until the substance has been rescheduled pursuant to the Article 2 treaty procedure. The treaty was not intended to hinder a party from adding new therapeutic products to its domestic armamentarium. The Article 2 procedure can be quite prolonged, and patients would be unjustly denied the benefits of a valuable medicine if that procedure were required to be completed before a specific pharmaceutical product could be made available. This would conflict with the treaty's basic premise. Hence, so long as a pharmaceutical product has met all of the party's standard regulatory criteria of quality, safety and efficacy, that specific product, at the least, can be rescheduled and made available for treatment and sale, subject to certain conditions. It is unclear whether the treaty would apply at all to cannabinoids that do not possess THC-type psychoactivity, such as cannabidiol. Cannabidiol, for example, is not a scheduled substance in the UK.

Special issues also arise in the case of cannabis, if cultivation for medical purposes is allowed. The Single Convention requires a government monopoly to take control of the stocks. However, an argument can be made that such a government monopoly need not be established if the cannabis is being supplied solely for clinical trials, rather than for trade. That question has been posed to the INCB, and an answer is being awaited. Furthermore, this governmental monopoly requirement does not apply if the cannabis is being cultivated and held by a manufacturer of medicinal preparations.

The domestic mechanisms by which a cannabis-based medicine could be made available to patients would vary somewhat in each country. In the US, for example, if the Food and Drug Administration (FDA) were to approve a specific cannabis product for marketing, that product would necessarily be removed from Schedule I, i.e. FDA approval signifies that the product has an accepted medical use. However, its placement in one of the CSA's remaining four schedules would depend on a number of factors relating primarily to its abuse potential and safety. If a cannabis product were initially placed in Schedule II, but over time there were little evidence of abuse or diversion, it might later be transferred through an administrative proceeding to a less restrictive schedule. This was the path taken by Marinol. A rescheduling action does not require congressional approval or legislation, although Congress can override (or directly make) a scheduling decision.

In the US system, only a specific formulated product would be approved and scheduled, not the active principle. For example, Marinol was placed in Schedule II, and later III, of the CSA as 'dronabinol (synthetic) in sesame oil and encapsulated in a soft gelatin capsule in a U.S. Food and Drug Administration approved product'. However, any other

THC product remains in Schedule I. Hence, even if a cannabis-based or cannabinoid pharmaceutical product were approved, cannabis itself would still remain in Schedule I.

Placement in Schedule I severely limits a substance's availability. Physicians cannot prescribe Schedule I substances, even for identified patients who have failed on all standard therapies. Schedule I substances can only be dispensed within the confines of a federally licensed research project. To be sure, researchers must obtain a license (registration) from the US Drug Enforcement Administration to conduct research on any controlled substances. However, securing a Schedule I research licence requires the applicant to undergo an often prolonged and onerous approval process.

A product's status as a Schedule I controlled substance is not the only impediment to its widespread use in medical treatment in the US. Even Schedule II status limits the number of patients who may be able to receive a medicine. Unlike in the UK, physicians cannot prescribe unlicensed medicines for any purpose. However, once a product is approved for some medical purpose, physicians may prescribe that product for both labelled and 'off-label' uses. But such off-label prescription is scrutinised more closely when it involves a substance that is classified in Schedule II.

UK law would also require a rescheduling procedure. In the UK, cannabis and cannabis resin are listed in Schedule 1 of the Misuse of Drugs Regulations 2001. If the Medicines and Healthcare Products Research Agency (MHRA) were to approve a cannabis product, the Home Office has indicated that it would move expeditiously to reschedule the product to allow its general prescription. However, the UK regulatory structure differs in some important respects from that of the US. In the UK, physicians may prescribe, on a named patient basis, an unlicensed medicine (or a licensed medicine for an unlicensed, 'off label' use) in Schedule 2 (or 'lower'), so long as an 'appropriate preparation' is available. Hence, if cannabis or cannabis resin were moved from Schedule 1 to Schedule 2, a suitable preparation could be made available to a limited number of patients on this basis. Such a change would also enable research on the substance to take place without a special licence from the Home Office.

In Canada, cannabis has not been placed in a uniquely restrictive schedule. Under the Controlled Drugs and Substances Act, cannabis is contained in Schedule II, the same category as morphine. Hence, if a cannabis product were approved for marketing under the Food and Drugs Act and the Food and Drugs Regulations, that product could be prescribed without the need for rescheduling. Furthermore, Canada's Special Access Programme would in theory permit a pharmaceutical-quality cannabis preparation to be prescribed by individual physicians to specific patients on a case-by-case basis. Finally, Section 56 of the Controlled Substances Act allows the Health Minister to exempt certain individuals, including patients, from the Act's prohibitions. This has been applied to enable a limited number of seriously ill patients to use cannabis lawfully.

Separating the issues of cannabis use

There appears to be wide agreement that the different strands of cannabis reform – medicinal, recreational, agricultural/industrial – should be considered and analysed separately. Otherwise, fear, confusion, and antipathy may prevent any single question from enjoying a full and objective assessment.

Opponents of cannabis commonly obscure the issues by contending that the campaign for medical use is merely a 'stalking horse' for the legalisation of recreational use. A vocal minority of legislators, policy-makers, law enforcement personnel, medical organisations and members of the general public also view the 'medical marijuana movement' with considerable suspicion. Advocacy organisations, by simultaneously arguing for recreational use, medical access and hemp production, have provided fuel to this attitude. Such suspicion merely hinders objective reasoning, obscures the genuine scientific and social issues, and in some cases, creates obstacles that impede the ability of researchers to pursue *bona fide* studies.

Had the medicinal cannabis movement begun earlier in the century and/or focused on cannabis extracts and tinctures, its separate identity would have been better established and maintained. This would have been particularly true if the medical profession had continued to employ and endorse such cannabis products during the time when recreational use of the smoked herb was on the rise.

Unsurprisingly, the strength of this perceived link is strongest in the US. As noted above, the medicinal cannabis movement became associated at its inception with advocacy groups seeking cannabis legalisation. The strategy of legalisation advocates, it has been suggested, is to convince the American public that cannabis has medical benefit, and to appeal to their sympathy for seriously ill persons. This greater acceptance of the use of cannabis for medical purposes will, in theory, gradually lessen resistance to its recreational use. That perception has been recently exacerbated by the fact that it was advocacy groups and their supporters – rather than healthcare and medical groups – that organised and funded the state initiatives authorising the use of medicinal cannabis. Indeed, many national organisations of patients and healthcare professionals, such as the California Medical Association and the American Medical Association, did not support or even opposed such initiatives.

However, there may be a less pronounced link in other countries between 'legalisation' advocates and the medicinal cannabis movement. In the UK, for example, the Alliance for Cannabis Therapeutics, an organisation composed of patients, physicians and politicians, has been one of the most visible supporters of medicinal cannabis. ACT contends that cannabis need not be legalised for recreational use in order for suitable cannabis preparations to be made available to seriously ill people (House of Lords Select Committee on Science and Technology, 1998). ACT's singleness of goal may explain in part why the UK appears more willing to isolate the medical from the recreational issues. The House of Lords Report clearly stated that the 'stalking horse' concern should not prevent reasoned discussion of the medical issues, nor be 'a reason to resist medical use if … it is justified by the evidence' (House of Lords Select Committee on Science and Technology, 1998).

Interests of pragmatism and compassion have also enabled some countries such as the UK to separate the issues. Failure to do so, it is said, unfairly punishes sick people, places law enforcement personnel in an untenable position, and brings the law into disrepute. Indeed, some believe that permitting the use of cannabis on prescription will, by creating 'a clear separation between medical and recreational use … make the line against recreational use easier to hold' (House of Lords Select Committee on Science and Technology, 1998).

By contrast, other countries, such as the US, are reluctant to permit any 'crack' in national campaign messages aimed at holding back the flood of drug abuse. In the US, it is feared, a pragmatic approach would 'send the wrong message' to young people and to the American public. In short, the US prefers to insist that if cannabis use is sometimes harmful, all cannabis use must be resisted.

A current example demonstrates the lengths to which the US will go to maintain a uniform cannabis prohibition. Despite the fact that the US Controlled Substances Act excepts from the definition of 'marihuana' the mature stalks, fibre made from such stalks, oil or cake made from cannabis seeds, any other compound, preparation, etc. from such oil or cake, and sterilised cannabis seeds, the Drug Enforcement Administration has recently sought to cleanse the US marketplace of any hemp-related products intended for human consumption. The DEA has issued a rule that places in Schedule I of the CSA all hemp-based food products containing any tetrahydrocannabinol, which is listed separately from marijuana in Schedule I, no matter how small the amount (DEA, 2003). This action unleashed the wrath of numerous interest groups, including hemp, environmental and natural foods organisations, as well as cannabis advocates.

Separating medicinal and recreational cannabis use

A country may wish to make medicinal cannabis available, but may conclude that, in light of its perceived treaty obligation, it cannot permit recreational use. There is precedent for a maintaining a legal separation between the medicinal use of a substance and its illicit recreational use. This has been true even if, as is the case with cannabis, the substance's 'reputation' as a drug of abuse has largely preceded its development as a medical product. As prescription drug abuse expands, countries must inevitably devise mechanisms to distinguish between the licit and illicit use of lawful pharmaceutical products. Hence, the historical distinction between 'licit' and 'illicit' drugs may become less relevant than the distinction between licit and illicit uses of drugs.

In some instances, the medical iteration has been formulated and packaged as a pharmaceutical product, whereas the 'street' version is less refined. For example, in the US, the illicit version of gamma hydroxybutyric acid (GHB) is a Schedule I substance. However, when formulated as an FDA-approved pharmaceutical product, it is classified in Schedule III. Dronabinol's regulatory treatment provides another example of such bifurcation. Marinol is contained in Schedule III of the CSA, whereas THC, when not formulated in such a product, remains in Schedule I.

In some cases, the separation is maintained through limitations on the numbers of physicians who may prescribe, or the types of healthcare facilities that can provide, the drug. The UK has utilised this type of system to permit the provision of diamorphine (heroin). A limited number of physicians are licensed to prescribe diamorphine and cocaine to addicts for maintenance. In addition, diamorphine can be used within a hospital for pain treatment. In the US, marketing approval for a new controlled substance product may be conditional on the use of patient and prescriber registries and the use of centralised pharmacies to prevent illicit use. Similar restrictions have been proposed for existing prescription analgesics, such as OxyContin.

What may drive a change in a nation's attitudes towards cannabis?

Patient and healthcare advocacy movements

The civil rights and anti-war movements in the US fostered changes across the Western world – promoting, on the one hand, greater respect for equality and individuality and, on the other, profound distrust of conventional values and authorities. In turn, the concept of individual empowerment took root in the Western culture. These developments spawned a virtual army of advocacy groups, some formally organised, others bound by loose affiliations of individuals, many overlapping in their goals and interests.

The patient self-help movement emerged out of these events. Fuelled by the rapidly expanding Internet, advocacy and support groups dedicated to particular types of medical conditions disseminate information and commentary and combat obstacles to treatment. 'Outliers' – the significant percentages of patients who do not benefit from standard medications – are no longer merely empty statistics. Able to keep abreast of new developments in science and medicine, patients communicate and exchange their views on a variety of relevant issues, demand innovative treatment, and mobilise support for changes in governmental laws or policies.

This change has not been lost on pharmaceutical companies. Within the US pharmaceutical industry, direct-to-consumer (DTC) advertising has become a well-accepted means of increasing patient demand and, therefore, of sales. It has become commonplace for patients to research published studies and other information relating to their conditions and to pressure their physicians to consider the newest treatment modalities.

Unsurprisingly, much of the recent demand for medicinal cannabis has emerged, not from the halls of science, but from the patient community. In light of the changes described above, such patient advocacy now has a far more powerful influence on governmental policymakers and the medical profession.

Renewed interest in herbs and alternative medicine

The natural foods movement, reinforced by patient advocacy and empowerment, has also given new vigour to the interest in botanical medicines and dietary supplements. Renewed support for botanical and other natural products has been accompanied by an increased distrust of the pharmaceutical industry and its new chemical entities.

Flooded by patient testimonials, both conventional physicians and regulatory authorities have become more receptive to the concept of botanical medicines. The US Food and Drug Administration recently issued draft guidance, setting forth the pathway for developing a botanical product into a prescription medicine. The US Government has established a well-funded centre – the National Centre for Complementary and Alternative Medicine – within the National Institutes of Health to conduct and support research into the effectiveness of botanical products and other alternative medical treatments. A recent US federal law, the Dietary Supplement Health Education Act (DSHEA), loosened regulatory controls over non-prescription botanical products and other dietary supplements.

In other countries, there is even greater acceptance of botanical products. In Germany, for example, herbal remedies are an integral part of mainstream medicine. Such countries, therefore, are more likely to be receptive to botanical products, particularly if they have been developed in accordance with international regulatory standards for quality, safety, and efficacy.

Cannabis, as a herb that has been used safely around the world for thousands of years, is the quintessential modern botanical medicine. In addition, there is widespread and renewed interest in the health and cosmetic benefits of hemp seed and oil products. Indeed, as indicated above, the DEA's recent efforts to suppress hemp food products and dietary supplements has brought it into conflict with new interest groups whose health-related goals have nothing to do with cannabis. There appears to be broad sympathy for the idea that, because of that history, pharmaceutical products prepared from standardised, whole plant cannabis extracts should not be subject to the same degree of scrutiny as new chemical entities that have never been tried in humans. Thus, the groundwork has now been laid for the development of a cannabis-based prescription medicine.

Scientific developments

As is more fully described elsewhere in this book, the identification of THC as the primary psychoactive component of cannabis and the discovery of the endocannabinoid receptor system has provided critical evidence of the active principles and modes of action of cannabis. Such information sparked a worldwide renewal of scientific interest in the therapeutic potential of cannabis and cannabinoids.

These new findings opened up a wide horizon of research opportunities. Anxious to explore the significance and potential of the receptor system, waves of researchers, many of them funded by grants from the US National Institute on Drug Abuse (NIDA), embarked on research programmes. Cannabinoid research organisations were formed, whose members conducted and published the results of rigorous and *bona fide* scientific studies. Such research has provided important – and incontestably valid – information relevant to the function of cannabis as a medicine.

Furthermore, the rapid progress in the UK toward a pharmaceutical-quality, non-smoked cannabis-based medicine has demonstrated that a commercial development process can control and standardise raw materials from the earliest stages of cultivation. This in turn has encouraged many mainstream physicians, researchers and pharmaceutical companies to step into the arena. The presence of such moderate voices, previously unconnected with cannabis or with cannabis advocacy movements, has helped to reduce the debate's previously vitriolic character.

The environmental and natural foods movements

During the past three decades, the environmental movement has grown in power and visibility. Many groups have conducted educational and political campaigns to target problems of soil pollution and depletion, poor air quality, destruction of natural resources, and loss of fragile and unique habitats. In the opinion of many environmental activists, hemp holds great promise for both agriculture and industry. Hemp cultivation has resumed with vigour in many parts of the world. Increased familiarity and comfort with hemp may promote greater interest in and receptivity toward cannabis, particularly its therapeutic potential.

A pressing need for harm reduction

A number of countries, breaking ranks with the prohibitionist approach exemplified by the US 'War on Drugs', have gravitated toward the concept of 'harm reduction' as a pragmatic means of addressing the drug abuse problem. This movement toward harm reduction has been fuelled by a number of serious concerns.

First, there is a pressing need to stem the rising tide of heroin addiction. Injection drug use brings with it a host of public health and safety issues. New cases of AIDS and hepatitis C are on the rise among i.v. drug users, and the ravaging effects of these diseases have had a devastating effect on public health resources. In addition, illicit injection drug use creates panoplies of other serious health consequences. It is also accompanied by criminal activity related to the addict's need to support his or her habit.

Many countries have begun to recognise that criminal penalties do not deter illicit drug use and that innovative measures are necessary. Some theories have suggested that heroin addiction is facilitated when individual drug users (1) are exposed to black market sources that offer a spectrum of drug choices and (2) are marginalised and isolated from the dominant culture by the threat (or fact) of criminal law enforcement. Therefore, some countries, such as the Netherlands, have sought to separate the markets of 'hard' drugs, such as heroin and cocaine, from those of 'soft' drugs, primarily cannabis, and to strip cannabis of its 'outlaw' character, thereby retaining its users within the mainstream culture.

Second, the sheer numbers of otherwise law-abiding young people arrested for the crime of cannabis possession has also fuelled an interest in another form of harm reduction. As a general rule, the adverse effects of law enforcement should not exceed the adverse impact of the criminal offence. Over the last several decades, more and more evidence has demonstrated that cannabis consumption causes harm of a far lesser type and magnitude than that resulting from the use of harder drugs. However, arrest, conviction and imprisonment – and even the mere existence of a criminal record – may destroy employment and other opportunities for a host of youthful 'offenders'. A strict prohibitionist policy also increases the contact of young cannabis users with the black market and increases the mystique of cannabis, and therefore, attractiveness to young users. Thus, pressure is building to reduce, or even eliminate, criminal sanctions for cannabis possession and use. The Australian Institute of Criminology in 1995 conducted an extensive analysis of the extent to which various cannabis control options reduce or produce harm (McDonald and Atkinson, 1995).

Finally, there is a growing concern that maintenance of the current prohibitions will ultimately bring the law into general disrepute. In many countries, cannabis laws are often not enforced according to their terms, e.g. offenders are released with a warning or caution rather than criminally prosecuted, or are enforced unevenly, e.g. juries refuse to convict patients being prosecuted for the medicinal use of cannabis. Hence, there is the dual need (1) to devise sanctions that more accurately reflect the nature of the transgression and are therefore enforceable; and (2) to determine whether or not cannabis has legitimate therapeutic value.

Some nations, without reducing criminal penalties, have in practice assigned a very low priority to the prosecution of cannabis possession/use offences or otherwise have applied greater leniency to such offences. In the Netherlands, for example, the principle of expediency, which allows the public prosecutor to refrain, on public interest grounds, from instituting a criminal prosecution, is deeply embedded in the structure of the criminal law. However, in other countries, such as the UK, such informal practices may be less acceptable, and actual changes in the law may be deemed more desirable. Even in the Netherlands, the current pragmatic approach is viewed as 'a policy in need of revision'. In a recent speech, the Dutch Minister of Justice remarked that 'the great discrepancy [in cannabis policies] between formal prohibition and informal acceptance ... not only obscures the policy, but is also detrimental to the government's authority' (Korthals, 2001).

As popular support grows for cannabis use (recreational or medical or both), the perceived legitimacy of prohibitive law dims accordingly. Recent polls indicate that large majorities of the populace in many countries support access to medicinal cannabis, and increasing percentages support cannabis decriminalisation. In order to be effective, prohibitions must affect only a small subgroup of the population. When a practice becomes endemic, the threat of sanctions cannot eradicate it. The Indian Hemp Commission recognised that reality in 1894 India. A recent report out of Jamaica has candidly acknowledged such endemic use in 2000 Jamaica (Chevannes, 2002). The Western world in general may almost have reached the point at which cannabis laws become essentially unenforceable. In order to maintain the general respect for the rule of law, then, such archaic prohibitions must fall.

Influence of the international community

International control bodies may influence a nation's attitudes toward cannabis and other drugs. In its annual reports, the International Narcotics Control Board (INCB) comments on the drug control programmes of countries around the world. In many cases, the INCB has sharply criticised nations either for their affirmative policy decisions or for their failure to take action to address a problem. For example, in its 2001 report, having noted that cannabis remains the most widely abused and trafficked drug in Europe, the Board stressed that the Netherlands' policy of tolerating the consumption and sale of cannabis products in 'coffee shops' is 'not in compliance with the international drug control treaties' (INCB, 2001). It further chastised the Netherlands for failing to create 'legal instruments' to deal with the problem of internet advertising and sales of high-THC cannabis seeds. By contrast, the Board congratulated Norway for its 'strict implementation of the international drug control conventions'.

The Board elsewhere indicated its concerns with countries in Western Europe that have decriminalised offences relating to, or that 'openly tolerate', the possession and abuse of cannabis and other drugs. Questioning whether such decriminalisation or toleration would be a 'proper strategy' for achieving a reduction in drug abuse, the Board remarked, 'None of these Governments ... have been able to provide ... information showing that the application of such measures reduces the demand for illicit drugs'. The report further deplored the 'growing gap' between developed and developing countries with regard to cannabis policy, which, it insisted, will impede effective international drug control efforts. The Board emphasised that developing countries have been devoting resources to the eradication of cannabis and to fighting illicit trafficking in the drug, while developed countries have 'decided to tolerate the cultivation of, trade in, and abuse of cannabis' (INCB, 2001).

Looking to the Americas, the Board cautioned Canada about its new medicinal cannabis regulations permitting access to medicinal cannabis. The report warned that 'there has been no reliable scientific evidence of the safety and efficacy of smoking cannabis herb for therapeutic purposes', and that 'the action was explicitly opposed by the Canadian Medical Association'. The Board also expressed concern about the 'widespread opinion in Jamaica that cannabis is not a harmful drug', and urged the nation to continue to impose criminal sanctions on cannabis possession and abuse 'in accordance with the international drug control treaties'. By contrast, the report applauded the US for having 'consistently applied strict measures in conformity with the provisions of the international drug control treaties' (INCB, 2001).

It is difficult to predict whether, or to what extent, a country may be influenced by the INCB's opprobrium or by the criticisms of neighbouring countries. If a changeover occurs in a nation's governing party, such influences may take on new importance.

The sheer passage of time

As time has passed, retrospective studies have demonstrated that in jurisdictions such as the Netherlands, South Australia and eleven US states during the 1970s that decriminalised cannabis possession, there has not been a resultant increase in cannabis abuse. Since opponents of decriminalisation generally argue that such measures will cause cannabis use to rise, such data will no doubt provide encouragement to countries considering the enactment of similar reforms.

After several decades of widespread cannabis use there is very little evidence that cannabis causes serious physical or psychological harm. While not completely benign, the harms of cannabis are less than those resulting from the heavy use of alcohol and tobacco. Indeed, to the extent that cannabis users substitute cannabis for alcohol, it can be said that cannabis is protective of individual and public health. Furthermore, a recent study of four of the remaining seven US IND patients who had used cannabis regularly for 11–27 years revealed no significant adverse effects of such long-term use (Russo *et al.*, 2002).

Time has also demonstrated that draconian sanctions do not serve to deter cannabis use. Despite the global enactment of prohibitory domestic criminal laws and the existence of international agreements, cannabis use (as well as other drug use) has continued to rise in many jurisdictions. Strident policy analyses contend that the 'War on Drugs' has been a failure and that only education and public health measures can achieve the desired outcome. Without deterrence as a defining rationale, cannabis prohibition cannot long survive.

In addition, the sheer numbers of cannabis users, particularly among young people, has imposed a serious drain on law enforcement resources. Numerous governmental commissions have recognised that these resources could be more effectively spent fighting violent crime. Indeed, many commentators have emphasised that law enforcement becomes virtually impossible when a prohibited activity becomes endemic in the population, and when the general public ceases to view the activity as criminal.

Over the past few decades, it has become apparent that cannabis users come from all professions and social classes. Most of these individuals are productive citizens, and many are highly respected in their fields. If such persons speak out about their cannabis use it may help further to dispel the negative stereotypes that previously surrounded the cannabis user. Greater support for decriminalisation may result.

Attitude of the medical profession

Ultimately, no substance can gain acceptance as a medicine unless its use enjoys the support of the medical profession. In order to recommend or prescribe a medicine, most physicians require that its safety and efficacy be 'evidence based', i.e. demonstrated through acceptable evidence – generally data from controlled clinical trials. This is particularly so for a substance, like cannabis, that carries considerable social stigma; however, it also holds true for other more 'innocuous' botanical products and dietary supplements. Physicians will never feel fully comfortable in recommending or prescribing such substances unless they have adequate assurance that they meet modern evidentiary standards and that, on balance, they are more likely to produce benefit than harm.

In general, the medical profession has entered the cannabis controversy with caution and trepidation. For example, as indicated above, in the US a number of major medical organisations opposed the state initiatives that legalised the use of medicinal cannabis. This opposition was founded in large part on their concern that the initiative or legislative processes, by circumventing state and federal regulatory requirements, would set a dangerous precedent for the approval of other medicines. Physicians feared that without such regulatory oversight, patients would be offered false hope, exposed to unknown risks, and encouraged to use a substance whose composition was unpredictable and uncontrolled.

In addition, physicians wish to be able to guide patients effectively through the informed consent process. In the absence of information from controlled clinical trials, they contend that they cannot inform patients about the likely risks and purported benefits, appropriate dosages and dosing strategy, method of administration, etc. of medicinal cannabis. On the basis of such concerns, the Canadian Medical Association has discouraged its members from advising patients about the use of medicinal cannabis.

Finally, fear of governmental sanctions may also discourage physicians from talking with patients about medicinal cannabis. In the US, the Federal Government vigorously asserted that a physician's mere 'recommendation' of cannabis violates federal law. In some cases, state medical boards have begun to investigate physicians who frequently recommend cannabis to their patients. Without the robust cooperation of the medical profession, the US state initiatives have had only limited effectiveness. This fear of sanctions may not be as dominant outside the US.

The antismoking movement

Since the 1960s, the dangers of smoking tobacco have become evident, and both governmental agencies and private organisations have initiated aggressive antismoking campaigns. Thus, as other myths about cannabis are gradually debunked, the dangers of pulmonary harm have taken on new visibility. In the Western world, smoking is the primary cannabis delivery method. While other modes of administration exist, they are not as popular, nor as easily accessible, as smoking. There appears to be general agreement that this concern has limited relevance for terminal patients suffering from unrelieved pain or other symptoms. However, if cannabis is to be smoked on a long-term basis, either by patients with a chronic disease or by recreational users, the risks of pulmonary damage take on greater significance.

In general, it is unlikely that cannabis in smoked form will ever garner acceptance from governments or the medical profession. In the US, for example, this issue played a significant role in the IOM report. Pointing to the risk of pulmonary harm, that report recommended against the long-term use of smoked cannabis for medical purposes. This is particularly true if there are significant sentiments against cannabis in general. In such countries, the risk of pulmonary harm will be viewed as the new 'objective' danger that replaces old, 'unscientific' fears of insanity and criminality. However, while there is no doubt evidence that long-term cannabis smoking may cause some degree of pulmonary damage, there is only tenuous evidence linking it to lung cancer or other devastating diseases.

Other countries may respond differently to this concern. The Canadian Government has agreed to fund clinical studies exploring the therapeutic potential of smoked cannabis in chronic conditions. Unlike the US, some nations may be more comfortable with the idea of permitting patients to use smoked cannabis on a compassionate basis, at least during the period of time required for a more suitable cannabis medicine to reach the pharmacies.

The availability of new medical products

The significance of the cannabinoid receptor system and its endocannabinoids has not been lost on the pharmaceutical industry. Once deterred by the stigma and bureaucratic difficulty of working with cannabis, these companies are now showing a renewed interest in developing synthetic cannabinoid or cannabimimetic compounds. For example, Pharmos is currently conducting Phase II and III clinical trials investigating the neuroprotective effect of dexanabinol, an apparently non-psychoactive synthetic isomer of THC, in traumatic brain injury victims. It recently reported the results of preclinical studies using other cannabimimetic molecules in the treatment of neuro-inflammatory conditions and disorders. Indevus Pharmaceuticals is investigating the anti-inflammatory and analgesic properties of adjulemic acid, a synthetic non-psychoactive THC derivative. Others are seeking to attempt to find more effective ways of delivering dronabinol (THC). For example, Unimed recently unveiled its intention to produce an inhaled version of Marinol. Oxford Natural Products is seeking to develop a suppository containing a prodrug ester of THC, dronabinol hemisuccinate.

Cannabis opponents may claim that the herbal material and its preparations should remain illegal for medical (and, *a fortiori*, recreational) use pending the outcome of these efforts. Indeed, as noted above, the US Government once believed that Marinol would obviate the need for medicinal cannabis. Although many patients dislike the effects of oral dronabinol, cannabis opponents continue to assert that herbal cannabis need not be authorised, since an approved cannabinoid medicine is available.

It is unlikely that the potential availability of additional synthetic products will significantly hamper efforts to make cannabis available for medical purposes. First, such products will not be available for a number of years, and seriously ill patients are no longer willing to suffer (or risk prosecution) while they wait. Second, with the increase in popular and scientific support for the use of botanical products, there is a strong sentiment in favour of a naturally derived cannabis medicine. Furthermore, encouraging evidence from current UK clinical trials with standardised whole plant extracts suggests that a cannabis medicine will be available in the very near future.

Prescription medicine abuse

Prescription drug abuse and diversion are on the increase. In the US, the OxyContin debacle has focused a spotlight on the issue. Regulatory authorities have expressed their growing concern about the abuse potential of new pharmaceutical products, particularly analgesics.

With regard to cannabis, this factor may be the proverbial knife that cuts both ways. On the one hand, there may be greater reluctance to allow an already-illicit drug to enter the pharmaceutical marketplace, out of fear that its diversion and abuse will be inevitable. Furthermore, prescription drug diversion and abuse have made it clear that both regulatory authorities and the medical profession must devise better ways to distinguish between legitimate patient use and illicit activities. In the US, a number of measures are currently under consideration.

On the other hand, some reports have suggested that the existence of a prescription will enable law enforcement to distinguish bona fide patients from recreational users. However, as the OxyContin situation has demonstrated, the mere possession of a prescription is not a sufficient touchstone, since doctor-shopping and prescription fraud may be common. Other antidiversionary measures, including better industry efforts to ensure that patients and physicians accurately understand the appropriate indications for a product, may be necessary in the future to prevent illicit use.

Relative influence of factors

The above list of factors is certainly not exhaustive. A country's cannabis policies will also be affected by such influences as: the strength of domestic antidrug advocacy organisations, particularly those that are affiliated with conservative religious groups; the government's perceived obligations to assist source nations with their efforts to eradicate drug production and trafficking; and the attitudes of public health and law enforcement agencies. For example, between 1968 and 1972 in the Netherlands, the Ministry of Justice had developed misgivings about the law's repressive approach to cannabis use and became receptive to psychological and sociological approaches, such as separating the hard and soft drug markets (De Kort, 1994).

Some of the above factors will affect more significantly the future of cannabis as a medicine, others its availability as a recreational substance. Even if the above factors support a general re-evaluation of cannabis, they do not necessarily suggest that efforts to decriminalise its recreational use will proceed in parallel with efforts to make it available for medical or industrial purposes. Again, depending on a country's unique character, such reforms may proceed down quite different paths. However, over time, one path's progress will inform and influence the others. Overall, the character of the debate appears gradually to be moving from strident diatribe to a more reasoned dialogue.

Where are we now?

For the first time since its re-introduction into Western medicine during the early part of the nineteenth century, the time may be ripe for cannabis to enjoy an objective evaluation. However, around the world, that evaluation may take place at a different pace, and with a different outcome, depending on a country's culture, political climate and perceptions of its international obligations. Some examples may illuminate this point.

The Netherlands

In 1976, the Netherlands, while technically retaining criminal prohibitions against cannabis possession, cultivation and supply, issued law enforcement and prosecutorial guidelines providing for non-prosecution under certain circumstances. Under this policy, possession of cannabis for personal use, and a small quasi-retail trade, is permitted. So-called 'coffee shops' are allowed to sell up to 5 g of cannabis, subject to strict conditions. Coffee shops cannot keep more than 500 g of cannabis in stock, sell hard drugs, admit or sell to minors, advertise or create a nuisance. A 'grey market' of illegally imported and domestically cultivated cannabis supplies the coffee shops.

The purpose of this policy was twofold: (1) to separate the markets for 'hard' and 'soft' drugs and (2) to remove cannabis's stigma as an illegal substance, thus keeping cannabis users integrated within the mainstream culture, rather than forcing them into criminal circles. The policy appears to have been successful. Rates of cannabis use in the Netherlands are mid-range in relation to other European nations, and considerably lower than in the US and Australia. Rates of heroin addiction are lower than in many countries, including the US. Despite the ostensible success of this approach, the Netherlands current ruling party has announced that it will seek to close many of the coffee shops.

The Netherlands has also taken a proactive position in the medicinal cannabis debate. Desiring to promote further research and recognising the need for a legal source of high-quality, standardised cannabis, the country in 2000 established a national agency, The Office of Medicinal Cannabis (OMC), to manage the necessary cultivation and/or importation. The OMC is responsible for licensing growers to cultivate medicinal grade cannabis, and will take control of the stock and supply cannabis and cannabis preparations for medical and scientific purposes. In March 2003, new legislation was enacted that enables physicians to prescribe, and pharmacies to supply, medicinal cannabis to patients.

Canada

Canada has recently taken a very active interest in the therapeutic potential of cannabis. In 1999, Health Canada indicated that it would support and fund controlled clinical trials investigating the potential role of cannabis as a therapeutic agent. In light of the pubic perception that smoked herbal cannabis was medically effective and the reality that patients in Canada were currently using cannabis in that form, Health Canada indicated that it wished to evaluate that use. Therefore, the investigation of the safety and efficacy of smoked research-grade cannabis in such trials was to be a priority. In July of 2001, Health Canada announced that the first trial, to be conducted at McGill Pain Centre and involving patients with chronic neuropathic pain, had been funded. The trial is underway. Proposals involving alternate preparations and novel delivery systems, as well as basic research, could also be considered 'in certain circumstances'.

Pending the development of a prescribed cannabis-based medicine, Health Canada has also authorised a limited number of seriously ill patients to use medicinal cannabis pursuant to Section 56 of the Controlled Drugs and Substances Act (CDSA). Under Section 56, the Minister of Health has discretionary power to grant an exemption from the application of any or all part of the CDSA or its regulations, if the Minister believes the exemption is necessary for medical or scientific purposes or is otherwise in the public interest.

In 2000, Health Canada awarded a 5-year CDN$5.8 million contract to Prairie Plant Systems to grow and produce research-quality cannabis. The first crop, which was grown underground in an abandoned copper mine, was available in early 2002 and was to be distributed to researchers and qualified patients. To satisfy its obligations under the Single Convention, Canada established a national agency – the Office of Marihuana Medical Access – to take control and supervise distribution of the crop.

In 2000, the Ontario Court of Appeal ruled that the law's blanket prohibition against personal possession and use of cannabis, even for medical purposes, was unconstitutional. The court ruled that a prohibition against possession and cultivation for medical use was not necessary to fulfil Canada's obligations under the Single Convention. It further ruled that the lack of an adequate legislated standard for determining medical necessity under Section 56 and the vesting of unfettered discretion in the Minister did not accord with principles of fundamental justice. As a result, the court declared invalid the entire prohibition against cannabis possession; however, the ruling was suspended for one year to allow the Government to develop a defined regulatory process through which patients could be authorised to use cannabis in cases of medical necessity.

Following that ruling, in 2001 Health Canada issued regulations (the Marihuana Medical Access Regulations) designed to make the medical exemption process more transparent. Under the regulations, patients with terminal diseases and other serious conditions qualify to use cannabis. In the case of terminal disease, the patient's personal physician must declare in writing that all conventional treatments have been tried or considered, that cannabis would mitigate the patient's symptoms, and that the benefits of cannabis use would outweigh the risks. For other conditions, an additional declaration from one, and in some cases, two specialists, and greater evidence of medical necessity, is required. Furthermore, the medical declaration must state the recommended daily dosage of dried cannabis, in grams, and the form and route of administration. If the recommended daily dose exceeds 5 g, the physician must declare that he or she has engaged the patient in a detailed discussion of potential risks and benefits. The regulations also authorise a patient, or person designated by the patient, to cultivate cannabis for the patient's personal medical use. With the promulgation of these regulations, Canada became the first country in the Western world to authorise patients to use cannabis for medical purposes. Several hundred patients have received approvals through this process.

Recent events suggest, however, that there may be obstacles to the fuller availability of medicinal cannabis, at least in its herbal, smoked form. For example, there is discontent within the medical profession, without whose cooperation the current access regulations cannot be implemented. The Canadian Medical Association has expressed concerns that physicians do not have sufficient information about cannabis to fulfil the obligations placed on them by the new regulations. The Alberta Medical Association has advised Canadian physicians to 'think carefully' before signing a medical declaration. An antismoking physician group, Physicians for a Smoke-Free Canada, has argued strongly against the use of smoked cannabis for medical purposes, particularly for patients with chronic diseases or disorders.

In addition, the current Minister of Health, in the face of a reprimand from the INCB and opposition from the US, expressed reservations about Health Canada's plan to distribute herbal cannabis to authorised patients. The Minister indicated that the Government would require more evidence of efficacy from clinical trials in order to satisfy its obligation under the Single Convention to restrict the use of cannabis to medical and scientific purposes.

Nevertheless, a recent court decision ruled that the access regulations were invalid under the Canadian constitution and essentially required Canada to devise a workable programme to provide medicinal cannabis to qualifying patients. Subsequently, a court of appeal reinstated the regulations, but loosened the stringency of the patient-qualification criteria and essentially paved the way for cannabis dispensaries to be licensed. Therefore, Canada's general criminal prohibition against cannabis possession is no longer in immediate peril. On 23 December 2003, the Supreme Court ruled that Parliament has the constitutional right to prohibit cannabis possession using the criminal law. In addition, in September 2002, a committee of the Canadian Senate called for the full legalisation of cannabis. As a result, the Canadian Government has begun seriously to review its laws governing the recreational use of cannabis and is currently considering a bill that would decriminalise the possession of small amounts. Such decriminalisation efforts have been vigorously opposed by the US, however, which has insisted that the liberalisation of cannabis laws would create serious border security problems and increase the flow of illicit cannabis into the US. With such a powerful neighbour, the future of significant cannabis reform within Canada remains uncertain.

The United Kingdom

Historically, the UK has had one of the 'most restrictive' cannabis control policies in Europe. As in the US, it refused to deviate from that position despite the contrary recommendations of respected commissions. For example, following a wave of debate about cannabis in Parliament and the press, in 1967, the Hallucinogens Sub-Committee of the Home Office Advisory Committee on Drug Dependence issued a report (the Wootton Report) that examined the misuse of cannabis and lysergic acid diethylamide (LSD).

The report concluded that cannabis use was widespread, reaching beyond the radical movement and across class barriers. It determined that cannabis did not lead to heroin addiction, cause violent crime or aggression, antisocial behaviour, or (in normal people) physical dependence or psychosis, and indeed, was much less dangerous than opiates, amphetamines and barbiturates, and less dangerous than alcohol. Therefore, while recommending that restrictions be maintained through the criminal law on the availability and use of cannabis, the report urged that cannabis legislation should be separated from that dealing with the harder drugs and that the current penalties for possession and supply should be reduced. The report specifically recommended that the possession of a small amount of cannabis should not normally be regarded as a serious crime leading to imprisonment. It urged that medicinal cannabis preparations should continue to be available on prescription.

The Wootton Report had virtually no impact. Indeed, in 1973 the medical use of cannabis preparations was prohibited. Little reform took place over the next two decades. However, late in the 1990s, a dramatic interest in cannabis reform surfaced. In 1997, the British Medical Association issued a report recommending that the Government amend the law to allow the prescription of cannabinoids to patients whose conditions are not adequately controlled by standard medications and called for further research into the use of cannabinoids for treatment of a number of conditions. The BMA noted that such prescriptions should not include either cigarettes or herbal preparations 'with unknown concentrations of cannabinoids or other chemicals' (BMA, 1998).

Following that report, in 1998 two significant events occurred. First, the UK Home Office licensed a British pharmaceutical company, GW Pharmaceuticals, to cultivate and possess cannabis for research purposes, and the company embarked on a full-scale pharmaceutical development programme to produce a range of non-smoked standardised medicinal cannabis extracts.

Second, the British House of Lords appointed a Select Committee on Science and Technology to consider the scientific and medical evidence relating to medicinal cannabis. After receiving extensive expert testimony, the Committee urged that clinical trials for the treatment of multiple sclerosis and chronic pain 'should be mounted as a matter of urgency', and that research should be supported into alternative modes of administration that would retain the benefit of rapid absorption offered by smoking, without posing the risk of pulmonary and other harm (House of Lords Select Committee on Science and Technology, 1998). The report also recommended that the Government should reschedule cannabis and cannabis resin in order to allow physicians to prescribe appropriate cannabis preparations. However, the Committee stressed that cannabis should continue to be a controlled drug, rejecting the argument that the absolute prohibition on its recreational use should be lifted.

The Government flatly rejected the rescheduling recommendation. However, it did make repeated assurances that if the quality, safety and efficacy of an appropriate cannabis preparation were established, the

Government would actively cooperate in permitting the medicine to be prescribed. In 2001, the House of Lords Select Committee on Science and Technology issued a follow-up report examining the current state of research into the therapeutic uses of cannabis, the roles of Government regulatory bodies in the licensing of cannabis-based medicines, and more recent issues relating to the prosecution of medicinal cannabis users. It stressed the undesirability of prosecuting patients who use or cultivate cannabis for their personal medical use. The House of Lords Select Committee on Science and Technology also urged a reconsideration of regulatory requirements that may unnecessarily delay the development of cannabis-based medicines.

In 1999, the Police Foundation issued its Report of the Independent Inquiry into the Misuse of Drugs Act of 1971 (Runciman, 1999). That report contained an entire chapter on cannabis. It concluded that cannabis was much less harmful that the other main illicit drugs, that there was little evidence that the law was effective as a deterrent to cannabis use, and recommended substantial reductions in sanctions for cannabis offences. It urged the Government to reclassify cannabis into Class C and to move it from Schedule 1 to Schedule 2 of the Misuse of Drugs Regulations to permit supply and possession for medical purposes. This proposal was again rejected.

Momentum for general cannabis reform continued to build. In March 2002, the Advisory Council on the Misuse of Drugs recommended that cannabis be moved from Class B to Class C in Schedule 2 of the Misuse of Drugs Act 1971. The Council explained that cannabis is less harmful than other substances within Class B, and therefore:

> The continuing juxtaposition of cannabis with these more harmful Class B drugs erroneously (and dangerously) suggests that their harmful effects are equivalent. This may lead to the belief, amongst cannabis users, that if they have had no harmful effects from cannabis then other Class B substances will be equally safe.

At this writing, Parliament is considering legislation that would, to a great extent, implement the Council's recommendations.

Other countries

Although the US continues to maintain a draconian prohibitionist system, it appears to be losing its influence on worldwide drug policy. Interest in medicinal cannabis is rapidly growing. Indeed, for the first time, a US Democratic presidential candidate, Dennis Kucinich, has endorsed the legalisation of medicinal cannabis, and in a recent gubernatorial recall election in the state of California, all the major candidates endorsed the concept of medicinal cannabis. Widespread publicity and attention has been focused on the work of GW Pharmaceuticals, a UK pharmaceutical company that is advancing on the largest clinical development programme ever undertaken into standardised, non-smoked, cannabis-based medicinal extracts. The company has reported that the results of its Phase II and Phase III trials are quite encouraging. GW submitted its first marketing approval application to the UK Medicines and Healthcare products Regulatory Agency at the end of March 2003. Now that there is a strong likelihood that a prescription medicine will soon become available, moderate voices, including those of physicians, researchers and other professionals, have entered the dialogue.

In November 2001, representatives from 10 European countries met to discuss and exchange information about medicinal cannabis developments within their borders. The participants indicated that their governments' interest was strong and clinical trials were being conducted, or at least seriously considered, in a number of jurisdictions; however, research has been hindered by the difficulty of obtaining access to lawful sources of standardised materials.

Similar developments are taking place in other parts of the world. In Australia, although the use of cannabis for medical (or non-medical) purposes is formally prohibited by law, a number of states have implemented or are considering significant reforms. In 2000 in New South Wales, the Working Party on the Use of Cannabis for Medical Purposes issued a report recommending, among other things, that Government either fund or otherwise facilitate research into the therapeutic efficacy of cannabis and cannabinoids and that the governing law be amended to remove obstacles to the conduct of such trials. It further urged the Government to establish a compassionate regime that would enable seriously ill patients to use smoked cannabis without fear of criminal sanctions, pending the development of more appropriate preparations and modes of delivery.

In many countries, parallel efforts are underway both to make cannabis available as a medicine and to decriminalise cannabis use and possession. In Switzerland, for example, significant changes are in the offing. Under changes contained in a pending proposal, Swiss drug policy would both decriminalise the cultivation, manufacture, possession and purchase of cannabis as preparatory acts for personal consumption. The draft legislation would also allow the Government to 'define priorities' for the enforcement of remaining cannabis-related offences, although the INCB contends that such reforms would contravene the provisions of the international drug control treaties (INCB, 2002). A research institute has been authorised to cultivate cannabis and to manufacture standardised cannabis extracts for research purposes, and the Swiss Government has approved clinical studies using Marinol, cannabis extracts and herbal cannabis.

Ending thoughts

It appears that the old cannabis myths are rapidly disappearing, and that objective evidence may at last become the foundation of new public policy. There is widespread support for various types of cannabis depenalisation or decriminalisation, some of which has been precipitated by judicial decisions. In Italy, Luxembourg, Portugal and Spain, personal consumption of cannabis already is not considered a criminal offence, and preparatory acts, including acquisition, transportation and possession, are subject only to administrative sanctions. Belgium is also considering decriminalisation measures. As demonstrated by the recent UK Advisory Council report, a critical mass of opinion seems to have formed around the conclusion that the harmfulness of cannabis, even when used recreationally, lies somewhere between that of caffeine and codeine. Evidence is rapidly demonstrating that medicinal cannabis – particularly when standardised, formulated and administered by means of a non-smoked delivery system – has an important place in medicine's armamentarium. A rational approach to cannabis seems to be at hand.

References

Abel E (1980). *Marihuana: The First Twelve Thousand Years*. New York: Plenum Press.

Adams R (1973). Marijuana. In: *Marijuana: Medical Papers 1839–1972*. Oakland: Medi-Comp Press: 345–374.

Baum D (1996). *Smoke and Mirrors*. New York: Little, Brown & Co.

BMA (1997). *Therapeutic Uses of Cannabis*. London: British Medical Association.

Bonnie R, Whitebread C (1970). The forbidden fruit and the tree of knowledge: An inquiry into the legal history of American marijuana prohibition. *Virginia Law Review* 56(6).

Bonnie R, Whitebread C (1974). *The Marijuana Conviction*. Charlottesville, VA: University of Virginia Press.

Chevannes B (2002). A Report of the National Commission on Ganja. Jamaica.

DEA (2003). 68 Fed. Reg. 14113 (21 March). US Drug Enforcement Administration.

De Kort M (1994). The Dutch cannabis debate, 1968–1976. *J Drug Issues* 24(3): 417–427.

Drug Policy Forum Trust (1997). Alternative systems of cannabis control in New Zealand. www.nzdf.org.nz/fulltext.htm (accessed 20 March 2002).

Hough M, Warburton H, Few B, May T, Man L, Witton J, Turnbull P (2003). *A Growing Market*. York: Joseph Rowntree Foundation.

House of Lords Select Committee on Science and Technology (1998) *Cannabis: The Scientific and Medical Evidence*. The House of Lords Session 1997–8, 9th report. London: Stationery Office.

International Narcotics Control Board (2001). Report. Vienna: INCB.

International Narcotics Control Board (2002). Report. Vienna: INCB.

Joy J E, Watson Jr S J, Benson Jr J A (1999). *Marijuana and Medicine: Assessing the Science Base*. Division of Neuroscience and Behavioral Research, Institute of Medicine. Washington, DC: National Academy Press.

Korthals A (2001). *European Cities Conference on Cannabis Policy*. Utrecht, The Netherlands: Ministry of Justice: 22–24.

Krajeski K (2000). How flexible are the United Nations drug conventions? *Int J Drug Policy* 10(4): 329–338.

Lupien J C (1995). Unraveling an American dilemma: The demonization of marihuana. Master's thesis presented to the Faculty of the Graduate School of Pepperdine University.

McDonald D, Atkinson L (eds) (1995). *The Social Impact of Legislative Options for Cannabis in Australia*. Canberra: Australian Institute of Criminology.

McDonald D, Moore R, Wardlaw G, Ballenden N (1994). *Legislative Options for Cannabis in Australia*, National Drug Strategy Monograph No. 26. Canberra: Australian Institute of Criminology.

Mikuriya T (1973). Introduction. In: *Marijuana: Medical Papers 1839–1972*. Oakland: Medi-Comp Press.

Musty R, Rossi R (2001). Effects of smoked cannabis and oral delta-9-tetrahydro-cannabinol on nausea and emesis after cancer chemotherapy: A review of state clinical trials. *J Cannabis Ther* 1(1): 29–42.

Nahas G G, Suciu-Foca N, Armand J P, Morishima A (1974). Inhibition of cellular mediated immunity in marihuana smokers. *Science* 183 (1974): 419–420.

Office of the UN Secretary General (1973). *Commentary on the Single Convention on Narcotic Drugs 1961*. New York: UN.

Office of the UN Secretary General (1976). *Commentary on the Convention on Psychotropic Substances 1971*. New York: UN.

Runciman V (1999). *Drugs and the Law. Independent Inquiry into the Misuse of Drugs Act of 1971*. London: Police Foundation: 14.

Russo E, Mathre M L, Byrne A, Velin R, Bach P J, Sanchez-Ramos J, Kirlin K A (2002). Chronic cannabis use in the compassionate investigational new drug program: An examination of benefits and adverse effects of legal clinical cannabis. *J Cannabis Ther* 2(1): 3–57.

Single E (1998). Options for cannabis reform. *Int J Drug Policy* 10(4): 281–290.

Sinha J (2001). The history and development of the leading international drug control conventions. Prepared for The Senate Special Committee On Illegal Drugs. Canadian Library of Parliament.

Stenchever M A, Kunysz T J, Allen M A (1974). Chromosomal breakage in users of marihuana. *Am J Obstet Gynecol* 118: 106–113.

Werner C (2001). Medical marijuana and the AIDS crisis. *J Cannabis Ther* 1: 17–33.

Whitebread C (1995). The history of the non-medical use of drugs in the United States. Speech to the California Judges Association.

14

Development of cannabis-based medicines: risk, benefit and serendipity

Brian A Whittle and Geoffrey W Guy

The development of novel medicines is a rewarding but risky business. The development process centres on the minimisation and management of the risk; it cannot be avoided entirely. The risks arise in several forms that fall broadly into scientific, social and legislative areas. The scientific and technical risk factors are common to the development of all new drugs but with the development of cannabis-based medicines there are other, less tangible, social, quasi-scientific and legislative factors that can affect the progress of a new drug to the market. The rate at which a new drug can be brought to fruition obviously affects the financial success of a private or public company early in its corporate life. This chapter examines, with particular reference to a cannabis-based medicine, the factors on which the various risks can be overcome or minimised.

Development of medicines is a highly controlled process and any new products need approval by the relevant regulatory authority. It is the process of putting together a credible dossier of information for consideration by regulatory authorities that is the driver throughout the development process. The work to produce a confident registration dossier involves careful planning. Most of the problems, when identified, can be addressed by well-targeted research and development. Quality and safety risks are important because they ultimately relate to the intrinsic marketability of the product and its survival on the market after launch. Delay in taking a product to the market in a timely fashion can be fatal to the financial prospects of a pharmaceutical company, particularly if it is in start-up mode. When the product reaches the clinical study phase, the risks of failure are reduced but are still considerable. There is also the risk of delay from the regulatory process itself, without which it is not possible to market new medicinal products. Add to these scientific risks, and the fact that there are less quantifiable but nevertheless real risks relating to the attitudes of patients, practitioners and shareholders. In the case of cannabis-based medicine there is the implication of working with a scheduled substance whereby the general legislative climate may affect the ultimate marketing of the product. Additionally, there are issues relating to protection of inventions surrounding the product, which will eventually allow the sponsor to reap the benefits of the investment in research.

In order to achieve timely registration and commercialisation, the various lines of research have to be dovetailed together. The regulatory authorities have the responsibility of balancing the safety risks and weighing these against the benefits of the new medicines as part of the evaluation process. In the UK, it is the Committee on Safety of Medicines (CSM), advised by the professional secretariat who then make the regulatory risk/benefit assessment. The CSM's primary remit is safety, which also takes into account efficacy in relation to safety. There are also considerable non-technical risks. Table 14.1 details some of the risks that are encountered when developing a cannabis-based medicine.

Cannabis as a medicine

Cannabis has a long history of use as a medicine, and also as a recreational and ritualistic substance. Then, as now, pain was probably the urgent stimulus that caused patients to seek treatment. Written records of the use of cannabis as a medicine span more than five millennia, and its use probably extends back to the time when humans first experienced pain, and looked for agents to treat it. The reasons for selection of particular plants to treat disorders are not known with certainty. However, a number of theories have been advanced.

The doctrine of signatures focused many early investigations into the uses for natural medicines, often leading to the use of inappropriate, and at times dangerous materials. According to this theory, the shape and form of natural products, particularly plants, and the locations where they were found gave a clue to their usefulness as treatments for disease. It is a document that appears frequently in history, and dies hard. In the process, it has led to the use of appropriate plants such as willow bark (*Salix alba*) for the treatment of fevers. It is now known that *Salix* contains salicylate esters that are antipyretic and which also modify the generation of inflammatory mediators.

However, more often than not, the doctrine of signatures has not been a guiding light to therapeutic utility, but has certainly enriched our language with names such as eyebright (*Euphrasia* spp.) and lungwort (*Pulmonaria* spp.). Regardless of the validity of the theory, it provided the impetus to test plants for the treatment of disease. There are no clues

Table 14.1 Risk factors in development of cannabis-based medicines

Risk	Strategies for evaluation and reduction of risk
Anecdotal evidence	Critical analysis of data to achieve a consensus opinion. Design protocols for generating objective data
Epidemiological data	Critical analysis and stratification to isolate confounding factors
Quality issues: botanical raw material	
Impurities and contaminants from field grown crops	Grow under glass in controlled conditions
Botanical drug substance	GMP methodology and control procedures
Botanical drug product	Innovative product design and GMP manufacture
Preclinical safety	
Adverse toxicology	Acute and repeat dose studies to international regulatory standards to define effects on target organs
Clinical safety	
Adverse events	Adverse event monitoring in the context of clinical studies
	Physical measurements
Peripheral effects	Functional tests
Cognitive effects	
Inappropriate pharmacokinetics	Enzyme inhibition and reduction studies
Interaction(s) with other drugs	
Efficacy	Dose evaluation studies: dose titration controlled clinical studies
Withdrawal due to lack of effect	Randomised placebo comparison of various ratios of cannabinoid
Demonstration of need required	Pharmacovigilance
Appearance of adverse events late in development	Submit dossier to NICE
Development of addiction liability abuse potential	Advanced Dispensing System (ADS)
Threshold effect	

GMP, Good Manufacturing Practice; NICE, National Institute of Chemical Excellence.

to the usefulness of cannabis from its 'signatures'. It is likely that trial and error will have played the major part in the investigation of plants for medicinal use, as has religious conviction and superstition based on empirical use.

The empirical approach to research and the uses of plant medicines led to the use of many worthless materia medica, but the successes are very important for modern rational medicine. Plants such as opium, belladonna, cannabis, colchicum, hyoscymus, willow and capsicum have all been used historically to treat the cardinal signs of inflammation: pain, swelling, redness and loss of function. This includes not only pain and other signs arising directly from trauma but also agents that modify the perception of pain, and relieve the associated anxiety. A few prepared plants are still official as Active Pharmacuetical Ingredients. However, it is estimated that about a quarter of all drug substances in the current pharmacopoeias owe their origins to active constituents from plants or closely related synthetic derivatives. It is significant that the relief of pain is a prime focus of empiricism and one that has driven the search for plant medicines historically, and up to the present date.

Cannabis was lastly the subject of a monograph in the 1914 British Pharmacopoeia, and was deleted from the BPC after the 1934 edition. The legislative reasons for the disappearance of cannabis preparations from the pharmaceutical armamentarium are dealt with by Alice Mead in Chapter 13. Fankhauser has suggested four reasons for the disappearance of cannabis-based medicines. These are the:

- development of novel chemical agents as active ingredients
- difficulties in ensuring consistent quality
- economic problems of production and importation from (principally) Asian production areas during the World Wars
- legal sanctions.

These points illustrate the problems that have beset the development of a cannabis-based medicine in the twenty-first century. The supply and economic problems are solvable, and the quality issues are now well understood. Recently, evidence on safety and efficacy against pain and other symptoms of multiple sclerosis has been generated for a regulatory dossier, but legal restrictions are still unresolved. These are a major hurdle in some principal pharmaceutical markets, although in the UK there is an enlightened attitude to the medicinal use of cannabis. In October 2000 the UK Minister of Health (Mr David Blunkett, now Home Secretary) stated of cannabis-based medicines: 'Should as I believe it will, this programme (of trials) be proved to be successful, I will recommend to the Medicines Control Agency that they should go ahead with authorising its medicinal use' (Government Response to the House of Lords Select Committee on Science and Technology's Report on the Therapeutic Uses of Cannabis, 2001).

The historical legacy

Safety and efficacy are not absolutes, but a medicine must be safe and effective enough for its purpose. Quality is not negotiable whether the medicinal product is a complex botanical or a new chemical entity. Development of a cannabis-based medicine takes account of these regulatory imperatives. The fact that humans have been exposed to cannabinoids for many thousands of years can be advanced to justify early entry into later stage clinical trials of an extract of the plant rather than pure chemical constituents. It is likely that the human repertoire of metabolic enzymes will recognise and deal with plant extracts more easily than novel synthetic molecules. This provides a degree of reassurance in that cannabis is active in humans and apparently free of gross toxicity. Anecdotal information of this type cannot be relied upon alone in a regulatory sense but at least it reduces the risk of failure in early Phase II trials, which is the fate of many new chemical entity-based drugs.

There is a wealth of anecdotal data on the medical uses of cannabis. The use of reports of clinical benefit by patients is viewed with scepticism in some quarters, but in the development of Sativex, a cannabis-based prescription medicine, feedback from patients has been informative and reliable. For any prescription product, health registration and marketing approval are based on a risk benefit analysis of quality, safety and efficacy data. For drugs based on new chemical entities, harmonisation of regulatory guidelines throughout Europe has resulted in a clear route for registration for this type of drug. Guidelines are available from the European Medicines Evaluation Agency (EMEA), which indicate the issues of concern to the regulatory authority.

In the case of botanicals, harmonisation is less complete, and there are national differences in the emphasis placed on particular aspects of the regulatory package. However, the basic principles are the same: evaluation to provide a risk benefit analysis based on quality, safety and efficacy. Increasingly, the question of need is introduced into the process of release of new products onto the market. For cannabis-based medicines these issues apply but others are also important. These relate to attitudinal, historical, legal and enforcement issues, which arise because in most countries cannabis is still regarded as a drug of abuse. The change to a prescription medicine therefore has to take account of not only traditional regulatory parameters but also these other factors.

Attitudes to cannabis have swung from acceptance as a galenical product in widespread use over 100 years ago, to prohibition as a drug of abuse in the mid-twentieth century. In the first edition of *Merck's*

Table 14.2 Therapeutic indications given in *Merck's Manual* (1899) for *Cannabis indica* (CI) as extract and cannabine tannate (CT)

Indication	Product	Comment
Albuminuria	CI	As diuretic in haematuria
Asthma	CI	Sometimes useful in chronic cases
Irritable bladder	CI	
Bronchitis	CI	In very chronic cases
Chordee	CI	
Chorea	CI	May do good; often increases the choretic movements
Climacteric disorders	CI	
Coughs	CI	
Cystitis	CI	
Delirium	CI	In nocturnal delirium with softening of the brain
Delirium tremens	CI	Useful and not dangerous
Diarrhoea	CI	
Dropsy	CI	As diuretic
Dysmenorrhoea	CI	Very useful
Dyspepsia	CI	
Dysuria	CI	In haematuria
Epilepsy	CI	
Exophthalmos	CI	
Gastralgia	CI	
Gastric ulcer	CI	
Gonorrhoea	CI	To relieve pain and lessen discharge
Headache	CI	In neuralgic headache
Haematuria	CI	
Hemicrania (migraine)	CI	
Hiccough	CI	
Hydrophobia	CI	
Hysteria	CI & CT	
Impotence	CI	
Inflammation	CI	In chronic types
Insomnia	CI & CT	Alone or with hyoscyamus (CI)
Labour	CI	
Locomotor ataxia	CI	
Mania	CI	
Melancholia		
Menorrhagia and metrorrhagia	CI	Sometimes very useful
Migraine	CI	
Nephritis, acute	CI	As diuretic especially in haematuria
Neuralgia	CI	
Opium habit	CI	
Ovarian neuralgia	CI	

(continued)

Table 14.2 *Continued*

Indication	Product	Comment
Ovaritis	CI	
Pain	CI	
Paralysis agitans	CI	
Phthisis (tuberculosis)	CI	
Sea sickness	CI	To $^1/_2$ grain of the extract to relieve headache
Tetanus	CI	Serviceable in many cases; best combined with chloral
Tic douloureux	CI	
Trismus	CI	
Uterine cancer	CI	

From Beers and Berkow (1899).

Manual (Beers and Berkow, 1899) a number of preparations of cannabis are listed. These galenical preparations were included in complex prescriptions intended as hypnotics and sedatives. Uses described are 'hysteria, delirium, nervous insomnia etc.'. Table 14.2 lists the therapeutic indications for *Cannabis indica* and Cannabine Tannate in *Merck's Manual*. Cannabine Tannate was a proprietary preparation of cannabis extract that is described as: 'A yellow or brownish powder; slightly bitter and strong astringent taste. Soluble in alkaline water or alkaline alcohol, very slightly in water or alcohol.' Its uses were listed as treatments for 'hysteria, delirium, nervous insomnia etc. Dose 8–16 grains (0.5–1.0 g) at bedtime in a powder with sugar. Maximum dose 24 grains (approximately 1.5 g).'

The therapeutic indications, which were not only current 100 years ago, but appear to have been a mainstay of practitioner prescribing at that time are shown in Table 14.2. The table highlights that the list of conditions historically treated by cannabis preparations was very wide and covers most of the therapeutic areas currently catered for by the benzodiazapenes, analgesics, antiepileptics and treatments for migraine.

Table 14.2 is remarkable for the wide range of conditions for which cannabis was considered suitable. Some of the therapeutic indications listed are ones that are tabled for examination in controlled trials currently in the programme of work being carried out by GW Pharmaceuticals plc. The small number of references to cannabine tannate probably reflects its relatively short-lived use, in contrast to galenical preparations that were used as components of extemporaneous prescriptions until the mid-twentieth century.

At the time that *Merck's Manual* was written it was thought that the active substance in cannabis was one or more alkaloids, and the names 'cannabinene' and 'cannabine' have been applied to what was thought to be a volatile, liquid alkaloid, resembling nicotine in odour. The method of preparation of cannabine tannate follows traditional methodology of the time for separation of alkaloids from plant material. The volatile 'aether oils', believed to be responsible for toxicity, were separated by distillation. The residue was extracted with water and what was presumably plant proteinaceous matter was precipitated using lead acetate. Tannic acid was added and the lead was removed by precipitation with hydrogen sulfide. The cannabine tannate was used as the active constituent in complex prescriptions. From what is now known of the chemical and physical properties of the active ingredients of cannabis, it is remarkable that cannabine tannate had any significant activity, unless of course it contained water-soluble constituents which have not been isolated to date. No attempt appears to have been made to obtain Intellectual Property Rights (IPR) on cannabine tannate other than registration of the trademark. The assumption that cannabis contained alkaloids led researchers 100 years ago to use models for extraction of active constituents that are now inappropriate. We know now that cannabinoids, which are the principal active constituents of cannabis, are virtually insoluble in water.

The non-medical use of cannabis early in the twentieth century caused a swing away from the use of cannabinoids as useful prescription medicines to the point where they were regarded as drugs of abuse. This attitude has become deeply entrenched in the minds of some professionals and regulators, and can only be changed by provision of cogent evidence that the balance of benefit to risk is strongly in favour of reinstatement of cannabis as a medicinal product.

One result of prohibition was the discouragement of serious research into the medicinal uses of cannabis from about 1970 onwards. The majority of research, funded by the National Institutes for Health (NIH) under the National Institute for Drug Abuse (NIDA) programme, was concerned primarily with investigation of the adverse effects of cannabis, not its clinical utility. Government-funded research focused on mode of action studies and the development of new chemical entities which would replace cannabis, or act as antagonists. The objective was to find new chemical entities with analgesic properties but without the psychotropic effects of tetrahydrocannabinol (THC), and also to find molecules that would antagonise the psychotropic effects of THC. There are a number of agonist and antagonist molecules that bind avidly to cannabinoid receptors under laboratory conditions, as is discussed in Chapter 5. However, medicines based on single cannabinoids or synthetic CB_1 agonists have been found to be less efficacious than products based on extracts of cannabis.

Parenthetically, the NIDA programme of research also led to the discovery of endocannabinoids – the endogenous compounds that also bind at receptors for phytocannabinoids in brain and other tissues. Although endocannabinoids are completely different in their chemistry from plant cannabinoids, molecular models of these compounds can be overlaid on the receptors for phytocannabinoids (Hurst *et al.*, 2001). The discovery of anandamides and related compounds has transformed our view of the importance of cannabinoids and indicated a physiological role for endocannabinoids as mediators of an intercellular signalling system in the brain. It has also been shown that endocannabinoids and cannabinoid receptors are present in most phyla. This prompts the question as to their teleological significance. A proposed primary function for endocannabinoids in mammals is the initiation of the suckling response in the newborn (Fride *et al.*, 2001). A humoral function for endocannabinoids is an interesting counterpoint to their role as mediators and signalling molecules.

There is always a risk that entrenched attitudes to cannabis and cannabis-based products will survive even in the face of evidence of clinical utility. Attitudes towards the toxicity of cannabis are even more difficult to shift. However, the discovery of the endocannabinoid system and its physiological role provide the basis for a rational reassessment. It is vital that cogent evidence provided on the safety and efficacy of both phyto- and endocannabinoids is used to put these two groups of substances into perspective.

The fact that there are cannabinoid receptors in the human brain and other tissues means that their role is a subject for legitimate research. The argument that permanent harm may be caused to brain cytoarchitecture by a single exposure to cannabis and should therefore be avoided at all costs (*The Observer*, 2002) seems hardly credible in view of the ubiquitous presence of endocannabinoids in many phyla. The identification of precursors and degradative enzymes suggests that endocannabinoids are mediators in a widely distributed neural control system.

Similar arguments could be advanced against tobacco smoking. Nicotine has a greater addiction potential than cannabis or ethanol.

Discussions on the adverse effects of cannabis should clearly distinguish the effects that are due to the method of administration (smoking) and critically compare the effects of active principles using similar methods and routes of administration.

The confounding of variables resulting from disparate routes of administration is a feature of many publications on the adverse effects of cannabis. Results that show cannabis in a negative light are easier to get published in peer-reviewed journals than are reports of clinical usefulness. Many reported studies have not been critically and comparatively evaluated. This represents yet another risk in development – the risk that research will be stifled and reporting of positive results will be suppressed. In the present editorial climate there is a presumption of toxicity and addictive liability against cannabis and cannabinoids, which can only be balanced by well-designed and competently executed trials.

It is inevitable that cannabis and cannabinoid-based products will be compared with other drugs of abuse. Availability and control should therefore be based on evidence and not presumption.

Cannabis is not the first street drug to be reinstated as a prescription medicine. Heroin is a drug of abuse but as diamorphine hydrochloride it is a useful prescription medicine. In the case of diamorphine there is clear evidence of addictive liability, yet it is available as a controlled drug on doctor's prescription in the UK and some other territories. When the removal of diamorphine from the therapeutic armamentarium was threatened the decision was reversed because of the action of concerned physicians. The decision to retain diamorphine as a prescription medicine was evidence based, and the campaign for its retention was mobilised by involved professionals. Doctors felt that their ability to practice medicine without diamorphine compromised the level of care that they wished to provide for seriously ill patients. There is an interesting parallel here; some physicians regard cannabis as a treatment that can alleviate pain in patients who would otherwise fail to obtain relief of symptoms with the best available existing therapy. Again, concerted action by concerned professionals, backed by evidence on efficacy and safety, is likely to provide justification for the restoration of cannabis as a prescription medicine.

Need is another factor that has been introduced into the regulatory equation. The UK government has already taken the initiative to refer an eventual prescription medicine based on cannabis to the National Institute for Clinical Excellence (NICE). This body was set up in 1999 as a Special Health Authority with the objective of improving the quality of care that is provided for patients by professionals in the NHS. NICE is required to consider clinical, quality of life issues as well as cost when formulating its advice. Its role and guidance are often controversial. Reference to NICE is an additional risk in development. The normal course of events is for NICE to consider the place of new medicines after they have received Marketing Authorisation. The referral of Sativex before authorisation is unusual but underlines the determination to establish an evidence-based assessment of need for a cannabis-based prescription product.

Unregulated use of cannabis by patients speaks of need from the patients' perspective. A survey of unregulated use of cannabis by patients for medicinal purpose was carried out. Of more than 3000 patients who responded, the majority suffered from multiple sclerosis (MS) or other neurological conditions. The next largest group of responders were sufferers of various forms of arthritis (see Chapter 6 for further details).

There is concern by government that the widespread use of cannabis by patients on their own initiative to treat serious disease is bringing the law into disrepute. Possession is still an offence in the UK, but few magistrates now pass sentences on those who can show a bona fide use for medicinal purposes. The law in the UK was changed in early 2003 to reclassify cannabis to a Class C drug. Since this law came into force in January 2004, people found in possession of a small amount of cannabis for personal use are not arrested. In some states of the USA law enforcement for possession of cannabis, regardless of any claim that it is used for medical purposes, is little short of draconian.

In 1997, the UK government set up the House of Lords Technical Subcommittee to advise on its future policy with regard to cannabis. Conscious that the law was being brought into disrepute, the options considered were:

- decriminalisation of all cannabis for medical use
- reinforcement of existing policies on possession more effectively
- the establishment of an evidence-based case for a medicinal product, which could be made available on prescription.

In the event, the House of Lords Committee recommended to the Government that clinical research to establish the place of cannabis in medicine should be encouraged (House of Lords Select Committee on Science and Technology, 1998). The committee also noted the start that had been made on this process by GW Pharmaceuticals, who had proposed to carry out clinical trials and scientific investigation of medicinal cannabis. In order for a cannabis-based product to be registered as a medicine it would be necessary for a sponsor to make an application for a Marketing Authorisation. For a confident submission to be made, a dossier of evidence on quality, safety and efficacy needs to be provided. In order to construct such a dossier, it is necessary to carry out clinical trials on material of proven quality with the assurance of safety. The Home Office granted GW Pharmaceuticals the necessary licence for possession of material in order to carry out this research.

Elsewhere in the world, the Canadian Government are under pressure to reform its medical marijuana policy (Beeby, 2003) and are considering a Dutch option whereby marijuana is made available at a 'corner' pharmacy to needy patients who are in receipt of a doctor's prescription. A law that became effective in the Netherlands on 17 March 2003 makes the Netherlands the first country to treat marijuana like an ordinary prescription drug.

Currently, Health Canada allows approved patients to smoke marijuana to relieve symptoms including nausea and pain, however, there is no direct legal supply of the substance to sufferers. Health Canada is currently revisiting the question of supply of cannabis and the type of pharmaceutical presentation that is most appropriate.

Regulatory route

Theoretically, it would be possible to register a cannabis-based medicine by either the new chemical entity or the botanical route. Technically, cannabis is a botanical drug and could be registered using the procedure outlined in current guidelines. However, the draft guidelines produced by the FDA relate primarily to products intended for general sale and cannabis is specifically excluded in the current draft. Cannabis-based medicines differ materially from some other botanicals in that the active constituents are well defined.

The new chemical entity regulatory route is familiar to the pharmaceutical industry and regulatory authorities. Consequently there should be relatively few surprises in this route of registration with its emphasis on quality, safety and efficacy data. In many countries it is necessary to demonstrate pharmaco-economic evaluation as a fourth criterion and in the UK NICE has been established to advise in this respect. In the case of a prescribable product containing cannabis-based medicinal extract (CBME), the argument for need is central to the debate on legalisation. Need is one of the factors that informs decisions on the liberalisation or tightening of the existing laws. Patients with chronic, intractable pain have no doubts on the question of need; opinion among professionals is divided, but rapidly moving towards acceptance of the usefulness of cannabinoids in the treatment of intractable diseases. Some of the reservations about need are based upon the lack of availability of suitable preparations with adequate procedures for surveillance and control. The question of need will therefore resolve itself when there is a suitable preparation, which has been evaluated and approved by a regulatory authority.

For new chemical entities, the principal items in the dossier are those defined in Directive 65/65/EEC and subsequent harmonised legislation. The choice of regulatory route is therefore:

- new chemical entity (NCE) based on a single substance. This can be either synthetic or purified from a plant biomass
- a rational mixture of NCEs, or
- a partially purified extract obtained from plant biomass.

Registration based on an extract as a drug substance, rather than an NCE, has been chosen by GW Pharmaceuticals after consideration of experience with dronabinol (Marinol) capsules. Dronabinol is synthetic THC, and is less effective than the same amount of THC administered as an extract of cannabis. The concept that botanicals are more efficacious than the sum of the parts, i.e. principal known constituents, is a basic tenet of phytomedicine. It is central to the justification for use of extracts in which not all of the constituents are known. This argument is viewed with scepticism in some quarters, but it is becoming increasingly clear that there is a scientific basis for the use of botanical extracts. The following factors may be important:

- *Potentiation* Ben-Shabat *et al.* (1998) have demonstrated that the entourage effect, which operates in connection with endocannabinoids, is also a feature of phytocannabinoids. Compounds which themselves do not bind to cannabinoid receptors and which have little pharmacological effect, when given together with cannabinoid agonists have a greater effect than the agonists alone. Antagonism of unwanted effects is seen when cannabidiol (CBD) is given in conjunction with THC (Karniol *et al.*, 1975).
- *Summation* Subclinical doses of minor cannabinoids given alone or in combination with one of the major cannabinoids have an effect greater than the major cannabinoid itself. This can be

regarded as summation rather than potentiation (Williamson and Evans, 2000).

- *Interactions*   The pharmacokinetic interactions between cannabinoids may explain some of these effects. Cannabidiol is an antioxidant and at a physical level may slow down the degradation of cannabinoid mixtures. At a cellular level, its interactions with other cannabinoids are complex. On the one hand it modulates the effect of THC and on the other it inhibits the hydrolysis of endo-cannabinoids (Zuardi *et al.*, 1982).
- *Entourage effects.*

For these reasons alone, there is sufficient evidence for useful interactions between cannabinoids to justify the use of extracts rather than a single cannabinoid or a defined mixture of purified cannabinoids. Another justification for using extracts, although at this stage difficult to prove rigorously, is the fact that humans have been exposed to cannabinoids in the form of extracts for thousands of years. They have probably developed detoxifying mechanisms for dealing with naturally occurring mixtures more efficiently than is the case for single, synthetic chemicals which are usually unknown in nature. The pharmacodynamic and pharmacokinetic bases for these interactions are dealt with in Chapters 7 and 8.

Regulatory attitudes towards botanicals

The attitudes of regulatory authorities and their method of dealing with regulatory evaluation of botanicals vary geographically. In territories where the majority of the population have access only to traditional medicines, the level of regulation of botanical drugs tends to be light. The monographs used to control the quality of materia medica in these countries are essentially based on botanical descriptions and simple chemical tests for identification. Assays for markers, not necessarily active substances, are present in a minority of monographs.

In Europe and the USA, there are monographs that are based on the same principles, but increasingly there is a move to more detailed and more precise assay methods in Western pharmacopoeial monographs. This is particularly the case where high-performance liquid chromatography-mass spectroscopy (HPLC-MS) and linked MS-gas liquid chromatography (MS-GLC) techniques can be applied to quantification of plant constituents.

In the USA, the guidelines on registration of botanicals apply particularly to general sale products. The emphasis is very much on quality, as for many of the agents that are in widespread use there is as yet no clear definition of the active principles. In many cases a number of structures have been proposed as the actives, but where there is a multiplicity of constituents, reliance is placed on the ratio of such constituents. This can be done using hyphenated chromatography techniques, thereby defining the relative abundance of constituents that have a characteristic retention time. Two-dimensional nuclear magnetic resonance (NMR) techniques provide additional information on markers that are characteristic of the herb. Although correspondence between batches is not exact, there is sufficient reproducibility to use the pattern of activity as a fingerprint for identification purposes. Comparison of area under the curve for selected chromatographic peaks gives a global overview of composition based on selected peaks. Multivariate analysis can be used to characterise complex mixtures of this type. Where an active component of a plant extract is not known, it provides data to show substantial similarity between consecutive batches of material used as a botanical drug substance. However, problems arise where the active species is unknown, and the pattern of peaks acts merely as a marker rather than an index of therapeutic activity. Where the active constituents are known, and validated assay methods are available, this approach is redundant. In the case of cannabis-based medicines it is known that cannabinoids are active constituents. Even though it is clear that the activity of cannabis extracts may be greater than the sum of the constituent cannabinoids, target cannabinoids can be used for identification and assay purposes. In writing a specification for the botanical drug substance, limits can be set for the percentage of 'target' cannabinoid. Alternate or other cannabinoids can be assayed individually if present in substantial quantity or grouped together as 'other cannabinoids'.

Where the active constituent of a botanical drug is clearly defined, as in the case of cannabis, it is thus possible to provide precise data on quality. Unfortunately, the current US guidelines specifically exclude marijuana as a botanical, although following discussions with the FDA, a rubric for defining the quality aspects of cannabis has been worked out, which is a hybrid between botanical and Active Pharmaceutical Ingredient (API) guidelines.

Whichever route of registration is followed, the key regulatory issues remain: quality, safety, efficacy and need.

Quality

Quality, whether the medicinal product is a botanical or based on an API, is not negotiable in the context of health registration. Quality is an important issue in determining the registerability of a botanical drug and represents an area of risk in drug development. The principal issues are consistency of the drug substance and stability of the eventual product. Quality control is an area where most risks can be minimised and problems solved by application of adequate resources. The relative importance of these issues depends on the specific drug, and whether the biomass is produced by field growing or under controlled conditions. Historically, cannabis has been grown in both environments. The important criteria are:

- Assurance on quality during growing and harvesting
- Reproducibility from batch to batch (genetic uniformity is ideal)
- Stability, based on objective criteria.

Field-grown crops

The Good Agricultural Practice (GAP) guidelines on medicinal and aromatic plants provide guidance on the production of plant materials used in food, animal feedstuffs, medicinal, flavouring and perfumery industries (Good Agricultural Practice, 1998). The guidelines apply to all methods of production including organic production, and contain provisions for avoiding damage to existing wildlife habitats where drugs are wild crafted. It also seeks to avoid the impact of collection on biodiversity. The main aim is to ensure that plant raw material provides biomass of the highest quality in terms of hygiene, lack of contamination and assurance that the active constituents are preserved. Seed materials are identified botanically, and an increasing amount of information is required on the plant variety, cultivar or chemovar and provenance. The keynote here is traceability. Although the regulations specifically refer to seed materials, the same principles of traceability apply to vegetatively propagated clones or cuttings and it is important to certify provenance of the starting material used in organic production. Growing under glass in a controlled environment and using clones are major steps in building in quality. Where conventional methods of growing are used the methods should be outlined and justified. Clearly, there are risks arising from lack of certainty in identification of plants, inclusion of other species, horticultural factors and adventitious contamination of field-grown crops. The key issues in the GAP guidelines are summarised in Table 14.3.

Table 14.3 Key issues arising from Good Agricultural Practice guidelines

Scope	Applies to growing and primary processing of all medicinal and aromatic herbs
Environment	Avoid damage to existing wildlife habitats
Seeds/propagation material	Material should be identified botanically and should be 100% traceable
Cultivation	Avoid environmental disturbances
Soil and fertilisation	Soil cannot be contaminated with sludge, heavy metals, residues of plant protection products and other not naturally occurring chemicals. Fertilisers should be applied sparingly
Irrigation	Should be minimised and water quality should meet national standards
Maintenance/protection	Pesticide and herbicide use should be avoided as far as possible, any use should be documented
Harvest	Should be carried out when plants are of best possible quality. Equipment should be clean and in perfect working order. Care should be taken to avoid toxic weeds mixing with harvested crop
Delivery	Freshly harvested plant material should occur as quickly as possible after harvesting
Primary processing	Includes: washing, freezing, distilling, drying
Packaging	After primary processing the product should be packaged in a preferably new, clean container
Storage	Storage should be in a dry, well aerated building in which the daily temperature fluctuations are limited
Documentation	All starting materials and processing steps must be documented. Batches should only be mixed if guaranteed to be homogeneous

Growing in a controlled environment

Crops grown in the field are exposed to a number of risks. These come from the attention of insects, other predators, vermin and birds, and even human operatives; all contribute to the microbial bioburden of the biomass. Pesticides used as control measures may also find their way into the harvested botanical. Variations in humidity are conducive to the appearance of mould metabolites. These risks can be minimised by adherence to GAP and good husbandry but the control of the variables in field-grown plants presents a demanding task for quality control (QC). Where it is economically feasible, as in the case of cannabis, it may be desirable to grow the plants under glass. This provides the ultimate in control of quality, and provides a higher level of assurance than can be provided even by strict adherence to the GAP guidelines.

Growing under glass allows for cultivation throughout the year by providing additional light and heat. Cannabis is a short day-length flowering plant and in the field produces one crop per year around the vernal equinox when day-length is changing most rapidly north of the Equator. When cannabis is grown under glass, the vegetative phase can be optimised by growing in 24-hour high-intensity light. The flowering phases can be compressed and arranged so that there is a succession of cropping. Flowering is induced by shortening the day-length and plants can be harvested at the optimum time for recovery of cannabinoids. Plants produced from cuttings have the same genotype and this extends to the qualitative and quantitative content of cannabinoids.

Horticulture

Plants are harvested when the flower heads are beginning to die back. There are a number of factors that can adversely affect the quality of cannabis, particularly during harvesting. If crops are allowed to lie on the ground without frequent turning they may be prone to mould attack and additional contamination from birds and vermin, resulting in a high bioburden. These risks are avoided when the crop is grown under glass. Prompt drying at low temperature in a low-humidity environment with protection from light appears to ensure that the dried biomass has the required quality. When moisture has been reduced to less than 10%, the material is stable and can be stored at low temperature without minimal loss of cannabinoid for several months. Chapter 2 provides detailed information on growing and harvesting cannabis.

Production of botanical drug substance

Where it is intended to use a plant extract as the active substance, it is necessary to ensure that the process for arriving at the extract from biomass is as consistent as possible. Cannabinoids are water insoluble but are readily extracted by lipophilic solvents. Historically, ethanol was used to prepare a tincture that could be used as a component of prescriptions. More frequently, ethanol was removed from the tincture to give a soft extract for conversion into solid dosage forms such as pills. Unfortunately this material, which is essentially an oleoresin, is an unpromising material for formulating modern, pharmaceutically acceptable products. Dissolved in a vehicle containing ethanol and propylene glycol the extract can be applied as a spray to the oromucosal epithelium. It is well absorbed and this product was used in the clinical trials described in Chapter 9.

It has been found that extraction with liquid carbon dioxide at high pressures provides an extract in which most of the colouring matter is left behind. The pressure and temperature of carbon dioxide determines its solvent characteristics. There is a trade off between total extraction at lower pressures, which is economically advantageous, and high selectivity at higher operating pressures. In some cases it is better to maximise extraction and carry out a secondary treatment to clean up the extracts (GW Pharmaceuticals, 2002). The liquid carbon dioxide extract can be purified by 'winterising' a solution of the extract in ethanol to precipitate waxes and other lipid constituents. The de-waxed extract is then suitable for the formulation of solutions for oromucosal administration.

Consistency and stability

Consistency and stability are two of the most important regulatory requirements for the drug substance and the finished product. There are a number of risks involved in obtaining a botanical drug substance (BDS) that has the required physical characteristics and stability. Generally, botanical drugs that have been properly harvested and dried are inherently stable. In the case of medicinal cannabis (botanical raw material) there is real time support for a shelf life of several months for well-dried biomass. Stability of the dried biomass can be enhanced by reduction of ambient humidity and protection from light and storage in an inert atmosphere. The degradative processes that are known to occur in cannabis BDS are conversion of the cannabinoid acids into free cannabinoids, oxidative changes and conversion to cannabinol.

The degradation of the carboxylic acids that are the precursors of THC and CBD is a process that is a function of time and storage temperature. It is not known whether all of the THCA and CBDA are converted into the cannabinoid before there is further conversion into cannabinol. It seems likely that cannabinol can be produced directly from THC when biomass is heated. High cannabinol levels in samples of cannabis drug substance are usually an indicator of exposure to heat. The nature of the oxidative changes taking place in cannabis biomass, or in solutions of pure cannabinoid for that matter, is not fully understood. The process does not appear to be linear and the possibility remains that there are substances present in extract of cannabis that trigger or retard the oxidation. It is possible that attempts to purify material free from these inhibitors results in more rapid oxidation. When botanical drug substance is stored in air it is less stable than material stored in an inert atmosphere. The zones on thin-layer chromatographs (TLC) have not been fully identified but would appear to be large molecular weight compounds, which stay near the origin on TLC and have long HPLC retention times.

The dosage form

Whereas most cannabis used for recreational purposes is either smoked or ingested orally as 'brownies', both methods of administration involve the application of heat which decarboxylates the cannabinoid acids. These acids are the storage form in the plant. Neither of these routes is the first choice for a medicinal product. Smoking cannot be justified by a pharmaceutical company as a method of administration for medicolegal reasons. Administration via the respiratory tract is a very effective way of getting cannabinoids into the systemic circulation very quickly, and has focused attention on non-smoked respiratory tract formulations.

Routes of administration

During the smoking of a typical marijuana cigarette (joint), 8–10 puffs are taken and it is interesting to consider the physics of this device as a guide to more pharmaceutically acceptable dosage forms. A typical joint contains approximately 1 g of cannabis biomass. The first portion of the cigarette is ignited to provide heat. Hot smoke drawn from the ember causes decarboxylation of THCA and CBDA (and the corresponding acids of minor cannabinoids). The cannabinoid acids are not volatile; free cannabinoids are vaporised at temperatures in the range 175–225°C, but have appreciable vapour pressure at temperatures below this range. A portion of the smoke is inhaled and this will contain cannabinoid vapour and cannabinoid condensed on smoke particles (Gieringer, 1996). A portion of the cannabinoid vapour will condense on cooler cannabis herb further down the cigarette. The next draw on the cigarette will increase the temperature (which may reach 700–1000°C locally), and repeating the process causes more cannabinoid to be generated from cannabinoid acid and be vaporised. There will also be revaporisation of cannabinoids that have condensed. This process will continue until the butt can no longer be managed (some officiandos hold the butt with a pin to extract the maximum utility from the cigarette). However a proportion of the total cannabinoid of the cigarette will remain in the butt.

Cannabinoid vapour may condense on dust or smoke particles, and in the high relative humidity of the respiratory tract it is possible that there will be an increase in size of the particles as they absorb water. In the lung, there is deposition of particulate matter high in the bronchial tree and studies have shown that there is also an increased incidence of inflammatory change in the short term in areas where particulates are deposited by eddies to the mainstream inspiratory current (Hardy *et al.*, 1993). In the long term, the same areas of lung are foci for neoplastic changes.

Attempts to produce a dosage form that can be administered into the respiratory tract have to accommodate the intractable physical properties of the cannabinoids. Pure CBD is a solid melting at 64–66°C; THC is liquid at room temperature. Liquid carbon dioxide extracts of decarboxylated cannabis contain lipid-soluble matter from cell contents. A proportion of this material can be removed by chilling an ethanolic solution. This process is referred to as 'Winterisation'. Winterised extracts of cannabis are viscous liquids at room temperature and are practically insoluble in water. These properties make it difficult to formulate cannabis extract as a conventional dry particle inhaler. Consequently, attention has been focused on other ways of administering cannabis as a vapour. Patent application GB0126150.2 (GW Pharmaceuticals, 2001b) describes a device in which a metallic or ceramic substrate coated with cannabis extract is heated by means of an electrical current. The current required to vaporise the charge of cannabis is computed in the first few milliseconds of the operational cycle. The appropriate amount of electrical energy is then applied and the vapour so produced is drawn into the inspiratory volume. The incorporation of a number of doses on a non-oxidisable, flexible ribbon allows a cartridge of doses to be prepared. The use of individual doses can then be controlled using the safe dispensing system described in patents GB2368061 and GB2368098 (GW Pharmaceuticals, 2001c, 2001d). When available, this delivery system will allow a critical reappraisal of any toxicological effects of inhaled cannabinoids free of pyrogenic substances and particulates that characterise smoked cannabis. It should then be possible to distinguish the effects of cannabinoids *per se* from smoked cannabis.

Other sites of administration that avoid the first pass effect are the distal rectum and oromucosal epithelia. Suppository formulations of Δ^9-THC hemisuccinate have been investigated (Brenneisen *et al.*, 1996; Nahas, 1999).

Oropharyngeal administration

Sublingual drops containing cannabinoids in a vehicle comprising ethanol and propylene glycol have been shown to be an effective dosage form. Application of small, metered volumes of solution allow patients to titrate the dose required up to a level which gives symptom relief. Figure 14.1 shows the plasma levels obtained by different methods of administration. Inhalation produces a T_{max} and a C_{max} which is similar to that produced by intravenous administration. C_{max} by sublingual or buccal administration of a spray is less rapid, but similar areas under the curve are produced by oromucosal administration.

Patients find that the oromucosal route of administration is convenient because, although slower than the respiratory route, the time course of absorption is such that the patient can judge whether they are likely to experience cognitive effects. Indeed, many patients have found that they are able to titrate, using partial doses in the form of iterations from the pump action sublingual spray, up to a level of efficacy that was achieved before they experienced cognitive effects. This feature of 'titration to criterion' has been built into subsequent clinical trial designs.

Titration of dose to give symptom relief at a point where the patient is comfortable with CNS effects can act as a safety feature. However, because patients may titrate up to a point that is limited by their personal level of tolerability, which is defined in terms of CNS effects, this may register as an increase in the number of adverse events, statistically.

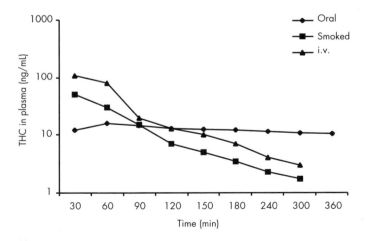

Figure 14.1 Mean plasma concentrations of Δ^9-THC after three routes of administration. Redrawn from Ohlsson *et al.* (1980).

Solid oromucosal dosage forms suitable for indications where it is desirable to have a more prolonged plasma concentration curve have been developed. These include rapidly dissolving tablets and gels that can be placed in the maxillary fosse. By varying the composition of the gels it is possible to have a formulation that provides delivery of a cannabinoid over a period of minutes to more than one hour (GW Pharmaceuticals, 2001a). This is particularly useful for those conditions where it is desirable to provide a higher concentration of a non-psychoactive cannabinoid over a prolonged period. Earlier studies have been carried out using the pump action spray that delivers a metered volume of typically 25–100 µL of solution as a spray. The material sprayed onto the sublingual or buccal mucosae is absorbed, and the small volume administered means that very little of the applied dose is swallowed, thus giving optimum conditions for oromucosal absorption.

With cannabis extracts there is a marked first pass effect. Oral administration of cannabis extracts means that material absorbed from the gastrointestinal tract is presented first to the liver where metabolism can occur. One of the metabolites detected in circulating blood is 11-hydroxy THC. This compound is also psychoactive and may contribute to the prolonged psychoactive effects noted after oral administration of cannabis formulations.

Security and the Advanced Dispensing System

Clearly, there are risks in making available an abusable drug in a patient-friendly dosage form for domiciliary use. To minimise the risk of diversion a secure dispensing system has been developed in parallel with the products. In addition to the operational characteristics of the various dosage forms, it is necessary to ensure that they are not easily diverted into unauthorised use. In order to do this it is necessary to have accessory packaging that will tread a careful line between security and patient convenience. Many of the patients for whom the medication is intended have impaired motor coordination and devices need to take this into account. Security requires that there is complete traceability of medication dispensed to patients. A secure dispensing system has been devised which incorporates a number of mechanical and electronic features. The algorithm used in the control part of the package has been designed to ensure that the medication is patient-specific. The history of use can be recorded and it is possible to transmit this information to a remote computer. This allows distance monitoring of usage and also allows communication with the patient, effectively allowing clinical trials to be monitored remotely. If the current trend to accept a cannabis-based product as a prescription item continues, then the secure dispensing system may not be required in all cases. However, it is available if required to de-risk this aspect of drug control.

Plate 11 shows the cartridge, device and docking station that make up the Advanced Dispensing System, and this is described in more detail in Chapter 9.

Safety

Registration of a botanical as a prescription medicine, as for any NCE, requires input of data on preclinical and clinical safety. Preclinical safety for botanicals may be inferred from the long history of safe use by patients and practitioners. However, such data are not regarded as sufficient for regulatory purposes. Cannabis has an exceptional record of safety (Grinspoon and Bakalar, 1993). It is virtually impossible to kill animals with acute oral doses, and there are no substantiated deaths from ingestion of cannabis. However, impressive as this record is, it can only be used as supportive data for more focused studies. It is remarkable that anecdotal evidence on toxicity of drugs is regarded as an acceptable basis for regulatory warning and, occasionally, withdrawal of marketing approval, but is discounted when it points to efficacy. The Yellow Card system for adverse event reporting and its counterparts in other countries is based on anecdote.

Cannabis has for many years been an illegal substance and its use presents regulatory authorities with a dilemma. In addition to these procedural difficulties, there is also the practical problem of comparing smoked versus non-smoked administration, and determining the composition of the cannabis used in the earlier studies. There is a basic programme of preclinical safety studies which are mandatory before clinical studies can begin.

Regulatory imperatives

All phases of development of new drugs are expensive in terms of resource. There are several setpiece studies that are required to meet regulatory requirements. The funding of these major regulatory studies imposes financial restraint and discipline on the R&D budget of a development company. From a practical point of view, any accommodation that can be arrived at in phasing the preclinical safety studies has to be seen as an advantage for registration by the botanical route. The long history of use of botanicals can be taken into account to allow an early start of the clinical programme for botanical drugs. It is clear that over decades, centuries or even in some cases millennia, a window of dosing has been defined which gives a presumption of safety and efficacy. Traditionally, botanical medicines were prepared using prescribed methods. Attempts to streamline methods of preparation by using radically different solvent systems may result in the extraction of toxic principles. In the case of cannabis, the availability of validated assay methods allows quality and safety to be monitored in a range of extracts and formulations. In the past, the quality of surveillance has not been as rigorous as is now required, but repeated trial and error will have defined doses and modes of administration that are effective and safe in treating patients. Efficacy and safety in this context are relative terms when viewed from a twenty-first century perspective. However in previous ages natural medicines were regarded as being fit for their purpose and the criteria were sufficient efficacy and safety.

The purpose of rigorous clinical trials is to build upon this presumption of safety and efficacy so that the regulatory authority can arrive at evidence-based decisions on risk and benefit. In the UK Medicines Act, Section 12 deals specifically with the way in which botanical drugs can be supplied and used without specific registration, but this accommodation afforded by the Medicines Act relates to supply in the course of a consultation. The botanical drugs which can be supplied in this way are mostly non-prescription drugs and this avenue of supply is not relevant in the case of cannabis. This section of the Medicines Act relates to the traditional use of botanical drugs and if a sponsor wishes to make more specific claims, then a Marketing Authorisation Application must be sought after presenting the results of clinical studies.

Perhaps the most important advantage of registration via the botanicals route is timing. The existence of a long history of 'safe enough' and 'effective enough' administration provides a platform from which further research can be planned. Essentially the clinical investigation of a botanical starts with the benefit of exposure in humans. In the case of NCEs, preclinical toxicity studies are required to gauge the doses at which a novel chemical, hitherto untried in humans, can be administered. It is necessary to carry out statutory toxicity studies in order to provide this data for a Clinical Trials Exemption (CTX – IND equivalent). In the case of botanicals, some studies, including mutagenicity and short-term animal safety studies are of course necessary before exposing patients to the new preparation of the botanical. With a botanical, the investigation essentially starts in Phase II. With a new chemical entity it is necessary to move forward from laboratory evaluation of safety and efficacy into human pharmacology (Phase I) and then into Phase II studies. The object of Phase II studies is to demonstrate that the new drug is probably effective in specific models of diseases. In Phase III studies a sufficient number of patients are treated to provide statistically valid evidence on this point. By using the botanical approach it is therefore possible to start the project effectively in Phase II and work in both directions, i.e. to extend preclinical safety and efficacy studies on the one hand and move forward into Phase III studies more rapidly on the other. This is part of the management of risk, and there are real savings to be made in the appropriate phasing of confirmatory preclinical safety studies.

A recurrent nightmare in drug development is the failure in early Phase II of drugs that were promising preclinical candidates. At this point the drug development company will have sunk a great deal of time and resources into demonstrating pharmacological activity in relevant preclinical models, and carried out regulatory toxicology. It is also likely to be stretched financially and is at its most vulnerable stage at this point. The risk is that the key piece of information, namely that the new medicine produces a therapeutic effect in humans, is missing. In the case of plant extracts that have a long history of use, this information is often known from traditional use.

The likelihood of late appearance of hitherto undetected side-effects is probably less of a problem in the case of plant extracts that have been widely used for centuries than in the case of synthetic molecules that are foreign to humans. Nevertheless, in addition to the preclinical studies, clinical trials include surveillance on adverse events and this is continued in long-term safety studies.

Occasionally, national agencies carry out studies on exceptional drugs. The toxicology of THC has been investigated by the NIH under the National Toxicity Program (NTP) and the NIH has also supported studies on aspects of CBD toxicity. The NTP report on THC gives a full description of the preclinical work carried out to provide assurance on the safety of synthetic THC (NTP Technical Report, 1996). Studies on CBD are less complete than for THC and for many years it was considered to be an inactive constituent of cannabis. Studies on the effect of CBD on male reproductive function (Rosenkrantz et al., 1978) showed that in this respect it had a small and reversible effect on sperm count similar to that of THC. The prospect of using CBD as a drug substance means it is necessary to carry out additional work on this component and any combination product. Studies carried out in the rat using an extract of cannabis containing CBD at doses up to 225 mg/kg per day in diet did not show any effect on sperm count or motility (GW Pharmaceuticals, unpublished data).

There is always a risk that even when preclinical studies have been carried out to reveal target organ toxicity, adverse events with a low frequency will appear when patient numbers are increased. With reference to this, Phase IV pharmacovigilance is essential.

Efficacy

Preclinical efficacy studies do not always predict the therapeutic indication for which a novel API will eventually prove to be most successful. However, in the case of new medicines that are based on plants with a very long history of effective use this is less likely to happen. The development of new medicines from cannabis has led to some surprises.

THC was formerly regarded as the most active and perhaps the only constituent of cannabis. The expectation was that it would be possible to separate psychotropic and other pharmacological effects by manipulation of the molecular architecture of THC or ligands for the same binding sites. The availability of synthetic compounds also fits in well with the established regulatory paradigms for registration of NCE-based medicines, and avoids the perceived problems in registration of botanical products. In publications as late as 1996 (Budavari, 1996), CBD is described as an inactive constituent of cannabis. Although it was known that it did not have the psychotropic effect of THC, the finding that it had intrinsic analgesic activity was surprising and was clinically significant.

Table 14.4 lists the pharmacological characteristics of THC and CBD. In a number of respects, the pharmacological activity of CBD differs from that of THC in sign. This raises the interesting possibility that products containing a mixture of two or more cannabinoids would have a pharmacological effect that is the summation of some properties and antagonism of others. This interaction now makes it possible to understand the anecdotal accounts of the effects of combinations of THC and CBD when taken for non-medical use. In the early 1990s it was discovered that endogenous compounds, chemically unrelated to phytocannabinoids, bind to CB receptors and mimic their effects. This opens up the possibility that endocannabinoids are mediators or modulators of other receptor systems within the CNS and peripherally.

The first endocannabinoid was named anandamide and has been found in a wide range of mammalian tissues. Interestingly, it is also found in most phyla (a notable exception being some insects) and as far down the phylogenetic tree as Hydra.

Table 14.4 Pharmacological and pharmacodynamic properties of THC and CBD

Effect	THC	CBD	Reference
CB$_1$ (Brain receptors)	++	±	Showalter et al., 1996; Pertwee, 1998
CB$_2$ (Peripheral receptors)	+	++	Showalter et al., 1996
CNS effects			
Anticonvulsant[a]	−−	++	Carlini et al., 1973
Antimetrazol	−	−	Unpublished GW clinical data
Anti-electroshock	−	++	Unpublished GW clinical data
Muscle relaxant	−−	++	Petro, 1980
Antinociceptive	++	+	Unpublished GW clinical data
Catalepsy	++	++	Unpublished GW clinical data
Psychotropic	++	−	Unpublished GW clinical data
Antipsychotic	−	++	Zuardi et al., 1991
Neuroprotective antioxidant activity[b]	+	++	Hampson et al., 1998
Antiemetic	++	−	Sallan et al., 1975
Sedation (reduced spontaneous activity)	+	+	Zuardi et al., 1991
Appetite stimulation	++	−	Mattes et al., 1994
Appetite suppression	−	+	
Anxiolytic	−	+	Unpublished GW clinical data
Cardiovascular effects			
Bradycardia	−	+	Smiley et al., 1976
Tachycardia	+	−	Laviolette and Belanger, 1986
Hypertension[c]	+	−	Singh et al., 1981
Hypotension[c]	−	+	Adams et al., 1977
Anti-inflammatory	±	±	Brown, 1998
Anti-inflammatory effects			
Rat paw oedema	−	++	Unpublished GW clinical data
COX 1	±	±	Unpublished GW clinical data
COX 2	−	−	Unpublished GW clinical data
TNFα antagonism	+	++	Strivastava et al., 1998
Glaucoma	++	+	Perez-Reyes et al., 1976

[a]THC is proconvulsant.
[b]Effect is CB$_1$ receptor independent.
[c]THC has a biphasic effect on blood pressure; in naïve patients it may produce postural hypotension and it has also been reported to produce hypertension on prolonged usage (GW Internal Report No. 002/000159).

In the USA, most of the cannabis has been grown from strains selected for high THC content and maximum psychotropic effect. European cannabis and cannabis from India, south-western Africa and South-East Asia contains THC but also a relatively high concentration of CBD. This may explain why it is sometimes difficult to compare and interpret historic data, even in peer-reviewed publications, where cannabis from different geographical locations has been used.

The confounding impact of variability in composition can be avoided by selection of appropriate chemovars. Propagation by cuttings ensures that the genotype is fixed and the proportion of the target cannabinoid is constant. In a study to define qualitative consistency in successive crops, the coefficient of variation (cv) of THC in replicate cuttings was shown to be less than 1.5% (Whittle *et al.*, 2001). The cv of CBD was similar, indicating consistency.

The wide range of pharmacological effects noted for the major cannabinoids may not be unrelated to the earlier use of these compounds in clinical medicine. A century ago, European varieties of cannabis were used to treat migraine, epilepsy and as a hypnotic (Table 14.2). It is possible that these effects may have been due in part to the CBD content, as a significant proportion of cannabis available in Europe originated in the Indian subcontinent (Indian hemp). Unfortunately it is difficult to establish at this distance in time the composition of the cannabis preparations used in these reports. As part of the development of cannabis-based medicines for specific indications, it is therefore necessary to reinvestigate the effects of preparations containing specific ratios of cannabinoids. Clinical work is being undertaken to evaluate the efficacy of medicines containing different ratios of cannabinoids.

Cannabinoid receptors and efficacy of cannabis-based medicines

In addition to receptor binding activity, cannabinoids may have other, non-cannabinoid-mediated effects. Cannabidiol is a case in point. In addition to its cannabinergic activity, its activity in models of stroke, and its antiepileptic activity appear to be mediated by non-cannabinergic mechanisms. Cannabinoid receptors on cell membranes are very close to vanilloid receptors, and allosteric effects may help to explain some of the effects of cannabis and its constituents. Cross-talk between cannabinergic, endorphin μ and κ, and vanilloid (VRI) receptors may help to understand the wide-ranging effects of cannabis on different modalities of pain.

Table 14.4 tabulates the differences in pharmacological activity for THC and CBD. Whereas THC is highly psychoactive, CBD is not. THC binds to, and is a potent agonist of CB_1 cannabinoid receptors; CBD is approximately 100 times less active in this respect. Both THC and CBD bind to CB_2 cannabinergic receptors, which are most abundant in tissues of the immune system.

A study funded by the Medical Research Council has recently been reported (Zajicek *et al.*, 2003). The study was a randomised, placebo-controlled comparison of Marinol and a cannabis extract (Cannador) at 33 UK centres and with 630 patients. The results of the study were mixed. Although there was no statistically significant change in overall spasticity (as measured by the Ashworth score), there were significant improvements for both treatments in subjective measures of spasticity, muscle spasm, pain and sleep, and in an objective measure of mobility. It was concluded that the study, combined with others, shows that cannabis may be clinically useful in treating symptoms of multiple sclerosis. This study is discussed fully in Chapter 9.

It is now apparent that cannabidiol has a pharmacological profile that differs from that of THC. It is useful as a therapeutic agent in its own right and as an adjuvant to THC. In addition to interaction at CB_1 and CB_2 receptors, there are a number of other effects of these cannabinoids, which are probably mediated by other receptors or by cross-talk with other receptor systems. In addition to its interaction with vanilloid receptors, cannabinoid receptors have been identified pre-synaptically at dopamine, gabaminergic, glutamate, 5-HT and cholinergically mediated synapses. The cross-talk between CB receptors and other receptors appears to be a feature, perhaps even a defining characteristic, of cannabinoids.

While it is satisfying to be able to classify the prime pharmacological actions of drugs, there is a risk if it deflects research and overlooks other actions which may be important toxicologically. Diseases are rarely due to a single pathological defect and it is likely that drugs to treat them need to be multifocal. There is also the possibility that drugs introduced for the treatment of one condition may find their true metier in another (propranolol and minoxidil for example).

One of the milestone pharmacological findings in cannabinoid research was the cloning of the CB_1 receptor. The original work was done in rat cerebral cortex (Matsuda *et al.*, 1990). This opened the way for detailed investigation of agonists and antagonists with the prospect of producing novel compounds, but also provided the basis for understanding the modes of action of cannabinoids. Chapter 5 deals with this in greater detail, and illustrates the fascinating interrelation between phyto- and endocannabinoids.

Discovery of the CB_1 receptor was followed in 1993 by recognition of the CB_2 receptor that is also a member of the superfamily of G protein-coupled receptors. The cannabinoid CB_1 receptor has the architecture shared by other G protein-coupled receptors, and the similarities and differences are now well documented (Matsuda and Bonner, 1995).

Many synthetic CB_1 agonists have been produced, some with very high affinity, but it has not so far proved possible to separate the analgesic effect of these compounds from their psychotropic effects; both effects appear to be related to activation of the CB_1 receptor. The work on receptor binding for other cannabinoids has nevertheless enlarged our understanding of the effects of cannabidiol.

The discovery that anandamide (arachidonoylethanolamide) binds to CB receptors and can mimic the effects of phytocannabinoids has sparked off research into structural relationships, and a whole new pharmacology of endocannabinoids. The mechanics of production of endocannabinoids, the ready availability of precursors and identification of the enzyme responsible for their destruction, and the existence of a transporter system strengthen the case for regarding them as naturally occurring mediators. The existence of a specific transport system is controversial, although it is possible that this class of mediator does not require the accoutrements of other classical mediators. It is entirely possible that a characteristic feature of endocannabinoids is that they are ubiquitous and are formed from components present in most cells and do not need specialised storage organs. Fatty acid amide hydrolase (FAAH), the enzyme that is responsible for destruction of anandamide, has been described in the literature (Deutsch and Chin, 1993). CBD is an inhibitor of this enzyme and the search is on for other inhibitors.

The significance of the discovery of endocannabinoids cannot be overestimated. Not only is a new area of pharmacology opened up for investigation using familiar structure–activity relationship methodology, but the possibility that endocannabinoids constitute an intracellular and intercellular communications system within the body is now established. Since the discovery of anandamide, the search for chemical analogues and other, related, structures has produced a new generation of compounds, some of which are being groomed as candidate drugs.

Pharmacological effects (particularly of CBD) that cannot be attributed to cannabinergic receptor activity include effects on tumour necrosis factor-alpha, interleukins, inflammatory cytokines, nitric oxide and antioxidant activity. The interaction between phytocannabinoids and endocannabinoids (including anandamides, 2-arachidonoylglycerol and noladin ethers) is also another complicating factor in understanding the multifaceted pharmacology of THC and CBD.

There is a clear parallel between plant opioids and endorphins on the one hand and phytocannabinoids and endocannabinoids on the other. The analogy is compelling and instructive. The more so since there is cross-talk between opioid and cannabinoid receptors (Salio *et al.*, 2001). It is becoming apparent that there is a hierarchy of receptors that may be operated by mediators, and there is the interesting possibility that some 'super mediators' have a supervisory role in modulating the effect of the more familiar primary mediators. A consequence of this work is that cannabinoids may now be regarded as a component part of an essential control system for the body. They may be mediators in their own right, or act as conductors of the mediator orchestra. A further consequence of the receptor binding by both phyto- and endocannabinoids is that there may be reciprocal interaction. The turnover of endocannabinoids provides the substrate for the concept of a tonic system that is responsible for mood. Phytocannabinoids can also act by displacing the endocannabinoid balance.

An intriguing feature of the fatty acid amides is the role of some of the less potent compounds in a 'supporting role'. Salio *et al.* (2001) showed that compounds based on long-chain fatty acids other than arachidonic acid have less intrinsic activity as cannabinoid ligands but appear to potentiate the effect of anandamide. This potentiation is referred to as an 'entourage effect' (Ben Shabat *et al.*, 1998), and it is interesting to speculate on its biological significance. The development of specific and potent antagonists of cannabinoids has provided tools that allow the investigation and analysis of the effects of plant and endocannabinoids. Indeed, there appears to be a degree of endocannabinoid tone that determines many somatic and mental functions. In some cases the effect is dramatic. Newborn animals given an endocannabinoid antagonist on day 1 of life never learn to suckle, fail to thrive and die (Fride *et al.*, 2003). There are other effects attributed to endocannabinoids that link to a variety of endocrine effects. Endocannabinoids may therefore be a humoral link between neural and hormonal control.

The possibility of abuse of cannabis has been used, consciously or unconsciously, to discourage research into its therapeutic benefits. The same arguments could be advanced against research into opioids or nicotine research. Both opioids and nicotine are addictive, but investigation of their pharmacology and pharmacodynamics has led to novel and useful new medicines. Research into cannabis has similar potential.

The fact that morphine and its derivatives can be abused does not interdict investigation of the activity of endorphins as ligands to receptors, and their modulating role on mediators within the nervous system. In the arena where research into the pharmacology of plant opioids and endorphins has led to an unravelling of the receptor binding, this is seen as a legitimate field of study. The same duality is seen in the case of cannabinoids and endocannabinoids, but the acceptance of medicines based on phytocannabinoids is only now being won. The clinical research that is now being carried out on cannabinoids and endocannabinoids may serve to crystallise attitudes towards these agents as useful medicines. Certainly the parallels between cannabinoid and morphinoid therapeutics are clear.

The diversity of actions of cannabis should not come as a surprise, in view of its long history of use. However the pharmacodynamic actions underlying these effects are truly remarkable, and have produced a flurry of research into related compounds. Anandamide itself and the closely related compounds based on arachidonic acid and other fatty acids have the short half-lives which would be expected of mediators. Longer lasting compounds such as the noladin ethers have been made synthetically and it is interesting that subsequently these were found to be naturally occurring compounds. A number of other synthetic programmes have produced endocannabinoid derivatives that have clinically useful half-lives. Compounds related structurally to endocannabinoids that have useful pharmacokinetic profiles are now under study as therapeutic agents. However, the CB_1 active endocannabinoids produced to date do not show separation of psychomimetic and other effects. Chapter 6 describes the results of Phase I clinical trials that indicate the activity of a high THC extract, a high CBD extract and Sativex – an approximately 50:50 mixture of THC and CBD. These results illustrate the risk of assuming that biological activity of a botanical medicine is attributable to only one constituent.

Conventional wisdom has previously equated the effects of cannabis with THC, but the effects of CBD, hitherto regarded as inactive, are remarkable, clinically useful – and surprising. In addition to analgesic activity *per se*, CBD interacts with THC to give clinical effects that are greater than those achieved by either compound itself. Discovery of these effects is important in two respects. It offers treatments for diseases refractory to existing medications and opens up a whole new area of pharmacology. Serendipity indeed.

Recent data from Phase III clinical trials are described fully in Chapter 7. Essentially, a double-blind parallel group study compared the efficacy of Sativex, the THC:CBD product, with placebo in the treatment of neuropathic pain in 66 patients with MS. Sativex provided highly statistically significant relief of pain in comparison with placebo and highly statistically significant reduction in sleep disturbance. In a double-blind parallel group study comparing the efficacy of Sativex with placebo in the treatment of chronic refractory pain in 70 patients with MS and other neurological conditions, Sativex provided statistically significant pain relief (as evidenced by the diminished use of analgesic rescue medication) and a statistically significant reduction in sleep disturbance. In a double-blind parallel group study comparing the efficacy of Sativex with placebo in the treatment of a number of symptoms in 160 patients with MS, Sativex provided a highly statistically significant improvement in the symptoms of spasticity. Positive trends were also observed in a number of other MS symptoms (providing useful additional support to significant results obtained in Phase II trials).

The benefits seen in these studies are all the more notable in that they represent clinical improvement over and above that which patients obtain with their standard prescription medicines (patients receiving both active and placebo medicines continued to take their standard prescription medicines during the trial). In addition, the trials have demonstrated that Sativex has a surprisingly broad spectrum of therapeutic effects and a reassuring safety profile. Self-titration (adjustment) of their dose enabled most patients to achieve improvement in their symptoms without incurring a level of unwanted effects that would interfere with day-to-day living.

Risks, benefits and serendipity

Many of the drugs currently in use were discovered by synthesis of new structures, preclinical testing and grooming as new medicines. New medicines in the late twentieth century were based on small molecular weight compounds that were screened in (mainly) *ex vivo* or *in vivo* models of the target disease. The models used for discovery are validated on compounds of known activity and it is therefore likely that the compounds that are discovered will have similar properties. Historically, the probability of a single synthetic molecule becoming a world-class drug is probably greater than 100 000:1.

The advent of high throughput screening, and the exploitation of genomic and proteomic methodology, has multiplied the number of compounds which can be tested. However, compounds which are shown to be active in *ex vivo* tests still have to pass the rigour of testing in living systems and eventually in the clinic. As information on a new chemical accumulates, the odds of its eventual emergence as a world-class drug shorten, but are still considerable. When new medicines are at the stage where pharmaceutical development companies feel confident in seeking partners for eventual marketing, approximately 1 in 8 products eventually emerge as world-class products (PJB Publications, personal communication).

The risk of failure for a medicine based on a natural product should be lower, as described by McPartland and Guy in Chapter 4. If the materia medica that are the active ingredients have been in use for thousands of years, it is likely that human metabolism will have adapted to these substances and dealt with them metabolically. Many of the substances that are present as active constituents of plant medicines fall into defined classes and the human liver has adapted to deal with groups of related molecules effectively. The presence of families of cytochrome P450 enzymes is testimony to the body's ability to deal with xenobiotica.

The pharmaceutical revolution is still young and in the second part of the twentieth century there was a move away from plant-derived medicines to single, synthetic molecules. Novel xenobiotic molecules are likely to be of types not encountered by the human metabolic systems and the organs responsible for metabolism must adapt quickly to deal with these compounds. The chances of commercial success for a new medicine are increased by novelty but the very novelty of xenobiotica imposes a strain on the metabolic capability of humans. This may lead to surprises in the form of new types of adverse effects attributable to the compound itself or its metabolites. During early clinical trials it is therefore imperative that careful observation for unexpected adverse events is a prime focus. Only relatively frequent adverse events will emerge, even in a well-executed clinical trials programme. It is also important to be aware of unexpected effects that may point to new indications. Paradoxically, new indications for novel medicines may only emerge after widespread use in the clinic, as for example in the case of sildenafil and minoxidil. These compounds are now primarily used for purposes quite other than those for which they were synthesised and clinically tested in the first instance – more serendipity!

Phase II confirmation of clinical activity of phytomedicines should not give surprises in terms of adverse events, since the materia medica have been used in traditional medicine for hundreds, if not thousands, of years. Their continued use in traditional medicine will have selected out those compounds that are unsafe, and perhaps those that are ineffective.

In this respect, the record of traditional medicine is less clear on questions of efficacy than safety. Safety is the prime concern of regulatory authorities and they have acted where necessary to ban certain traditional drugs (e.g. The Medicines (Aristolochia and Mu Tong etc.) (Prohibition) Order, 2001). Recent clinical trials of phytomedicines have focused on safety primarily. If it is shown that the treatment can be administered with confidence and safety, clinical studies can then re-explore efficacy and optimum dosage regimes for treatment of human disease. Protocols for early clinical trials address the primary aspects of the disease but well-written protocols will allow for investigators to note the unexpected. Even after many years of traditional use, re-examination of established materia medica may reveal additional indications that can be developed into new medicinal products.

Most human diseases are multifactorial and are characterised by complex symptomatology. It is not unreasonable to use medicines that have multifactorial actions. Instead of magic bullets, perhaps we need a well-directed broadside! Inclusion of a number of defined end-points in clinical studies allow for the possibility that some of the symptoms may be more amenable to treatment than others.

One of the benefits of detecting unexpected effects is that IPR can be established if the discovery is novel and non-obvious. Thus the early clinical research should aim to confirm the traditional use of the phyto-medicine target. One of the features of recent research in cannabinoids is that there have been a number of totally unexpected discontinuities that have completely altered the prospects for medicinal products based on cannabis. From the 1960s onward, cannabinoid research sponsored by government agencies has been directed towards investigation of the mode of action of cannabinoids, the problems associated with un-regulated use, and discovery of novel compounds with cannabinergic activity. The latter have investigated both synthetic agonists and antagonists of THC.

In the last 40 years, research into cannabinoids has changed focus dramatically. It has moved from a search for reasons to prohibit the use of cannabis, to an investigation of its medicinal use. Along the way it has opened up the possibility that endocannabinoids have a physiological role and are very important 'super mediators', which have a supervisory oversight of a number of other mediators. The physiological implications of endocannabinoid tone in health and disease have still to be fully explored.

In the future it can be expected that in addition to the work on phytocannabinoids, there will be further development of compounds

Table 14.5 Botanical medicines and their endogenous receptors

Botanical drug	Endogenous receptor	Mediators
Opium	Mu, kappa, delta	Endorphins
Capsaicin	Vanilloid	Substance P
Salix	LOX, COX	Prostanoids
Cannabis	CB_1, CB_2, vanilloid	Endocannabinoids

related to the endocannabinoids already known. The principal chemovars currently in use for preparation of extracts of cannabis are THC and CBD. The precursors and metabolic products of these cannabinoids can also be extracted, and although they are currently thought to be inactive pharmacologically, refinement of testing methodologies may reveal intrinsic activity.

Inflammation and pain are the signs and symptoms that cause most patients to seek medical help. It is remarkable that in at least four cases, botanical medicines used since antiquity have been mirrored by systems within the body that control inflammation and pain (Table 14.5).

Cannabis and preparations derived from it were once highly regarded as useful medicines. In the last part of the twentieth century their use was banned because of perceived problems with abuse. Re-examination of risk and benefit mean that the time has now come for cannabis and cannabinoids to be re-evaluated, and to take their place as useful medicines for the treatment of pain and other symptoms that are refractory to other drugs. Their multiplicity of pharmacological actions is initially surprising to the modern pharmaceutical mind, but we are now beginning to understand it in terms of interaction with endocannabinoid-mediated neural function. This means that eventually they can be evaluated for use in other therapeutic conditions.

Cannabis, once used as a phytomedicine, was outlawed, but is now being re-evaluated as a truly remarkable and safe prescription medicine, from a renewable source.

References

Adams M D, Earnhardt J T, Martin B R *et al.* (1977). Cannabinoid with cardiovascular activity but no overt behavioural effects. *Experientia* 33: 1204–1205.

Beeby D (2003). Canadian Press. http://www.cannabisnews.com/news/thread16079.shtml (accessed 27 April 2003).

Beers M H, Berkow R (1899). *Merck's 1899 Manual of the Materia Medica*. New York: Merck and Co.

Ben-Shabat S, Fride E, Sheskin T et al. (1998). An entourage effect: inactive endogenous fatty acid glycerol esters enhance 2-arachidonoyl-glycerol cannabinoid activity. Eur J Pharmacol 353: 23–31.

Brenneisen R, Egli A, Elsohly M A et al. (1996). The effect of orally and rectally administered delta 9-tetrahydrocannabinol on spasticity: a pilot study with 2 patients. Int J Clin Pharmacol Ther 34: 446–452.

Brown D T (1998). The therapeutic potential for cannabis and its derivatives. In: Brown D T, ed. Cannabis. The Genus Cannabis. London: Harwood Academic Publishers.

Budavari S, ed. (1996). Merck Index, 12th Edition. New Jersey: Merck and Co.

Carlini E A, Leiter J R, Tannhauser M, Berardi A C (1973). Cannabidiol and Cannabis sativa extract protect mice and rats against convulsive agents. Pharm Pharmacol 25: 664–665.

Deutsch D G, Chin S A (1993). Enzymatic synthesis and degradation of anandamide: a cannabinoid receptor agonist. Biochem Pharmacol 46: 791–796.

Fride E, Ginzburg Y, Breuer A et al. (2001). Critical role of the endogenous cannabinoid system in mouse pup suckling and growth. Eur J Pharmacol 419: 207–214.

Fride E, Foox A, Rosenberg E et al. (2003). Milk intake and survival in new born cannabinoid CB1 receptor knock out mice; evidence for a 'CB3' receptor. Eur J Pharmacol 461: 27–34.

Gieringer D (1996). Why marijuana smoke harm reduction? Bull Multidisciplinary Assoc Psychedelic Stud 6(3).

Good Agricultural Practice (GAP) (1998). Guidelines for Good Agricultural Practice (GAP) of Medicinal and Aromatic Plants (5th August 1998). Final Europam Version. Interactive European Network for Industrial Crops and their Applications (IENICA).

Government Response to the House of Lords Select Committee on Science and Technology's Report on the Therapeutic Uses of Cannabis (2001). 2nd Report, HL Paper 50, Session 2000–01.

Grinspoon L, Bakalar J B (1997). Marihuana, the Forbidden Medicine, rev and exp edn. New Haven: Yale University Press.

GW Pharmaceuticals (2001a). Patent Application Number GB0103638.3.

GW Pharmaceuticals (2001b). Patent Application Number GB0126150.2.

GW Pharmaceuticals (2001c). Patent Number GB2368061.

GW Pharmaceuticals (2001d). Patent Number GB2368098.

GW Pharmaceuticals (2002) Patent Application Number GB0222077.0.

Hampson A G, Grimaldi M, Axelrod J, Wink D (1998). Cannabidiol and (−) Δ^9-tetrahydrocannabinol are neuroprotective antioxidants. Proc Natl Acad Sci USA 95: 8268–8273.

Hardy J G, Newman S P, Knoch M (1993). Lung deposition from four nebulizers. Respir Med 87: 461–465.

House of Lords Select Committee on Science and Technology (1998). Cannabis: The Scientific and Medical Evidence. The House of Lords Session 1997–8, 9th report. London: Stationery Office.

Hurst D, Norris J, Guarnieri, Reggio P (2001). Conformational requirements for CB1/endocannabinoid interaction. Poster, page 11. 2001 Symposium on the Cannabinoids, International Cannabinoid Research Society, El Escorial, Spain, 28 June.

Karniol I G, Shirakawa I, Kasinski N *et al.* (1975). Cannabidiol interferes with the effects of delta-9-tetrahydrocannbinol in man. *Eur J Pharmac* 28: 172–177.

Laviolette M, Belanger J (1986). Role of prostaglandins in marihuana-induced bronchodilation. *Respiration* 49(1): 10–15.

Matsuda L A, Bonner T I (1995). Molecular biology and the cannabinoid receptor. In: Pertwee R G, ed. *Cannabinoid Receptors*. London: Academic Press: 117–143.

Matsuda L A, Lolait S J, Brownstein MJ *et al.* (1990). Structure of a cannabinoid receptor and functional expression of the cloned cDNA. *Nature* 346: 561–564.

Mattes R D, Engelman K, Shaw L M, ElSohly M A (1994) Cannabinoids and appetite stimulation. *Pharmacol Biochem Behav* 49(1): 187–195.

Nahas G G (1999). Delta-9-THC hemisuccinate in suppository form as an alternative to oral and smoked THC. In: Sutin K M, Harvey D J, eds. *Marihuana and Medicine*. New Jersey: Humana Press: 123–135.

NTP Technical Report (1996). Toxicology and carcinogenesis studies of 1-*trans*-delta^9-tetrahydrocannabinol in F344/N rats and B6C3F$_1$ mice. Bethesda, MD: National Institutes of Health.

Ohlsson A, Lindgren J-E, Wahlen A *et al.* (1980). Plasma delta-9 tetrahydrocannabinol concentrations and clinical effects after oral and intravenous administration and smoking. *Clin Pharmacol Ther* 28(3): 409–416.

Perez-Reyes M, Wagner D, Wall M E, Davis K H (1976). Intravenous administration of cannabinoids and intraocular pressure. In: Braude M C, Szara S, eds. *The Pharmacology of Marihuana*. New York: Raven Press: 829–832.

Pertwee R G (1998). Advances in cannabinoid receptor pharmacology. In: Brown D T, ed. *Cannabis. The Genus Cannabis*. London: Harwood Academic Publishers: 125–174.

Petro D J (1980). Marijuana as a therapeutic agent for muscle spasm or spasticity. *Psychosomatics* 21(1): 81–85.

Rosenkrantz H, Fleischman R W, McCraken D *et al.* (1978). Toxicity effects, testicular morphology and serum hormone profiles of rhesus monkeys and fischer rats treated orally with cannabidiol for 30–90 days. Report number MRI-DA 02-78-19. Mason Research Institute.

Salio C, Fischer J, Franzoni M F *et al.* (2001). CB1-cannabinoid and mu-opioid receptor co-localization on postsynaptic target in the rat dorsal horn. *Neuroreport* 12: 3689–3692.

Sallan S E, Zinberg N E, Frei E (1975). Anti-emetic effect of delta^9-tetrahydrocannabinol in patients receiving cancer chemotherapy. *N Engl J Med* 295: 795–797.

Showalter V M, Compton D R, Martin B R, Abood M E (1996). Evaluation of binding in a transfected cell line expressing a peripheral cannabinoid receptor (CB2): identification of cannabinoid receptor subtype selective ligands. *J Pharmacol Exp Ther* 278: 989–999.

Singh N, Vrat S, Ali B, Bhargava K P (1981). An assessment of biological effects of chronic use of cannabis in human subjects. *Q J Crude Drug Res* 19: 81–91.

Smiley K A, Karber R, Turkanis S A (1976). Effect on cannabinoids on the perfused rat heart. *Res Commun Mol Pathol Pharmacol* 14: 659–675.

Strivastava M D, Strivastava B I, Brouhard B (1998) Delta⁹-tetrahydrocannabinol and cannabidiol alter cytokine production by human immune cells. *Immunopharmacology* 40(3): 179–185.

The Observer (2002). The real danger of cannabis. http://www.observer.co.uk/comment/story/0,6903,776394,00.html (accessed 11 November 2002).

Whittle B A, Guy G W, Robson P J (2001). Prospects for new cannabis-based prescription medicines. *J Cannabis Ther* 1(3/4): 183–205.

Williamson E M, Evans F J (2000). Cannabinoids in clinical practice. *Drugs* 60: 1305–1314.

Zajicek J, Fox P, Sanders H et al. (2003). Cannabinoids for treatment of spasticity and other symptoms related to multiple sclerosis (CAMS study): multicentre randomised placebo-controlled trial. *Lancet* 362: 1517–1526.

Zuardi A W, Shirakawa I, Finkelfarb E, Karniol I G (1982). Action of cannabidiol on the anxiety and other effects produced by delta 9-THC in normal subjects. *Psychopharmacology (Berl)* 76: 245–250.

Zuardi A W, Rodrigues J A, Cunha J M (1991). Effects of cannabidiol in animal models of antipsychotic activity. *Psychopharmacology (Berl)* 104: 260–264.

Glossary

Accession   an item added to a collection

Achene   a dry, single-seeded fruit that does not open to release its seed

Aetiology   the set of factors that contribute to the occurrence of a disease

Aflatoxin   a toxic compound produced by a mould fungus in agricultural crops

Agonist   a drug, hormone or other substance that triggers a response in a specific body tissue or group of cells by binding to specific receptor molecules on or inside cells

Allele   one of two or more alternative forms of a gene, occupying the same position (locus) on paired chromosomes and controlling the same inherited characteristic

Antagonist   a substance, often a drug, that reduces or nullifies the effect an agonist has on the body

Biotype   a naturally occurring group of individuals with the same genetic makeup

Botanical drug substance   an extract derived from the dried raw material of a plant through some process of extraction

Bract   a modified leaf that arises from the stem at the point where the flower or flower cluster develops

Calyx   the group of sepals, usually green, around the outside of a flower that encloses and protects the flower bud

Cannabinoid   molecules found only in the cannabis plant

Catalepsy   actual or apparent unconsciousness while muscles become rigid and remain in any position in which they are placed

CBME cannabis-based medicine extract

Chemovar plants within a given botanical species defined by the metabolites they produce rather than their morphology

Chiral a molecule whose arrangement of atoms is such that it cannot be superimposed on its mirror image

Claude A group of organisms believed to comprise all the evolutionary descendants of a common ancestor

Clone a collection of organisms, cells or molecular segments that are genetically identical direct descendants of a single parent by asexual reproduction, for example, plant cuttings or grafts

Cognition process of acquiring knowledge by the use of reasoning, intuition or perception

Cultivar a variety of a cultivated plant that is developed by breeding and has distinctive morphology and a designated name

Decoction the extraction of an essence or active ingredient from a substance by boiling in water

Dimorphism the occurrence of two different forms of flowers, leaves, etc., on the same plant or on different plants of the same species

Dysmenorrhoea severe pain or cramps in the lower abdomen during menstruation

Dysphoria a state of feeling acutely hopeless, uncomfortable and unhappy

Endocannabinoid endogenous cannabinoid

Epidural a local anaesthetic injected into the space between the outer membrane covering the spinal cord and the spine

Exon a discontinuous sequence of DNA that codes for protein synthesis and carries the genetic code for the final messenger RNA molecule

Founder effect The reduced genetic diversity which results when a population is descended from a small number of colonising ancestors

Full-sib a progeny from a cross between two, known, single parents, therefore, the individuals of the progeny are full siblings (true brothers and/or sisters)

Gamete   a specialised male or female cell with half the normal number of chromosomes that unites with another cell of the opposite sex in the process of sexual reproduction

Genome   the full complement of genetic information that an individual organism inherits from its parents, especially the set of chromosomes and the genes they carry

Genotype   the genetic content of an organsism

Genus   a category in the taxonomic classification of related organisms, comprising one or more species

Germ plasm   the hereditary material that is transmitted from one generation to another

Heterosis (hybrid vigour)   the increased growth, disease resistance and fertility seen in hybrid species

Heterotic   the ability to acquire properties or characteristics which are not always individually present in an organism

Heterozygous   used to describe a cell or organism that has two or more different versions (alleles) of at least one of its genes

Homozygous   having two identical genes at the corresponding loci of homologous chromosomes

Hydroponic   the growing of plants without soil in a nutrient liquid with or without gravel or another supporting medium

Immunomodulation   modification of some aspect of the immune system as part of a treatment

Indigenous   originating in and typical of a region or country

Inflorescence   flowering structure that consists of more than one flower and usually comprises distinct individual flowers

Intraplantar   within or introduced into the sole of the foot

Ischaemia   an inadequate supply of blood to a part of the body, caused by partial or total blockage of an artery

Isoenzyme   one of two or more enzymes that are different chemically but function in the same way

Labile   readily or frequently undergoing chemical or physical change

Laminotomy a surgical procedure involving the cutting of one or more of the thin plates behind the body of a vertebra

Ligand an atom, molecule, group or ion that is bound to a central atom of a molecule, forming a complex

Locus the position of a gene on a chromosome

Metabolite a substance that is involved in or is a by-product of metabolism

Monoclonal antibody (MAb) a highly specific antibody produced in large quantities by clones of an artificially created cell

Monoecious a plant that has separate male and female flowers on the same plant

Neuropathic damage to the peripheral or central nervous system as a result of injury, disease or dysfunction of the nervous system itself

Nociceptive a stimulus that causes pain

Phenotype the visible characteristics of an organism resulting from the interaction between its genetic makeup and the environment

Photoperiod the daily cycle of light and darkness that affects the behaviour and physiological functions of organisms

Phototropism the tendency of an organism to grow toward or away from a source of light

Phyllotaxy study of the factors that determine the growth patterns and arrangement of plant leaves

Phylogeny the development over time of a species, genus or group, as contrasted with the development of an individual

Pistil a carpel or group of fused carpels forming the female reproductive part of a flower and including the ovary, style and stigma

Polygene any in a group of genes where the number of those genes present collectively determines the extent of a characteristic

Polygenic the heredity of complex characters that are determined by a large number of genes, each one usually having a relatively small effect

Progeny an offspring of a person, animal or plant

Psychometric branch of psychology dealing with the measurement of mental traits, capacities and processes

Psychosis a psychiatric disorder such as schizophrenia or mania that is marked by delusions, hallucinations, incoherence and distorted perceptions of reality

Psychotomimetic used to describe a drug or other factor that produces a condition resembling psychosis

Ruderal plant that grows in wasteland or disturbed ground

Sinsemilla a very strong form of marijuana obtained from unpollinated female hemp plants

Staminate used to describe plants that have stamens, especially flowers with stamens but without female parts

Taxon denotes any group or rank in the classification of organisms, e.g. class, order, family

Trait a quality or characteristic that is genetically determined

Transduction conversion of stimuli detected in receptor cells to electrical impulses that are then transported by the nervous system

Triploid possessing three representatives of each chromosome, usually sterile

Index

Page numbers in *italic* refer to figures or tables.

Abu al-Fadl Radi ad-Din al-Ghazzi al-'Amiri, 3
accession, 467
acetylcholine, 106–107
achene, 467
addiction, 251–253, 286
  beliefs about, 375–376, 377
  increasing concern with, 372
adenylate cyclase, 104, 105
administrative expediency principle, 395, 410
adolescents, cannabis-related psychosis, 254
Advanced Dispensing System, 245, 449–450,
  Plate 11
adverse effects
  cannabis-based medicines, 242, *243*, 256, *256*
    acute, 292
    patient counselling, 285–286
    route of administration and, 436
    surveillance, 452, 453
  criminal penalties, 409
  recreational cannabis use, 253–254, 370, 379,
    384, 412
  see also safety
Advisory Committee on Drug Dependence,
  Hallucinogens Subcommittee report *see*
  Wootton Report
Advisory Committee on Traffic in Opium,
  388–389
Advisory Council on the Misuse of Drugs
  (ACMD), 301, 422
advocacy movements, patient and healthcare,
  229, 406
aetiology, 467
Afghani No. 1, 77
aflatoxin, 49, 467
aflatoxin B1, 166
aggressive behaviour, 168, 180–181
agonist, 467
agricultural use, declining, 371–372
AIDS *see* HIV infection/AIDS
'air hunger', 261
ajulemic acid (CT-3), *109*, *124*, 125–126, 415
Akkadian medicine, 1–2
alcohol (ethanol)
  Cannabis plant extracts, 444
  dependence, 178–179, *179*, 186

driving impairment, 329–330, 331–333, 339
alkaloids, plant, 91, 467
allele, 467
Alliance for Cannabis Therapeutics (ACT), 229,
  404
allodynia, 290–291
alternative medicine, 407
Alzheimer's disease, 235
AM251, *121*, 123
AM281, *109*, *121*, 193–194
AM374 (palmitylsulfonyl fluoride), 113–114, *114*
AM381 (stearylsulfonyl fluoride), 113–114, *114*
AM404, *109*, 112–113, *113*
AM630, *110*, *121*, 123–124
American Medical Association (AMA), 376
'amotivational syndrome', 379
amputation, phantom limb pain after, 171,
  233–234
analgesic effects, 169–171
  animal models, 170
  future research, 260–261
  history, 6, 272–274
  human studies, 170–171
  in multiple sclerosis, 144–145
  perioperative, 260–261
  THC/CBD interaction, 167
  see also pain
analgesics, 271, 467
analysis, forensic *see* forensic analysis
anandamide, 107–108, 454, 457, 459
  analgesic activity, 234
  antitumour effects, 240
  CB receptor affinity, 108, *109*
  deficiency syndrome, 91–92
  discovery, 9
  enzymic hydrolysis, 111–112
    inhibitors, 113–114, *114*
  functions, 111–112, *112*
  receptor coevolution, 86, 87
  structure, *108*
  surreptitious mimic theory, 84
  transport (uptake) inhibitors, 112–113, *113*
    antispastic activity, 148–149
  transporter, 148
  VR1 receptor actions, 111

animal models
    analgesic activity, 170
    multiple sclerosis, 141–142
animals
    preclinical safety studies, 450, 451–453
    receptors with plant ligands, 84–85
Anslinger, Harry J, 375–376, 389
antagonist, 467
anthelminthic activity, possible, 240
anther, 467
anticoagulants, 285
antidepressants, 365
antiemetic properties, 230–231
antihistamines, 365
anti-inflammatory effects, 191–195, 235
    animal models, 193–195
    in-vitro models, 191–193
antioxidant effects, 154, 187–191, 239
anti-parkinsonism drugs, 284
antipsychotic drugs, 182, 183–184
antismoking movement, 414
antitumour effects, 240
anxiety, 172–177, 237
    animal models, 172–173, *173, 174, 175*
    human studies, 173–177
apigenin, anti-inflammatory effects, 192
apomorphine, 180, 184
appetite stimulation, 91, 234–235, 261–262
Arabic medicine, 3
arachidonoyl ethanolamide *see* anandamide
2-arachidonoyl glycerol (2-AG), 87, 107–108
    CB receptor affinity, 108, *109*
    enzymic hydrolysis, 112, 114
    functions, 111–112
    structure, *108*
arachidonyl-2′-chloroethylamide (ACEA), *109,*
    118, *118*
arachidonyl glyceryl ether (noladin ether), 108,
    108
    CB receptor affinity, 108, *109*
arachidonylcyclopropylamide (ACPA), *109,* 118,
    118
arachnid pests, 50
Arizona, 383
aroma, cannabis, 23–24, 80
arthritis, 437
    collagen-induced (CIA), 194–195, *196,* 235
    rheumatoid, 261
Ashworth Scale, 259–260
asthma, 236–237
atomic absorption spectroscopy (AAS), 311–312
attitudes to cannabis control, 229–230,
    369–426
    1960s to present day, 379–385
    drivers of change, 406–416
    in specific countries, 417–424
    United States case study, 370–377
Australia, 399, 423
Ayurvedic medicine, 2

back pain, chronic, 289, *290*
bacterial bioburden, 49
Belgium, 334–335, 424
benzo[α]pyrene, 166
benzodiazepines, 365
bhang, 2, 323
bioavailability
    cannabidiol, 220
    cannabinol, 220
    δ^9-THC, 216, 218, 219–220
biotypes, 74–78, 467
    cannabinoid profiles, 78–80
    geographical origins, 72
    see also varieties, *Cannabis*
bladder function, in multiple sclerosis,
    144–145
body fluids, forensic analysis, 312–316
botanical drug substances (BDS), 428–430,
    467
    clinical trials, 461–462
    consistency and stability, 445–446
    historical use, 462–463, *463*
    production, 53, 444–445
    quality, 442–446
    regulatory attitudes, 440–441
    regulatory route, 431, 438–440
    renewed interest in, 407
    safety issues, 451–452
    see also cannabis-based medicinal extracts
botanical raw material
    Good Agricultural Practice guidelines *see* Good
        Agricultural Practice
    harvesting and drying, 42, 444
    processing, 42
    production, *31,* 37–42, 442–444
Botrytis cinerea, 50, 51, 53, *53*
Bowery, Thomas, 4
brachial plexus injury, 254–255, *257,*
    257–258
bract, 467
brain injury, 239–240, 415
breeding, *Cannabis* plant, 35–36, 55–69
    current achievements, 63–67
    future developments, 67–68
    germ plasm sources, 60–63
    goals and strategies, 56–59
    spectrum, 55–56
British Medical Association (BMA), 12, 229, 274,
    421
British Pharmacopoeia, 430
bronchodilator activity, 236–237
buccal, 468
Bureau of Narcotics and Dangerous Drugs
    (BNDD), 380
burglary risk, 286

calcium channels, 104
California, 383, 385
calyx, 23, *24,* 468

Canada
  attitudes to cannabis, 387, 411, 414
  legalisation of medicinal cannabis, 394, 399,
    402–403, 418–420, 438
  US relations, 388, 419–420
Canadian Commission of Inquiry into the Non-
  Medical Use of Drugs (LeDain Commission)
  (1970), 331, 378–379
Canadian Medical Association, 411, 413, 419
cancer
  antidepressant effects, 178
  antiemetic effects, 230–231
  legalisation of cannabis use, 382
  pain relief, 171
  tumour growth inhibition, 240
Cannabaceae, 9, 73–74
cannabichromene (CBC)
  antidepressant activity, 177
  plant breeding and, 61–62, 64
  plant metabolism, 79
cannabichromevarin (CBCV), 62–63
cannabidiol (CBD), 205
  abnormal, 127, 127–128
  actions, 90, 196, 455
  in alcohol withdrawal, 179
  analgesic activity, 170, 171, 261, 283
  antidepressant activity, 177, 178
  antiepileptic activity, 186, 187, 236
  anti-inflammatory effects, 194–195, 196, 235
  antioxidant activity, 189, 239
  antispastic effect, 148, 179–182
  anxiolytic activity, 172–177, 173, 174, 175,
    237
  cannabis medicinal extracts, 245–246
    chronic pain, 283, 287
  CB receptor interactions, 87, 168–169, 456
  effects on endocannabinoid system, 92
  immunosuppressive activity, 151
  induction of drug-metabolising enzymes,
    214–215
  inhibition of drug-metabolising enzymes,
    213–214
  interactions with other cannabinoids, 440
  legality of medical use, 401
  metabolism in humans, 208–216
    in vitro, 210–211
  in multiple sclerosis, 232
  pharmacokinetics, 207, 220
  pharmacological effects, 453–455, 454, 456,
    457
  in plants, 10, 61, 165
    cloned vs seed-sown, 33, 34, 34–35
    different biotypes, 79–80
    different varieties, 11, 27, 28
    distribution in tissues, 20, 20
    metabolism, 79
  in schizophrenia, 183–185
  stereoselectivity, 110, 119–120, 120
  structure, 206

THC interactions see under δ⁹-tetrahydrocannabinol
THC ratio, 165, 196
toxicity studies, 452–453
cannabidiol-7-oic acid, 209
cannabidiolic acid (CBDA), 445, 446
cannabidivarin (CBDV), 62–63, 79
cannabielsoic acid, 313, 313
cannabigerol (CBG), 39
  anti-inflammatory effects, 192
  cloned vs seed-sown plants, 34–35
  plant breeding programmes, 62
  plant metabolism, 79
cannabigerol-monomethyl ether (CBGM), 79
cannabigerovarin (CBGV), 62–63
cannabine tannate, 432–433, 433–434
cannabinoid (CB) receptor agonists, 107–117
  aminoalkylindole, 115, 116
  chirality, 117–120
  classical, 115, 115, 116
  eicosanoid, 115
  inverse, 123–124
  in multiple sclerosis, 151–152
  non-classical, 115, 116
  see also CB₁ receptor agonists; CB₂ receptor
    agonists
cannabinoid (CB) receptor antagonists, 120–124
  see also CB₁ receptor antagonists; CB₂ receptor
    antagonists
cannabinoid (CB) receptors, 103–139
  coevolution with phytocannabinoids, 84–93
  discovery, 9
  effects of phytocannabinoids, 92–93
  efficacy of cannabis-based medicines, 455–460
  evolution, 80–84, 82, 87
  ligands, 107–125, 109–110
    chirality, 117–120
    endogenous, 107–114
      see also endocannabinoids
    other, 124–125
      see also cannabinoid (CB) receptor agonists;
      cannabinoid (CB) receptor antagonists
  other/novel types, 125–128
  reason for existence in animals, 84–85
  as vestigial receptors, 92–93, 94
  see also CB₁ receptors; CB₂ receptors
cannabinoids, 468
  biological function, 27–28, 80–81, 435
  chirality, 117–120
  coevolution with CB receptors, 84–93
  forensic analysis see forensic analysis
  in herbal cannabis, trends, 304–306, 305, 306
  identification methods, 303–304
  interactions and effects, 165–204
  metabolism, 208–216
  monoterpene and dibenzopyran numbering
    systems, 10, 205, 320, 321
  pain and, 275–278, 283
  pharmacodynamics, 103–139

cannabinoids (*cont'd*)
  pharmacokinetics *see* pharmacokinetics
  in plants
    breeding programmes, 56–57, 60–63
    cloned *vs* seed-sown, *33, 33–34, 34*
    different biotypes, 78–80
    different varieties, 11, 27, *28*
    distribution, 10, *20,* 20–22, *21*
  stability in botanical products, 445–446
  structure–activity relationships, 206–207
  structures, *206*
  terminology, 78–79
  yield components, 57–58
  see also endocannabinoids; phytocannabinoids;
    specific compounds
cannabinol (CBN), 79, 147, 205
  analgesic activity, 170, 171
  anti-inflammatory effects, 191–192
  CB receptor affinity, *110,* 117
  metabolism, 208–216
  pharmacokinetics, *207,* 220
  structure, *115, 206*
cannabis
  forensic control, 301–328
  international control, 369–426
  medicinal *see* medicinal cannabis
  see also marihuana
Cannabis, 18, 71–101
  biotypes *see* biotypes
  coevolution with humans, 84–94
  evolution, 73–74
  origin of association with man, *72,* 72–73
  plants *see* plants, *Cannabis*
  species debate, 74–78
  taxonomy, 73–74
Cannabis afghanica, 74
Cannabis indica (Indian hemp), 4–5, 9, 36
  biotypes, 75–78
  cannabinoid content, 79–80
  extract, therapeutic indications, *432–433,* 433
  origins, 72
  species debate, 74, 78
  ssp. *afghanica,* 76–77, 79, 80, Plate 1
  ssp. *chinensis,* 77–78, 79
  ssp. *indica,* 76, 79, 80
  ssp. *kafiristanica,* 75–76, 79
Cannabis ruderalis (wild hemp), 9, 74–75,
    Plate 1
  cannabinoid content, 80
  distribution, *72, 75*
Cannabis sativa, 9, 18, *19*
  forensic control, 307–312
  geographical origin, *72, 75,* 310–312
  growth and morphology, 17–54
  species debate, 74, 78
  ssp. *indica see Cannabis indica*
  ssp. *sativa,* 36, *72, 75,* 79
  ssp. *spontanea, 72, 75*
  see also plants, *Cannabis*

cannabis-based medicinal extracts (CBME), 230,
    274
  acute side-effects, 292–294
  anxiolytic activity, 177
  cannabinoid content, 205, 245–246, 283
  choosing, for clinical research, 245–246
  chronic pain studies, 171, 282–295
  consistency and stability, 445–446
  contraindications, 284–285
  delivery systems, 242–245
  dosing, 246, 248–250, 286–288
  driving fitness, 296
  future research, 260–262
  long-term use, 294–295
  pain management, 296, *297*
  preparation, 444–445
  recent clinical research, 254–260
  regulatory route, 438–440
cannabis-based medicines
  changing attitudes, 229–230, 380–385
  chronic pain, 271–299
  clinical studies, 229–269
  contraindications, 284–285
  delivery systems, 242–245, 447, 449–450,
    Plate 11
  development *see* development of cannabis-
    based medicines
  dose titration, 249, 286–288, 448
  driving and, 250, 363–365
  efficacy, 453–460
  factors affecting attitudes to, 406–416
  growth and morphology, 17–54
  long-term use, 294–295
  new synthetic products, 414–415
  safety issues, 250–254
  see also medicinal cannabis
Cannador, in multiple sclerosis, 259
cannflavin A, anti-inflammatory effects, 193
canvas, 18
capillary electrochromatography (CEC), 308
capillary zone electrophoresis (CZE), 308, 309
capsaicin, 111, *111, 463*
carbon dioxide, liquid, 445
carboxy-tetrahydrocannabinol (carboxy-THC)
  forensic analysis, 314–315, 316
  forensic interpretation, 317–318, 322
carrageenan-induced hyperalgesia/hypersensitivity,
    193–194
β-caryophyllene, anti-inflammatory effects, 192
catalepsy, 184, 468
catatonia, 167, 180
CB receptors *see* cannabinoid receptors
CB$_1$ receptor agonists, 104–117, 456–457
  anti-inflammatory effects, 193–194
  in multiple sclerosis, 145, 146–147, 149, 151,
    154
  selective, *109,* 118, *118*
CB$_1$ receptor antagonists, 120–124, *121*
  in multiple sclerosis, 146

CB₁ receptors, 81, 104–107, 456
  effector functions, 104–107
  evolution, 87
  expression pattern, 105–106
  human *vs* rat brain, 88–89
  knockout mice, 83, 104
  ligands, 107–114, *109–110*
  mutant, 92
  presynaptic, 105–106
  single nucleotide polymorphisms (SNPs), 87
  splice variant (CB₁ₐ), 104
CB₂ receptor agonists, 104–117
  anti-inflammatory effects, 193–194
  in multiple sclerosis, 146, 151
  selective, *110*, 118–119, *119*
CB₂ receptor antagonists, 120–124, *121*
CB₂ receptors, 81, 104, 456
  effector functions, 107
  knockout mice, 104
  ligands, 107–114, *109–110*
  in nociception, 275, *275*
CB₂-like receptor, 125–126
CBC *see* cannabichromene
CBD *see* cannabidiol
CBG *see* cannabigerol
CBME *see* cannabis-based medicinal extracts
CBN *see* cannabinol
Center for Medicinal Cannabis Research
  (CMCR), 383
cerebral palsy, 231–232
chemovars, 9–10, 20, 454, 468
  see also varieties, *Cannabis*
children, antiemetic effects, 231
China, 17
  ancient, 1, 17, 18, 77
  opium problem, 386–387
Chinese hemp, 77–78, 79
Chinese immigrants, 373
chiral, 468
chirality, CB receptor ligands, 117–120
chronic obstructive airways disease, 261
chronic relapsing allergic encephalomyelitis
  (CRAE), 181
cigarettes, cannabis
  cannabinoid pharmacokinetics, 216–218, 220,
    446–447
  trends in potency, 304–306, *305*
  see also smoking, cannabis
1,8-cineole, 166
citronellol, anxiolytic activity, 172
climbing rope test, 167–168
clinical research, 12, 229–269
  chronic pain, 282–295
  delivery systems, 242–245
  future directions, 260–262
  GW Pharmaceuticals database, 241–242,
    243
  practical issues, 245–254
  publication issues, 436

recently completed, 254–260
  review of published, 230–240
clinical trials, 245–254, 459–460
  choice of extract, 245–246
  design, 246–248
  patients, dosing and outcome measures,
    248–249
  phytomedicines, 461–462
  safety issues, 250–254, 451–452
Clinical Trials Exemption (CTX), 451–452
clones, 468
  see also cuttings
cocaine, 372, 373–374, 405–406
coevolution, 71–72
  cannabis and humans, 84–94
  see also evolution
coffee shops, Dutch, 417
cognition, 468
  effects on, 250–251
  laboratory studies, 330–336
collagen-induced arthritis (CIA), 194–195, *196,
    235*
Commission on Narcotic Drugs (CND), 389–390,
    400
Committee on Safety of Medicines (CSM), 428
compassionate use, 381–382
complex regional pain syndrome, 290–291
compound 59, 114, *114*
conjunctivae, reddened, 317
consistency, cannabis-based medicines, 445–446
contraindications, medicinal cannabis, 284–285
Controlled Drugs and Substances Act (CDSA)
  (Canada), 402–403, 418
Controlled Substances Act (CSA) (USA, 1970),
  11, 379
  exemptions, 404–405
  medicinal cannabis use, 382, 401–402
  overriding nature, 383–384, 385
  rescheduling actions, 380–381, 401
Convention Against Illicit Traffic in Narcotic
  Drugs and Psychotropic Substances (1988
  Trafficking Convention), 392–393, 394
Convention on Psychotropic Substances (1971
  Convention), 391–392, 393–394,
    400–401
corneal reflex, nictitating membrane, 167
cortisol, plasma, 176–177
CP50,556 *see* levonantradol
CP55,940, 115, *116*, 120
  CB receptor affinity, *109*, 117
  in multiple sclerosis, 146, 147
criminal behaviour, 373–374, 377
criminalisation, 377, 391, 392–393
  adverse effects, 409–410
  see also decriminalisation
crops
  field-grown, 50–53, *52, 53*, 442, *443*
  grown in controlled environment, 42–45, *44,
    443–444*

crude marijuana extract (CME), analgesic activity, 170
Culpepper, Nicholas, 4, 20
cultivar, 468
cuttings (clones)
  advantages of growing, 29–34, *33*
  forensic control, 307
  potting up rooted, 38
  taking, 37–38, *40–41*
  vs seed-sown plants, *33*, 33–34
cyclooxygenase-2 (COX-2), 126
p-cymene, 166
cytochrome P450 enzymes (CYPs), 166, 210, *210*
  inhibition/induction, 212–216, *213*
  phase I metabolism by, 211–212, *212*
cytokines, 107, 150

dagga, 387
Dangerous Drugs Act (1925), 388
database, GW Pharmaceuticals patient, 241–242, *243*
day length, 22, 39
decarboxylation, 468
decoction, 468
decriminalisation, 378, 380–381, 395, 396
  de facto, 397
  in specific countries, 417, 420
  trends in cannabis use after, 412
  see also criminalisation
delivery systems, cannabis-based medicines, 242–245, 447, 449–450, Plate 11
delta⁹-tetrahydrocannabinol *see* δ⁹-tetrahydro-cannabinol
demonisation, cannabis, 375–376
depenalisation, 395–396
dependence, 251–253, 286
  see also addiction
depression, 177–178
  animal models, 177
  in chronic pain, 280
  human studies, 178
developing countries, 411
development of cannabis-based medicines, 427–466
  dosage form, 446–450
    oropharyngeal administration, 448–449
    routes of administration, 446–447
    security issues, 449–450
  efficacy, 453–460
  historical legacy, 431–438
  quality, 442–446
    consistency and stability, 445–446
    field-grown crops, 442
    grown in controlled environment, 443–444
    horticulture, 444
    production of botanical drug substance, 444–445
  regulatory attitudes to botanicals, 440–441
  regulatory route, 438–440

risk factors, 427, *429*
risks, benefits and serendipity, 460–463
safety, 450–453
dexanabinol (HU-211), 239–240, 415
diamba, 76
diamorphine *see* heroin
dibenzopyran numbering system, 10, 205, 320, *321*
5'-dimethylheptyl-cannabidiol (5'-DMH-CBD), *109*, 119, *120*
dimorphism, 468
Dioscorides, Pedacius, 2, 18
disease control, plant, 49–50
dispensaries, US state, 383, 385
doctrine of signatures, 428–429
dopamine, 106–107, *107*
dorsal horn, 276
dosage forms, 446–450
dosing, 246, 248–249, 286–288
driving, 296, 329–368
  alcohol *vs* cannabis-related impairment, 329
  forensic control, 324, 329–330
  laboratory studies, 330–336
  medicinal cannabis use, 250, 363–365
  prospective studies, 344–362, *345–359*
  retrospective analyses of traffic collisions, 336–343, *340–341, 342*
dronabinol (Marinol), 242–243, 439
  alternative delivery methods, 415
  in Alzheimer's disease, 235
  driving and, 363
  introduction, 382
  legality of use, 12, 382, 392, 401, 405
  in multiple sclerosis, 259
  use, *vs* illicit cannabis use, 323
dropping out, 379
drowsiness, driving and, 363
drug abuse, 436
  'hard' *vs* 'soft' drugs, 417
  harm reduction approach, 408–410
  history in US, 372–377
  legislation *see* legislation
  prescription, 415–416
Drug Abuse Prevention and Control Act (USA, 1970), 301
drug development *see* development of cannabis-based medicines
Drug Enforcement Agency (DEA), 363, 380–381, 405
drug testing, mandatory, 379
dry mouth, 294
drying, plant material, 42, 444, Plate 9
Duckfoot leaves, 64
Duquenois colour test, 303
Durban landrace, 76
dysmenorrhoea, 468
dysphoria, 168, 293, 468
dystonias, 181–182
dystonic (dt) mutant rats, 179–180

ear-swelling assay, 194
efficacy, cannabis-based medicines, 453–460
Egypt, 1, 387
emotional changes, chronic pain, 295
endocannabinoid deficiency syndrome (EDS),
    91–92
endocannabinoid system, 104, 457–458
    effects of phytocannabinoids, 92–93, 457–458
    in multiple sclerosis, 149–150
endocannabinoid tone, 93, 277–278, 458
endocannabinoids, 78–79, 107–114, 457–459,
    468
    CB receptor affinity, 108, 109–110
    discovery, 9, 435
    enzymic hydrolysis, 111–112
    modulation of nociception, 276–277, 277
    structures, 108
    see also specific compounds
endogenous, 468
endorphins, 455, 457
entourage effect, 10, 166, 458
    botanical medicines, 439, 440
    FAAH inhibition and, 114
enuresis, 468
environmental movement, 408
enzyme immunoassays (EIA), 314
enzyme-linked immunosorbent assay (ELISA),
    309–310
epidural, 469
epilepsy, 185–187, 236
    animal models, 186
    human studies, 187
essential fatty acids (EFAs), 10
essential oils, terpenoid, 10, 23–26, 80
ethanol see alcohol
Ethiopia, 2
ethnic minority groups, cannabis use, 374, 375
euphoria, 293
Europe, 12, 411, 423–424
    history of medicinal use, 1, 2–6, 369–370
    regulation of botanicals, 440
    road traffic laws, 333–335
European hemp (Cannabis sativa ssp. sativa), 36,
    72, 75, 79
European Medicines Evaluation Agency (EMEA),
    431
evolution
    Cannabis, 73–74
    CB receptors, 80–84, 82, 87
    receptors, 82–84
    see also coevolution
evolutionary arabesque concept, 82–84, 85
exogenous, 469
exon, 469
expediency principle, administrative, 395, 410
experimental allergic encephalomyelitis (EAE),
    142
    immunomodulation, 150–152
    neuroprotection, 153, 154

symptom control, 144, 145, 146, 232
experimental models see animal models

FAAH see fatty acid amide hydrolase
fatalities, cannabis-related, 323
fatigue, driving and, 363
fatty acid amide hydrolase (FAAH), 111–112,
    457
    endogenous inhibitors, 114
    inhibitors, 113–114, 114
        antispastic activity, 150
        in cannabis, 148
FDA see Food and Drug Administration
Federal Bureau of Narcotics (FBN), 375–376,
    377, 380
female flowers, 22, Plate 3, Plate 4
    cannabinoid content, 20, 20
    parts, 23, 24
female plants, 22, 23, Plate 4
    breeding programmes, 58–59, 59
    male floret production, 28–29
    pollen, 29
fertility, plant breeding programmes and, 64, 66,
    66–67
fibre hemp
    breeding, 55
    cultivation, 10
    harvesting, 22–23
    industrial uses, 18, 371–372
    strains, 61–62
Finola, 22
flavonoids, 165, 166
    anti-inflammatory effects, 193
    antioxidant activity, 190–191
flowering, 39, 444
    day length and, 22
    induction, 39
    light levels, 45
flowers see inflorescence
Food and Drug Administration (FDA), 372
    approval of cannabis products, 382, 401
    guidance on botanicals, 407, 438, 441
forensic analysis, 302
    cannabinoids in body fluids, 312–316
        development of techniques, 313–316
        methodology, 313
    geographical origin, 310–312
    interpretation, 316–323
    present situation in UK, 303–304
    quality control, 324
    techniques, 306–312
forensic control, 301–328
    analytical aspects see forensic analysis
    driving and cannabis, 324, 329–330
    legal aspects, 301–302
    trends in cannabis potency, 304–306, 305, 306
    see also international cannabis control
c-fos, 182–183, 277
FOXP2 gene, 88

France, 4, 5, 369
free radical-associated disease, 188
free radicals, 187–188
full-sib, 469
fungal contamination
    outdoor crops, 51, 52, 53, 53
    regulatory requirements, 49

G protein-coupled receptors (GPCRs), 81, 82–83, 104
G proteins, 81, 104–105
G1 variety (high THC), 20, 20, 34, Plate 1
    breeding program, 35–36
    cloned vs seed-sown, 33, 33–34, 35
    M1 clone, 65, 65
G5 variety (high CBD), 20, 20
    breeding program, 36
    cloned vs seed-sown, 33, 33–34, 34
    M16 clone, Plate 1
    outdoor cultivation, 51–53, 52, 53
G116 variety (high THC), Plate 7
GABA (γ-aminobutyric acid), 106–107
Galen, 2
galenical preparations, 431–434, 432–433
gamete, 469
gamma hydroxybutyric acid (GHB), 405
ganja, 9, 76
gas chromatography with flame ionisation
    detectors (GC-FID), 324
gas chromatography–mass spectrometry
    (GC/MS), 303, 304, 314, 315, 316
Gayer Test, 167
gene duplication, 83, 87
genetically modified cannabis, 67–68
Geneva Conventions
    1925, 387–388
    1931 and 1936, 388–389
genome, 469
genotype, 469
genus, 469
geographical origin, cannabis samples,
    310–312
germ plasm, 469
    sources, breeding programmes, 60–63
Germany, 334
glaucoma, 237–238, 261, 382
Gloria variety, Plate 1
glutamate, 106, 107, 189
glutathione peroxidase, 188–189
glutathione reductase, 189
glycine, 106
Good Agricultural Practice (GAP), 48–50, 442,
    443, 443, 469
Good Clinical Practice, 469
Good Laboratory Practice, 469
Good Management Practice, 469
Greece, Ancient, 2, 18
grey mould, 50
'GV point', 31–33, 32

GW Pharmaceuticals, 230, 421, 423
    clinical trials, 12, 246–254
    drug delivery systems, 244–245, 447, 449–450,
        Plate 11
    legal issues, 437–438
    patient database, 241–242, 243
    plant breeding programme, 55–68
    regulatory issues, 439
GW405833, anti-inflammatory effects, 193–194

Hague Convention, 1912, 386–387
hair analysis, 316
haloperidol, 182, 183–185
harm reduction approach, 408–410
Harrison Narcotics Act, 1914, 373
harvesting, 42, 444
hash/hashish, 10, 24, 77
hashish landraces, 61–62
Haze, 76
head injuries, 240, 415
Health Canada, 418, 419, 438
heart disease, ischaemic, 285
heat exposure, 445, 446
hemp, 369
    changing attitudes, 408
    fibre see fibre hemp
    lignified stems, 23
    plants see plants, Cannabis
    seeds see seeds
    see also Cannabis
hepatitis C, 409
herbal remedies, 407
Herodotus, 2, 72, 75–76
heroin (diamorphine), 405–406, 436
    addiction, 409, 417
heterosis (hybrid vigour), 57, 65, 469
heterotic, 469
heterozygous, 469
'high', 292–294
    forensic aspects, 317
    patient preparation, 285–286
    THC/CBD interactions, 168
high-performance liquid chromatography
    (HPLC), 308, 309
high-performance liquid chromatography
    (HPLC)-radioimmunoassay (HPLC-RIA),
    313–314
Hindu Kush, 77
history
    botanical medicines, 428–430, 462–463, 463
    hemp cultivation, 17, 71–72, 72
    hemp use, 18
    medicinal use see under medicinal cannabis
HIV infection/AIDS, 152, 191
    appetite stimulation, 234–235
    injection drug users, 409
    legalisation of cannabis use, 382
    pain syndromes, 279
Hodges, Clare, 12

Home Office Central Research Establishment, 313–314
homologues, 469
homozygous, 469
horizontal gene transfer (HGT), 84–85
HortaPharm B.V., 56
horticulture, 444
hot plate test, 167, 170
House of Lords Select Committee on Science and Technology, 12, 229, 274, 421–422, 437–438
HU-210, 115, *116*
  anti-inflammatory effects, 193–194
  CB receptor affinity, *109*, 117
HU-211 (dexanabinol), 239–240, 415
HU-243, *116*, 117
HU-308, *110*, 118–119, *119*
Humulus, 9, 73, 78
Huntington's disease (HD), 180–181, 232
hybrid vigour (heterosis), 57, 65, 469
hydroponic, 470
7-hydroxy-5'-dimethylheptyl-cannabidiol (7-OH-5'-DMH-CBD), *109*, 119, *120*
11-hydroxy-δ⁸-tetrahydrocannabinol (11-OH-δ⁸-THC), 207
8α-hydroxy-δ⁹-tetrahydrocannabinol (8α-OH-THC), 208, 212, *212*
8β-hydroxy-δ⁹-tetrahydrocannabinol (8β-OH-THC), 208, 212, *212*
11-hydroxy-δ⁹-tetrahydrocannabinol (11-OH-δ⁹-THC), 207, *207, 320*
  metabolism in humans, 208–209, 211, *212*
  pharmacokinetics, 217, 218, 219
7-hydroxy-cannabidiol (7-OH-CBD), 209, 211
5-hydroxytryptamine (5-HT; serotonin), 106, 239
hyperalgesia, 193–194, 276
hypertension, 285
hyphenated techniques, forensic analysis, 313–316
hypotension, postural, 294

identification, cannabinoids, 303–304
immigrants, United States, 372–373, 374–375
immune cells, 107, 150
immunoassay, 309–310, *310*, 470
immunomodulation, 107, 150–152, 470
INCB *see* International Narcotics Control Board
incontinence, 145
Indevus Pharmaceuticals, 415
India, 2, 4–5, 370
Indian hemp *see Cannabis indica*
Indian Hemp Commission Report (1894), 370, 410
indigenous, 470
induction, hepatic cannabinoid metabolism, 212–213, *213*, 214–216
industrial uses, 18, 371–372
inflammation, 275–276, 462–463
  see also anti-inflammatory effects

inflammatory disorders, 235
inflorescence, 470, Plate 3, Plate 4, Plate 8
  anatomy, 23, *24*
  manicuring, *20, 21*, 42
inhalational route of administration, 244, *244*, 274, 447
  see also smoking, cannabis
injection drug use, 409
insanity, cannabis, 370, 377
insect pests, 49, *50*
insomnia, 237
INSPIRE, 229
Institute of Medicine (IOM) report (USA, 1999), 235, 274, 384, 399, 414
intellectual property
  protection, plant cultivars, 57
  rights (IPR), 462, 470
interactions, pharmacological, 165–169
  botanical extracts, 440
  via hepatic enzyme inhibition/induction, 212–216, *213*
interferon-γ (IFN-γ), 191–192
international cannabis control, 369–426
  1960s and new symbolism, 378–385
  current situation, 417–424
  drivers of change, 406–416
  influence on individual nations, 410–411
  international legislation/conventions, 385–394
  legality of medicinal cannabis under, 398–403
  possible reforms, 395–398
  separating cannabis uses, 403–406
  United States case study, 370–377
  see also forensic control
International Narcotics Control Board (INCB), 301–302, 392, 424
  influence on individual nations, 410–411, 419
  legality of medicinal cannabis, 398, 399–400, 401
intoxication *see* 'high'
intraocular pressure (IOP), 237–238
intraplanar, 470
intravenous administration, 219, 220
investigational new drug (IND), 381–382
6-iodopravadoline (AM630), *110, 121*, 123–124
ion channels, 104
Ireland, 5
ischaemia, 470
ischaemic heart disease, 285
isoenzyme, 470
Italy, 397, 424

Jamaica, 76, 410, 411
joints *see* cigarettes, cannabis
Jun proteins, 183
JWH-133, *110*, 118–119, *119*

L-759633, *110*, 118–119
L-759656, *110*, 118–119, *119*
labile, 470

LaGuardia Committee Report (1944), 377
laminotomy, 470
language, emergence of, 88
LeDain Commission (Canada, 1970), 331, 378–379
legalisation
    medicinal cannabis, 380–385, 397, 400–403,
        437–438
    recreational cannabis, 396–397
    separation of issues involved, 403–406
legislation, 301–302
    effects on research, 11–12, 434–435
    history, 6, 8, 372, 373–376, 377, 379
    international, 385–394
    possibilities for reform, 395–398
    road traffic, 333–335, 364
    in specific countries, 417–424
    see also decriminalisation; forensic control;
        prohibition
levodopa, 284
levonantradol (L-nantradol; CP50,556), 115, 116
    analgesic activity, 171
    antiemetic effects, 231
licking for water behaviour, 172, 174
ligand-gated ion channels (LGICs), 82
ligands, 470
    exogenous, 86–87
    plant, with animal receptors, 84–85
    receptor coevolution, 84–85, 87–88, 89–91
lighting, 43–45, 44
    effects on yield, 45, 46, 47
    flowering phase, 39, 45
    mother plants, 37
    vegetative growth phase, 39
limonene, 166, 172
linalool, anxiolytic activity, 172
lipophilicity, 207, 207–208
lipopolysaccharide (LPS), 191–192
liquid chromatography, 316
locus, 470
Luxembourg, 424
LY320135, 109, 121, 123

M77 variety, Plate 1
male flowers, 20, 22
male plants, 22, 23, Plate 2
    pollen, 29
manicuring, 20, 21, 42
marihuana (marijuana), 76
    in experimental model of multiple sclerosis, 147
    prohibition in US, 374
    smoking see smoking
    trends in potency, 304–306, 305, 306
Marihuana Medical Access Regulations, 419
Marijuana and Medicine: Assessing the Science
    Base see Institute of Medicine report
Marijuana Tax Act (USA, 1937), 11, 373, 376
Marijuana/AIDS Research Service (MARS), 382
Marinol see dronabinol
Marshall, C R, 292

mass spectrometry (MS), 314
    hyphenated techniques, 314, 315–316
mass spectrometry–mass spectrometry (MS/MS),
    314, 315–316
mast cells, 275, 275
McCaffrey, General Barry, 384
'medical necessity' defence, 381, 385
medical profession
    attitude to cannabis, 371, 413, 419, 436
    criminal law sanctions, 383–384, 385, 413
medicinal cannabis, 428–430
    history, 1–16, 272–274
        drug development and, 431–438, 432–433
        time line, 7–8
        in USA, 5, 369–370, 371
    legal aspects, 11–12, 302, 369–424
        status in individual countries, 417, 418–420,
            421–422
    vs other uses of cannabis, 403–406
    see also cannabis-based medicinal extracts;
        cannabis-based medicines; clinical research
Medicines Act (UK, 1968), 451
Medicines and Healthcare Products Research
    Agency (MHRA), 402, 423
Medicines Control Agency, 12
Mediterranean fever, familial, 171
medulla, rostro-ventro-medial (RMV), 105, 276,
    276–277
memory deficits, 251
Merck's Manual, 431–434, 432–433
metabolism, cannabinoids, 208–216
    forensic aspects, 317–323
    induction/inhibition of CYP in liver, 212–216,
        213
    P450 isoforms responsible, 211–212, 212
    in vitro in humans, 209–211
metabolite, 470
metals, trace, 311–312
methanandamide, 109, 118, 118
Mexican Americans, 374, 375
microbiological safety, plant material, 49
microsomal aldehyde oxygenase (MALDO),
    211–212
migraine, 3, 5, 239, 277
Misuse of Drugs Act (UK, 1971), 6, 11, 301, 422
Misuse of Drugs Regulations (UK, 1985), 302,
    399, 402, 422
mitogen-activated protein kinase, 104
monoclonal antibody (MAb), 309–310, 311, 470
monoecious, 470
monomethyl cannabidiol (ME-CBD-2), 172
monoterpene numbering system, 10, 205, 320,
    321
Moraceae, 73–74
Moreau de Tours, Dr Jacques-Joseph, 369
Moroccan cannabis, 11
morphine, 170, 372, 373
motor performance, laboratory studies, 330–336
MS Society, 229

multiple sclerosis (MS), 12, 141–163, 437
  antioxidant activity, 154, 188–189
  bladder dysfunction, 144–145
  cannabis as a therapeutic, 142–143
  clinical studies, 231–232
  clinical trial methodology, 248–250
  depression, 178, 280
  disease progression, 295
  experimental models, 141–142
  GW Pharmaceuticals database, 241–242
  immunomodulation, 150–152
  neuroprotection, 152–155
  pain (including neuropathic pain), 258, 272,
    273, 459–460
    characteristics, 279, 279
    experimental models, 144–145
    'n of 1' studies, 288–289, 289, 290
  recent clinical studies, 254–257, 255, 256, 258,
    259–260
  spasticity
    animal studies, 146–150, 181, 232
    clinical studies, 231–232, 256–257, 259–260,
      460
  symptom control, 143–150, 232
  tremor, 145–146, 232
musculoskeletal pain, 171
mutualism, 71
myrcene, 169–170

'n of 1' trials, 247–248
  chronic pain, 283, 288–291, 289, 290, 291
nabilone, 242–243
  analgesic use, 273–274
  anti-anxiety effects, 237
  antiemetic effects, 231
L-nantradol see levonantradol
narcotics, 470
  cannabis classification, 375–376, 377
  US legislation, 373–374
National Cancer Institute (NCI), 382
National Center for Complementary and
  Alternative Medicine, 407
National Commission on Marihuana and Drug
  Abuse (Shafer Commission) (1972), 378, 380
National Institute for Clinical Excellence (NICE),
  436–437, 438
National Institute of Drug Abuse (NIDA), 6, 408
  cannabis product, 11, 171
  medicinal cannabis supply, 381–382
  research by, 11–12, 434–435
National Institutes of Health (NIH), 407, 452
National Organization for the Reform of
  Marijuana Laws (NORML), 380
National Toxicity Program (NTP), 452
natural foods movement, 408
needs, patients', 436–437
Negms test, 303
Netherlands, 416, 417, 438
  INCB attitude, 411

legislation, 397, 410
  road traffic law, 333–334
neurofibromatosis, 254–255
neuroleptic drugs, 182, 183–184
neurological disorders, 231–232, 437
  clinical trial methodology, 248–250
neuromodulators, 111–112
neuropathic, 470
neuropathic pain, 231–232, 233–234, 273,
  278–279
  in multiple sclerosis see under multiple sclerosis
  recent clinical research, 257, 257–258
neuroprotection, 189–190, 239–240, 261
  in multiple sclerosis, 152–155
neuropsychological testing, 250–251
neurotransmitters
  CB$_1$ agonist actions, 105–107
  endocannabinoids as, 111–112
new chemical entities (NCE), 431, 471
  regulatory route, 438–439
  safety issues, 451–452
new drug development see development of
  cannabis-based medicines
New Orleans, 375
nicotine, 435, 458
NIDA see National Institute of Drug Abuse
night vision, 362
nitric oxide (NO), 191–192
nociception, 275–278, 276, 277
nociceptive, 471
nociceptive pain, 278–279
nociceptors, 275–276
noladin ether see arachidonyl glyceryl ether
noradrenaline, 106
Northern Lights No. 1, 77
nuclear factor kappa B (NF-κB), 190–191
nuclear magnetic resonance (NMR), 441
nucleus accumbens, 106–107, 107

O-689, 109, 118, 118
O-1184, 109, 124, 124–125
O-1238, 109, 124, 124–125
O-1602, 127, 127–128
O-1812, 109, 118, 118
'off label' prescribing, 402
Office of Marihuana Medical Access, 418
Office of Medicinal Cannabis (OMC), 417
Old English Herbarium Manuscript V, 2–3
onion thrip, 50
open-field test, 168
opiates (opioids), 458, 471
  international legislation, 386–387
  US legislation, 373–374
  withdrawal, 240
  see also heroin; morphine
opioid receptors, 455, 457
opium, 372, 373, 386–387, 463
Opium and Narcotics Drug Act (Canada, 1929),
  388

oral administration, 242–244, 448–449
    δ^9-THC, 216, 218–219
    cannabidiol, 220
oropharyngeal administration, 448–449
    see also sublingual administration
O'Shaughnessy, W B, 4–5, 272, 369
outcome measures
    clinical trials, 248–250
    pain management, 281
ovary, 23, *24*
Oxford Natural Products, 415
oxidative associated diseases, 187–188
OxyContin, 415, 416
oxytocic activity, possible, 240

pain, 274–280, 462–463
    assessment, 280–281
    cannabinoid physiology and, 275–278
    chronic, 171, 233–234, 271–299
        aetiology, 277–279
        management, 281, *281, 282*
        clinical research experience, 282–295
            acute side-effects, 292–294
            cannabinoids used, 283
            contraindications, 284–285
            long-term follow-up, 294–295
            patient preparation, 285–286
            patient selection, 283–284
            results of 'n of 1' studies, 288–291, *289,
            290, 291*
            study design, 282–283
            titration, 286–288
    neural pathways, 275–277, *276, 277*
    neuropathic *see* neuropathic pain
    nociceptive, 278
    possible indications, 297
    postoperative, 260–261
    psychogenic, 278
    psychosocial factors, 280
    quality of life aspects, 280–281
    see also analgesic effects
palmitoylethanolamide (PMEA), *114*, 125
    analgesic activity, 234
    anti-inflammatory effects, 193
palmitylsulfonyl fluoride (AM374), 113–114, *114*
paper, 18
parkinsonism, tetrabenazine (TBZ)-induced, 180
patients
    advocacy movements, 229, 406
    GW Pharmaceuticals, database, 241–242, *243*
    legalisation campaigns, 381–382
    needs, 436–437
periaqueductal grey (PAG), 105, 239
Permanent Central Opium Board (PCOB), 389
pest control, 49
pesticides, 48, 49, 50, 443
phantom limb pain, 171, 233–234
pharmaceutical industry, 414–415
pharmacodynamics, 103–139

pharmacokinetics, 205–208, *207*
    forensic aspects, 317–323
    by route of administration, 216–220
Pharmos, 414–415
phencyclidine (PCP), 182–183
phenotype, 471
phenylmethylsulfonyl fluoride (PMSF), 113
photonastism, 47, *48*
photoperiod, 471
phototropism, 45–47, 471
phylogeny, 471
phylotaxy, 471
    decussate, 31, *32*
    'GV point', 31–33, *32*
physicians *see* medical profession
phytocannabinoids, 10, 79, 115, *115*
    biological function, 27–28, 80–81
    coevolution with CB receptors, 84–93
    different biotypes, 79–80
    effects on endocannabinoids, 92–93, 457–458
    interactions and effects, 165–204
    psychoactivity, 80
    reason for animal receptors, 84–85
    see also cannabinoids; *specific compounds*
phytomedicine, 471
    see also botanical drug substances
pilot studies, 246–247
α-pinene, anti-inflammatory effects, 192
Pinnatifidofillia, 64
2-pinyl-5-dimethylheptyl resorcinol (PR-DMH),
    172
pistil, 23, *24*, 471
plant-based medicines *see* botanical drug sub-
    stances
plants, *Cannabis*, 9–11, *19*
    biological function of cannabinoids and ter-
        penes, 27–28
    breeding *see* breeding, *Cannabis* plant
    cannabinoid distribution, 10, 20–22, *21*
    chemovars *see* chemovars
    crop quality, safety and efficacy, 48–50
    cross-breeding, 9
    cultivation for industrial uses, 302
    cultivation for personal use, 397
    cuttings *see* cuttings
    female *see* female plants
    flowering *see* flowering
    flowers *see* inflorescence
    forensic control, 307–312, *311*
    geographical origin, 310–312
    growth and morphology, 17–54
    growth in controlled environment, 42–45, *44,
    443–444*
    'GV point', 31–33, *32*
    harvest and drying, 42, 444, Plate 9
    history of cultivation, 17
    legality of cultivation for medical use, 401
    life cycle, 22–23
    male *see* male plants

mother, 37, *37*
optimising cannabinoid production, 23–26
outdoor cultivation, 50–53, *52, 53*, 442, *443*
phototropy and photonasty, 45–47, *48*
potting up of cuttings, 38
processing, 42
propagation of medicinal, 29–42, *31*
selecting and cloning seedlings, 29–36, *30*
sinsemilla technique *see* sinsemilla
uses, 17–18
varieties *see* varieties, *Cannabis*
vegetative form, 31, *32*
vegetative growth period, 39
see also Cannabis sativa
plasma concentrations
forensic analysis, 312–316
forensic interpretation, 317–323
by route of administration, 216–220, 448, *448*
Pliny, 2
Police and Criminal Evidence Act (1984), 301
Police Foundation, 422
policies, possible cannabis, 395–398
polygene, 471
polygenic, 471
Portugal, 424
postoperative pain, 260–261
postural hypotension, 294
potassium channels, 104, 105
potency of cannabis, trends, 304–306, *305, 306*
potentiation, botanical extracts, 439
powdery mildew, 50
preclinical safety studies, 450, 451–453
prescribing, 'off label', 402
prescription medicine abuse, 415–416
prochlorperazine, 365
progeny, 471
prohibition, 471
    cannabis, 374, 375–376, 388, 390–392, 434
        with administrative expediency principle,
        395, 410
        changing attitudes, 412
    narcotics, 373–374
    partial, 397
    see also decriminalisation; legislation
propagation, plant, 29–42, *31*
protein binding, 207–208
Protocol Amending the Single Convention, 1972,
    392
psychiatric conditions, 237
psychoactive drugs, other, 285
psychogenic pain, 278
psychometric, 471
psychosis, 471
    cannabidiol (CBD) therapy, 237
    cannabis-associated, 185, 253–254
    contraindicating medicinal cannabis, 284
    see also schizophrenia
psychosocial factors, chronic pain, 280
psychotomimetic, 471

publication, clinical research, 436
pulegone, 166
pulmonary damage, 414
pulse rate, 317
pump action spray (PAS) formulations, *244,*
    244–245
Pure Food and Drug Act (PDFA) (USA, 1906),
    372
Purple Haze, 36
L-pyroglutamate, 180–181

quality control (QC)
    analytical procedures, 324
    cannabis-based medicines, 442–446
quality of life
    improvements, 291
    pain and, 280–281
quantitative trait loci (QTL), 67
quercetin, 190–191

Randall, Robert, 381
randomised controlled trials (RCTs), 246–247
rapid eye movement (REM) sleep deprivation test,
    168
raw material, botanical *see* botanical raw material
reactive oxygen species (ROS), 187–188
receptors, 471
    animal, with plant ligands, 84–85
    coevolution with ligands, 84–85, 87–88
    endogenous, *463*
    evolution, 82–84
    see also cannabinoid (CB) receptors
recreational cannabis use
    adverse effects, 253–254, 370, 379, 384, 412
    dependence, 252
    legalisation, 396–397
    medicinal cannabis use after, 285, 286
    plant breeding, 55–56
    separation from medicinal use, 403–406
rectal administration, δ⁹-THC, 219–220
reefers *see* cigarettes, cannabis
reform of cannabis control, possibilities for,
    395–398
regulation
    cannabis, 396–397
    development of cannabis-based medicines,
        438–440
    safety of cannabis-based medicines, 450–453
regulatory authorities (medicines), 428
    attitudes towards botanicals, 440–441
research
    clinical *see* clinical research
    effects of legislation, 11–12, 434–435
    future, 462
restriction profiling, 308
Reynolds, Sir John Russell, 5
rheumatoid arthritis (RA), 261
riamba, 76
road tracking ability, 360, 361, 364–365

road traffic
 collisions, retrospective analyses, 336–343,
  340–341, 342
 legislation, 333–335, 364
 see also driving
Road Traffic Act (1988), 333
Rome, Ancient, 2, 18
rope, 18
rostro-ventro-medial (RMV) nucleus, brainstem,
  105, *276,* 276–277
routes of administration, 446–447, *448*
 δ⁹-THC, 216–220
 CBD and CBN, 220
Royal Pharmaceutical Society, 12, 229
ruderal, 472
Rumpshaker mice, 145

Sabur ibn Sahl, 3
safety, cannabis-based medicines, 250–254,
  450–453
 regulatory imperatives, 450–453
 see also adverse effects
sail cloth, 18
saliva, analysis of cannabinoids, 315
Salix alba, 428, 463
Santhica cultivar, 62
Sativex, 431, 437, 459–460
schizophrenia, 92, 182–185
 animal models, 182–184
 cannabis-associated, 185, 253–254
 human studies, 184–185, 261
 see also psychosis
scientific developments, 407–408
Scythians, 2, 72, 75–76
security, cannabis-based medicines, 286, 449–450
seedlings
 leaf, Plate 5
 selecting and cloning, 29–36, *30*
seeds
 commercial uses, 10, 17–18
 plants grown from, 29–35, *32, 33*
seizure disorders, 236
 alcohol withdrawal, 179
 epileptic, 185–187, 236
self-fertilisation (self-pollination), 29
 plant breeding programmes, 58–59, *59*
self-titration, 472
serotonin (5-hydroxytryptamine), 106, 239
Severity of Dependence Scale (SDS), 252
Shafer Commission, 378, 380
Shen Nong Ben Cao Jing, 1
Shiverer mice, 145
side effects *see* adverse effects
signatures, doctrine of, 428–429
Single Convention on Narcotic Drugs (United
  Nations, 1961), 11, 390–391
 legality of medicinal cannabis, 302, 398–401
 national interpretations, 393–394
single nucleotide polymorphisms (SNPs), 87

sinsemilla, 9, 28, 472
 trends in potency, 306, *307*
Skunk no. 1, 35–36, 77
sleep, effects on, 237
 CBME, 258–259, 289–290, *291*
 driving performance and, 363
smell, cannabis, 23–24, 80
smoking, cannabis
 analgesic activity, 171
 antidepressive effect, 178
 antismoking movement and, 414
 cannabinoid pharmacokinetics, 216–218, 220,
  446–447
 in glaucoma, 238
 GW Pharmaceuticals patient database,
  241–242, *243*
 medicinal cannabis delivery via, 242, 274, 446
 passive, forensic aspects, 318–319
 see also cigarettes, cannabis
smoking, tobacco, 414, 435
social upheavals, chronic pain study, 295
solid-phase extraction, 314–315
solid-phase microextraction (SPME), 315
Spain, 424
spastic mutant mice, 145
spasticity, 179–182
 animal models, 179–181
 human studies, 181–182, 231–232
 in multiple sclerosis *see under* multiple sclerosis
Sphaerotheca macularis, 50
spider mites, 50
spinal cord
 dorsal horn, 276
 injuries (SCI), 178, 231–232, 254–255
SR141716A, *109, 121,* 121–124, *122*
 in inflammation, 192, 194
 in schizophrenia, 183
 in spasticity, 149
SR144528, *110, 121,* 121–122
 in inflammation, 193–194
stability, cannabis-based medicines, 445–446
'stalking horse' concerns, 403, 404
staminate, 472
'stash', *21*
stearylsulfonyl fluoride (AM381), 113–114, *114*
stepping stone thesis, 377, 390
stroke, 239–240
sublingual administration, 274, 448–449
 chronic pain study, 282–295
 pharmacokinetics, *244,* 244–245
 side-effects, 294
substance misusers, 285
substitution theory, 374
Sumerian medicine, 1–2
summation, botanical extracts, 439–440
supercritical fluid chromatography with atmospheric pressure chemical ionisation mass
  spectrometry, 307–308
superoxide dismutase (SOD), 188–189

support groups, patient, 229, 406
surreptitious mimic theory, 84
Switzerland, 423–424
synaptic messengers, retrograde, 111–112, *112,* 144
synaptic neurotransmission, 144

tail suspension test, 177
taxon, 472
taxonomy, 73–74
temperature, *Cannabis* plant growth, 37, 43
terpenoids/terpenes, 23–24, 80, 472
  actions, 90, 166
  analgesic activity, 169–170
  anti-inflammatory effects, 192
  anxiolytic activity, 172
  biological function, 27–28
  pharmacological interactions, 165–167
α-terpineol, 166, 172
4-terpineol, 190
δ⁸-tetrahydrocannabinol (δ⁸-THC), 115, *115,* 205
  analgesic activity, 170
  antiemetic effects, 231
  CB receptor affinity, *110,* 117
  metabolism, 210–211
  pharmacokinetics, *207*
  structure, *206*
  THC interaction, 147
δ⁹-tetrahydrocannabinol (δ⁹-THC), 6, 103, 205
  administration by smoking, 216–218
  in alcohol withdrawal, 179, *179*
  analgesic activity, 170, 171, 233
  analysis in body fluids, 314–316
  antidepressant activity, 178
  antiemetic properties, 230–231
  antiepileptic activity, 186, 187
  anti-inflammatory effects, 191, 192
  antioxidant activity, 190
  antitumour effects, 240
  anxiogenic effects, 173–174
  appetite stimulation/weight gain, 234–235
  bronchodilator activity, 236–237
  CB receptor affinity, 87, *110,* 115–117, 456
  CBD ratios, 165, 196
  in CBME, 245–246
    chronic pain, 283, 287
  driving performance and, 330–331, 332–333, 337–339, 365
  effects on endocannabinoid system, 92
  forensic analysis, 317, 318–323, 324
  in glaucoma, 237–238
  in herbal cannabis, trends, 304–306, *306, 307*
  immunosuppressive activity, 151–152
  induction of drug-metabolising enzymes, 215–216
  inhibition of drug-metabolising enzymes, 214
  intravenous administration, 219
  legal status, 11–12, 402, 405

metabolism in humans, 208–216
  P450 isoforms responsible, 211–212, *212*
  Phase I hepatic, 210–211, *211*
in multiple sclerosis, 147, 232
numbering systems, 10, 205, 320, *321*
oral administration, 216, 218–219, *448*
pharmacokinetics, *207,* 207–208, 216–220
pharmacological effects, 453–455, *454, 456*
pharmacological interactions
  CBD, 147, 165, 167–169, 195–196, 213–214
  terpenoids and flavonoids, 165–167
in plants, 10
  breeding programmes, 60–61, *63,* 64–66, *65*
  cloned *vs* seed-sown, *33,* 33–34, *34–35*
  different biotypes, 79–80
  different varieties, 11, 27, *28*
  distribution in tissues, 20, *20*
  metabolism, 79
  psychosis induction, 185
  rectal administration, 219–220
  rodent responsiveness, 89
  structure, *115, 206*
  toxicity studies, 452
tetrahydrocannabinol carboxylic acid (THCA), 445, 446
δ⁹-tetrahydrocannabinol-11-oic acid (THCCOOH), 207, 208, 211
  pharmacokinetics, 217, 218–219
tetrahydrocannabinolic acid synthase, 79
tetrahydrocannabivarin (THCV), 205
  analgesic activity, 169
  cloned *vs* seed-sown plants, *33*
  licit *vs* illicit cannabis users, 323
  metabolism, 208–216
  plant breeding programmes, 62, *63, 64, 64*
  plant content, 10
  plant metabolism, 79
  structure, *206*
Tetranychus spider mites, 50
THC *see* δ⁹-tetrahydrocannabinol
THCV *see* tetrahydrocannabivarin
Theiler's mouse encephalomyelitis virus (TMEV) model, 142
thin-layer chromatography (TLC), 303–304, 446
  hyphenated techniques, 314–315
  two-dimensional, 304
Thrips tabaci, 50
time, passage of, 412
time line, cannabis, 7–8
titration, medicinal cannabis, 249, 286–288, *448*
tobacco smoking, 414, 435
tobacco thrip, 50
tolerance, 252
Tourette's syndrome, 240
trace metals, 311–312
traditional medicines, 461–462
Trafficking Convention, 1988, 392–393, 394
trait, 472

transduction, 472
'trash', *21*
tremor
    alcohol withdrawal, 179, *179*
    multiple sclerosis, 145–146, 232
trichomes, 23–26, *25–26*, 472
    peltate (sessile; unstalked), 24–26, *26*, Plate 5,
        Plate 6
    stalked glandular, 23, 24, *25–26*, 27
tricyclic antidepressants (TCAs), 365
triploid, 472
triploid hybrids, *66*, 66–67
tumour necrosis factor (TNF)-α, 192, 261

ultraviolet spectroscopy–Fourier-transform
    infrared spectroscopy (UV/FTIR), 315
Unimed, 415
United Kingdom (UK), 420–422
    attitude to cannabis-based medicines, 430
    clinical research, 12
    forensic analytical techniques, 303–304
    history of hemp use, 18
    history of medicinal use, 2–3, 4, 5–6
    legalisation of medicinal cannabis, 399, 402,
        405–406, 437–438
    legislation, 6, 301, 388, 397
    medical *vs* recreational cannabis use, 404
    road traffic laws, 333, 335
    trends in cannabis potency, 304–306, *305*
United Nations
    Commission on Narcotic Drugs (CND),
        389–390, 400
    International Narcotics Control Board *see*
        International Narcotics Control Board
United States of America (USA), 422–423
    antismoking movement, 414
    cannabis rescheduling case, 380–381
    history of cannabis control, 370–385
        1960s to present day, 378–385
        association with ethnic/unpopular groups,
            374
        decline in industrial/agricultural use,
            371–372
        expanding illicit use, 374–375
        Federal Government involvement, 375–376
        increasing concerns with addiction, 372
        loss of support within medical profession, 371
        opiate/cocaine threat and, 372–374
        stepping stone thesis, 377
        substitution theory, 374

history of medicinal use, 5, 369–370, 371
international legislation and, 385–387,
    389–390
legality of medical cannabis use, 397, 399,
    401–402, 405
medical profession and cannabis, 383–384,
    385, 413
medical *vs* recreational cannabis use, 404–405
prescription medicine abuse, 415–416
regulatory attitudes towards botanicals, 440,
    441
research, 11–12
road traffic legislation, 335
trends in cannabis potency, 304–306, *306, 307*
urinary cannabinoids, 208–209
    forensic analysis, 314, 316
    forensic interpretation, 317–320, 322, 323
    pharmacokinetics, 217, 218–219
Urticaceae, 73–74

vanilloid receptors (VR1), 86, *86*, 87, 455
    agonist activity of cannabinoids, 111, 120
varieties, *Cannabis*, 78
    cannabinoid content, 11, 27, *28*
    selection for cannabinoid production, 29–36,
        30
    see also biotypes; chemovars; G1 variety; G5
        variety
VDM-11, 113, *113*
vestigial receptor hypothesis, 85
vestigial receptors, 92–94
vision, 362
visual analogue scale (VAS), 280
volume of distribution, 207

War on Drugs, US Government, 379, 382, 412
weight, body, 234–235
WIN55212, 115, *116*, 120
    anti-inflammatory effects, 191–192, 194
    CB receptor affinity, *110*, 117
winterisation, 445, 447
withdrawal symptoms, cannabis, 252, 286
Woodward, Dr William, 376
Wootton Report (1968), 378–379, 388, 420–421
World Health Organization (WHO), 302, 390,
    392, 400

yield, cannabinoid, 57–58, *65*, 65–66

zopiclone, 365